THE GUIDE TO CARDIOLOGY
SECOND EDITION

Edited by

Robert A. Kloner, M.D., Ph.D.
Director of Research
The Heart Institute
The Hospital of the Good Samaritan
Professor of Medicine
University of Southern California
Section of Cardiology
Los Angeles, California

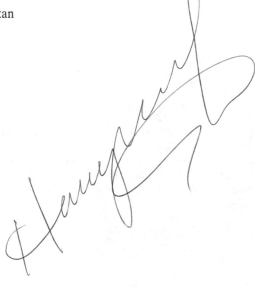

Le Jacq Communications
New York

Preface

Cardiology is a rapidly evolving field in terms of diagnostic techniques, pharmacologic therapy, catheter intervention techniques, and surgical therapeutic options. Since 1984, when the first edition of *The Guide to Cardiology* was published by John Wiley and Sons, there have been tremendous advances in the field. Doppler echocardiography is used for diagnosing and, in some cases, quantitating degrees of valvular abnormality. Electrophysiologic testing has become standard in many medical centers for aiding in diagnosis and treatment of arrhythmias. Thrombolytic therapy is now standard therapy for acute myocardial infarction. Control of lipid levels may help arrest or perhaps even reverse coronary atherosclerosis. New and powerful lipid-lowering drugs have been tested and made available since 1984. Interventional cardiology has progressed with the use of angioplasty for not only isolated coronary lesions, but for treating multi-vessel coronary artery disease as well. Percutaneous balloon valvuloplasty appears promising for treating certain cases of valvular stenosis without having to subject the patient to a thoracotomy. Coronary atherectomy devices and lasers are undergoing clinical trials. Thus, it seems an important and opportune time to update *The Guide to Cardiology*.

A number of large and comprehensive cardiology texts offer detailed information about the ever-broadening knowledge base of cardiology. Realizing that many clinicians do not have the time to read these texts thoroughly, we undertook *The Guide to Cardiology* to provide a selective, concise, current, and practical handbook on the fundamentals of the specialty. As in the previous edition, the first half of the book reviews diagnostic techniques and procedures. Besides updating the existing chapters, we have added chapters on Doppler echocardiography, electrophysiologic testing, and newer imaging modalities. The second half of the book presents chapters on specific problems in cardiology that the clinician is likely to encounter, such as hyperlipidemia, myocardial infarction, angina pectoris, cardiac arrhythmias, conduction abnormalities, valvular heart disease, cardiomyopathy and myocarditis, heart failure, hypertension, and congenital heart disease. Many of these chapters have been entirely rewritten to take into account recent advances. The hyperlipidemia chapter details the approach to treatment and discusses the new and potent agents available for treating lipid abnormalities; the hypertension chapter has been revised to reflect the recent changes in pharmacologic therapy. The treatment section on myocardial infarction now details the use of the various thrombolytic agents and post-infarct therapy. New sections that have been added include chapters on silent myocardial ischemia, interventional cardiology, and pacemaker therapy. There are chapters that deal with the approach to patients with noncardiac or cardiac surgery, which the cardiology consultant may find especially useful. New therapies for pulmonary embolism are presented. There is a new section on cor pulmonale. Also included are chapters on related areas such as the effect of exercise on the heart, cardiopulmonary resuscitation, heart disease in pregnancy, diseases of the aorta, and cardiac problems in systemic diseases, including AIDS.

Thanks to the support of E.R. Squibb & Sons, Inc., sections of this book have also appeared in the journal *Cardiovascular Reviews and Reports*. My hope is that physicians will find the text a useful guide for clinical practice. It may also be a useful review-text for physicians preparing for board examinations and for trainees who are participating in rotations on Cardiology services.

The drugs, indications for drugs, and drug dosages referred to throughout this book are those commonly used by practicing cardiologists and suggested by the authors. However, not all drugs, doses, and indications mentioned are Food and Drug Administration approved. Therefore, it is suggested that the package inserts or Physicians' Desk Reference be consulted as well for drug indications, contraindications, side effects, and dosages as recommended by the Food and Drug Administration. While the procedures and treatments in the text are based upon current standard practices, they should serve as a guide and not as the sole reference or sole determinant for practice and therapy of individual patients.

I wish to acknowledge the excellent help and advice of Melissa Culverwell, who served as an editorial consultant throughout the preparation of this book. I would also like to thank Margaret Inman and Kathryn Clark for their editorial work, Elizabeth Janice for her work on the book sections published in *Cardiovascular Reviews and Reports*, and Judith A. Kloner for her helpful suggestions.

Robert A. Kloner, M.D., Ph.D.
Los Angeles, CA
April 1990

Contributors

Elliott M. Antman, M.D.
Associate Professor of Medicine
Harvard Medical School
Director, Samuel E. Levine Cardiac Unit
Cardiovascular Division
Brigham and Women's Hospital
Boston, Massachusetts

Damian A. Brezinski, M.D.
Department of Medicine
Beth Israel Hospital
Boston, Massachusetts

Edward J. Brown, M.D.
Assistant Professor of Medicine
Director, Cardiovascular Research Laboratory
Stony Brook Medical Center
Stony Brook, New York

Ricardo G. Cigarroa, M.D.
Research Fellow, Cardiovascular Division
Department of Internal Medicine
University of Texas Southwestern Medical Center
Dallas, Texas

Victor J. Dzau, M.D.
William G. Irwin Professor of Medicine
Chief, Division of Cardiology and Vascular
    Medicine
Stanford University School of Medicine
Stanford, California

Andrew C. Eisenhauer, M.D.
Director, Acute Myocardial Intervention Program
Co-Director, Pacemaker Service
The Heart Institute
The Hospital of the Good Samaritan
Los Angeles, California

Peter L. Friedman, M.D., Ph.D.
Assistant Professor of Medicine
Harvard Medical School
Director, Clinical Electrophysiology and
    Arrhythmia Service
Associate Physician
Brigham and Women's Hospital
Boston, Massachusetts

Samuel Z. Goldhaber, M.D.
Associate Professor of Medicine
Harvard Medical School
Associate Physician and Staff Cardiologist
Brigham and Women's Hospital
Boston, Massachusetts

Lee Goldman, M.D.
Professor of Medicine
Harvard Medical School
Vice Chairman and Chief of the Division
    of Clinical Epidemiology
Brigham and Women's and Beth Israel Hospitals
Boston, Massachusetts

Thomas B. Graboys, M.D.
Assistant Professor of Medicine
Harvard Medical School
Associate Physician
Brigham and Women's Hospital
Boston, Massachusetts

Maleah Grover-McKay, M.D.
Assistant Professor of Medicine and Radiology
Department of Internal Medicine
University of Iowa Hospitals and Clinics
Iowa City, Iowa

James M. Hagar, M.D.
Clinical Instructor
Section of Cardiology
University of Southern California
School of Medicine
Los Angeles, California

Haim Hammerman, M.D.
Senior Lecturer
Technion, Israel Institute of Technology
Department of Cardiology
Rambam Medical Center
Haifa, Israel

Donald P. Harrington, M.D.
Associate Professor of Radiology
Harvard Medical School
Director, Cardiovascular and
    Interventional Radiology Section
Department of Radiology
Brigham and Women's Hospital
Boston, Massachusetts

L. David Hillis, M.D.
Professor of Internal Medicine
University of Texas Southwestern Medical Center
Director, Cardiac Catheterization Laboratory
Parkland Memorial Hospital
Dallas, Texas

Joseph P. Ilvento, M.D.
Director, Cardiac Pacing and Electrophysiology
The Heart Institute
The Hospital of the Good Samaritan
Assistant Clinical Professor of Medicine
University of California, Los Angeles
School of Medicine
Los Angeles, California

Robert A. Kloner, M.D., Ph.D.
Director of Research
The Heart Institute
The Hospital of the Good Samaritan
Professor of Medicine
University of Southern California
Section of Cardiology
Los Angeles, California

Sherif B. Labib, M.D.
Instructor of Medicine (Cardiology)
Tufts University School of Medicine
Cardiology Fellow
New England Medical Center Hospital
Boston, Massachusetts

Joel S. Landzberg, M.D.
Research Fellow in Cardiology
Brigham and Women's Hospital
Boston, Massachusetts

Richard A. Lange, M.D.
Assistant Professor of Internal Medicine
University of Texas Southwestern Medical Center
Associate Director, Cardiac Catheterization
    Laboratory
Parkland Memorial Hospital
Dallas, Texas

Thomas H. Lee, M.D.
Assistant Professor of Medicine
Harvard Medical School
Brigham and Women's Hospital
Boston, Massachusetts

Richard R. Liberthson, M.D.
Associate Professor of Medicine and Pediatrics
Harvard Medical School
Assistant Physician and Pediatrician
Massachusetts General Hospital
Boston, Massachusetts

Leonard S. Lilly, M.D.
Assistant Professor of Medicine
Harvard Medical School
Cardiologist
Brigham and Women's Hospital
Boston, Massachusetts

Sylvia A. Mamby, M.D.
Senior Associate Consultant
Cardiovascular Diseases
Mayo Clinic
Scottsdale, Arizona

James D. Marsh, M.D.
Associate Professor of Medicine
Harvard Medical School
Associate Physician
Brigham and Women's Hospital
Boston, Massachusetts

Gilbert H. Mudge, M.D.
Associate Professor of Medicine
Harvard Medical School
Director of Clinical Cardiology Service
Associate Physician
Brigham and Women's Hospital
Boston, Massachusetts

Allen J. Naftilan, M.D., Ph.D.
Assistant Professor of Medicine
The University of Alabama at Birmingham
Division of Cardiovascular Disease
Hypertension Program
Birmingham, Alabama

Stephen Oesterle, M.D.
Director, Cardiac Catheterization
    and Coronary Intervention Laboratories
The Heart Institute
The Hospital of the Good Samaritan
Los Angeles, California

Carl E. Orringer, M.D.
Clinical Assistant Professor of Internal Medicine
Division of Cardiology
University of Michigan Medical Center
Ann Arbor, Michigan

Natesa G. Pandian, M.D.
Associate Professor of Medicine and Radiology
Tufts University School of Medicine
Director, Noninvasive Cardiac Laboratory
New England Medical Center Hospital
Boston, Massachusetts

Priscilla Peters, B.A.
Clinical Specialist
Section of Cardiology
Harper Hospital
Detroit, Michigan

Marc A. Pfeffer, M.D., Ph.D.
Associate Professor of Medicine
Harvard Medical School
Brigham and Women's Hospital
Boston, Massachusetts

Joseph F. Polak, M.D.
Assistant Professor of Radiology
Harvard Medical School
Brigham and Women's Hospital
Boston, Massachusetts

LeRoy E. Rabbani, M.D.
Research Fellow in Medicine
Cardiovascular Division
Harvard Medical School
Brigham and Women's Hospital
Boston, Massachusetts

Shereif Rezkalla, M.D.
Assistant Clinical Professor of Medicine
University of Wisconsin
Madison, Wisconsin
Cardiologist
Marshfield Clinic
Marshfield, Wisconsin

Steven L. Schwartz, M.D.
Instructor of Medicine (Cardiology)
Tufts University School of Medicine
Cardiology Fellow
New England Medical Center Hospital
Boston, Massachusetts

Thomas L. Shook, M.D.
Director, Coronary Care Unit
The Heart Institute
The Hospital of the Good Samaritan
Los Angeles, California

David J. Skorton, M.D.
Professor of Medicine and Electrical and
    Computer Engineering
Associate Chair for Clinical Programs
Department of Internal Medicine
University of Iowa Hospitals and Clinics
Iowa City, Iowa

Neil J. Stone, M.D.
Associate Professor of Medicine
Section of Cardiology
Northwestern University School of Medicine
Chicago, Illinois

Peter H. Stone, M.D.
Assistant Professor of Medicine
Harvard Medical School
Associate Director, Samuel E. Levine Cardiac Unit
Cardiovascular Division
Associate Physician
Brigham and Women's Hospital
Boston, Massachusetts

Howard Waldman, M.D.
Instructor in Medicine
Harvard Medical School
Clinical Assistant in Medicine
Massachusetts General Hospital
Boston, Massachusetts

Richard F. Wright, M.D.
Clinical Instructor
University of California, Los Angeles
School of Medicine
Director of Research
Pacific Heart Institute
Santa Monica, California

Joshua Wynne, M.D.
Professor and Chief
Division of Cardiology
Wayne State University
Detroit, Michigan

Eliot Young, M.D.
Assistant Clinical Professor of Medicine
Harvard Medical School
Chief, ECG Laboratory
New England Deaconess Hospital
Boston, Massachusetts

Contents

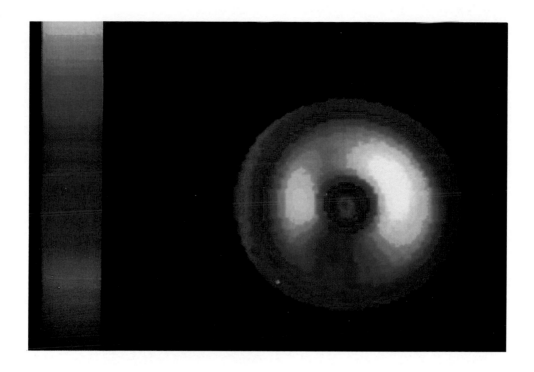

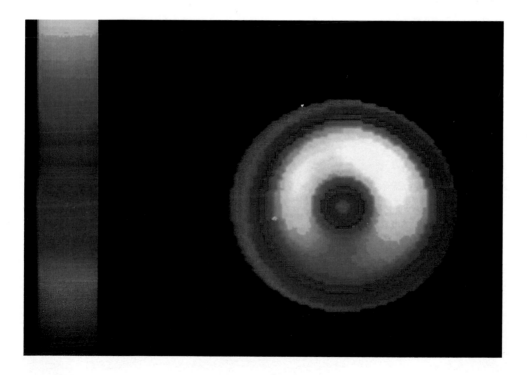

Figure 5. *Thallium-201 bullseye plot. These short-axis SPECT images are a superimposition of quantitative information contained on multiple short-axis views. Maximal uptake of thallium-201 for each point in the short axis is obtained as shown in Figures 3 and 4 (see Chapter 5). The data are then displayed as a series of concentric, color-encoded circles. The more central circle corresponds to the apex and the larger one to the left ventricular base. A significant stenotic lesion in the inferior wall appears in the top image as a region of decreased thallium uptake (blue). This image is compared with a resting (redistribution) view (bottom image) in the same patient. This confirms that the defect corresponds to ischemic yet viable myocardium.* **From Chapter 5.**

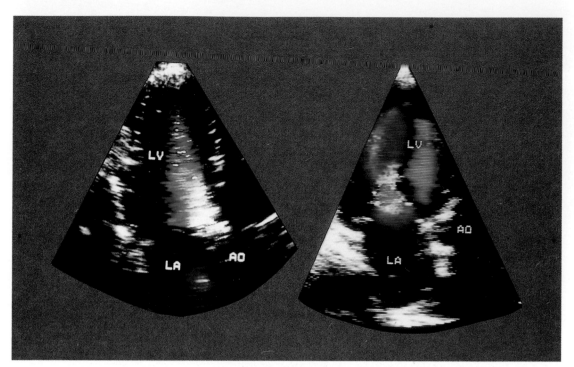

Figure 2. *Color-flow Doppler mapping of normal left ventricular flows as recorded from the apical long-axis view. The systolic frame (left) illustrates left ventricular outflow. The flow is going away from the transducer and is encoded with a bright blue color. In the diastolic frame (right), flow is seen going from the left atrium (LA) to the left ventricle (LV). The blood is traveling toward the transducer and is encoded as red. The center of the flow jet, which is near the mitral annulus, contains flow velocity exceeding the Nyquist limit, and aliasing is noted. There are progressively brighter shades of red with color reversal to blue in the central core. Also seen is vortex flow, or blood that has hit the apex and is turning toward the outflow tract. This is seen as faint blue. Ao = aorta.* **See Chapter 8 for this and following color figures.**

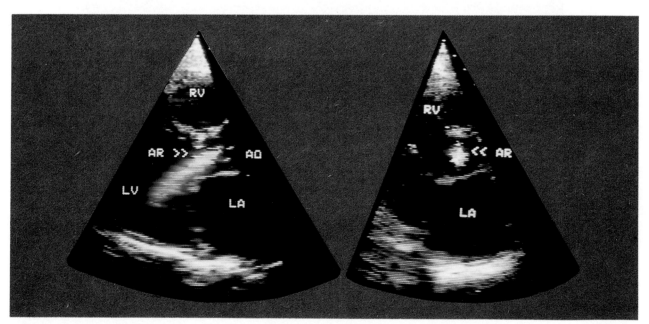

Figure 7. *Color Doppler images of aortic insufficiency from the parasternal long-axis (left) and short-axis (right) views. In the parasternal long-axis view, the regurgitant flow is seen as a blue jet going from the left ventricular outflow tract toward the mitral valve and posterior wall. In the short-axis view, the jet is seen as a bright blue circle within the outflow tract. Ao = aorta; AR = aorta regurgitant; LA = left atrium; LV = left ventricle; RV = right ventricle.*

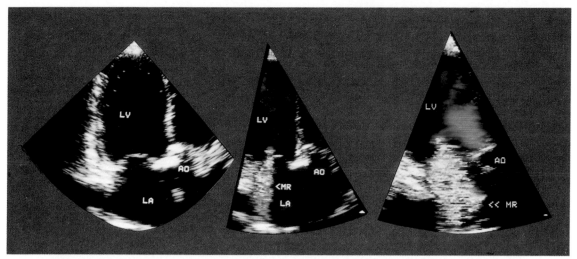

Figure 9. Color Doppler images recorded in the apical long-axis view from two patients with mitral regurgitation (MR). On the left is a two-dimensional echo image for orientation. The mitral regurgitant jets are seen as bright mosaic patterns in the left atrium due to high-velocity turbulent flow. The frame in the center is from a patient with moderate MR, the image on the right from a patient with severe MR. Note that the regurgitant jet occupies a larger portion of the left atrium (LA) in the latter. LV = left ventricle; Ao = aorta.

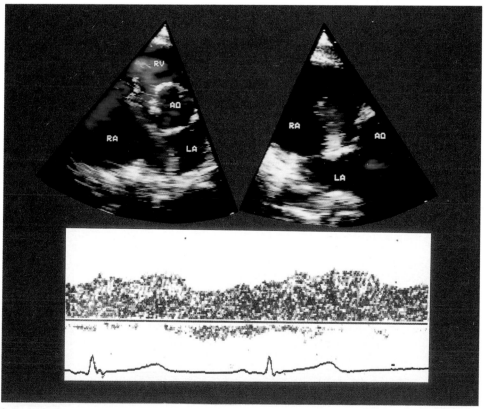

Figure 11. Color Doppler and CW Doppler recordings from a patient with an atrial septal defect. The image at top left was recorded from a parasternal short-axis view. The frame at top right was recorded from a low right parasternal position; the interatrial septum lies almost perpendicular to the ultrasound beam in this orientation. In both images, the shunt flow is visualized as an orange jet traveling from the left atrium (LA) to the right atrium (RA). Ao = aorta; RV = right ventricle. The CW tracing (bottom) illustrates the typical continuous low-velocity flow profile of an interatrial shunt.

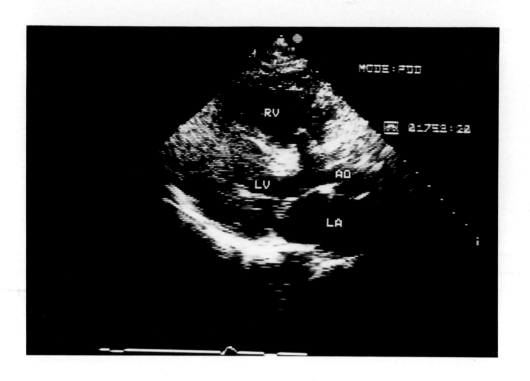

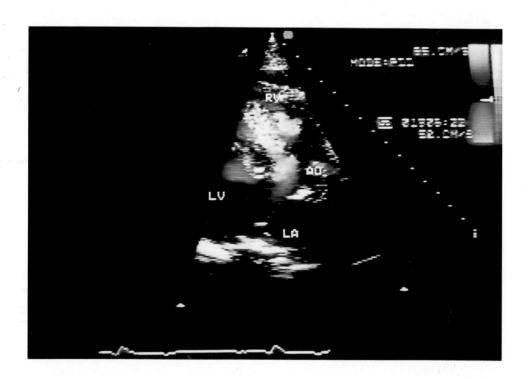

Figure 12. *Two-dimensional and color Doppler images from a patient with a congenital membranous ventricular septal defect and an aneurysm of the membranous septum, as recorded from the parasternal long-axis view. The 2D echo image at top is for orientation. The color Doppler image on the bottom shows a bright red mosaic jet traveling from the left ventricle (LV) to the right ventricle through the defect. LA = left atrium; Ao = aorta.*

1

The Cardiac History

Robert A. Kloner

Despite the recent surge in cardiac diagnostic technology, the history and physical examination remain the cornerstones of the patient work-up. This chapter discusses the cardiac history and reviews the major symptoms directly related to the heart: chest pain, shortness of breath (dyspnea), syncope, edema, palpitations, cough, hemoptysis, cyanosis, and fatigue.

CHEST PAIN

In most cases the cause of chest pain can be derived from an adequate history. The patient should be questioned as to the quality, duration, radiation, exacerbating and ameliorating factors, and frequency of the pain. Chest pain due to angina pectoris is typically a dull, substernal pain or pressure that radiates down the arms and up into the jaw; typically lasts a few to 15 minutes; is exacerbated by exertion, anxiety, and cold; and is relieved by rest and nitroglycerin. Patients often will not refer to angina as pain but will describe it as an uncomfortable sensation or discomfort. Other descriptions include a ''burning,'' ''squeezing,'' or ''tight'' sensation. When angina is suspected, the patient should be questioned regarding the presence of cardiac risk factors such as smoking, hypertension, hyperlipidemia, and diabetes.

The chest pain of myocardial infarction may be similar to that of angina but is usually more severe, is not relieved by rest or nitroglycerin, and lasts longer. A careful history of drug use should be obtained, given recent data implicating cocaine as a cause of myocardial infarction. Pericardial chest pain tends to be sharper than angina, positional (worse when the patient is lying down and often relieved by sitting up), and exacerbated by inspiration.

Several cardiac conditions cause chest pain that may mimic the pain of angina, such as hypertrophic cardiomyopathy, mitral valve prolapse, pulmonary hypertension, and myocarditis. The pain of mitral valve prolapse is often of shorter duration and may not be related to exertion.

Many noncardiac causes of chest pain may be confused with cardiac chest pain. Noncardiac causes of chest pain and their differentiating features are listed in Table 1.

DYSPNEA

Dyspnea is defined as an uncomfortable awareness of breathing, with a need for increased ventilation. When dyspnea is due to chronic organic heart disease, it is typically exacerbated by exertion and develops gradually over weeks to months.

Dyspnea at rest is more common in lung disease but is also exacerbated by exertion, making the distinction between cardiac and pulmonary dyspnea difficult. Further differentiating features between these two types of dyspnea will be discussed in later chapters. Both cardiac and pulmonary dyspnea should be differentiated from functional dyspnea, which occurs at rest, may not be exacerbated by exertion, and is often accompanied by anxiety. Normal persons experience dyspnea upon exercise. Sudden onset of dyspnea at rest may be due to a variety of causes, including pneumothorax, pulmonary embolism, and pulmonary edema. End-stage heart disease is associated with chronic dyspnea at rest.

Orthopnea is dyspnea that occurs while the patient is recumbent. It is due to redistribution of fluid from dependent parts of the circulation to the thorax. It occurs in patients with heart failure and is relieved by standing or sitting. Paroxysmal nocturnal dyspnea is an extreme form of orthopnea in which the patient wakes from sleep with a sense of severe breathlessness and suffocation. This symptom is due to interstitial pulmonary edema.

Table 1. Noncardiac Causes of Chest Pain that May Mimic Cardiac Pain

DISEASE ENTITY	DIFFERENTIATING FEATURES
Musculoskeletal	Pain tends to be exacerbated by motion of certain extremities and certain postures; often follows a nerve route distribution; point tenderness may be present in costochondritis.
Herpes zoster	Chest wall pain occurs several days before development of typical rash; pain follows dermatome distribution.
Pulmonary	
Pleuritis, pneumonitis	Pain is sharp, worse with inspiration, associated with fever, cough.
Pulmonary embolism	Pain is pleuritic when there is an associated infarction; shortness of breath is typically present; massive pulmonary embolus associated with cardiovascular collapse may be confused with myocardial infarction.
Gastrointestinal	
Esophageal	Esophagitis and esophageal spasm often mimic angina; the latter may be relieved by nitroglycerin; patient may complain of regurgitation of food and have relief with antacids.
Gastric and duodenal (gastritis, ulcers)	Epigastric discomfort typically is exacerbated by aspirin, alcohol, and relieved by food, antacids.
Gall bladder (cholecystitis)	Right upper quadrant cramping; pain exacerbated by fatty foods, occurs after eating; there may be associated ECG abnormalities
Pancreatitis	Mid- and epigastric abdominal pain; possible history of associated alcohol ingestion; exacerbated by ingestion of food.
Functional	Nonexertional chest tightness often associated with anxiety, hyperventilation and perioral paresthesia; "panic attack."
Aortic dissection	Pain typically is sharp, tearing in nature, may radiate to the back; onset of pain is often as severe as pain ever becomes, in contrast to myocardial infarction, in which the pain has a crescendo-like onset.

SYNCOPE

Syncope is a temporary loss of consciousness associated with muscle weakness and inability to stand upright. Common cardiac causes include arrhythmias (both tachyarrhythmias and bradyarrhythmias, including atrioventricular block and sick sinus syndrome). Stokes-Adams attacks are episodes of loss of consciousness due to asystole or ventricular fibrillation in the setting of high degrees of atrioventricular block. One form of cardiac syncope results from episodic ventricular fibrillation associated with prolonged QT interval, and may be familial. In this condition, ventricular fibrillation may spontaneously revert to sinus rhythm.

Other causes of cardiac syncope include valvular heart disease (especially aortic stenosis), hypertrophic obstructive cardiomyopathy, congenital heart disease (especially tetralogy of Fallot), atrial myxoma, cardiac tamponade, acute myocardial infarction, mitral valve prolapse, vasovagal attacks, and orthostatic hypotension, which is often associated with administration of certain antihypertensive medicines.

Cerebrovascular disease and subclavian steal syndrome may also result in syncope. A rare cause of syncope is excessive sensitivity of the carotid baroreceptor to pressure. In this condition—carotid sinus syncope—slight pressure to the neck (tight collar, rapid turning of the head) causes extreme bradycardia coupled with peripheral vasodilatation and hypotension.

Another rare cause is associated with excessive coughing, resulting in increases in intrathoracic pressure large enough to reduce systemic venous return. Other causes of syncope are hypoglycemia, hyperventilation, migraine headache, and micturition. Loss of consciousness may also occur with seizures and should be differentiated from syncope of cardiac origin.

The history may be extremely useful in differentiating the causes of syncope, especially if a witness observed the patient during the event. For example, if the patient was observed to develop loss of consciousness associated with typical epileptiform movements and incontinence, then seizure is more likely to be the diagnosis. However, Stokes-Adams attacks may be associated with a few clonic jerks due to reduced perfusion to the brain. Patients should be questioned about the presence of an aura before the loss of consciousness, which suggests seizures as a diagnosis. Also, recovery of consciousness tends to occur more slowly in patients with seizure disorders than with syncope due to cardiac disease.

Abrupt loss of consciousness suggests Stokes-Adams attacks, other cardiac arrhythmias, or seizures as a cause. Gradual onset of syncope is more suggestive of a vasodepressor reaction or syncope due to a metabolic cause, such as hypoglycemia or hyperventilation. The patient should be questioned about the presence of palpitations before syncope, which may suggest arrhythmias as a cause.

A history of syncope associated with a change in body position from lying to standing suggests orthostatic hypotension. Syncope associated with a change in body position, such as bending over or leaning forward, is suggestive of left atrial myxoma or ball-valve thrombus of the left atrium. Syncope independent of changes in body position occurs with arrhythmias, asystole, and hyperventilation; seizures also occur independent of body position. Syncope occurring after exertion of the upper extremities may suggest subclavian "steal" syndrome as a cause. The patient should be questioned in detail about antihypertensive drug use, which may contribute to orthostatic hypotension as a cause of syncope.

Vasodepressor syncope—the common faint—typically occurs in persons undergoing emotional or physical stress (such as pain). These patients often have a chronic history of such episodes. The episodes are accompanied by peripheral vasodilatation and bradycardia, and can be terminated by having the patient lie down.

The syncope of hypertrophic obstructive cardiomyopathy typically occurs after cessation of exercise, while the patient is in an upright position or maintaining an erect posture for a long period, when standing suddenly, or after coughing. A family history of syncope is not uncommon.

A detailed history is especially important. The patient should be questioned as to history of known valvular or congenital heart disease; history of transient ischemic attacks, which might suggest a cerebrovascular cause for syncope; epilepsy; migraine headaches; anxiety; and use of insulin, which might suggest a hypoglycemic episode.

Many of the same conditions that can cause syncope may cause dizziness, light-headedness, or faintness (sense of impending loss of consciousness, sometimes referred to as presyncope). Vertigo due to disturbances of the inner ear is associated with a sense of "the room spinning" but rarely is associated with loss of consciousness.

PALPITATIONS

The term palpitation refers to an uncomfortable awareness of the heart beat, usually associated with an arrhythmia. The patient may complain of a forceful pulsation of the heart, often with an increase in frequency of heart beats, with or without irregular rhythm. If patients describe a skipped beat or the heart stopping for an instant, they may be sensing the compensatory pause after a premature beat; it is not uncommon for patients to sense the postextrasystolic beat as a forceful contraction. After strenuous exercise, palpitations due to rapid sinus tachycardia are common and normal.

Palpitations with sinus tachycardia at rest or with mild exertion may indicate a disease state, such as high cardiac output states due to thyrotoxicosis, AV fistulas, anemia, beriberi, and heart failure. Palpitations that come on suddenly and end abruptly may indicate paroxysmal atrial tachycardia, atrial fibrillation, atrial flutter, or paroxysmal junctional tachycardia, whereas a gradual onset and end is more likely to reflect sinus tachycardia. The patient should be asked whether the palpitations feel like a regular fast rhythm or irregular rhythm, as the latter is more suggestive of atrial fibrillation. Palpitations may also be felt with very slow rates, as in AV block.

Patients should be questioned about concomitant symptoms. With very rapid heart rates of supraventricular tachycardias, patients may describe lightheadedness or presyncope. Syncopal episodes after palpitations suggest asystole or severe bradycardia after a tachycardia (as in sick sinus syndrome) or may be due to a Stokes-Adams attack. If the patient has angina with rapid palpitations, the chest pain is probably ischemic in origin and due to an increase in oxygen demand greater than oxygen supply to the heart.

EDEMA

Edema is a perceptible accumulation of fluid in the tissues. Questioning the patient on the location of the edema may be important in determining whether the edema is due to a cardiac or noncardiac cause. Common cardiac causes of edema include right- or left-sided heart failure, biventricular failure, constrictive pericarditis, restrictive cardiomyopathy, and tricuspid valvular disease. Peripheral edema due to a cardiac cause is usually distributed from the ankles upward; but in patients who are bedridden, the edema is more prominent in the presacral area. In patients who are upright during the day, edema of the lower extremities typically becomes more severe in the evening, a feature also common to peripheral edema due to venous insufficiency. Edema of the lower extremities associated with a history of prominent neck veins is suggestive of a cardiac cause rather than venous insufficiency alone.

In adults, edema of the face and upper extremities without edema of the lower extremities is more suggestive of a noncardiac cause, such as superior vena caval syndrome (obstruction of this vessel due to carcinoma of the lung, lymphoma, or aortic aneurysm) or angioneurotic edema. Periorbital edema with edema of the face often accompanies acute glomerulonephritis, the nephrotic syndrome, and myxedema; it is not uncommon in children with cardiac edema. When edema of one extremity occurs, local problems, such as thrombophlebitis, lymphatic obstruction, or varicose veins, are probably the cause.

Patients should be questioned about accompanying symptoms, such as dyspnea, ascites, and jaundice. Cardiac edema associated with dyspnea may result from mitral stenosis, left ventricular failure, and cor pulmonale due to chronic obstructive lung disease. Cardiac edema without a history of dyspnea is more suggestive of constrictive pericarditis, tricuspid stenosis or regurgitation, or right heart failure. The patient will describe ascites as an increase in abdominal girth or a swelling of the abdomen. When ascites is of cardiac origin, the patient often has a history of peripheral edema before the development of ascites. Conversely, if the history of ascites occurs before peripheral edema, and especially if jaundice is present, the diagnosis is more likely hepatic dysfunction.

COUGH AND HEMOPTYSIS

Cough is defined as a sudden explosive expiration, initiated by an effort to expel mucus or foreign material from the tracheobronchial tree, while hemoptysis is defined as coughing up blood. Causes of cough due to cardiac disorders include pulmonary edema, pulmonary hypertension, pulmonary emboli leading to infarction, and aortic aneurysms compressing the tracheobronchial tree. Cough associated with dyspnea may be due to cardiac or pulmonary disease. Determining which of these is the cause may be difficult. A long history of productive cough in a patient who is a heavy smoker or a history of cough associated with wheezing in a patient with known allergic (extrinsic) asthma suggests a pulmonary cause. A cough that produces pink, frothy sputum is likely associated with acute pulmonary edema; a cough that produces thick yellow sputum is more likely of an infectious nature.

Hemoptysis may be due to a number of noncardiac causes, including pulmonary tuberculosis, pneumonia, bronchiectasis, carcinoma of the lung, and chronic obstructive lung disease. Cardiovascular causes include mitral stenosis, pulmonary emboli leading to infarction, Eisenmenger's physiology, pulmonary arteriovenous fistulas, and rupture of an aortic aneurysm into the tracheobronchial tree. Large amounts of blood (more than $1/2$ cup) due to brisk bleeding are more likely to be due to focal ulceration, as in bronchogenic carcinoma, bronchiectasis, presence of a foreign body, and rupture of an arteriovenous aneurysm; less often, it may occur in mitral stenosis and pulmonary infarction. Exsanguinating hemoptysis suggests rupture of an aortic aneurysm into the bronchi.

Associated symptoms may clarify the cause. Hemoptysis associated with pleuritic chest pain suggests pulmonary infarction; hemoptysis associated with chronic cough and grey sputum in a patient who smokes suggests chronic bronchitis; hemoptysis associated with purulent sputum suggests pulmonary infection, including abscess; hemoptysis associated with dyspnea on exertion or during pregnancy may be associated with mitral stenosis; episodes of hemoptysis in an otherwise healthy young woman may be due to pulmonary adenoma.

OTHER SYMPTOMS OF CARDIAC DISEASE

Although fatigue and weakness are not specific symptoms of cardiac disease, they do occur with decreased forward cardiac output, as in heart failure. These symptoms may occur after massive diuresis with orthostatic hypotension and hypokalemia. In addition, fatigue and weakness are side effects of some antihypertensive medications, such as alpha methyldopa and, occasionally, beta blockers.

Either the patient or the patient's family may note cyanosis, but cyanosis often goes unnoticed. Cyanosis indicates that 5 g or more of reduced hemoglobin is present. Cyanosis occurs in certain forms of congenital heart disease with right to left shunts, pulmonary embolism, peripheral vascular disease, and low output states.

Gastrointestinal symptoms such as anorexia, nausea, and vomiting may occur in right-sided heart failure and may be secondary to digitalis toxicity.

Epigastric distress is not uncommonly associated with left ventricular inferior wall infarction or ischemia. Indigestion may occur as the sole symptom of angina pectoris or myocardial infarction. Hiccups may occur in patients with myocardial infarction or after cardiac surgery.

Bibliography

Braunwald E: The history. In: Braunwald E, ed. *Heart Disease: A Textbook of Cardiovascular Medicine.* Philadelphia: Saunders; 1988, p. 1.

Fowler NO: The history in cardiac diagnosis. In: Fowler NO, ed. *Cardiac Diagnosis and Treatment.* Hagerstown: Harper & Row; 1980, p. 23.

Fuster V: The clinical history. In: Brandenburg RO, Fuster V, Giuliani ER, McGoon DC. *Cardiology. Fundamentals and Practice.* Chicago: Year Book Publishers, Inc; 1987, p. 185.

Hurst JW, Morris DC, Crawley S, Dorney ER: The history: Past events and symptoms related to cardiovascular disease. In: Hurst JW, ed. *The Heart.* New York: McGraw Hill; 1986, p. 109.

Wood P: *Diseases of the Heart and Circulation*– 3rd ed. Philadelphia: Lippincott; 1968.

CHAPTER 2

The Physical Examination

Robert A. Kloner

GENERAL APPEARANCE AND VITAL SIGNS

A useful approach to the cardiovascular physical examination is to begin by recording the general appearance and vital signs, followed by examination of the patient from the head downward.

The general appearance of the patient may provide helpful clues as to the nature and severity of cardiac illness. For example, cachexia is not uncommon in end-stage heart disease. If the patient appears short of breath at rest or when walking from one end of the examining room to another, significant disease is suggested. Body habitus should be noted; long extremities and an arm span exceeding height, kyphoscoliosis, and pectus excavatum or pectus carinatum suggest Marfan's syndrome. Extreme obesity, somnolence, and cyanosis suggest Pickwickian syndrome.

Vital signs (pulse rate, respiratory rate, blood pressure, and temperature) are crucial parts of the cardiovascular physical examination. Pulse rate should be determined by palpating the radial pulse for a full minute, noting the strength of the pulse and irregularities in rhythm. The apical rate should be determined by cardiac auscultation.

Blood pressure is recorded with a sphygmomanometer and a stethoscope over the brachial artery. The standard-size blood pressure cuff is designed for the average adult arm. In patients with large or obese arms, a standard cuff will overestimate arterial pressure; therefore, a leg cuff should be used to measure pressure in their upper extremities. As the cuff is deflated, the first appearance of clear tapping sounds (phase I of Korotkoff sounds) is the systolic pressure. Most physicians record the disappearance of sounds (phase V of Korotkoff sounds) as the diastolic pressure, but if phase IV (a sudden muffling of sounds before their disappearance) is heard and is more than 10 mm Hg from phase V, then it should be recorded

as well. An auscultatory gap is a period of silence occurring after phase I and before phase II of Korotkoff sounds. (Phase II is the period in which the clear tapping sounds of phase I are replaced by soft murmurs.) If the reappearance of sound is read mistakenly as systolic pressure, then this pressure is underestimated. The auscultatory gap occurs where there is reduced velocity of blood flow through the arms (i.e., aortic stenosis) or venous distention of the arms.

To determine blood pressure in the basal state, multiple readings must be obtained. Blood pressure should be measured in both arms, as differences between extremities greater than 15 mm Hg may signify obstructive lesions in the arterial tree. It is useful to measure both supine and standing blood pressures, especially in patients who have symptoms suggesting orthostatic hypotension and who are taking antihypertensive medicines. Normally, there is only a small, transient decrease in systolic arterial pressure of 5-15 mm Hg and a rise in diastolic pressure when a person assumes upright posture. Systolic blood pressure in the legs may be up to 20 mm Hg higher than in the arms, but diastolic pressure should be the same. In patients with hypertension, pressures in the legs should be recorded to rule out coarctation of the aorta, in which case pressures are lower than in the arms.

Pulsus paradoxus is a fall in arterial pressure greater than 10 mm Hg during inspiration. It is associated with pericardial tamponade, but may also occur in chronic lung disease, asthma, pleural effusions, and pneumothorax. It may be appreciated by feeling the radial pulse diminish or disappear during inspiration. Pulsus alternans occurs during a regular rhythm when every other heart beat has a higher systolic pressure. This phenomenon is associated with end-stage left ventricular failure and can occur for several beats after a premature contraction.

EXAMINATION OF THE HEAD AND FACE

Facial edema may occur in myxedema, constrictive pericarditis, tricuspid valve disease, and superior vena caval syndrome. Several structural facial abnormalities are associated with various congenital cardiac diseases, as in Down's, Turner's, Hurler's, and Noonan's syndromes. In Down's syndrome, which is usually associated with endocardial cushion defect and ventricular septal defect, there is a prominent medial epicanthus and large protruding tongue. Turner's syndrome is associated with coarctation of the aorta, bicuspid aortic valve, and other congenital cardiac abnormalities; these patients characteristically have webbing of the neck and widely set eyes (hypertelorism). In Hurler's syndrome, in which aortic and mitral regurgitation, cardiomyopathy, and coronary artery disease may be present, the facies exhibit coarse features and there is corneal clouding. Patients with Noonan's syndrome, in which a characteristic cardiovascular abnormality is pulmonic stenosis, have hypertelorism, webbing of the neck, small chin, low-set ears, epicanthal folds, and ptosis. Patients with a nonfamilial form of supravalvular aortic stenosis may have a so-called "elfin facies," with a prominent, high forehead; low-set ears; hypertelorism; a small, pointed chin; epicanthal folds; overhanging upper lip; upturned nose; and dental abnormalities.

Examination of the eyes should include assessment for exophthalmos and stare, which occur in both hyperthyroidism and advanced right-sided heart failure. Arcus is a light-colored ring around the iris associated with hypercholesterolemia in young adults; this may be a normal finding in the elderly. Xanthelasma are lipid-filled plaques that surround the eyes and also are associated with hypercholesterolemia.

Blue sclera can be seen in Marfan's syndrome, osteogenesis imperfecta, and Ehlers-Danlos syndrome; they are associated with aortic dilatation and dissection. Cataracts occur in a number of diseases associated with cardiovascular disorders, including Marfan's syndrome, myotonic dystrophy, homocystinuria, and rubella. Argyll Robertson pupils (small, unequal pupils that do not react to light but do react to accommodation) are classic for central nervous system syphilis and may be associated with luetic aortitis.

Fundi should be examined for the presence of hypertensive and atherosclerotic arterial changes. Roth's spots are hemorrhages with a white center, which are observed on funduscopic examination; they are usually due to infective endocarditis. Conjunctival hemorrhages also may be seen in endocarditis.

A deep vertical crease in the earlobe in young patients is associated with premature atherosclerosis, but this is a nonspecific finding.

EXAMINATION OF THE NECK

Examination of the neck includes assessing the jugular venous pressure and pulse, carotid pulse, and thyroid gland.

JUGULAR VENOUS PULSE

The internal jugular vein should be examined for determination of jugular venous pressure and is more reliable for this purpose than the external jugular vein. The pulsations caused by this vein are best visualized with a flashlight shining tangentially across the neck. Jugular venous pulses are effectively examined with the patient lying at a 45° angle, but if venous pressure is high, a greater inclination is desirable (60-90°). If it is low, the patient should be positioned at a 30° angle. To estimate central venous pressure, the patient is placed at 45° and the height of the oscillating meniscus of the jugular pulse is determined. Normally the height of the pulse wave is less than 4 cm above the sternal angle. Since the sternal angle is approximately 5 cm above the right atrium, central venous pressure is normally less than 9 cm H_2O (4 cm above the sternal angle plus 5 cm above the right atrium). Thus, to determine central venous pressure (in cm H_2O), one adds (in cm) the height of the jugular pulse above the sternal angle to 5.

The wave form of the jugular venous pulse yields important information. (Details of the components of the pulses are described in Chapter 7.) With the unaided eye, two waves per heart beat are visible: the *a* and *v* waves. The a-wave reflects atrial contraction and occurs before the carotid pulse. After the a-wave, pressure drops; this is called the x descent, due to atrial relaxation, and occurs just before the second heart sound. The v-wave follows and results from a rise in right atrial pressure as blood flows into the right atrium while the tricuspid valve is closed. The v-wave occurs just after the carotid pulse. After the v-wave, there is a smaller fall in pressure, the y descent, which is due to the fall in right atrial pressure as the tricuspid valve opens; it ends just after the second heart sound.

When the jugular venous pressure is elevated, the v-wave becomes higher and the y descent more prominent. Conditions in which jugular venous pressure increases reflect an increase in right atrial pressure, as occurs in right heart failure, pericardial disease (cardiac tamponade and constrictive pericarditis), and restrictive cardiomyopathies. The jugular venous pressure is also elevated in superior vena caval obstructions.

With cardiac tamponade, the x descent is prominent and the y descent is small; with constrictive pericarditis the y descent is prominent and deep. Large a-waves are observed in pulmonary stenosis, tricuspid stenosis, right ventricular hypertrophy, pulmonary hypertension, and ventricular septal hypertrophy. In conditions of atrioventricular (AV) dissociation, when the atrium contracts against a closed tricuspid valve, giant or cannon a-waves are observed. A prominent regurgitant v-wave and absence of an x descent suggest tricuspid regurgitation. In tricuspid stenosis, the y descent is typically gradual.

THE CAROTID PULSE

Normally, the carotid pulse has a rapid rise to a rounded peak followed by a less rapid decline, which is interrupted in its early phase by an incisura or dicrotic notch (a sharp downward deflection representing closure of the aortic valve). As the pulse wave is transmitted from the ascending aorta to the peripheral vessels, the systolic upstroke becomes steeper and its amplitude higher; the incisura or dicrotic notch becomes smoother in configuration.

The carotid pulse contour is abnormal in a number of disease states. A delayed systolic peak (pulsus tardus) is typical of aortic stenosis, in which there may also be an accentuated anacrotic notch (a pause on the ascending limb of the pulse). A bisferiens pulse occurs when there are two systolic peaks; it is associated with aortic regurgitation, a combination of aortic regurgitation and aortic stenosis, and hypertrophic obstructive cardiomyopathy (formerly called idiopathic hypertrophic subaortic stenosis). Pulsus paradoxus and pulsus alternans, described earlier, are appreciated by palpation of the pulse. Pulsus alternans, which occurs with a regular rhythm, should be distinguished from pulsus bigeminus, which occurs with ectopic bigeminal rhythm, usually ventricular. In this latter condition, the weaker beat follows a shorter interval. Pulsus parvus refers to a weak pulse and can be encountered in any condition in which left

ventricular stroke volume is reduced. The arterial pulse may be accentuated or bounding in patients with high cardiac output states (e.g., hyperthyroidism and arteriovenous fistulas), aortic regurgitation, or rigid, sclerotic arteries. Excessive carotid pressure during the physical examination should be avoided in elderly patients, who may have atherosclerosis.

All peripheral pulses should be examined. Reduced, unequal pulses or bruits may signify significant obstructive disease due to atherosclerosis or other causes (dissection, aneurysm, aortitis, embolism). Further discussion of carotid pulses appears in Chapter 7.

EXAMINATION OF THE LUNGS

Bilateral rales that are fine and crackling (like crackling cellophane) and that are often more prominent at the bases of the lungs occur in congestive heart failure. Rales, however, may be due to noncardiac causes (e.g., pneumonia), in which case the rales have a coarser sound and are unilateral. Auscultation of the lungs after deep breathing and coughing decreases false-positive findings. Pleural effusions secondary to heart failure are usually bilateral; when they are unilateral, they tend to occur on the right side. The physical findings of pleural effusion include dullness to percussion and reduced or absent vocal fremitus.

EXAMINATION OF THE HEART

Inspection and palpation of the precordium provides information concerning the location and quality of the left ventricular impulse. The examiner should palpate the precordial movements of the heart with the patient both in the supine and the left lateral decubitus position. This latter maneuver increases the ability to palpate the left ventricle. The apex beat is the lowest and most lateral point on the chest at which the cardiac impulse can be felt. Normally, it is superior to the fifth left intercostal space and within the left midclavicular line. It is often, but not always, the point of maximal impulse, since pulsations arising from other structures may be more forceful.

The normal precordial pulse is an outward systolic motion felt during isovolumetric contraction as the left ventricle rotates and strikes the anterior chest wall, followed by retraction of the left ventricle as blood is ejected from the cavity. With left ventricular hypertrophy, the outward systolic motion is exaggerated and sustained. Displacement of the left ventricular impulse downward and to the left suggests left ventricular dilatation, as occurs in chronic aortic regurgitation or chronic congestive heart failure.

Aneurysms of the left ventricle result in a large systolic bulge, which is felt above and often medial to the apex beat. Left ventricular dyskinesis may be appreciated as two impulses separated by several centimeters. A presystolic impulse is felt when the atrial contribution to left ventricular filling is increased (in myocardial ischemia, left ventricular hypertrophy due to hypertension, aortic stenosis, or myocardial fibrosis) and is associated with a fourth heart sound.

Double systolic impulses plus a presystolic impulse typically are felt in hypertrophic obstructive cardiomyopathy. Parasternal lifts usually are due to right ventricular or left atrial enlargement in the setting of mitral regurgitation. Systolic retraction of the chest is associated with constrictive pericarditis. Prominent systolic pulsations in the left second intercostal space represent pulmonary hypertension or increased pulmonary blood flow. Finally, thrills may be palpated in association with loud murmurs (such as those resulting from aortic stenosis, ventricular septal defect, and pulmonary stenosis).

AUSCULTATION

First Heart Sound

There has been controversy as to the origin of the first heart sound (S_1). The classic theory holds that it is due to closure of the mitral and tricuspid valves. An alternative explanation holds that it is due to movement and acceleration of blood in early systole. The S_1 is often split, with the first component representing mitral and the second component representing tricuspid valve closure. The two components are separated by a narrow interval of 0.02-0.03 sec. The S_1 is heard best in the mitral area.

Conditions that increase the intensity of the S_1 include mitral stenosis (in cases where the valve is not extensively calcified and is still pliable), exercise, thyrotoxicosis, systemic hypertension, and a short PR interval, which results in the AV valves being widely separated at the beginning of ventricular contraction. Conditions that decrease the intensity of the S_1 include a prolonged (>0.20 sec) PR interval (AV valves have partially closed before a later onset of ventricular contraction), aortic insufficiency (also due to premature mitral valve closure), mitral insufficiency, and

cases of mitral stenosis in which the valve is severely calcified and rigid. The intensity of the S_1 varies in complete heart block and in atrial fibrillation. Abnormally wide splitting of the S_1 is unusual, but may occur in Ebstein's anomaly when associated with right bundle branch block; occasionally in right bundle branch block alone; and in tricuspid stenosis.

Second Heart Sound

The second heart sound (S_2) consists of two components: A_2, representing closure of the aortic valve, and P_2, representing closure of the pulmonic valve (Figure 1A). The two components normally fuse with expiration and are separated (by 0.02-0.06 sec) with inspiration. Wide splitting of S_2 with preservation of respiratory variation occurs when P_2 is delayed relative to A_2. This situation occurs with complete right bundle branch block, occasionally in Wolff-Parkinson-White syndrome, with ventricular premature beats arising from the left ventricle, with pacing from the left ventricle, in pulmonic stenosis, and in severe mitral regurgitation in which the left ventricular ejection time is shortened. Broad fixed splitting of S_2 occurs in atrial septal defect, with an average splitting interval of 0.05 sec (range, 0.03-0.08 sec). Fixed splitting may also occur in right ventricular failure due to any cause, although the splitting interval is not usually wide in this situation.

Reversed or paradoxical splitting of the S_2. When aortic valve closure is delayed, the A_2 and P_2 are separated during expiration and come together during inspiration. Thus, the splitting is said to be reversed (Figure 1A). The two most common causes of reversed splitting of the S_2 are left bundle branch block and aortic stenosis. Other causes include right ventricular paced and ectopic beats, hypertrophic obstructive cardiomyopathy, patent ductus arteriosus, and, less often, systemic hypertension and ischemic heart disease. The S_2 is single in tetralogy of Fallot, pulmonary atresia, hypoplastic left heart syndrome, and truncus arteriosus. The S_2 may appear single when the P_2 is very faint due to obesity and emphysema.

Intensity of the S_2. The A_2 is best heard in the second right intercostal space and the P_2 in the second left intercostal space. In adults, the A_2 is normally louder than the P_2. Hypertension within the aorta or pulmonary artery results in a loud A_2 or P_2 respectively. Dilatation of these vessels may also cause the S_2 to be accentuated. In thin-chested persons the S_2 may be louder. The A_2 is also accentuated in coarc-

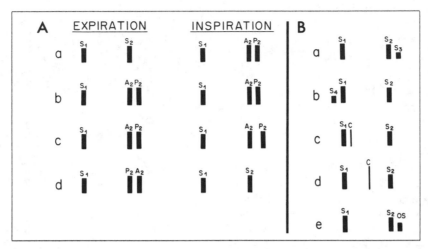

Figure 1. *A: Respiratory variation of the second heart sound. S_1 = first heart sound; S_2 = second heart sound; A_2 = aortic component of S_2; P_2 = pulmonic component of S_2. (a) Normal splitting of S_2 in inspiration. (b) Fixed splitting of S_2, as in atrial septal defect. (c) Splitting in expiration enhanced with inspiration, as in right bundle branch block. (d) Paradoxical splitting. Splitting in expiration but not in inspiration, as in left bundle branch block and aortic stenosis. B: Timing of the extra heart sounds in relationship to S_1 and S_2. S_3 = third heart sound; S_4 = fourth heart sound; C = click; OS = opening snap. (a) S_3. (b) S_4. (c) Early systolic ejection click. (d) Midsystolic ejection click. (e) Opening snap.*

tation of the aorta and corrected transposition of the great arteries.

The A_2 is reduced in intensity in aortic stenosis, when the valve is rigid secondary to calcification; it may also be reduced in intensity in aortic regurgitation. The P_2 is reduced in both valvular and infundibular stenosis. In patients with a greater distance between the origin of the S_2 and chest wall, due to either a thoracic deformity or lung disease, especially emphysema, the intensity of the S_2 is reduced.

Third Heart Sound

The third heart sound (S_3) is a low-pitched sound occurring approximately 0.15 sec (range, 0.1-0.2 sec) after the S_2. It is probably due to rapid expansion and filling of the left or right ventricle in early diastole (Figure 1B). An S_3 may be a normal finding in young persons; but when it is associated with a pathologic condition, it is also termed a protodiastolic gallop or an S_3 gallop. Left-sided S_3's are heard best at the apical area with the bell of the stethoscope.

Frequent causes of an S_3 gallop are high cardiac output states, as in anemia or thyrotoxicosis; mitral insufficiency, in which there is increased ventricular filling in early diastole; and congestive heart failure

with a dilated ventricle. Other causes include atrial septal defect, ventricular septal defect, patent ductus arteriosus, and aortic insufficiency. An S_3 should be differentiated from an opening snap of mitral stenosis, which tends to be a higher frequency sound and occurs 0.03-0.12 sec—that is, earlier—after the S_2. An S_3 also may be confused with the pericardial knock of constrictive pericarditis, which tends to have a somewhat higher frequency, occurs earlier than an S_3 (0.09-0.12 sec after A_2), and radiates more widely over the precordium.

Fourth Heart Sound

The fourth heart sound (S_4), or presystolic gallop, is a low-frequency vibration that occurs when the atrium contracts into a ventricle (left or right) with reduced compliance. An S_4 occurs when the ventricular walls are stiff due to hypertrophy, fibrosis, or ischemia. Thus, an S_4 is a common feature of systemic hypertension and aortic stenosis with left ventricular hypertrophy, hypertrophic obstructive cardiomyopathy, and coronary artery disease. A left-sided S_4 is best heard with the bell of the stethoscope at the apex; placing the patient in a left lateral decubitus position accentuates it. An S_4 originating from the right ventricle occurs with pulmonary hypertension and pulmonary stenosis.

When heart rates are very rapid, an S_3 and S_4 may merge to produce a "summation gallop."

Ejection Sounds and Clicks

Ejection sounds and clicks are high-frequency sounds that arise from the aortic or pulmonic valve areas and occur in early systole (Figure 1B). Aortic ejection sounds occur in association with congenital aortic stenosis, bicuspid aortic valve, and acquired aortic stenosis; they imply that the valve is mobile and not heavily calcified. When due to an abnormal aortic valve, the sounds may radiate over the entire precordium. Ejection sounds also occur when the aortic root is dilated, as in systemic hypertension. Pulmonic ejection clicks are heard in cases of valvular pulmonic stenosis, pulmonary hypertension, and, occasionally, idiopathic dilatation of the pulmonary artery. In cases of pulmonary stenosis, the earlier in systole the ejection sound is heard, the more severe the stenosis. Pulmonary ejection sounds are absent in subvalvular pulmonic stenosis or when valvular stenosis is caused by severely immobilized valves. The pulmonic ejection sound is typically louder during expiration, unlike most other right-sided cardiac sounds. It tends to be localized to the left upper sternal border, in contrast to aortic ejection sounds, which are heard more widely over the precordium. Pulmonic ejection sounds also tend to occur slightly earlier than aortic ejection sounds, and, as noted earlier, vary with respiration, while aortic ejection sounds do not.

Midsystolic Clicks

A midsystolic click or multiple clicks that may be accompanied by a late systolic murmur occur in patients with mitral valve prolapse (Figure 1B). Simultaneous echocardiographic and phonocardiographic studies show that the click or clicks correspond to the point of maximal prolapse of the valve.

Opening Snap

The opening snap (OS) is a high-frequency sound heard in early diastole in patients with mitral or tricuspid stenosis and results from the stiff valve snapping into its respective ventricle during the early filling phase (Figure 1B). The S_2-OS interval is important, in that severe stenosis is associated with a shorter S_2-

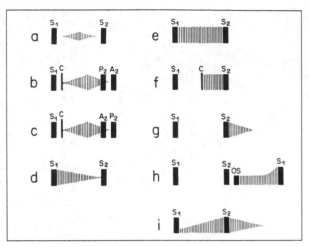

Figure 2. *Principal cardiac murmurs. (a) Short mid-systolic murmur as in innocent murmer. (b) Aortic stenosis. Aortic ejection click, mid- to late-peaking systolic murmur, delayed A_2. (c) Pulmonic stenosis. Pulmonic ejection click, systolic ejection murmur stops before P_2 but extends through A_2. (d) Holosystolic murmur decreases in late systole as in acute mitral regurgitation. (e) Pansystolic regurgitant murmur as in mitral regurgitation. (f) Midsystolic murmur due to mitral valve prolapse. (g) Diastolic decrescendo murmur due to semilunar valve insufficiency. (h) Diastolic murmur of mitral stenosis. (i) Continuous murmur as in patent ductus arteriosus.*

OS interval. The OS due to mitral stenosis is heard best between the mid-left sternal border and apex. Those due to tricuspid stenosis are heard at the lower left sternal border.

MURMURS

Murmurs are a series of vibrations due to turbulence of blood flow (Figure 2). The intensity of a murmur depends upon blood velocity and volume of blood flowing across the sound-producing area and the distance from the sound-producing area to the stethoscope. The intensity of murmurs is graded on a scale of 1 to 6. Grade 1 is the faintest murmur that can be heard; grade 2 is faint but slightly louder; grade 3 is moderately loud; grade 4 is a loud murmur associated with a palpable thrill; grade 5 is a very loud murmur but still requires a stethoscope to be heard; a grade 6 murmur is so loud that it can be heard without use of a stethoscope. Radiation of murmurs depends on the direction of blood flow responsible for the murmur, site of origin, and intensity of the murmur. Duration depends on the duration of the pressure gradient that causes the murmur. Timing of murmurs during systole or diastole is aided by simultaneous palpation of the carotid pulse.

Systolic Murmurs

Systolic murmurs are classified as midsystolic ejection murmurs or as pansystolic regurgitant murmurs (Figure 2). Midsystolic, diamond-shaped, crescendo-decrescendo ejection murmurs occur as a result of the forward ejection of blood into the root of the aorta or pulmonary arteries. They begin after the S_1 and end before the S_2. Pansystolic (or holosystolic) regurgitant murmurs occur due to backward flow of blood through the mitral or tricuspid valve or through a ventricular septal defect and have a more even intensity. They begin with the first heart sound and proceed to the second sound on their side of origin.

Systolic ejection murmurs. Causes of systolic ejection murmurs include physiologic or functional ejection murmurs (not associated with any cardiac abnormality), aortic stenosis, pulmonic stenosis, hypertrophic obstructive cardiomyopathy, ejection of blood through a normal valve into a dilated aorta or pulmonary artery, and increased rate of ejection of blood in otherwise normal persons due to anemia, fever, thyrotoxicosis, and exercise. An ejection murmur originating from one side of the heart always stops before closure of the semilunar valve on that side, but may continue through closure of the semilunar valve on the other side of the heart. Thus, the murmur of pulmonic stenosis continues through A_2 but stops before P_2. It is now believed that functional murmurs are probably aortic in origin. They tend to peak in early systole (<0.20 sec after the QRS complex). Murmurs caused by high grades of aortic stenosis or pulmonic stenosis tend to be prolonged and peak in mid- to late systole (>0.24 sec after the QRS complex). In tetralogy of Fallot, the systolic ejection murmur becomes shorter with increased severity of the pulmonic stenosis, as less blood crosses the pulmonary valve and more is ejected through the ventricular septal defect.

Pansystolic murmurs. Causes of pansystolic regurgitant murmurs include blood flowing retrogradely through the mitral and tricuspid valves and ventricular septal defect. The even intensity and long duration of the murmur correspond to the duration of the pressure difference across the orifice producing the murmurs.

These murmurs tend to have a higher frequency and a "blowing" quality compared with systolic ejection murmurs, which in general tend to be harsher. The murmur of tricuspid regurgitation increases with inspiration, whereas that of mitral regurgitation does not.

Early systolic murmurs. Early systolic murmurs may be heard in acute mitral regurgitation due to rupture of a chordae tendineae or papillary muscle or in infective endocarditis. The murmurs may be confined to early and midsystole and taper off in late systole. Since a large volume of blood enters a small, previously normal left atrium during systole, the ventricular and atrial pressures equalize during the second half of systole, suppressing the murmur. Tricuspid regurgitation due to disease of the valve itself rather than related to pulmonary hypertension can cause an early systolic murmur. Early systolic murmurs are heard in very small ventricular septal defects or ventricular septal defects once Eisenmenger's complex (pulmonary hypertension) develops. The murmur of patent ductus arteriosus becomes confined to early systole once pulmonary hypertension develops.

Late systolic murmurs. Late systolic murmurs are most frequently due to mitral valve prolapse and often begin with a midsystolic click or clicks. These murmurs begin in mid- to late systole, continue to the S_2, and tend to be of relatively high frequency. Sometimes, late systolic murmurs are musical in nature and sound like a honk or a whoop. Late systolic murmurs are rarely due to ventricular septal defect or coarctation of the aorta.

Diastolic Murmurs

Diastolic murmurs occur due to regurgitation of blood across the aortic or pulmonic valves or to forward flow across the mitral or tricuspid valves (Figure 2). When the cause is regurgitation across the semilunar valves, the murmurs begin in very early diastole, just after S_2; when the cause is flow across the AV valves, they tend to occur in mid-diastole.

Diastolic murmurs due to insufficiency of the semilunar valves. These murmurs begin with an S_2; they are high frequency, blowing, and decrescendo. When the aortic cusps are torn or perforated, the murmur of aortic regurgitation may have a musical or cooing quality. These murmurs are heard best with the diaphragm of the stethoscope in the third or fourth intercostal space at the sternal edge, while the patient is sitting upright and leaning forward. Aortic insufficiency due to disease of the valve leaflets typically radiates to the left sternal border, while that due to aortic root dilatation radiates to the right sternal border. It may be difficult to differentiate the murmurs of aortic from those of pulmonary regurgitation; however, inspiratory augmentation favors the latter. The pulmonary regurgitant murmur due to pulmonary hypertension (Graham Steell murmur) has a higher pitch and may be heard earlier in diastole than the murmur of pulmonary regurgitation due to primary valvular disease.

Diastolic murmurs due to forward flow through the mitral and tricuspid valves. Diastolic murmurs originating from the AV valves occur when forward flow through these valves is increased or when these valves become stenotic. These murmurs begin in early to mid-diastole, when ventricular pressure has fallen below atrial pressure and the valve opens, which may be associated with an opening snap. The murmur is low-pitched and rumbling and may intensify during atrial contraction just before the S_1 of the next beat. This presystolic accentuation typically is absent in atrial fibrillation. Occasionally, however, mild accentuation of a mitral diastolic rumble occurs in the absence of atrial systole due to closer coaptation of the diseased mitral leaflets toward end-diastole.

The murmur of mild mitral stenosis is relatively short and may disappear in mid-diastole and reappear with atrial contraction in late diastole, while the murmur of severe mitral stenosis tends to be longer in duration and more even in intensity. Mitral stenosis murmurs are best heard at the apex with the bell of the stethoscope and with the patient in the left lateral decubitus position. The murmur of tricuspid stenosis has similarities to that of mitral stenosis, but is augmented with inspiration, is higher in frequency, is best heard at the left lower sternal border, and occurs slightly earlier in diastole. Murmurs due to left atrial myxoma often mimic those due to mitral stenosis but tend to change in quality and intensity with alterations in body position.

Diastolic murmurs that occur with increased blood flow across the mitral valve have a number of causes: mitral regurgitation, ventricular septal defect, and patent ductus arteriosus. Increased flow across the tricuspid valve may result in a diastolic murmur as in tricuspid regurgitation and atrial septal defect.

An Austin Flint murmur is an apical diastolic rumbling murmur heard in aortic insufficiency due to "functional mitral stenosis," when the anterior leaf-

let of the mitral valve partially closes due to the regurgitant stream.

Continuous Murmurs

Continuous murmurs begin in systole and extend through the S_2 into all or part of diastole. They occur when there is a continuous pressure difference between areas. Abnormal connections between the systemic arterial and systemic venous systems or between the systemic and pulmonary systems may cause such murmurs. Continuous murmurs may be caused by patent ductus arteriosus, rupture of a sinus of Valsalva into the right side of the heart, systemic or pulmonary AV fistulas, and man-made fistulas (Blalock, Potts procedure, shunts for hemodialysis). Abnormalities in arteries may cause such murmurs, as occur in constriction of a peripheral systemic artery, constriction of a pulmonary artery, and coarctation of the aorta. The venous hum is a continuous murmur originating over the great veins of the lower part of the neck; it is a normal finding. It can be obliterated by recumbency, pressure over the veins of the neck, and by Valsalva maneuver.

MANEUVERS TO DIFFERENTIATE TYPES OF HEART SOUNDS AND MURMURS

Various physiologic and pharmacologic maneuvers may be useful in differentiating murmurs and sounds with similar characteristics.

Respiration

Inspiration results in increased right ventricular filling and stroke volume and decreased left ventricular filling and stroke volume. In general, the intensity of murmurs arising from the right side of the heart increases during inspiration, while the intensity of murmurs originating from the left side either does not change or decreases. In mitral valve prolapse, however, inspiratory decrease of left ventricular cavity size increases the redundancy of the valve, and the click occurs earlier and the murmur may become accentuated. An S_3 and S_4 originating from the right side are increased during inspiration.

Valsalva Maneuver

This maneuver involves forced expiration against a closed glottis. During phase I of the Valsalva maneuver, intrathoracic pressure rises and there is an increase in left ventricular output and blood pressure. During the strain phase (II), venous return is impaired with a reduction in right ventricular filling followed by a reduction in left ventricular filling, and there is a fall in stroke volume and blood pressure. During this strain phase, almost all murmurs and heart sounds diminish in intensity except the murmur of hypertrophic obstructive cardiomyopathy, which increases in intensity due to the reduction in left ventricular volume, and occasionally the murmur of mitral prolapse, which increases or occurs earlier due to more severe prolapse. During phase III (release of respiratory pressure), flow to the right side of the heart increases first, followed by increased flow to the left side. Thus, murmurs originating from the right side of the heart return to normal (or may actually temporarily increase) one to two cardiac cycles after release of the maneuver, while murmurs from the left side require four to 11 cardiac cycles to recover their intensity. Therefore, the Valsalva maneuver may aid in differentiating right-sided from left-sided murmurs.

When the cardiac cycle length varies, as in atrial fibrillation or with compensatory pauses after a premature contraction, systolic ejection murmurs after the pause are increased in intensity, whereas there is no change in left-sided pansystolic regurgitant murmurs or systolic murmurs due to ventricular septal defect. Therefore, this sign may be helpful in differentiating aortic stenosis from mitral regurgitation. There is, however, increased intensity after longer cycles in the murmur of tricuspid regurgitation.

Isometric Exercise

Isometric exercise consisting of hand grip for 30-40 sec causes an increase in systemic blood pressure and heart rate, cardiac output, and left ventricular filling pressure. This maneuver should be avoided in patients with myocardial ischemia and ventricular arrhythmias. Isometric exercise helps differentiate systolic murmurs due to valvular aortic stenosis and hypertrophic obstructive cardiomyopathy, which decrease during hand grip, from those due to mitral insufficiency and ventricular septal defect, which increase with this maneuver. The diastolic murmur of aortic insufficiency increases with hand grip. The murmur of mitral stenosis increases with hand grip due to increased cardiac output. The systolic murmur and click of mitral prolapse are delayed by hand grip.

Squatting

Squatting increases systemic venous return; at the same time, it increases arterial blood pressure. The systolic murmur of hypertrophic obstructive cardiomyopathy characteristically is reduced by squatting; the murmur of aortic insufficiency is accentuated. Third and fourth heart sounds are augmented during squatting.

Changes in Posture

Rapid changes in posture alter venous return; lying down from a standing position and elevation of the legs increase right ventricular filling and, hence, right ventricular stroke volume, followed by an increase in left ventricular stroke volume. Murmurs of aortic and pulmonic stenosis, functional systolic murmurs, mitral and tricuspid regurgitation, and ventricular septal defect are increased by maneuvers that increase venous return, while the murmur of hypertrophic obstructive cardiomyopathy is diminished and that of mitral prolapse is delayed or reduced. Gallop sounds are increased and splitting of the S_2 is widened with increased venous return.

Venous return is decreased by sudden standing, which has the opposite effect on murmurs. Specifically, the murmur of hypertrophic obstructive cardiomyopathy is increased by sudden standing.

Pharmacologic Maneuvers

When amyl nitrite is inhaled, there is marked systemic vasodilatation with a fall in blood pressure and reflex tachycardia. This is followed by an increase in venous return and cardiac output. Because of the increase in forward flow, systolic murmurs of hypertrophic obstructive cardiomyopathy, aortic stenosis, pulmonic stenosis, functional flow murmurs, and the diastolic murmurs of tricuspid and mitral stenosis are increased. The systolic murmur of tetralogy of Fallot, however, is reduced in intensity. Blood flowing through the pulmonary outflow tract decreases in favor of increased flow through the right to left shunt, due to reduced systemic arterial pressure. The fall in systemic arterial pressure results in diminution of the systolic murmur of mitral insufficiency, ventricular septal defect (less left-to-right shunting), patent ductus arteriosus, and the diastolic murmur of aortic insufficiency. Increased pressures on the right side of the heart and a slight increase in pulmonary artery pressure cause the murmur of tricuspid and pulmonic insufficiency to increase. The murmur of mitral valve prolapse occurs earlier, and is thus longer; however, the intensity of the murmur may have a variable response to amyl nitrite.

Amyl nitrite is especially useful in differentiating the murmur of mitral insufficiency (decrease) from aortic stenosis (increase); differentiating the murmur of rheumatic mitral stenosis (increase) from an Austin Flint murmur due to aortic insufficiency (decrease); differentiating right-sided regurgitant murmurs (increase) from left-sided regurgitant murmurs (decrease); and differentiating small ventricular septal defects (decrease) from pulmonary stenosis (increase).

Vasopressors may be used to assess murmurs including phenylephrine (0.5 mg IV) and methoxamine (3-5 mg IV). These drugs increase systemic and vascular resistance, increase systolic and diastolic arterial pressure, and increase systolic pressures within the ventricles. Phenylephrine is preferred because it elevates pressure for only 3-5 minutes; methoxamine has a duration of action of up to 15-20 minutes. The increased systemic pressure causes an increase in regurgitant flows, thus increasing the diastolic murmur of aortic insufficiency and the systolic murmur of mitral regurgitation. The systolic murmurs due to left to right shunts through ventricular septal defects and patent ductus arteriosus also are increased. Because these agents cause an increase in left ventricular size, they reduce the systolic murmur of hypertrophic obstructive cardiomyopathy and delay the onset of the click and murmur of mitral prolapse.

OTHER HEART SOUNDS AND RUBS

Artificial cardiac valves are associated with various heart sounds not normally heard. The caged-ball or disc valve has opening and closing sounds. Early evidence of valve dysfunction may result in a change in intensity or timing of these sounds. Pacemakers may produce a presystolic extra sound due to skeletal muscle contraction; and occasionally, the pacemaker wire causes a late systolic musical murmur due to its position across the tricuspid valve.

Pericardial friction rubs are described as scratching, grating, or squeaking sounds heard between the left sternal border and apex of the heart. The quality of the sound has been likened to the noise produced when two pieces of leather are rubbed together. These sounds may be inconstant, appearing or disappearing depending on the patient's position. They are easiest to hear with the diaphragm of the stethoscope pressed tightly against the chest while the patient is sitting up and leaning forward. Since the sound occurs as the heart moves within an inflamed pericardium, the rubs often have three components, reflecting movement of the heart during atrial systole, ventricular systole, and ventricular diastole. Three-component rubs are diagnostic of pericarditis; however, pericardial rubs may only have one or two components, in which case they may be confused with systolic or to-and-fro murmurs, respectively.

THE ABDOMINAL EXAMINATION

Valuable clues to the cardiac status may be derived from the abdominal exam. The liver may be enlarged and tender to palpation, due to venous congestion in cases of right heart failure or constrictive pericarditis. Pulsation of the liver occurs in severe tricuspid regurgitation, but can also be due to transmitted pulsations, as occurs in aortic aneurysms. Palpation of the spleen may reveal enlargement when there is concomitant hepatomegaly. The abdomen should be palpated for the presence of aortic aneurysms; if these are found, their width should be estimated. Auscultation should be performed to assess for bruits, which can be heard in cases of renovascular hypertension.

EXAMINATION OF THE SKIN AND EXTREMITIES

Reduction of blood flow may result in cool, cyanotic extremities. Cyanosis is particularly marked in the nailbeds. The term peripheral cyanosis refers to cyanosis in this setting of reduced flow secondary to peripheral vascular disease or heart failure. Central cyanosis refers to that which occurs with intracardiac or intrapulmonary right-to-left shunting and is more prominent in the conjunctiva and mucous membranes. Differential cyanosis is cyanosis in the lower but not the upper extremities and is associated with patent ductus arteriosus with right-to-left shunting.

Raynaud's phenomenon is recognized as the presence of cold-induced pallor of the fingers or toes, followed by intense cyanosis and pain. During the recovery period, there may be a hyperemic phase, in which case the digits appear bright red. Raynaud's phenomenon is associated with certain collagen vascular diseases, atherosclerosis, and primary pulmonary hypertension.

With long-standing arterial vascular insufficiency, atrophic skin changes include a thin, shiny appearance to the skin, loss of hair on the backs of the hands and feet, and dry, brittle nails containing transverse ridges. Small round scars, ulcers, and, in severe cases, gangrene of the skin develop. Venous insufficiency is associated with varicose veins, edema, brownish pigmentation and induration of the skin, and stasis ulcers. Stasis ulcers due to chronic venous insufficiency of the lower extremity typically occur in the area of the internal malleolus.

The skin should be examined for the presence of petechiae and the nailbeds for splinter hemorrhages, both of which are signs associated with bacterial endocarditis. Xanthomas are cholesterol-filled nodules located subcutaneously or along extensor surfaces of tendons and occur in certain types of hyperlipidemias.

Clubbing of the fingers and toes is seen with right-to-left shunts, pulmonary disease, and endocarditis as well as a number of noncardiac conditions.

A number of congenital heart diseases are associated with bony abnormalities. Patients with Holt-Oram syndrome have a thumb with an extra phalynx and atrial septal defect. Ellis-van Creveld syndrome includes polydactyly, hypoplastic fingernails, and atrial or ventricular septal defects. Long, thin, spiderlike fingers—arachnodactyly—are seen in Marfan's syndrome.

Bibliography

Braunwald E: The physical examination. In: Braunwald E, ed. *Heart Disease: A Textbook of Cardiovascular Medicine.* Philadelphia: Saunders; 1988, p. 13.

Constant J: *Bedside Cardiology*—3rd ed. Boston: Little, Brown & Co.; 1985.

Criscitiello M: Physiologic and pharmacologic aids in cardiac auscultation. In: Fowler NO, ed. *Cardiac Diagnosis and Treatment.* Hagerstown: Harper & Row; 1975.

Dohan MC, Criscitiello MG: Physiological and pharmacological manipulation of heart sounds and murmurs. *Mod Conc Cardiovasc Dis* 39:121, 1970.

Evans TC, Giuliani ER, Tancredi RG, Brandenburg RO: *Physical Examination in Cardiology: Fundamentals and Practice.* Chicago: Year Book Medical Publishers; 1987, p. 200.

Harvey WP: Gallop sounds, clicks, snaps, whoops and other sounds. In: Hurst JW, ed. *The Heart.* New York: McGraw-Hill; 1978, p. 255.

Leatham A, Leech GJ, Harvey PW, deLeon AC Jr.: Auscultation of the heart. In: Hurst JW, ed. *The Heart.* New York: McGraw-Hill; 1986, p. 157.

Levine SA, Harvey WP: *Clinical Auscultation of the Heart.* Philadelphia: Saunders; 1959.

Perloff JK: Systolic, diastolic and continuous murmurs. In: Hurst JW, ed. *The Heart.* New York: McGraw-Hill; 1978, p. 268.

Perloff WP: *Physical Examination of the Heart and Circulation.* Philadelphia: Saunders; 1982.

Tavel ME: *Clinical Phonocardiography and External Pulse Monitoring.* Chicago: Yearbook Medical Publishers, Inc.; 1978.

Eliot Young

Electrocardiography

Many aspects of electrocardiography are easy to understand and are quickly learned. Nevertheless, some criteria for clinical diagnosis are nondiagnostic or controversial. Poorly recorded tracings and the use of only one or a limited number of leads may also make interpretation difficult.

P WAVE

The P wave represents the spread of depolarization throughout both atria. The sinus node does not directly contribute to the electrocardiogram (ECG), but its activity is deduced from the presence of a normal P wave. Cramer et al. used a transvenous catheter to record sinus node potentials in the intact canine heart. This technique may prove to be clinically useful in the future.

The normal P wave is positive in leads 1, 2, aV_F and left precordial leads. It is negative in aV_R and variable in leads 3, aV_L and V_1. P-wave amplitude should not exceed 2.5 mm in any lead.

Electrocardiographic criteria for atrial enlargement are not always associated with such a morphologic change. Many laboratories prefer using the nonspecific term *atrial abnormality*. Nevertheless, certain P-wave changes are useful in suggesting left atrial enlargement (LAE) or right atrial enlargement (RAE).

The criteria for LAE are (1) P-wave duration of 0.12 sec or longer, (2) notched P wave with the duration between peaks more than 0.04 sec (Figure 1), or (3) biphasic P wave in V_1, with the late deflection negative and at least 1 mm deep and 0.04 sec wide.

Criteria for LAE are associated with conduction delay between right and left atria; left atrial dilatation, hypertrophy, or increased pressure in the left atrium may or may not be present (Josephson et al.). If LAE criteria are present in V_1, however, they may be the result of a very enlarged right atrium (Marriott). This "pseudo-LAE" pattern may be due to the right atrium enlarging to the left and anteriorly.

Criteria for RAE include (1) P wave is positive, peaked, and at least 2.5 mm in lead 2, 3, or aV_F (Figure 2), (2) the initial positive deflection of the P wave in V_1 or V_2 is at least 1.5 mm, or (3) P-wave axis is greater than $+75°$. Criteria for RAE may not necessarily be associated with right atrial hypertrophy, dilatation, or increased pressure in the right atrium. It may be due only to vertical heart position, sinus tachycardia, low potassium, or even hypertensive heart disease (Chou and Helm, 1965). The term *P congenitale* has been used to describe prominent P waves that are tallest in lead 1 rather than in lead 3, an axis that is more leftward than in the usual RAE.

Criteria for biatrial enlargement (BAE) include one or more of the criteria for both RAE and LAE.

ATRIAL ARRHYTHMIAS

Junctional rhythm with retrograde atrial conduction usually results in negative P waves in leads 2, 3, and aV_F (Figure 3), and biphasic (negative-positive) or positive P waves in V_1. Occasionally, retrograde P waves may even be biphasic (negative-positive) in leads 2, 3, and aV_F. The initial negative part of the P wave may be buried within the preceding QRS, simulating a normal upright P wave. The diagnosis of upper, middle, or lower AV nodal rhythm is not based solely on the P wave's appearing before (with short PR interval), within, or after the QRS. The PR or RP interval also depends on the difference in conduction antegradely into the ventricles and retrogradely into the atria. Recent evidence indicates that cells in the more proximal parts of the AV node (AN and N regions) show no inherent automaticity. As described by Cranefield et al., so-called junctional rhythms arise from the low atria, low AV nodal re-

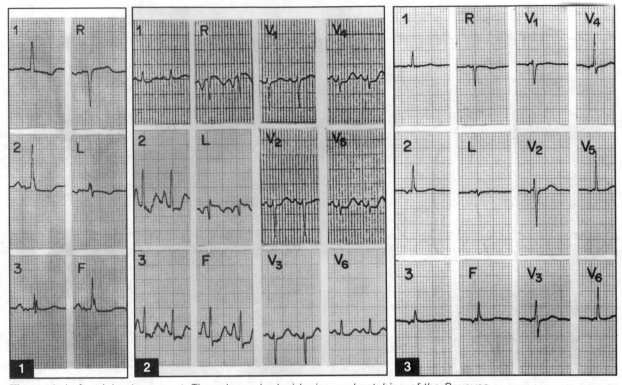

Figure 1. *Left atrial enlargement. There is marked widening and notching of the P waves.*
Figure 2. *Right atrial enlargement. The P waves in leads 2, 3, and aV$_F$ are very tall and peaked.*
Figure 3. *AV junctional rhythm. The P wave is negative in 2, 3, aV$_F$ and the PR interval is 0.10 sec.*

gion (NH), His bundle, or coronary sinus. Thus, it is now customary to use the less specific term *AV junctional* rather than *AV nodal* rhythm.

The mechanism of atrial flutter is controversial, but it is generally believed to be due to reentry. Atrial flutter rates usually range from 220-350 beats/min, but generally are about 300 beats/min. A supraventricular tachycardia with an apparent rate of about 150 beats/min should be carefully evaluated in order to rule out atrial flutter with 2:1 AV block. The F wave is biphasic (negative-positive) or entirely negative in 2, 3, aV$_F$ in 85% of cases and entirely upright in 15%. Electrophysiologic differences in these two types of flutter have not been completely delineated. Atrial flutter may be precipitated by rapid atrial pacing or stimulated atrial premature beats. It may also be terminated by rapid atrial pacing or multiple stimulated atrial premature beats, but not by a single stimulated atrial beat. Rapid atrial pacing may partially change the contour of flutter waves (fusion). This suggests that atrial flutter, although it may be due to reentry, may involve a small circuit and may not circulate around the orifices of the venae cavae (macro-reentry), as Sir Thomas Lewis concluded (Waldo). The

most common AV conduction ratio in the untreated patient is 2:1; 3:1 block is rare. Higher degrees of block may also be seen. Frequently, flutter waves may not be apparent, especially when 2:1 or even 1:1 AV conduction is present. Often, flutter will reveal itself spontaneously or by carotid pressure or drugs causing a higher degree of AV block and separating F waves from the QRS and T waves. The sinus P waves are often wide and notched (LAE) after flutter converts to sinus rhythm.

The mechanism of atrial fibrillation is not confirmed, but multiple reentry circuits is the most popular theory. Distinct and similar type f-waves and regular f-f intervals are not present. Atrial activity is represented by f-waves of varying rate, amplitude, and morphology that cause an oscillatory baseline (Figure 4). At times some of these f-waves may be quite prominent and somewhat regular, so-called flutter-fibrillation. If f-waves in V$_1$ measure 1.5 mm or more from top to trough, LAE is a possibility. Generally, flutter-fibrillation may also be distinguished from pure flutter by causing an irregular ventricular response. However, it has been shown that pure atrial flutter may be associated with an irregular ventricular

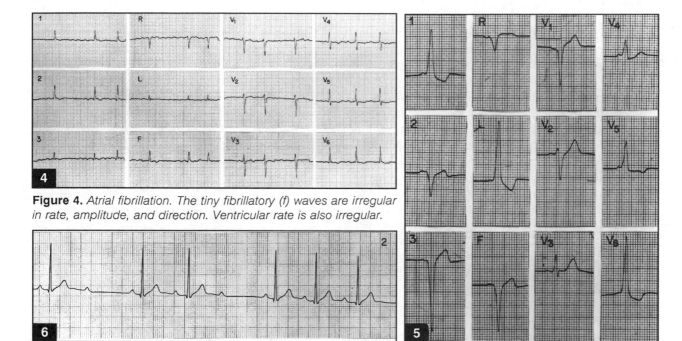

Figure 4. *Atrial fibrillation. The tiny fibrillatory (f) waves are irregular in rate, amplitude, and direction. Ventricular rate is also irregular.*

Figure 5. *Wolff-Parkinson-White (WPW) syndrome. The PR interval is very short and there is a marked delta wave on V$_4$-V$_6$, 1, and aV$_L$. Note similarities to left ventricular hypertrophy and inferior infarction.*
Figure 6. *Type I second-degree AV block (Wenckebach). The first two cycles show 2:1, 3:2 AV block.*

rate in 12% of cases and thus may simulate flutter-fibrillation (Besoain-Santander et al.).

Multifocal atrial tachycardia, also called chaotic atrial tachycardia, is characterized by constantly changing P waves of three or more waveforms at rates of 100 or more. There is no dominant P pacemaker, and P-P and PR intervals are variable. Some P waves may not be conducted. At the onset and offset of this arrhythmia the overall rate may be less than 100 beats/min. Although it is usually associated with pulmonary disease, it may be found in other types of heart disease, especially in the elderly and in diabetics. It is infrequently due to digitalis.

PR INTERVAL

The PR interval is measured from the beginning of the P wave to the beginning of the QRS. It is usually measured in the standard leads. It is derived by subtracting the earliest onset of the QRS in any one of these simultaneously recorded leads from the earliest onset of the P wave in any one of these leads. Lead 2 is most apt to show the earliest onset of the P wave and particularly, if a Q wave is also present in this lead, it will accurately display the PR interval. The PR interval represents the sum of conduction time

from upper right atrium through the AV node, bundle of His, bundle branches, and distal Purkinje fibers.

The normal PR interval in the adult varies from 0.12-0.20 sec. The PR interval usually shortens slightly with exercise because of catecholamine stimulation, which causes faster conduction in the AV node. A short PR interval with normal P and QRS may be due to posterior internodal tract bypass, atrio-His bypass, or congenital small or absent AV node. Short PR interval with anomalous QRS is most likely due to bundle of Kent bypass or Wolff-Parkinson-White (WPW) syndrome (Figure 5), but may be due to one of the above causes of short PR associated with Mahaim fibers. Both short PR interval with normal or anomalous QRS may be associated with supraventricular tachycardia. The former has been popularly called the Lown-Ganong-Levine (LGL) syndrome.

A prolonged PR interval may be due to excessive vagal tone and occurs in athletes or during sleep. It may also be due to drugs (digitalis), as well as disease of the AV node, His bundle, or simultaneous involvement of both bundle branches.

AV block is classified as first-degree (prolonged PR interval), second-degree (some P waves are not conducted), or third-degree (no P waves are conducted into the ventricles). In type I second-degree

AV block (Wenckebach), consecutive P waves are associated with a progressive increase in the PR interval until a P wave is not conducted (Figure 6). Usually only one P wave is dropped. This type of block generally occurs in the AV node. However, in about 10% of cases, type I AV block occurs in the His bundle or bundle branches. Type II second-degree AV block (dropping of P wave without progressive increase in PR interval) occurs in the His bundle or bundle branches. In type II AV block, it is common for two or more consecutive P waves to be dropped, causing syncope. Two to one AV block may be due to type I or II AV block. Three to one AV block may be due to 3:1 AV nodal block or type II block in the His-Purkinje system. The former is due to concealed conduction of two consecutive P waves in the AV node, but only the third P wave is conducted into the ventricle (Langendorf et al.). However, it is not the *type* of block, but *where* the block occurs that determines whether a pacemaker is necessary to prevent syncope. For example, patients with type I block of the His-Purkinje system usually require a pacemaker; patients with type I block in the AV node usually do not.

QRS, ST SEGMENT, T WAVE

The QRS represents depolarization of the ventricular myocardium. It does not include depolarization of the His-Purkinje system. If the first deflection of the QRS is negative, it is called a Q wave. If the QRS is entirely negative, it is a QS. The first positive deflection is an R wave. A negative deflection after the R wave is an S wave. Subsequent positive and negative deflections following R and S are R′ and S′, R″ and S″, etc. A capital letter indicates a deflection of large amplitude; a small letter, a deflection of relatively small amplitude.

The normal QRS duration varies in the adult from 0.05-0.10 sec. The QRS is usually measured in the limb lead that shows the widest QRS and may be 0.02 sec or so longer in the precordial leads. A wide QRS, 0.12 sec or longer, may be normal in duration in a given lead because a portion of its vectors are perpendicular to that lead. The QRS may be widened by hypertrophy, bundle branch block, hyperkalemia, myocardial infarction (peri-infarction block), and drugs, especially type IC antiarrhythmics.

QRS voltage is greater in children. Adult criteria for left ventricular hypertrophy in either limb or precordial leads apply to normal persons up to 35 years or even older. In the normal adult, the S wave in V_2-V_3 may be 25-30 mm because the dipole has twice as much strength in these leads as in lead V_6. Therefore, use of leads V_2 and V_3 in diagnosing left ventricular hypertrophy is less specific than using lead V_1.

Low voltage—5 mm or less—in the standard leads is most often found in normal persons but may be seen in obese persons and in those with pulmonary, myocardial, or pericardial disease.

The ST segment and T wave represent repolarization of the ventricles. The U wave is believed to represent repolarization of the His-Purkinje system. Repolarization is effected by many causes, both functional and organic.

The QT interval represents the duration of electrical systole. QT interval is determined in the lead that shows the longest measurement but with a T wave that has a distinct end point. The normal QT interval $= K\sqrt{R\text{-}R}$, where K is a constant and is equal to 0.37 for men and children and 0.40 for women, and R-R is the interval in seconds between two consecutive QRS cycles (Bazett formula). The QT interval corrected for heart rate (QTc) may be obtained by dividing the QT interval by the square root of the R-R interval. The upper limit for men is 0.39 sec and for women, 0.41 sec. Because of difficulties in obtaining an exact measurement of QT interval, it is customary to consider a QTc interval of more than 0.44 sec as abnormal. A prolonged QTc interval may be caused by ischemia, hypertrophy, electrolyte disturbance, surdocardiac syndrome (congenital prolonged QT interval with deafness), and drug effect, especially quinidine and similar type I drugs (Figure 7). A short QTc interval may be due to very early acute ischemia, electrolyte abnormalities (such as hypercalcemia), and drugs (especially digitalis).

ST elevation may be due to normal early repolarization, which may be as much as 3-4 mm in some precordial leads (Figure 8). Often, a fast heart rate will normalize these changes. Acute pericarditis may also cause ST-segment elevation and its contour is similar to normal early repolarization, forming an upward directed concavity (Figure 9). Ischemic current of injury forms a convex upward ST segment; but during its very early onset, it may simulate pericarditis or normal early repolarization. Atrioventricular junctional rhythm with retrograde P waves in 2, 3, and aV_F may cause ST-segment elevation due to abnormal atrial repolarization occurring at the time of the ST segment.

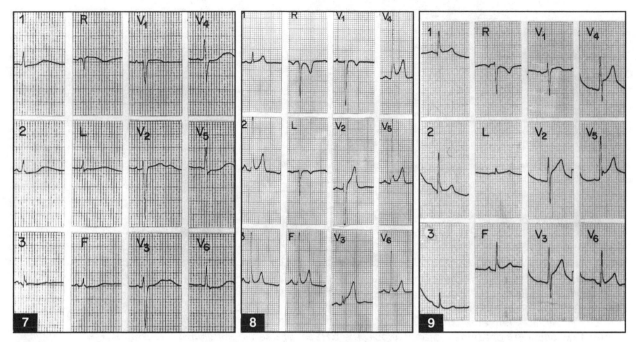

Figure 7. *Prolonged QT-U interval. The U waves fuse with the T waves in some leads, making it difficult to determine where the T wave ends. This patient had a potassium level of 2.7.*

Figure 8. *Normal early repolarization. The patient was a thin and tall normal 19-year-old man. ST elevation is present in all leads except aV$_L$, where it is isoelectric, and aV$_R$, where it is depressed.*

Figure 9. *Acute pericarditis. The ST segment is elevated in all leads except aV$_R$, in which it is depressed below the baseline.*

Other causes of ST-segment elevation include hyperkalemia, hypothermia, cardiac tumor, and acute cor pulmonale (ST-segment elevation in inferior and anteroseptal leads).

ST-segment elevation due to ischemic current of injury may be due to coronary artery spasm as well as obstructive organic coronary artery disease. If ST-segment elevation persists for more than two weeks after acute myocardial infarction, it is probably due to an extensive infarction (aneurysm) as described by Mills et al.

The ST segment may be depressed by hypertrophy, ischemia, drugs (especially digitalis), electrolyte imbalance, and sinus and ectopic tachycardias. The reference point for determining ST depression and elevation is the end of the PR segment. This reference point is especially important in evaluating an exercise test in order to avoid making a false diagnosis of ischemia.

LEFT VENTRICULAR HYPERTROPHY

The fact that there are so many QRS voltage criteria for LVH suggests that all of these criteria have limitations. Scott, who has devoted much time to the correlation of ECG with autopsy findings, favors the following criteria: R in 1 + S in 3 >25 mm, R in aV$_L$ >7.5, R in aV$_F$ >20, S in aV$_R$ >14, R in V$_5$ or V$_6$ + S in V$_1$ or V$_2$ >35, R in V$_5$ or V$_6$ >26, R + S in any precordial lead >45. These criteria apply only to adults. In LVH the ST-T may be directed opposite to the QRS and, in some cases, may not be associated with increased QRS voltage. In the presence of left anterior hemiblock, an S in III of 15 mm suggests LVH. However, LVH is often masked by left anterior hemiblock. It is difficult to diagnose LVH in the presence of left bundle branch block (LBBB). There is some evidence that (R-S in I) + (S-R in III) = 19 mm or more indicates LVH in the presence of LBBB. A very deep S wave in V$_1$-V$_3$ may be found in uncomplicated LBBB and should not be used in diagnosing LVH. However, a tall R wave, >25 mm or even less in V$_5$-V$_6$, indicates LVH in the presence of LBBB.

RIGHT VENTRICULAR HYPERTROPHY

The most common criteria used for diagnosing RVH are incomplete right bundle branch block (RBBB)

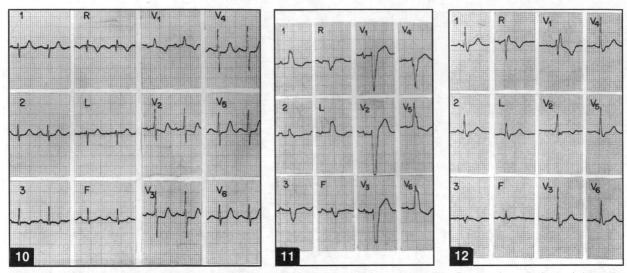

Figure 10. *Right ventricular hypertrophy. There is marked right axis deviation. The R wave is entirely upright and the T wave is negative in V₁. The ST segment is depressed in leads V₁-V₅.*

Figure 11. *Complete left bundle branch block. There is a notch near the summit of the R wave and the QRS is 0.13 sec in duration. Left atrial enlargement is present.*

Figure 12. *Complete right bundle branch block. The QRS is 0.12 sec in duration. There is an RSR' complex in V₁ and the intrinsicoid deflection is delayed to 0.09 sec.*

pattern with QRS between 0.08 and 0.1 sec, right-axis deviation of $+110°$ or more, R/S ratio in $V_1 >1$, qR in V_1, and R in $V_1 \geq 7$ mm (Figure 10). The first three criteria may be found as normal variants. In RVH, ST-T may be directed opposite to the QRS, especially in inferior leads and lead V_1.

BUNDLE BRANCH AND FASCICULAR BLOCKS

Complete bundle branch block is usually diagnosed if QRS is 0.12 sec or longer. However, in contrast to incomplete RBBB, incomplete LBBB may be present even when the QRS is as long as 0.15 sec. It is not the duration of the QRS but the contour that characterizes complete LBBB.

Sodi-Pallares described three degrees of LBBB. In first-degree LBBB, the initial Q wave may or may not be present and there is a slur confined to the lower part of the R wave in left ventricular leads. The intrinsicoid deflection is delayed by more than 0.04 sec. In second-degree LBBB, an initial Q is always absent; the slur involves most of the R wave, which is slightly rounded and the intrinsicoid deflection is further delayed. In third-degree (complete) LBBB, there is a notch on the summit of the R wave (Figure 11). The notch is supposed to occur during spread of ex-

citation across the septal barrier from the right ventricle to the left ventricle.

In RBBB, the right precordial leads show a late R wave with the intrinsicoid deflection at least 0.03 sec (Figure 12). Incomplete RBBB may occur with the duration of QRS between 0.08-0.11 sec.

In complete bundle branch block, the ST and T waves are opposite the R wave (secondary changes). If these ST-T changes do not occur (primary changes), ventricular disease in addition to conduction disease should be considered. Right bundle branch block tends to accentuate the axis that was present before development of block. There is evidence that LBBB with an axis more negative than $-30°$ indicates underlying ventricular muscle disease. In the presence of RBBB, voltage criteria for RVH (or posterior infarct) based on height of the R wave in right precordial leads is unreliable.

Uncomplicated left anterior hemiblock (LAH) and posterior hemiblock should not have a QRS duration of more than 0.10 sec. If the QRS is more than 0.10 sec, underlying infarction, LVH, or further peripheral conduction disease should be considered. Both the characteristic sequence of depolarization and axis must be considered in diagnosing hemiblock.

In LAH there is usually a qR in 1, aV_L, and an rS in 2, 3, aV_F. Mean axis is more negative than $-30°$. If RBBB is associated with LAH, there may not be

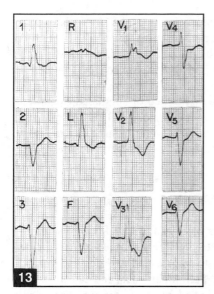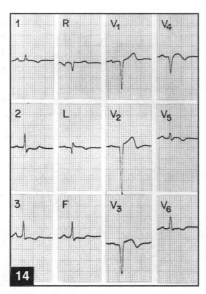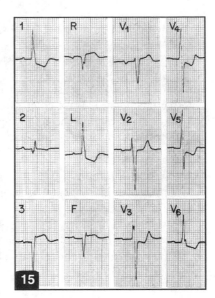

Figure 13. *Left anterior hemiblock masking right bundle branch block in standard and unipolar limb lead. There is no S wave in 1 or aV$_L$, but V$_1$ shows right bundle branch block.*

Figure 14. *Acute extensive anterior infarction. There are QS waves with ST elevation in V$_1$-V$_4$ and negative T waves V$_4$-V$_6$. The R wave is small in V$_5$-V$_6$.*

Figure 15. *Acute inferior infarction. There are Q waves and ST elevation in 2, 3, and aV$_F$. Also present is left ventricular hypertrophy by voltage criteria and marked ST-T changes in V$_2$-V$_6$, suggesting active ischemia.*

a late S in 1, aV$_L$ (masquerading pattern, Figure 13); and in the case of incomplete RBBB, there may be no late R in V$_1$. In posterior hemiblock, there is an rS in 1, aVL, and qR in 3 and aV$_F$. Mean axis is +110° or more. The diagnosis of posterior hemiblock should not be made without clinical correlation. RVH, vertical heart position, and extensive anterior infarct may simulate posterior hemiblock.

Hemiblock may mask or simulate myocardial infarction or ventricular hypertrophy.

MYOCARDIAL INFARCTION

When a patient with acute myocardial infarction is first examined, the ECG may show any combination of changes in the QRS, ST, or T wave. Changes in any of these, particularly in the QRS, may not appear for hours or days. In some cases the ECG may never show distinctive changes. The QRS changes generally last longer than ST and T changes and may remain for the rest of the patient's life. In the laboratory, the earliest change is T-wave inversion (ischemic), followed by elevation of RS-T segment (current of injury) and tall, upright T waves. Sometimes the very earliest change in the nonanesthetized closed-chest dog may be tall upright T waves, thus resembling the tall upright T waves (hyperacute changes) seen in

patients as described by Bayley et al. As the process in the laboratory progresses, changes occur in the QRS with development of Q waves that are indicative of myocardial necrosis.

It is difficult to diagnose myocardial infarction in the absence of Q changes because ST and T changes may only be due to reversible ischemia. These reversible changes have been shown to occur in the laboratory. Nevertheless, when they are associated with a suggestive history or elevated enzyme levels, they may be accepted as evidence that myocardial infarction has occurred.

Subendocardial infarction is usually associated with ST or T changes that persist for more than 24 hours. Data are insufficient to justify the use of the term *intramural infarction* in the presence of T changes. Large nontransmural infarctions (extending from one-half to three-fourths of the distance from endocardium to epicardium) may be associated with QRS changes (abnormal Q waves) that are often found in transmural infarction, as described by Cook et al.

Diagnostic Q-wave criteria for transmural myocardial infarction are often lacking even when such an infarction is present. It is common practice to diagnose infarction by the ST-T changes that are associated with any Q wave, even though the latter may be within normal limits. It has been shown that nondiagnostic Q waves may occur in up to 50% of infarctions. In some cases of extensive infarction with very poor ejection fraction, Q waves may not even be present (Young et al.).

Despite the lack of sensitivity of the ECG in diagnosing infarction, Q-wave criteria for infarction may be useful in the clinic. The following are suggested criteria for nomenclature of infarcts.

Anteroseptal Infarction. (1) QS is seen in V_1-V_2, occasionally also in V_3. (2) QS is seen in V_1 with QR or QRS in V_2-V_3.

Occasionally a qrS may be seen in any of these three leads. QS in V_1-V_2 and even in V_3 may be occasionally seen as a normal variant, especially in women and in pulmonary disease.

Anterior Infarction. (1) QS or QR is seen in V_2-V_4 with Q wave 0.04 sec or longer and magnitude more than 25% of the R wave. Patients with left ventricular hypertrophy may also show some of these changes. (2) Poor R-wave progression or even reversed R-wave progression is seen in V_1 or V_2 to V_3 or V_4. Poor R-wave progression may be seen as a normal variant, especially in women and in patients with pulmonary disease or LVH.

Anterolateral Infarction. Q waves in V_4-V_6 are at least 0.04 sec in duration and 15% or more of the total amplitude of the QRS.

Extensive Anterior Infarction. Abnormal Q waves and loss of R wave are seen in leads V_1-V_5 and even in V_6 (Figure 14).

High Lateral Infarction. (1) Q in aVL is at least 0.04 sec in duration and amplitude is 50% or more of the R wave. If the P wave is negative and even if the T wave is also negative, this rule cannot be used. (2) Q in lead 1 of 0.04 sec or longer and more than 10% of the total QRS voltage.

Inferior Infarction. Q wave in aV_F is at least 0.04 sec and amplitude 25% or more of the R wave (Figure 15). Any Q wave criterion applied to lead 3 is not specific enough to be useful by itself. Ten percent to 15% of inferior infarctions may have an initial r-wave in lead 3 or aV_F.

Posterior Infarction. Initial R in V_1-V_2 is at least 0.04 sec and R/S ratio is greater than 1. These criteria may be fulfilled by normal subjects, especially in the younger age group, and by right ventricular hypertrophy.

Infarction may be masked or simulated by left anterior or posterior hemiblock, LBBB, WPW syndrome, and left or right ventricular hypertrophy. It may also be simulated by hypertrophic obstructive cardiomyopathy.

SIGNAL AVERAGING

Signal averaging has been shown to be useful for recording late QRS potentials. These voltages are believed to be due to fragmented and delayed ventricular conduction. Preliminary data indicate that they are often present in patients with coronary disease and myopathy who have had or will have ventricular tachycardia or sudden death. This technique, together with other variables such as ventricular function, may especially be helpful in identifying high-risk patients (Zipes).

Ventricular arrhythmias are described in detail in later chapters.

Bibliography

Bayley RH, LaDue JS, York DJ, et al: Electrocardiographic changes (local ventricular ischemia and injury) produced in the dog by temporary occlusion of a coronary artery, showing a new stage in the evolution of a myocardial infarction. *Am Heart J* 27:164, 1944.

Besoain-Santander M, Pick A, Langendorf R, et al: AV conduction in auricular flutter. *Circulation* 2:604, 1950.

Chou T, Helm R: *Clinical Vectorcardiography*. New York: Grune & Stratton; 1967.

Chou TC, Helm R: The pseudo P pulmonale. *Circulation* 32:96, 1965.

Constant J: *Learning Electrocardiography*—1st ed. Boston: Little Brown; 1973, p. 321.

Cook RW, Edwards JE, Pruitt RD: Electrocardiographic changes in acute subendocardial infarction. I. Large subendocardial and large nontransmural infarcts. *Circulation* 18:603, 1958.

Cramer M, Hariman PJ, Boxer RA, et al: Catheter recordings of sinoatrial node potentials in the in situ canine heart. *Am J Cardiol* 41:374, 1978.

Cranefield PE, Wit AL, Hoffman BF: Genesis of cardiac arrhythmias. *Circulation* 47:24, 1973.

Josephson ME, Kastor JA, Morganroth J: Electrocardiographic left atrial enlargement. Electrophysiologic, echocardiographic, and hemodynamic correlates. *Am J Cardiol* 36:967, 1977.

Josephson ME, Wellens HJJ, eds.: *Tachycardias. Mechanisms, Diagnosis, Treatment*. Philadelphia: Lea & Febiger; 1984.

Langendorf R, Cohen H, Gozo EF: Observations on second degree atrioventricular block, including new criteria for differential diagnosis between type I and type II block. *Am J Cardiol* 29:111, 1972.

Lengyel L, Caramelli Z, Monfort J, et al: Initial electrocardiographic changes in experimental occlusion of the coronary artery in nonanesthetized dogs with closed thorax. *Am Heart J* 53:334, 1957.

Levine JH, Michael JR, Guarnieri T: Treatment of multifocal atrial tachycardia with verapamil. *N Engl J Med* 312:21, 1985.

Lown B, Ganong WF, Levine SA: The syndrome of short PR interval, normal QRS complex and paroxysmal rapid heart action. *Circulation* 5:693, 1952.

Marriott HJ: *Workshop in Electrocardiography*. Oldsmar, FL: Tampa Tracings; 1972.

Mills RM, Young E, Gorlin R, Lesch M: Natural history of ST segment elevation after acute myocardial infarction. *Am J Cardiol* 35:609, 1975.

Puech P: *Cardiovascular Clinics*, vol 6, no. 1. Philadelphia: FA Davis; 1974, p. 58.

Scott R: *Cardiovascular Clinics*, vol 5, no. 3. Philadelphia: FA Davis; 1974.

Sodi-Pallares D: *New Basis of Electrocardiography*. St. Louis: CV Mosby; 1956, p. 254.

Waldo A: Entrainment and interruption of atrial flutter with atrial pacing. Studies in man following open heart surgery. *Circulation* 56:737, 1977.

Young E, Cohn PF, Gorlin R, et al: Vectorcardiographic diagnosis and electrocardiographic correlation in left ventricular asynergy. *Circulation* 51:467, 1975.

Zipes DP: Genesis of cardiac arrhythmias: Electrophysiologic considerations. In: Braunwald E, ed. *Heart Disease*. Philadelphia: WB Saunders; 1988, p. 581.

4 Chest Radiograph in the Evaluation of Acquired Cardiac Disease

Donald P. Harrington

After the discovery of x-rays by Konrad Roentgen, the chest radiograph was rapidly incorporated into evaluation of cardiac disease and became an essential component of that evaluation. For many years, all diagnostic efforts in cardiac disease were based on the triad of clinical examination, electrocardiogram, and chest radiograph. Beginning with the era of cardiac catheterization and followed by the widespread use of echocardiography, the usefulness of the plain film has been questioned, but chest radiography survives despite technologic advances. This chapter reviews the basic principles of plain chest film examination in cardiac disease and looks at this safe, inexpensive, and reproducible screening procedure in the context of other tests that are more sophisticated but often more invasive.

PLAIN FILM EXAMINATIONS

Plain films may be separated into three categories. The first is the posteroanterior (PA) and lateral chest radiograph, which represents the most basic and useful examination of the heart by plain radiographic means; in both positions the patient is upright with deep inspiration (Figure 1). The second examination, four views of the heart with barium, is an extension of the first; the presence of barium within the esophagus provides a posterior cardiac marker, and the right and left oblique views of the heart (Figures 2 and 3) provide a greater appreciation of cardiac structures. This examination is also made with the patient in the upright position during deep inspiration. The third examination is the supine chest radiograph, which is sometimes confused with the portable film. The term *portable* refers to the x-ray equipment that is used to perform the study. In fact, the portability of this equipment limits the power and flexibility of the system, and portable film examinations may not be as useful as the standard PA chest radiograph, particularly if the patient is very obese. The term *supine* refers only to the position of the patient when the radiograph is taken. The limitation of this study is the heightened position of the diaphragm because of the lessened ability of the patient to take a deep breath. By necessity, the view is anteroposterior (AP) in direction, which also tends to widen the mediastinal and cardiac outline as compared to the PA upright chest. In a portable x-ray examination the PA position cannot be achieved, but the patient can be seated upright for an AP radiograph. The position in which the examination is performed should always be clearly identified on the film itself.

CARDIAC CONTOURS AND OVERALL SIZE

For the most part, the heart itself appears totally homogeneous on the film; muscle and blood are indistinguishable. Calcium deposits within the heart shadow can be distinguished from soft tissue, as can concentrations of normal fat around the heart; both may be significant clues to pathology. The contours of the heart are seen most readily in relationship to the air-filled lungs that surround it on two sides. We are easily able to distinguish the heart from aerated lung. This, in turn, allows a preliminary judgment about heart size, as a first step in the evaluation of the heart.

The simplest method for assessing overall heart size involves the use of the *cardiothoracic ratio* (Figure 1). The cardiothoracic ratio is generally expressed as a percent, with any value below 50% considered to be within normal limits; some authors suggest that 55% is a better limit of normal. The result is that while the number of true positives increases with a higher cardiothoracic ratio, so does the rate of false negatives. This value should be increased to 60% for children and infants.

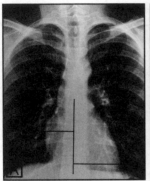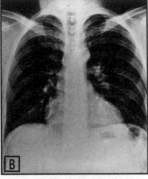

Figure 1. *Normal posteroanterior (PA) chest radiographs. (A) Inspiration film with markings for calculation of the cardiothoracic ratio. The vertical reference line is established using the spinous processes. The numerator of the cardiothoracic ratio is established by adding the longest distance to the right and left heart borders from the reference line. The denominator is the longest length between the inner aspects of the rib cage. Note also the normal distribution of the pulmonary vacularity, with pulmonary venous vessels seen in the lower lung fields but none in the upper lung fields. (B) Normal expiration film for comparison with A. The normal value of 50% cardiothoracic ratio is not valid with an expiration film.*

Care must be taken in the use of the cardiothoracic ratio in several common situations. The heart appears larger in both the supine and the AP positions in comparison with the standard upright PA positioning. There may also be a 1.0- to 1.5-cm difference in heart size between systole and diastole in the same patient. Abnormalities of the spine, such as kyphosis and scoliosis, and of the sternum, as in pectus excavatum, preclude the use of the cardiothoracic ratio as a measure of cardiac size. Finally, the established norms for the cardiothoracic ratio assume a deep inspiration on the part of the patient, so that an expiration film will tend to overestimate heart size (Figure 1B). This fact affects the supine radiograph as well because of the difficulty with a standardized deep inspiration in this position.

Several other methods of evaluating cardiac size have been developed, but those that provide the most precise measurements of heart volume also require complex analyses of both PA and lateral projections. They are seldom used in routine clinical work, and no method has received the same wide acceptance as the cardiothoracic ratio.

Lesions associated with moderate to severe cardiomegaly include the volume overload lesions of mitral, aortic, and tricuspid regurgitation, as well as congestive cardiomyopathy and pericardial effusion. Those acquired cardiac diseases in which the patient is not in heart failure and which show normal or only slight enlargement of the heart include all pressure overload lesions, such as mitral and aortic stenosis and systemic hypertension. Other disease processes in this group include acute myocardial infarction, hypertrophic cardiomyopathy, and constrictive pericarditis. Left ventricular failure from any of these or other causes results in cardiomegaly with left ventricular enlargement, left atrial enlargement, and pulmonary venous changes. An exception is if left ventricular failure is acute, as in acute myocardial infarction; then, hours are needed for ventricular and atrial dilatation, whereas the pulmonary vasculature changes can be seen acutely.

CARDIAC CONFIGURATION AND HEART BORDERS

Our next step in assessment of the heart is related to cardiac configuration and individual chamber enlargement. As previously stated, it is important to look at changes at the interface between the heart and the lung. These can be seen more readily at the points where the right and the left borders are outlined by the lungs. The PA radiographs in Figures 1 and 2 will serve as the visual reference for evaluation of the normal heart contours, since the first is normal and the second is an example of mild aortic stenosis, which only slightly alters cardiac configuration. Beginning at the left cardiophrenic angle, the apex of the heart is gently rounded and sharply delineated. Fat, a normal finding, can be seen in this area because fat is less dense than the heart and more dense than the lung (Figure 2A). The presence of fat at the cardiophrenic angle may blunt the distinction between these organs and falsely increase the cardiothoracic ratio. An extension of the cardiac contour outward and downward suggests left ventricular enlargement; when enlargement is severe, the air bubble within the stomach will be indented by the heart, since an enlarged left ventricle will press through the diaphragm. This can be best evaluated in the lateral projection. When the right ventricular chamber is enlarged, there may also be leftward extension of the ventricular contour, but the apex tends to be deviated upward rather than

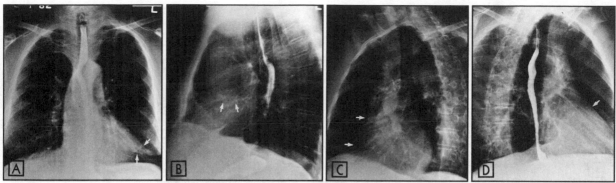

Figure 2. *Four views of the heart with barium from a patient with mild aortic stenosis. (A) PA radiograph. The heart size is normal. A fat pad is present at the cardiac apex, accentuated by the density of the overlying left breast (arrows). Some rounding of the left ventricular contour is present, consistent with left ventricular hypertrophy. The ascending arch and descending portions are dilated and ectatic due to a combination of aortic stenosis and aging. If post-stenotic dilatation were the only factor, the arch and descending portion of the aorta would be normal. (B) Lateral radiograph. Minimal aortic calcification is seen (arrows). This calcification was better seen fluoroscopically at the time of cardiac catheterization but was identified first by plain film examination. The ascending aorta is prominent above the aortic valve. The retrosternal space is clear. The left ventricle does not extend beyond the inferior vena cava, and the esophagus is not significantly displaced posteriorly. (C) Left anterior oblique (LAO) radiograph. Aortic calcification is obscured by overlying lung markings. The right atrial and right ventricular margin has a normal straight line configuration (arrows). The normal clear space is present between the right atrium and the left mainstem bronchus. (D) Right anterior oblique (RAO) radiograph. No deviation of the esophagus is present, and the right ventricular outflow tract is normal (arrow).*

downward, giving the appearance of a boot-shaped heart.

Localized bulging of the cardiac contour on the left lateral and posterior aspects of the cardiac border is seen frequently in aneurysms of the left ventricle. Ascending toward the pulmonary hilum, the left heart border rises diagonally as a line which either remains straight or becomes slightly concave in the region of the left atrial appendage before reaching the main pulmonary artery segment. A bulging of the segment is noted when the left atrium and its appendage are dilated (Figures 3 and 4).

In assessing the right heart border, we begin at the cardiophrenic angle on the right. A small portion of the right side of the heart is usually seen beyond the vertebral bodies; this represents the right atrium. Enlargement of either the right atrium or the right ventricle causes extension of the right border further to the right of the spine so that it appears more prominent than normal (Figure 5). Advancing further up the right side of the heart, the junction between the right atrium and the superior vena cava may be noted as a change in direction of these structures as they form a small niche. The superior vena cava is the only border-forming element above this level. Just

above the mainstem bronchus and right hilum lies the azygos vein, which is seen as a small mass density in supine radiographs (or in the upright radiograph when there is systemic venous distention). There are no absolute normal values for the extensions of these structures to the right or the left of the heart shadow; experience teaches how to differentiate normal from abnormal.

PULMONARY VASCULARITY

An understanding of the radiographic changes and their functional significance has only come about since the widespread use of cardiac catheterization. Thus, a more invasive, more sophisticated procedure has actually enhanced the plain film examination rather than replacing it.

The main pulmonary artery segments should be evaluated first, followed by the right and left pulmonary arteries and hilum, continuing into the smaller, more peripheral veins and arteries, and ending with the pulmonary parenchyma and pleural space. Enlargement of the main pulmonary artery segment is generally caused either by increased flow through the pulmonary artery, as in a left-to-right shunt, or by

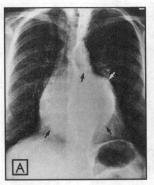 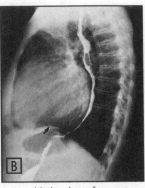 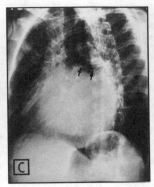 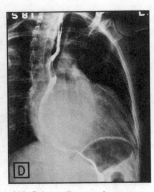

Figure 3. *Four views of the heart with barium from a patient with severe mitral stenosis. (A) PA radiograph. Cardiothoracic ratio is just above 50%. The left atrium is massively enlarged, causing a double density with the cardiac contour (lower black arrows). The left atrial appendage is dilated (white arrow). The left mainstem bronchus is markedly elevated by the left atrial enlargement (upper black arrow). Upper lobe vascularity on the right is easier to visualize than on the left because it is not obscured by the heart. In this case, the heart contour is displaced to the right by the left atrial enlargement and not right ventricular or right atrial dilatation. (B) Lateral radiograph. There is marked posterior deviation of the esophagus by the enlarged left atrium. The retrosternal clear space is still present despite the distortion caused by the enlarged left atrium, suggesting that right-sided enlargement is not present. Calcification (black arrow) is noted in the wall of the left atrium. (C) LAO radiograph. The left mainstem bronchus (arrows) is in contact with the enlarged left atrium and elevated. No vascular calcification is seen. (D) RAO radiograph. Further illustration of the size of the left atrium and deviation of the trachea. This series of films illustrates how the cardiothoracic ratio may underestimate the extent of cardiac enlargement, particularly when the dilatation is in the posterior direction with the left atrial enlargement.*

pulmonary hypertension. A third and uncommon cause of arterial prominence is post-stenotic dilatation of this segment due to pulmonary stenosis. Idiopathic dilatation of the pulmonary artery without pulmonary stenosis may occasionally be seen in women younger than 30. Increased blood flow or increased pressure can also cause enlargement of the right and left pulmonary artery segments. The vascularity in the more peripheral portions of the pulmonary arteries is helpful in differentiating between these two causes. This vascularity is best evaluated by covering over the hilum and proximal pulmonary arteries and viewing only the vessels in the outer two thirds to one half of the lung. Normal pulmonary vascularity is defined by experience; but except in the base of the lungs, only small, well-delineated vessels are seen. Increased vascularity or larger peripheral vessels are seen in high-flow shunt lesions (Figure 6), whereas no vessels are seen in pulmonary hypertension because of pruning of the peripheral pulmonary vessels.

Differentiation between arterial and venous vascularity is difficult at first. In the normal patient in the upright projection, an increased number of vessels may be seen in the lower lung fields. These are both arterial and venous, and the difference will become apparent on close inspection. The arterial vessels tend to be vertical, while the venous tend to be horizontal in their passage into the left atrium. The normal upper lobe has less arterial and venous vascularity than the lower lobe (Figure 1). As pulmonary venous pressure rises (15-20 mm Hg), no matter what the cause, the visible vascularity in the upper and lower lungs tends to equalize (Figure 7). As pressure rises further in the venous system (20-25 mm Hg), the lower lobe veins tend to disappear while upper lobe veins become more prominent (Figures 3 and 4A). This change occurs entirely on the venous side of the pulmonary circulation. Differentiation between arterial and venous vascularity is somewhat more difficult in the upper lung than in the lower; but here, too, the arteries tend to have a more vertical orientation than the veins, as in the lower lung fields. *Warning:* pulmonary vascular changes are accurately interpreted only if recorded in the upright position.

As pressure rises within the pulmonary venous bed, the capillary oncotic pressure is exceeded and pulmonary edema occurs above 25 mm Hg. The first manifestation of this is generally a bilateral haziness and confluence of structures within the pulmonary hila. Normally, the structures in the hila are distinct.

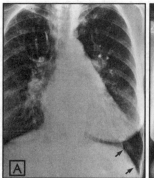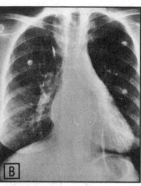

Figure 4. *Radiographs before and after replacement of the mitral valve in a patient with mitral stenosis. (A) PA radiograph preoperatively shows mild cardiomegaly, double density of enlarged left atrium, and prominent left atrial appendage. The left mainstem bronchus is only minimally elevated. The pulmonary vascular changes also demonstrate the classic changes of this disease process. Pulmonary vascularity is shifted to the upper lung fields, with diminution of the venous pattern in the lower lungs. There is diffuse blurring of the pulmonary hila. Kerley B lines (arrows) are noted at the left costophrenic angle. Increased density throughout both lung fields indicates early pulmonary edema. (B) Postoperative PA chest radiograph after replacement of the mitral valve. The previously noted pulmonary changes have been reversed. Overall heart size and slight prominence of the left atrial appendage remain.*

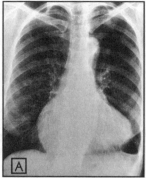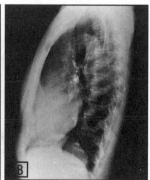

Figure 5. *Radiographs from a patient with combined mitral and tricuspid valvular disease, in whom tricuspid disease is the major component. (A) PA radiograph. Cardiomegaly is present with prominence of the right heart border. No double density of left atrial enlargement is present. Pulmonary vascularity is normal. (B) Lateral radiograph. Filling in of the retrosternal clear space, with no abnormal posterior displacement of the left ventricle or left atrium. The findings are specific for right-sided enlargement due to the patient's predominant tricuspid valvular disease.*

A second sign is the appearance of short, horizontal lines at the costophrenic angles, representing interstitial edema; these are the classic Kerley B lines (Figure 4). The next step in the process is haziness throughout the lung fields with frank pulmonary edema, also indicated by the so-called alveolar pattern and pleural effusion. Pulmonary edema of cardiac origin is usually associated with an increase in the cardiothoracic ratio, caused by left ventricular dilatation. This is not true when edema is rapid in onset, such as in an acute myocardial infarction, or when it is noncardiac in origin, as in the case of drowning or overhydration.

CARDIAC CALCIFICATION

Calcification within the left ventricular muscle is associated with injury and repair after myocardial infarction (Figure 8). In general, this calcification is more localized than pericardial calcification and may be associated with a bulging of the ventricular contour in aneurysm formation.

Cardiac calcification is useful in delineating specific pathologic processes within the heart. Calcification occuring within the pericardium, as shown in Figure 9, is indicative of pericarditis. In this example, calcification involves the entire pericardial space, whereas the calcification is usually seen in only parts of the pericardium. Calcification is a good indication of old pericarditis; only half the patients with constrictive pericarditis have evidence of calcification. Tuberculous pericarditis is the most common cause of pericardial calcification.

Calcification of the aortic and mitral valves is another common pathologic and radiologic phenomenon. Frequently, these valves are not seen clearly in the PA projection because they overlap the spine and tend to be superimposed on one another. The lateral and oblique projections are more useful in delineating valvular calcifications. In the lateral projection, the calcified aortic valve tends to be horizontally located in the middle third of the cardiac shadow, whereas the calcified mitral valve is in the posterior third and obliquely oriented. C-shaped calcification is frequently seen in the mitral annulus and, while the mitral valve is not directly calcified, mitral insufficiency

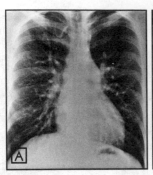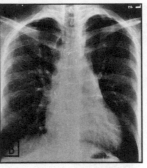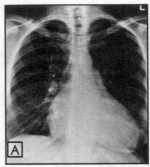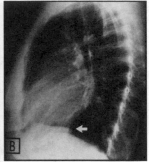

Figure 6. *PA and lateral chest radiographs from a patient with an atrial septal defect (ASD). (A) Normal heart size in a patient with a large ASD. The increased pulmonary arterial vascularity is evident in both lungs, as is prominence of the main pulmonary artery segment. Note the vertical orientation of the vessels. (B) PA radiograph after surgical closure of the ASD. The sternal sutures and slightly larger heart size are consistent with the preceding surgical procedure. The pulmonary vascularity is now normal and in striking contrast to that seen in panel A.*

Figure 7. *Chest radiographs from a patient with hypertrophic cardiomyopathy and clinical evidence of intermittent congestive heart failure. (A) PA radiograph. Cardiomegaly with left ventricular and left atrial dilatation. The pulmonary vasculature has normal to slightly increased upper lobe vascularity. (B) Lateral radiograph. The retrosternal clear space is still present. The enlarged left ventricle is displaced posteriorly to the inferior vena cava (arrow).*

is associated with this phenomenon. Valvular calcification itself is usually irregular and spiculated and is more extensive in the aortic as opposed to the mitral valve. Calcification of any cardiac structure is better appreciated using fluoroscopy rather than films because the motion of the calcified structure enhances visualization. Pathologic calcification of cardiac valves is far more frequent than radiologically evident calcification.

Calcification of the coronary arteries is frequently associated with atherosclerotic coronary artery disease. However, the calcium deposits are usually too small to be seen on the plain chest radiograph. When calcification is seen, its linear arrangement and railroad-track configuration are good indications of its origin.

OTHER CARDIAC DENSITIES

Fat densities within the heart are normal findings; for example, in the lateral film, a radiolucent stripe of epicardial fat can frequently be seen in the retrosternal area, or the slight radiolucent density of a cardiac fat pad may be found at the left cardiophrenic angle. The retrosternal fat stripe is indicative of pericardial effusion if it lies well within the cardiac shadow in the lateral projection and away from the normal retrosternal location. As the pericardial fluid accumulates,

it does so outside the epicardium, thus displacing the fat into a more central location in the overall cardiac shadow.

SPECIFIC CHAMBER ENLARGEMENT

The pathophysiologic response of the heart to a volume overload, such as aortic insufficiency, is cham-

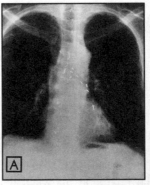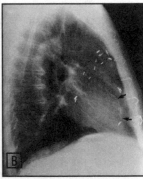

Figure 8. *Chest radiographs from a patient who had a previous myocardial infarction and coronary artery bypass graft. (A) PA radiograph. Postoperative changes and normal heart size are present. No calcification or abnormalities of the left heart border are present. (B) Lateral radiograph. An area of left ventricular infarction (arrows) shows calcification. At the time of cardiac catheterization, a contrast left ventriculogram demonstrated an aneurysm in the region of calcification. This calcification is more centrally located than in patients with pericardial calcification.*

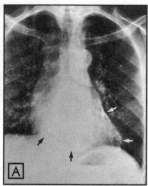 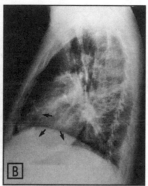

Figure 9. *Chest radiographs from a patient suspected of having constrictive pericarditis. (A) PA radiograph. Marked calcification of the entire pericardium (arrows). The overall heart size is normal, as is the pulmonary vascularity. Diffuse pulmonary parenchymal disease is noted. (B) The lateral film confirms the previous findings of extensive pericardial calcification. Cardiac catheterization did not demonstrate evidence of pericardial constriction, and no other cardiac abnormalities were noted. The calcification is unequivocal evidence of previous pericarditis, but it is not specific for the present activity of the disease process or its cause, although most cases of calcific pericarditis are tubercular in nature.*

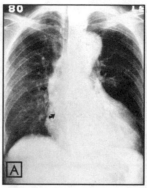 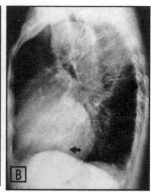

Figure 10. *Chest radiographs from a patient with signs and symptoms of aortic insufficiency. (A) PA radiograph. The heart is enlarged, with outward and downward displacement of the left heart border. The right heart border appears normal. The aortic knob is prominent, which may relate to patient age or preexisting chronic hypertension, but the dilatation of the ascending aorta (arrows) suggests aortic valve disease (although an aneurysm involving the ascending aorta is a possibility). Equalization of the upper and lower pulmonary vascularity is present. (B) Lateral radiograph. The retrosternal clear space is maintained, with marked enlargement of the heart posteriorly beyond the inferior vena cava, where it passes through the diaphragm (arrow). No calcification of valves or of the ascending aorta is noted. Blunting of the posterior angle of the left diaphragm is incidentally noted. The overall cardiac enlargement and configuration of the ventricles indicate left ventricular dilatation. Prominence of the ascending aorta suggests aortic valve disease. Together these observations suggest that aortic regurgitation is the predominant element. Increased pulmonary venous pressure is indicated by the shift of venous vascularity.*

ber dilatation; the response to a pressure overload, such as aortic stenosis, is myocardial hypertrophy. Dilatation of the ventricles will result in cardiomegaly and an abnormal cardiothoracic ratio, whereas ventricular hypertrophy generally only rounds out the left ventricular contour. Isolated dilatation of the left atrium does not result in cardiomegaly. Right atrial enlargement is difficult to distinguish from right ventricular enlargement; the two phenomena are usually considered together as right-sided dilatation. Ventricular hypertrophy subtly changes the cardiac contour but does not increase the size of the heart or of the cardiothoracic ratio (Figures 2, 10).

Differentiation between right and left ventricular enlargement is somewhat difficult. One must first establish whether or not the right ventricle is enlarged (Figure 5). If it is, it is seen as abnormal displacement of the cardiac shadow to the right of the ventral bodies and as a filling in of the retrosternal clear space in the lateral projection. There is also extension of the heart upward and to the left into the shape of a boot. The left anterior oblique (LAO) projection can also be used to evaluate the right ventricle. In this projec-

tion, the right border is seen as a relatively vertical line as it rises to meet the superior vena cava (Figure 2). If there is a step formed between the right side of the heart and the superior vena cava, right-sided enlargement is present. Right ventricular enlargement can mimic all the signs of left ventricular enlargement, so the latter cannot be adequately determined. If right ventricular enlargement is *not* clearly shown, evaluation of the left ventricle can proceed. Extension of the ventricle downward and outward to the left is one indication of enlargement. Another radiographic sign involves extracardiac organ relationships. In the lateral projection, one normally sees the posterior wall of the inferior vena cava as it rises from the abdomen.

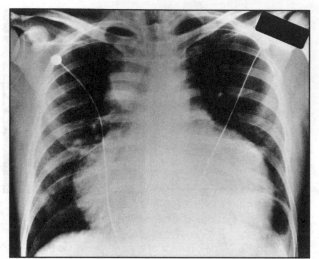

Figure 11. *Portable AP chest radiograph from a patient with pericardial effusion and mediastinal mass lesion. Obvious cardiomegaly is present, with uniform distribution that has been termed the* water bottle heart. *The pulmonary vascularity is normal in distribution, but the hila of the lung are obscured by the enlarging pericardial space. Cardiomegaly, other than from pericardial effusion, will not obscure the pulmonary vessels and hila. The mediastinal mass lesion is just above the right mainstem bronchus. This mass was a mediastinal tumor with pericardial metastasis, which led to the pericardial effusion.*

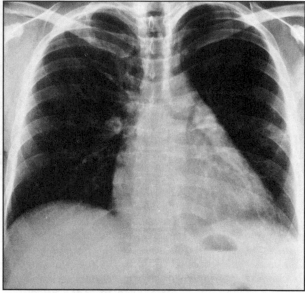

Figure 12. *PA chest radiograph from a patient with idiopathic pericardial effusion. The overall heart size is only slightly larger than normal, but the left hila and pulmonary vessels are totally obscured and the right hila is partially obscured. The pulmonary artery and pulmonary vascularity are normal.*

This is seen as a vertical structure arising from the diaphragm into the heart, and normally no cardiac shadow will be seen posteriorly. However, left ventricular enlargement will cause a portion of the left ventricle to extend beyond this vertical line (Figure 7). The outward and downward expansion of left ventricular dilatation will also encroach on the left diaphragm and, in extreme cases, indent the gastric air bubble.

Of all radiographic signs of chamber enlargement, those involving the left atrium are the most reliable. Left atrial enlargement is indicated in the PA projection by formation of a double density as the left atrium expands posteriorly and by prominence of the left atrial appendage on the left heart border (Figures 3 and 4). As the left atrium enlarges, it tends to encroach upon and elevate the left mainstem bronchus. This encroachment is especially clear in the LAO projection, where there is normally a clear space between the upper portion of the cardiac shadow and left main-

stem bronchus (Figure 2C). As the left atrium increases in size, this space is encroached upon by the cardiac silhouette until finally the left mainstem bronchus is displaced upward by the cardiac mass (Figure 3C). The LAO projection is also useful for separating the calcified mitral and aortic valves.

SPECIFIC PATHOLOGIC PROCESSES

A number of specific diseases may be identified on chest radiograph. Aortic valvular disease can present as aortic stenosis, as aortic insufficiency, or as a combination of these two. When aortic stenosis is the predominant lesion, the overall cardiac size is not increased. The result is a pressure overload of the left ventricle, which leads to myocardial hypertrophy. Myocardial hypertrophy may cause subtle changes in cardiac contour, but it does not lead to an increased cardiothoracic ratio. Calcification of the aortic valve frequently accompanies aortic stenosis, whether the underlying process is rheumatic heart disease or a congenital bicuspid aortic valve. Isolated dilatation of the ascending aorta, which results in an apparent increased density of the retrosternal space above the heart and a deviation of the superior vena cava to the right, is a further indication of aortic stenosis. This post-stenotic dilatation is caused by turbulent blood flow through the stenotic valve (Figure 2).

Dilatation of the ascending arch and descending portion of the aorta may result from the normal aging process or from sustained systemic hypertension.

When aortic regurgitation is the predominant lesion, there is volume rather than pressure overload of the left ventricle. This results in dilatation of the left ventricle and an increase in the cardiothoracic ratio.

Mitral valve disease is another example of a process that is usually a combination of stenosis and insufficiency. When stenosis predominates, the left atrium dilates because of pressure overload, while the left ventricle tends to remain normal-sized. Left atrial enlargement is indicated by prominence of the left atrial appendage along the left heart border density in the PA projection with posterior extension of the left atrial chamber, and — in the most severe cases — elevation of the left mainstem bronchus in the PA projection. In the LAO projection, the clear space between the cardiac shadow and the left mainstem bronchus is obliterated, with ultimate elevation of the mainstem bronchus. Also in the most severe enlargement, the left atrium can extend beyond the right heart border and give the impression of right-sided enlargement (Figure 3). With left atrial hypertension, the pressure is transmitted into the pulmonary venous bed, and there is a shift of pulmonary venous vascularity from the lower lung fields to an equal balance between upper and lower vessels, finally giving marked prominence to those in the upper lobe (Figures 3 and 4). In the presence of mitral regurgitation, left ventricular enlargement is added to these findings, reflecting the volume overload of the left ventricle by the regurgitation.

Tricuspid valve disease, regardless of its etiology, is usually not associated with radiographically identifiable calcification, as is mitral or aortic valve disease; rather, it is indicated by enlargement of the right side of the heart without evidence of pulmonary arterial or venous hypertension (Figure 5).

When any valvular disease is combined with ventricular failure, or when multiple valves are involved, the previously noted distinctions are blurred and generally unreliable. The greatest value of the chest x-ray in these cases is its ability to delineate the progressive physiologic and pathologic changes that accompany ventricular failure.

In patients with coronary artery disease, the chest radiograph is usually normal. This is true for both acute and chronic myocardial ischemia. Cardiomegaly, left ventricular and left atrial enlargement, and the accompanying signs of increased pulmonary venous hypertension are evident when ventricular failure results from myocardial ischemia. Infarction may lead to aneurysm formation, which may be identifiable on chest radiographs as a localized bulging of the left ventricle and may calcify. Other complications of infarction, such as papillary muscle infarction and acute mitral regurgitation or septal infarction with ventricular septal defect formation, are evident radiographically, although congestive heart failure is often the most obvious finding in these complications.

Myocarditis can only be identified as the myocardium fails with resultant left ventricular dilatation. This is a late sign, and such a limitation in radiographic identification also holds for cardiomyopathy, whether restrictive or hypertrophic (Figure 7).

Pericardial disease processes may be identified if calcification is present in pericarditis (Figure 9) or, in the case of pericardial effusion, when the effusion is large enough to give identifiable cardiomegaly and to displace the retroperitoneal fat stripe (Figures 11 and 12). Echocardiography has superseded all other diagnostic methods for identifying pericardial effusion, especially if the effusion is small. Once pericardial effusion has been established, the chest radiograph can be used to follow resolution of this process by changes in cardiac size.

SUPINE AND PORTABLE FILMS

The supine chest film is used to evaluate patients in the intensive care area and recovery room, when standard radiographic views cannot be obtained. As noted earlier, one limitation of this technique is that the standard cardiothoracic ratio cannot be used. Despite this, the serial nature of the film provides much diagnostic information. First, it shows increasing or decreasing cardiac size on a day-to-day basis; second, it shows change in the pulmonary venous vascularity, which can indicate cardiac function and/or pulmonary venous pressure. Portable chest films taken in the intensive care unit are limited by the variations in technique, patient positioning, and the respiratory cycle from one film to the next. However, when this drawback is taken into account, the chest film can provide a good anatomic and physiologic study.

Bibliography

Baron MG: Radiological and angiographic examination of the heart. In: Braunwald E, ed: *Heart Disease: A Textbook of Cardiovascular Medicine,* vol. I. Philadelphia: WB Saunders; 1988, p. 140.

Battler A, Karliner JS, Higgins CB, et al: The initial chest x-ray in acute myocardial infarction: Prediction of early and late mortality and survival. *Circulation* 61:1004, 1980.

Higgins CB, Lipton MJ: Radiography of acute myocardial infarction. *Radiol Clin North Am* 18:359, 1980.

Newell JD, Higgins CD, Kelley MJ: Radiographic-echocardiographic approach to acquired heart disease: Diagnosis and assessment of severity. *Radiol Clin North Am* 18:387, 1980.

Ravin CE: Pulmonary vascularity: Radiographic considerations. *J Thorac Imag* 3:1, 1988.

5 Nuclear Cardiology

CHAPTER

Joseph F. Polak

Nuclear medicine procedures designed to evaluate the heart continue to evolve as newer instrumentation and radiopharmaceuticals become available. Selecting the most useful diagnostic procedure is difficult, even for the nuclear medicine specialist. Since local experience with a test and its availability varies, clinicians should consult their nuclear cardiology specialists before ordering the tests described herein.

In this chapter, noninvasive examinations requiring intravenous administration of a radiopharmaceutical and using standard imaging and processing instrumentation are discussed.

MYOCARDIAL IMAGING: OVERVIEW

INSTRUMENTATION

The basic instrument used in nuclear medicine imaging is the Anger gamma camera. This device encodes information on the spatial distribution of a radioisotope onto a two-dimensional image. It can resolve objects separated by 1-2 cm. Combined with a computer interface, a gamma camera may be used to acquire electrocardiographically gated images of the cardiac blood pool; computer software then determines right and left ventricular ejection fractions. Newer software is available that measures thallium myocardial distribution and kinetics. This capability reduces the variability of the examination and improves the sensitivity and specificity of the technique.

Over the last few years, rotating gamma cameras capable of performing single-photon emission computed tomography (SPECT) have become a common feature in most nuclear medicine departments. This imaging approach does not significantly contribute to the evaluation of cardiac function. When combined with myocardial perfusion tracers, however, it offers improved sensitivity and specificity in the diagnosis of coronary artery disease. It also improves spatial localization and helps to delineate the size of ischemic or infarcted myocardium.

Although use of positron emission tomography (PET) is spreading, the technique remains available in only a few specialized centers throughout the country. Cyclotrons and specialized radiochemistry are needed to image O-15-, C-11-, or N-13-labeled compounds. The availability of inexpensive on-site rubidium-82 generators makes it possible to perform perfusion imaging without a cyclotron. Whether use of this technology will increase is unclear.

RADIOPHARMACEUTICALS

Radiopharmaceuticals and procedures available to aid in assessment of both the functional and metabolic integrity of the heart are categorized as: (1) myocardial perfusion and viability studies with thallium-201 and newer technetium-99m complexes; (2) cardiac function studies with gated or first-pass ventriculography; (3) detection and sizing of myocardial infarction using Tc-99m pyrophosphate or antimyosin antibody complexes; and (4) evaluation of myocardial metabolism with iodine-123 fatty acid analogs or positron emitters.

PERFUSION/VIABILITY IMAGING

Table 1 summarizes the characteristics and uses of perfusion imaging agents.

THALLIUM-201

Thallium-201 is a potassium analog. Its administration yields a lower radiation dose and improved spatial resolution compared with potassium analogs such

Table 1. Perfusion Imaging Agents

ISOTOPE	HALF-LIFE	COMPLEX	PRINCIPLE	USE
Tl-201	73 hr	Thallous chloride	Potassium analog; extraction	Perfusion imaging; intravenous injection
Tc-99m	6.03 hr	Hexakis isonitrile	Myocyte uptake and trapping	Perfusion imaging; intravenous injection
Rb-82	75 sec	Dissolved in saline	Potassium analog; extraction	Perfusion imaging; intravenous injection *Positron emitter* obtained from on site generator
N-13	10 min	Ammonia	Extraction, but retention affected by local metabolism	Perfusion imaging; intravenous injection *Positron emitter* generated from cyclotron

as rubidium and cesium. It is used clinically for assessment of regional myocardial perfusion.

Pathophysiology

Immediately after intravenous injection of thallium, the pattern of myocardial uptake reflects regional blood flow. Cardiac muscle has an extraction efficiency of 80-90% for this cation. Approximately 4% of the administered dose is captured by the myocardium.

In a normal subject at rest, local myocardial uptake of Tl-201 depends on blood flow and is therefore homogeneously distributed throughout the left ventricle. With exercise, increased myocardial perfusion causes increased uniform myocardial uptake of the tracer. In the presence of coronary artery disease, thallium uptake is unchanged if regional blood flow is normal. Areas of exercise-induced ischemia show a decrease in thallium uptake since regional delivery of the isotope is compromised.

Soon after intravenous administration of thallium, a phenomenon called *redistribution* occurs. This is a transition between early thallium distribution, proportional to blood flow, and a later steady state during which thallium uptake reflects the size of the local potassium pool, i.e., viable cardiac muscle. Clinically, the transition begins soon after injection. If the tracer is injected at the time of exercise, the myo-cardial segments supplied by stenosed coronary arteries have decreased thallium uptake. After the patient stops exercising, the redistribution phase begins and is usually completed in 3-5 hours (Figure 1). Areas with persistent thallium defects are thought to represent irreversibly damaged myocardium or scar. In some patients, local perfusion is so reduced that a repeat rest study must be performed if the size of resting metabolically active myocardium is to be assessed.

Procedure

A gamma camera (Anger type) with either medium-sensitivity or high-resolution collimators is used. Images of the heart are obtained from the anterior and at least two other left anterior oblique (LAO) projections (40° and 70°) so that all the cardiac segments are well visualized (Figure 2). SPECT image acquisition is performed with either 180° or 360° rotations of the gamma camera. Correction for attenuation due to tissue in the thorax is often performed, although it probably does not improve the efficacy of the test. After computer reconstruction of the images, analysis can be performed either on the transaxial images or on images reformatted to give long- and short-axis views.

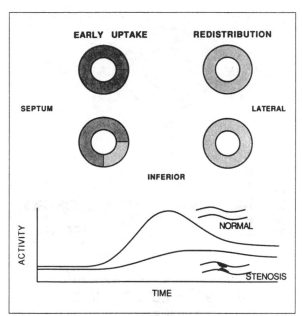

Figure 1. *Difference in myocardial kinetics for thallium-201 uptake in normal (top) and ischemic (bottom) myocardium. In these idealized short-axis images of the left ventricle, the section at bottom left shows a relative decrease in uptake in the inferolateral segment due to a circumflex stenosis. This is also seen on the time-activity graph of myocardial uptake drawn below. With redistribution (section at bottom right), uptake will become more homogeneous, so that the ischemic segment and normal segments will be indistinguishable.*

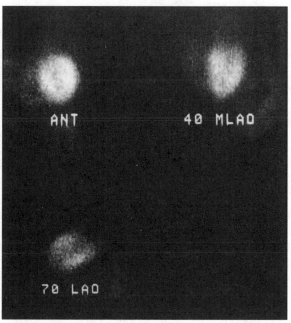

Figure 2. *Myocardial perfusion scintigraphy. Activity is normal throughout the left ventricular wall. ANT = anterior; 40 MLAO = 40° modified left anterior oblique; 70 LAO = 70° left anterior oblique. See color plate, p. xvii, for ischemic thallium image.*

When thallium imaging is performed during stress or exercise, the patient should reach a maximal exercise point (usually 85% of maximal predicted heart rate on the Bruce protocol) before being injected with a dose of approximately 2 mCi. He or she should also continue to exercise for 1-2 minutes or until the tracer has cleared the blood. For best results, imaging should start 5 minutes after injection. Redistribution images are also obtained at 3-5 hours after injection. If necessary, a repeat resting study can be ordered over the next week.

An alternate means of assessing coronary perfusion is with the use of dipyridamole. This vasodilating agent can be given intravenously or orally (IV formulation of dipyridamole is not yet commercially available) to patients who are unable to exercise, e.g., those with peripheral arterial disease. It is normally given intravenously over 4 minutes (0.56 mg/kg). Thallium is injected 10 minutes later and imaging begins another 5 minutes later. A moderate increase in heart rate normally occurs. Arrhythmias or chest pain due to the coronary steal induced by dipyridamole can be reversed with aminophylline. Oral administration of dipyridamole requires larger doses (300-400 mg); thallium is injected 45 minutes later. The incidence of arrhythmias is lower than with IV administration.

Patterns of Myocardial Uptake

A consistent scoring system must be used to describe the results of a thallium scan. A normal study shows either a homogeneous distribution of the isotope in the ventricle walls or a small apical defect, best seen in the anterior and 30° LAO views. This apparent apical thinning is due to both ventricular geometry and motion during the cardiac cycle. Localized areas of decreased uptake can be related to the territories of diseased coronary arteries. Multiple focal defects that fail to conform to these distributions may represent involvement by other processes such as sarcoidosis. Diffuse decreases in uptake suggest the presence of a cardiomyopathy. When attempting to

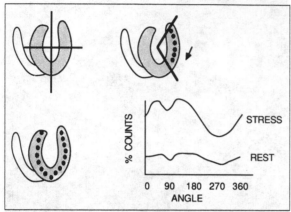

Figure 3. *The principle of quantitative thallium-201 scintigraphy. As a computer searches the left ventricular contour (normal myocardium), points of maximal uptake are plotted as percentage counts vs. the angular location. Such profiles can be acquired for stress and rest studies. Interpretation is more commonly made by comparing uptake curves for the patient's study to a library of normal values.*

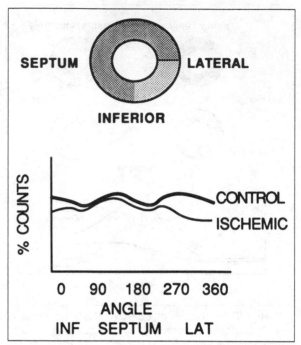

Figure 4. *A similar quantitative approach can be used to quantify uptake on single-photon emission computed tomographic (SPECT) short-axis slices of the ventricle. Here, uptake of the isotope is lower in the inferolateral segment than in normals (control).*

diagnose coronary artery disease, indirect evidence of myocardial dysfunction such as ventricular dilation or increased lung uptake should be reported.

Accuracy of the thallium study is increased if proper contrast enhancing schemes are used. Decreases of 10% in uptake that affect 20-30% of the circumference of the heart are usually considered abnormal. Most computer-assisted methods of analysis rely on measurements of isotope uptake along the circumference of the heart (Figure 3). These methods can be used on planar as well as on tomographic (SPECT) images. They have improved the sensitivity and specificity of the test for detecting coronary artery disease (Figures 4 and 5; see p. *xvii* for Figure 5).

TECHNETIUM-99m COMPLEXES

Technetium-99m complexed to isonitrile derivatives is being investigated as an alternative to Tl-201. The better imaging characteristics of Tc-99m as well as the improved dosimetry of the complexes suggest that they may soon replace Tl-201.

Pathophysiology

These compounds show high extraction efficiency by the myocardium. Their exact site of localization within the myocyte is unclear. Once within the cell, they are, for practical purposes, irreversibly bound.

Their uptake parallels myocardial blood flow. However, since they are not subject to redistribution effects, two separate injections are needed when stress/rest image pairs are needed.

Procedure

Because of the more favorable characteristics of the Tc-99m isotope, a gamma camera with a high-resolution collimator can be used. Imaging is similar to that described for thallium. Experience with these complexes is limited. Repeat rest injections are needed if rest images are to be compared to stress images.

Patterns of Myocardial Uptake

Analysis of Tc-99m complexes is similar to that of Tl-201. The sensitivity and specificity of myocardial imaging with these compounds should prove similar to those of Tl-201.

POSITRON EMITTERS

N-13 ammonia and rubidium-82 are used in conjunction with a positron camera. They both have a short half-life and are more useful for determining perfusion than myocardial mass.

Pathophysiology

Uptake of N-13 ammonia and Rb-82 is proportional to blood flow. Rb-82 is not metabolized, whereas uptake of N-13 ammonia is modified if local metabolic changes affect the glutamine synthetase pathway.

Procedure

Imaging requires a positron camera. With N-13 ammonia, a cyclotron is needed. With Rb-82, an Sr-82m generator is used. Concurrent dipyridamole injection offers the best opportunity for stress imaging.

MYOCARDIAL CONTRACTILITY

Table 2 summarizes the characteristics and uses of imaging agents for assessing myocardial contractility. Both left and right ventricular function can be assessed with either first-pass or gated equilibrium radionuclide angiocardiography (Figure 6). The widespread use of computer packages for data processing and the ease with which the blood pool can be labeled using Tc-99m red blood cells now favor the gated equilibrium approach.

Pathophysiology

Radionuclide angiography can be used to measure several indices of ventricular performance. Ejection fraction is a sensitive index of the contractile state of the left ventricle. Detection and quantification of regional changes in contractility correlate well with contrast ventriculography and with the absence of contracting myocardium, either when it is replaced by scar or when ischemia is present.

With exercise, patients with hemodynamically significant coronary artery stenoses usually have changes suggesting decompensation of normal myocardial contractility, global decreases of left ventricular ejection fraction, or the appearance of new wall motion abnormalities.

Procedure

Rest studies are more often performed with the patient supine. In a first-transit study, a rapid bolus is injected so that the bolus remains compact when it reaches the left ventricle. The multicrystal camera is the instrument of choice for such a study because it possesses a high count rate capability and permits extraction of statistically significant information during the short transit time of the injected bolus. Since most of the isotope is in the ventricular cavity during the critical imaging period, there is minimal interference from the small amount distributed to adjacent anatomic structures such as the lungs. The patient can therefore be positioned in the anterior, LAO, or right anterior oblique (RAO) position.

Table 2. Myocardial Contractility

ISOTOPE	HALF-LIFE	COMPLEX	PRINCIPLE	USE
Tc-99m	6.03 hr	Labeled red cells	Blood volume change synchronized to ECG	RV and LV ejection fraction; regional function; peak filling rate; ventricular volumes
Tc-99m	6.03 hr	Varied (DTPA) pertechnetate	First-pass transit	RV and LV ejection fraction; regional function; peak filling rate; ventricular volumes Shunt lesions
Kr-81m	13 sec	Dissolved in saline from generator	First-pass transit	Mostly RV function
Ir-191m	4.7 sec	Dissolved in saline from generator	First-pass transit	Mostly RV function
Au-195m	30.5 sec	Dissolved in saline from generator	First-pass transit	Mostly RV function Shunt lesions

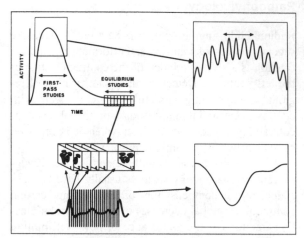

Figure 6. *Difference between first-pass and gated radionuclide angiocardiography. The first-pass angiocardiogram can be done without gating. The amount of activity over either the right or left ventricle is measured. Ejection fraction is normally calculated for the three to five cardiac cycles located near the point of maximal activity in the ventricular region of interest. The gated blood pool ventriculogram is the summation of activities detected during 100-300 cardiac cycles. The acquisition is synchronized to the electrocardiogram and is made when the activity in the blood pool is in a quasi-steady state.*

The equilibrium radionuclide angiocardiogram requires a greater degree of sophistication. First, the contents of the heart chambers must be labeled and remain so for the duration of the study. Technetium-99m-labeled red blood cells are the agent of choice. Second, patient radiation exposure must be kept to a minimum. This is achieved by synchronizing individual cardiac beats to the R wave of the electrocardiogram and by summing many individual cycles into a representative cardiac cycle. This is easily done if the cardiac rhythm is regular and without serious ectopy. Quantitative assessments of ejection fraction are more reproducible in the LAO projection; there is minimal overlap of the left ventricle with other cardiac chambers (Figure 7). Supplementary projections are used for additional qualitative interpretations (anterior, RAO, left lateral, or left posterior oblique positions).

With exercise, the first-pass study can be performed with the patient either supine or upright in the RAO, anterior, or LAO projections. When the predefined exercise level is attained, a repeat injection of radionuclide is given and a study acquired. This approach is difficult to use for graded levels of exercise because repeat injections are necessary. Using gated blood pool imaging, a widely used protocol increases the exercise state every 3 minutes. Imaging is conducted in the last 2 minutes of each stage.

With both first-pass and equilibrium techniques, regional wall motion abnormalities are assessed qualitatively during dynamic display of a reconstructed representative cardiac cycle or with computer-processed images of ejection fraction or paradox. Global ejection fraction is determined using a validated analysis package. There is some gain in accuracy over planar imaging reported with the use of SPECT at rest for measuring ventricular volumes. However, the time available for image acquisition during exercise ventriculography is too short for the use of SPECT.

Patterns of Contractility

The lower limit of ejection fraction for the left ventricle is 45-55% and that for the right ventricle is 40-50%, depending on the laboratory. The criteria for an abnormal exercise response also vary. Frequently cited criteria include either a fall of global ejection fraction, a failure to increase global ejection fraction by 5%, or the development or worsening of regional wall motion abnormalities. A depressed global left-ventricular resting early diastolic peak-filling rate is a more sensitive criterion of ventricular dysfunction than any other variable measured at rest. Early diastolic dysfunction has been measured in patients with coronary artery disease, with hypertrophic cardiomyopathy, and with hypertension.

MYOCARDIAL NECROSIS

Table 3 summarizes the characteristics and uses of imaging agents for assessing myocardial necrosis.

TECHNETIUM-99m PYROPHOSPHATE

Technetium-99m pyrophosphate, a bone scanning agent, is but one of many pharmaceuticals that concentrate at the site of recent myocardial necrosis. It is readily available and shows good tracer concentration within the infarct.

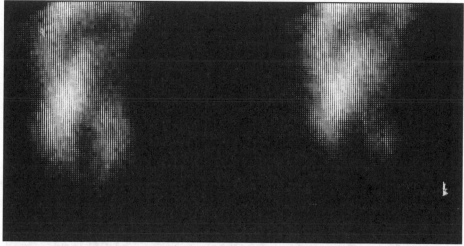

Figure 7. *Gated radionuclide angiocardiogram in the LAO projection. (Left) The diastolic image shows the ventricles maximally dilated. (Right) The systolic image shows strong uniform contraction of the left ventricle.*

Pathophysiology

The distribution of pyrophosphate uptake parallels the amount of calcium present in the region of recently damaged myocardium. Adsorption to crystalline hydroxyapatite, amorphous calcium phosphate, and calcium linked to myofibrils accounts for most of the uptake of this pharmaceutical. Pyrophosphate deposition is also dependent on persistent perfusion to the site of ischemic damage. Highest myocardial concentration of tracer occurs at 20-50% of the normal resting blood flow. Experimentally, the smallest infarct that can be visualized is 3 g. In the clinical setting, these factors result in an optimal imaging time of 36-72 hours after transmural infarction. Increased myocardial uptake can be seen as early as 4 hours after infarction, however.

Procedure

A standard gamma camera is used. SPECT imaging has shown higher sensitivity for non-transmural infarcts. Optimal imaging time is at least 3 hours after IV injection of Tc-99m. Anterior, LAO, and lateral projections are taken.

Patterns of Myocardial Uptake

Various scoring systems have been used to quantify the amount of pyrophosphate uptake in the myocar-

Table 3. Myocardial Necrosis

ISOTOPE	HALF-LIFE	COMPLEX	PRINCIPLE	USE
Tc-99m	6.03 hr	Pyrophosphate	Uptake by necrotic myocytes	Confirming infarct when ECG non-diagnostic Measuring infarct size
I-131	8.04 days	Iodinated to anti-myosin antibody	Binding to exposed myosin	Infarct sizing and confirmation
In-111	67 hr	DTPA chelate to anti-myosin antibody	Binding to exposed myosin	Infarct sizing and confirmation

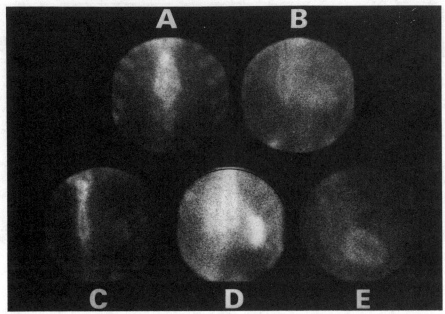

Figure 8. *Scintigraphic classification of myocardial uptake of Tc-99m pyrophosphate. (A) Normal. (B) Difuse. (C, D) Focal. (E) Massive.*

dium. In the classification we use, the scintigraphic patterns reflect the extent of abnormal uptake. Focal accumulations or diffuse massive uptake are unequivocal for myocardial infarction. Diffuse patterns of uptake, if they are as intense as the bones of the sternum, are suspicious for an infarct. A pattern of diffuse uptake that is less intense than the ribs is less likely to result from an infarct (Figure 8).

When myocardial uptake is focal, it can be localized to one or more segments of the myocardial wall by analysis of the scintigrams obtained in multiple projections. The inferior and lateral segments of the wall are perpendicular to the detector in the anterior projection, whereas the inferior, true posterior, and anterior segments are perpendicular to the detector in the lateral projection. Frequently, contiguous segments are involved, especially with inferior infarcts extending into the right ventricle. SPECT alleviates uncertainties in localization of the infarct and has been shown to be superior to planar imaging.

ANTIMYOSIN ANTIBODIES

Labeled antibodies to myosin localize at the site of recent myocardial infarcts. These agents are still under investigation. Although iodine (I-131) is normally labeled to the antibody, indium-111 chelates are gaining popularity.

Pathophysiology

The myosin protein is exposed after disruption of the cell membrane in the zone of an infarct. Labeled antimyosin antibodies, normally excluded by the intact membrane, can now reach and bind to the protein.

Accumulation is best in zones of lowest flow. Long intervals (24 hours) are needed to build up concentration sufficient for imaging.

Procedure

Although planar scintigraphy can be used, SPECT imaging is best suited. For example, after injection of 1-2 mCi of (DTPA)-coupled Fab fragment, imaging is performed at 24 and 48 hours.

Patterns of Myocardial Uptake

As with pyrophosphate imaging, zones of infarction can be clearly shown. False positives are less likely since many of the causes of pyrophosphate uptake (bones, fractures) do not affect labeled antimyosin. The approach is still investigational.

Table 4. Myocardial Metabolism

ISOTOPE	HALF-LIFE	COMPLEX	PRINCIPLE	USE
I-123	13.3 hr	Fatty acid analog (heptadecanoic acid)	Uptake in myocytes capable of metabolizing fatty acids	Cell viability
F-18	108 min	Glucose analog	Uptake in ischemic myocytes	Detection of ischemic but viable myocytes
C-11	20.3 min	Fatty acid analog (palmitate)	Oxidation of fatty acid	Decreased oxidation i.e., retention in ischemia
N-13	10.0 min	Ammonia	Perfusion Uptake in metabolically active cells	In combination with C-11 palmitate or F-18 deoxyglucose

MYOCARDIAL METABOLISM

Table 4 summarizes the characteristics and uses of imaging agents for assessing myocardial metabolism. Two categories of agents can be used to estimate myocardial metabolism: (1) single-photon emitters such as I-123 bound to fatty acids (heptadecanoic acid) and (2) positron emitters.

Pathophysiology

Myocardial metabolism is an interplay between the use of carbohydrates, fatty acids, and amino acids as substrates. Glucose uptake and metabolism predominate during ischemia. Increased uptake of an analog such as F-18 fluorodeoxyglucose reflects ischemic but viable myocardium. N-13–labeled amino acids (glutamate, leucine, alanine, aspartate, glutamine) show a prolonged early phase of clearance in ischemic myocardium. C-11 palmitate is cleared more slowly in ischemic myocardium due to impaired free fatty acid oxidation. Labeled heptadecanoic acid (methyl-C-11 or I-123) extraction is decreased in ischemia.

Procedure

These approaches are still investigational. Their high cost and the equipment required for acquisition and analysis of data relegate them to experimental purposes.

Table 5. Sensitivity and Specificity for the Detection of the Presence of Coronary Artery Disease

METHOD	SENSITIVITY (%)	SPECIFICITY (%)
Stress radionuclide ventriculography (early experience)	85%	81%
Stress radionuclide ventriculography (current values)	85-95	49-61
Stress thallium (planar, subjective)	85	85
Stress thallium (planar, quantitative)	93	86
Stress thallium (SPECT, subjective)	97	68
Stress thallium (SPECT, quantitative)	95	74

DETECTION OF CORONARY ARTERY DISEASE

With the proliferation of noninvasive diagnostic tests aimed at evaluating coronary artery disease, the clinician must keep very clearly in mind the questions he or she wishes answered by the test used and the population on which the test has been validated. Application of decision-making theory and, more important, Bayes' theorem, gives us insight into the limitations of the screening procedures. Consider, for example, the patient with a finite pretest likelihood of disease (determined by integrating all of the available clinical data). After a positive or negative test, the likelihood of disease depends not only on the sensitivity and specificity of the procedure, but also on this pretest likelihood of disease. If the patient has a high pretest likelihood, it is almost impossible to rule out disease with a negative test, whereas a low pretest likelihood of disease makes it very difficult to confirm disease with a positive test.

If we apply this logic to standard exercise electrocardiographic testing, there is no doubt that the test will yield accurate information in a group of symptomatic patients. In asymptomatic patients, however, the test is a poor discriminator between presence or absence of disease.

ROLE OF THALLIUM STRESS IMAGING

For detection of coronary artery disease, a set of "sensitive" criteria can be used, in the same way that the presence of resting Q waves on an ECG improves the detection sensitivity of an ECG exercise treadmill test. When either a stress-induced decrease in thallium uptake or a decrease in uptake during rest is used as the measure, the sensitivity of an abnormal test is 85% and specificity is 81%. For similar populations, the exercise test is 65% sensitive and 85% specific.

More specific criteria can be introduced if the clinical question is assessment of ongoing ischemia in patients suspected of having significant coronary artery disease. Many of these patients have resting Q waves or resting thallium defects. Appearance of a new thallium defect or worsening of a previous defect on exercise is 73% sensitive and 90% specific for the presence of significant coronary artery disease. The appearance of ST-segment changes is 77% sensitive and 86% specific in sample populations when acceptable ECG exercise tolerance tests are reviewed.

Thallium studies play an important role in assessment of patients with an unsatisfactory ECG stress test. Rest ECG abnormalities (left bundle branch block, ST-segment depression secondary to digitalis effect) or inability to reach established exercise end points occur in 5-20% of the populations commonly screened.

Under these circumstances, the stress thallium test can be 77% sensitive and 78% specific for detection of coronary artery disease.

The sensitivity and specificity of thallium-201 imaging are improved when computer-assisted analysis is used on the standard planar images. With the introduction and use of single photon emission computed tomography (SPECT) imaging, sensitivity and specificity have improved further (Table 5).

ROLE OF EXERCISE VENTRICULOGRAPHY

For detection of coronary artery disease, sensitive criteria include the presence of a reduced resting ejection fraction, with or without regional wall motion abnormalities; with exercise, appearance of new or the worsening of old regional wall motion abnormalities, and failure of exercise ejection fraction to rise by 0.05 rest EF units or 4% of the resting ejection fraction. Sensitivity is above 90% and specificity is 58% when this method is used to distinguish patients with coronary artery disease among the total group presenting with chest pain. An abnormal response is, however, rarely seen in normal, asymptomatic subjects.

More specific criteria can be introduced if assessment of the functional status of the left ventricle is desired. These include failure to increase ejection fraction by the appropriate amount or the appearance of new or worsening of old areas of regional wall motion abnormality. Sensitivity is estimated at 84%, compared with 94% when less specific criteria are used. Because of its poor specificity, ventriculography has lost favor as a screening test for detection of coronary artery disease.

LIMITATIONS OF RADIONUCLIDE METHODS

Thallium Scintigraphy

Right ventricular (RV) involvement secondary to coronary artery disease cannot be assessed by thallium-201 scintigraphy because the RV walls are not normally seen. By inference, rest or exercise defects seen in the inferior wall of the left ventricle may suggest right coronary disease. The sensitivity for detection of significant right coronary artery one-vessel disease (54-63%) or inferior myocardial infarction (88%) is poorer than that for anterior wall ischemia (71-85%) or infarction (100%). Similarly, one-vessel disease involving the circumflex artery is detected less reliably (33-44%). Detection accuracy has improved slightly with SPECT.

Although the overall detection efficiency is good, planar thallium imaging does not offer increased specificity in assessing the extent of significant coronary artery disease (Table 6). For example, a perfusion defect in the territory of the left anterior descending artery (anterolateral left ventricular wall) is seen in 80% of cases with solitary involvement of this vessel but in only 50% of cases with concomitant involvement of the other coronary arteries. This rate is improved with SPECT imaging. With left main disease, only 15% of patients show a typical perfusion defect involving the anteroseptal and posterolateral walls. Most of the remainder have high-risk Tl-201 scans, characterized by acute dilatation of the ventricle, increased lung uptake of thallium, and multiple defects in two or more coronary territories. Patients with left main equivalent disease show similar patterns.

The value of thallium uptake as a predictor of operative response to saphenous aortocoronary bypass surgery is twofold. Preoperatively, it confirms the physiologic significance of a coronary artery lesion. Postoperatively, it is a noninvasive means of assessing graft patency and surgical effectiveness. For example, areas in which preoperative perfusion defects were first detected (at rest or exercise) and then revascularized typically show normal perfusion response to exercise.

In combination with dipyridamole, thallium scanning can be used for risk stratification of patients undergoing vascular surgery. A normal Tl-201 dipyridamole scan predicts intra- and postoperative periods free of cardiac events.

Radionuclide Ventriculography

Radionuclide ventriculography has poor specificity when used to screen patients presenting with chest pain. Global and regional left ventricular function can also appear abnormal (false-positive) in patients with valvular disease, cardiomyopathies, and left bundle branch block; if it does appear abnormal, assessment by another imaging modality such as echocardiography is needed. Radionuclide ventriculography is also of limited value when arrhythmias are present.

Interpretation of exercise ventriculograms should take into account the distinction between screening for presence of coronary artery disease and assessing its physiologic importance. The rest study should serve

Table 6. Detection Accuracy for Thallium-201 Changes in Specific Coronary Territories

METHOD	ARTERY TERRITORY	SENSITIVITY (%)	SPECIFICITY (%)
Planar (subjective)	LAD	69%	91%
	Circ	38	92
	RCA	68	92
Planar (quantitative)	LAD	80	85
	Circ	63	94
	RCA	94	82
SPECT (qualitative)	LAD	76	92
	Circ	68	93
	RCA	75	90
SPECT (quantitative)	LAD	81	85
	Circ	86	85
	RCA	90	87

as a first step. A low ejection fraction with regional wall motion abnormalities suggests ischemic heart disease. The results of exercise testing more sensitively reflect the physiologic state of the ventricle. For example, patients with previously abnormal ventriculographic responses to exercise often have a normal exercise ejection fraction early after aortocoronary bypass surgery. In patients with valvular disease, development of exercise-induced left ventricular dysfunction can be used as an indicator for valve replacement.

Propranolol should be withdrawn 48 hours before stress thallium imaging and stress radionuclide ventriculography for detection of coronary artery disease, because it decreases the accuracy of both tests. Administration of nitroglycerin can also reverse areas of decreased thallium uptake or areas of regional dysfunction as detected by ventriculography.

MYOCARDIAL INFARCTION

TECHNETIUM-99m PYROPHOSPHATE

The overall sensitivity for detection of acute myocardial infarction varies from 51% to 100%, depending on the patient population and the interpretive criteria. When transmural myocardial infarction is suspected, sensitivity approaches 100% in patients imaged sequentially up to six days after the estimated acute event. If focal uptake is required for a scan to be considered positive, sensitivity is 82%. False positives are usually due to previous infarction. False-negative results occur in 6-7% of cases (75% of which are inferior infarcts), yielding a specificity of 93%.

With nontransmural infarcts, a focal pattern of uptake is 43% sensitive. SPECT imaging increases the sensitivity of pyrophosphate infarct imaging so that these subendocardial/nontransmural infarcts should almost always be detected.

Pyrophosphate imaging can assist in the clinical problem of documenting recent myocardial damage in a patient presenting with an equivocal electrocardiogram (left bundle branch block) or presenting too late in the clinical course for serial evaluation of cardiospecific enzymes.

Abnormal pyrophosphate uptake occurs in one third of patients with unstable angina. Positive scans have been shown to correlate with myocardial damage as documented by serum creatine kinase (MB) elevation in two thirds of these cases. Of the other third, almost half show uptake at the site of old infarcts. Pathologic correlations suggest that subclinical ongoing myocardial necrosis probably occurs in a large proportion of these cases.

Technetium-99m pyrophosphate imaging has also been used to delineate any associated extension of inferior infarcts into the right ventricle. This phenomenon occurs in more than one third of the cases of inferior infarction and can easily be seen by radionuclide imaging.

Infarct-avid scintigraphy is a sensitive and specific means of establishing whether myocardial infarction occurred perioperatively. Addition of a preoperative scan increases the accuracy of the examination, especially in patients undergoing saphenous aortocoronary bypass grafting.

The pattern and intensity of pyrophosphate uptake also holds prognostic significance. The amount of pharmaceutical taken up by the infarcted myocardium correlates with mortality and morbidity in the early period after hospital discharge. The "doughnut" pattern of uptake is also associated with a high mortality rate in the year after acute myocardial infarction. The failure of pyrophosphate uptake either to resolve or to decrease in intensity within 30 days of the first examination identifies patients with an increased death rate in the year after infarction. A high incidence of concomitant left ventricular dysfunction is seen in these patients.

THALLIUM-201

Imaging with thallium-201 detects both infarction and regions of peri-infarct ischemia. The overall sensitivity in acute (within 6 hours) events is 100%; for events occurring between 6 and 24 hours before imaging, sensitivity decreases to 88%. When imaging is carried out at more than 24 hours after the onset of symptoms, it decreases to 72%. The overall detection rate for transmural events is 88% and that for nontransmural infarctions is 63%. When infarct size is measured using enzymatic criteria, the sensitivity for large infarcts is 94% and for small areas of damage, 57%. The test is not specific enough to be of use in screening patients with acute chest pain, i.e., infarct versus noninfarct. There has, however, been increased use of the test for documenting the value of acute interventions aimed at preserving myocardium at risk. Thallium-201 can be used to assess the efficacy of thrombolysis or of balloon angioplasty. Successful thrombolysis is associated with a normalization of thallium-201 uptake in the re-opened coronary artery. Although intracoronary Tl-201 defines the abnormality best, follow-up intravenously administered Tl-201 studies can similarly document the success of the intervention.

Thallium-201 can be used to detect the presence of previous myocardial infarction. Blood et al. reported that the detection rate of a rest thallium study for previous infarction is 54%, while that for an abnormal exercise study with poor redistribution is more than 90%.

In patients with completed infarction, early exercise Tl-201 stress testing is being performed to document the presence of persistent ischemia, which may suggest a still-active stenosis near the culprit artery or a second significant stenosis. A normal response predicts the absence of cardiac events in the subsequent six to 12 months.

Thallium imaging is used in patients after aortocoronary bypass surgery when graft patency is questionable. Exercise and redistribution thallium images are obtained pre- and postoperatively. The graft patency rate is over 80% if no new defects are seen on rest-redistribution images or if transient defects are present on the postoperative study. A persistent defect suggests graft occlusion (73%) and, by inference, myocardial damage. In patients with unstable angina or with angina refractory to medical treatment, bypass surgery appears to normalize thallium uptake in those regions showing late redistribution on preoperative scans (77%). Persistent defects represent either new damage in a previously ischemic region or a site of myocardial scarring.

Right ventricular infarction cannot be appreciated on thallium images unless abnormally increased uptake is seen in the RV wall. This is possible only in patients with RV hypertrophy. The finding is most common in patients with chronic elevation of pulmonary artery pressures.

RADIONUCLIDE ANGIOGRAPHY (FIRST-PASS OR EQUILIBRIUM)

This imaging modality is used to identify alterations in regional or global ventricular function during and after ischemic damage.

Using global left ventricular ejection fraction as a criterion, the sensitivity for anterior transmural infarction is high (96-100%), whereas that for inferior infarction is 66%. The lack of sensitivity in the latter group can be understood if these patients are separated into subgroups, one without ST-segment depression on the precordial leads (sensitivity 14%) and one with ST depression (sensitivity 94%).

Serial evaluation of both global left ventricular ejection fraction and regional wall motion abnormalities in the postinfarction period show that regional and global asynergy improve slowly, with little change at two weeks after infarction and more dramatic results at two to four months.

Measurement of global left ventricular ejection fraction identifies patients with increased mortality risk in the postinfarction period; presence of both a low ejection fraction (less than 40%) and complex arrhythmias define a subclass of high-risk patients.

Inferior wall infarction is associated with depressed resting RV ejection fraction in approximately 50% of cases. This concomitant compromise of RV function reflects extension of the infarct zone into the RV wall. The rare case of right-sided congestive failure, low cardiac output, and relatively preserved left-sided function seen with RV infarction can thus be identifed by radionuclide angiography and appropriate therapy with fluids can be instituted.

Previous Infarction

Previous myocardial infarction can be documented from thallium or radionuclide ventriculographic studies. Abnormal myocardial uptake of pyrophosphate diminishes in the first two to three weeks after in-

farction in most patients, while defects on thallium-201 scintigraphy diminish more slowly after infarction, and by seven months have disappeared in 25% of patients with previous infarction. The wall motion abnormalities measured by radionuclide angiocardiography do not change significantly in the first four to six weeks after infarction. The detection rate is more than 80%.

MISCELLANEOUS CARDIAC DISORDERS

THALLIUM-201

Areas of absent or decreased myocardial uptake may result from an invasive process that replaces cardiac muscle with fibrous tissue, granulomas, or tumor. Thus, focal areas of decreased thallium uptake may be seen in patients with myocardial sarcoidosis, amyloidosis, or other infiltrative processes (as described by Strauss et al. 1975).

In patients with asymmetric hypertrophic cardiomyopathy, the relative asymmetry of uptake between the septum and left ventricular free wall can confirm its presence. Patients with symmetric hypertrophy secondary to pressure overload show relatively normal ratios of left ventricular and septal wall uptake.

Right ventricular hypertrophy and concomitant elevations in pulmonary arterial pressures can be estimated by comparing the uptake of right and left ventricular free walls. Kaaja et al. confirmed the presence of significant pulmonary artery pressure elevations (>30 mm Hg) in 28 of 33 patients when uptake of the RV wall was comparable to that of the left ventricular free wall. The amount of RV wall uptake also appears to correlate with pulmonary artery pressure elevation and increased pulmonary vascular resistance.

Patients with congestive cardiomyopathy can be expected to have large areas of decreased left ventricular uptake (>40% circumference) when an underlying ischemic cause is responsible (sensitivity 100%). Idiopathic cardiomyopathies more often present with an inhomogeneous diffuse pattern of decreased uptake; large focal areas are less common (incidence 25%).

VENTRICULOGRAPHY

Pohost et al. demonstrated the feasibility of using gated ventriculography to detect atrial myxomas; these patients have an area of decreased uptake in the area

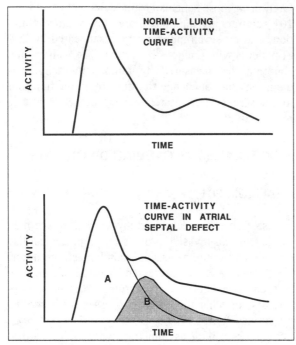

Figure 9. *Measurement of the time-activity curve over the lung normally shows a high-amplitude peak as the bolus or intravenously administered radioisotope passes through the lung. A second, smaller peak is due to systemic recirculation. In the case of a left-to-right shunt, as in an atrial septal defect, an early recirculation peak is detected. The area corresponding to this second peak is representative of the shunt lesion; A-B represents systemic flow.*

of the valve plane. These tumors must be large—usually more than 80 cm³—to be detected.

The therapeutic effects of calcium antagonists or inotropic agents can be monitored using either exercise or rest indices of ventricular function. A large experience has been gained for diastolic dysfunction in hypertrophic cardiomyopathies.

Left ventricular aneurysms can be detected during first-pass or gated studies. Although no large series are available, differentiation between true and false aneurysm is possible, more by the typical location of false aneurysms in the posterolateral wall than by any other criteria. Postoperative success of ventricular aneurysmectomy can be predicted based on residual ejection fraction of the portion of the left ventricular wall not involved in the aneurysm.

Congestive cardiomyopathy can be diagnosed and evaluated using radionuclide angiocardiography. Ejection fraction is decreased at rest (<40%) and the left ventricular cavity is enlarged. Coronary artery disease is the likely cause if contraction of the basal portions of the left ventricle is the last to be compromised, if regional asynergy involves a large, contiguous portion of the ventricular contour (>40%), and if the right ventricle is spared. Generalized hypokinesis with occasional areas of dyskinesia is more common in idiopathic cardiomyopathy. Depressed right ventricular function (<35% ejection fraction) also provides prognostic information in patients with severe left ventricular dysfunction.

Diastolic dysfunction of the left ventricle has been observed in patients with coronary artery disease, hypertrophic cardiomyopathy, and hypertension despite normal systolic function. Of the two parameters commonly measured, peak early-diastolic filling rate (PFR) and time to peak-diastolic filling rate, the former more accurately predicts early ventricular dysfunction. In coronary artery disease, the sensitivity of PFR is 50% given normal global regional left ventricular function. Improvement in this measure of ventricular function has been shown after coronary bypass surgery in patients with coronary artery disease and after calcium antagonist therapy in patients with hypertrophic cardiomyopathy.

Confirmation of left-sided valvular regurgitation and left ventricular volume overload in the absence of concomitant right-sided valvular regurgitation is possible for cases of significant (regurgitant fraction >0.20) valvular incompetence. The method most frequently used relies on good geometric separation of both ventricles and atria and considers the ratio of left-to-right ventricular stroke volume counts:

$$\frac{\text{LV stroke volume} - \text{RV stroke volume}}{\text{LV stroke volume}}$$

$$= \text{regurgitant fraction}$$

Abnormal blood pool increase in the liver during systole can also be used to document tricuspid regurgitation.

CENTRAL CIRCULATION

The transit of an intravenously injected bolus of a non-diffusible radiopharmaceutical can be followed and recorded, providing qualitative information about the anatomy of the heart chambers and the major vessels. This angiocardiogram can also be used to estimate the size of the heart chambers and the patency of the major veins and of the aorta and to detect and quantify physiologic shunts.

This technique can be used to provide gross anatomic and functional information in patients with suspected congenital anomalies. Tricuspid atresia and Ebstein's anomaly are identified by a right-to-left shunt through their atrial septal defect. With pulmonary atresia, either a right-to-left shunt is seen through an open ventricular septal defect or, if this shunt is absent, the bolus persists in the right atrium. The bolus persists in either the right atrium or right ventricle if tricuspid stenosis or pulmonic stenosis is present. On the left side of the heart, the left atrium is enlarged in the presence of mitral stenosis; in addition, pharmaceutical transit into the left ventricle and aorta is delayed. In severe aortic stenosis at birth or in hypoplastic left heart, a right-to-left shunt through a patent ductus arteriosus may also be detected. In transposition of the great vessels, cardiac activity disappears quickly; only the right heart and aorta can be identified.

Right-to-left shunts are measured using either of two techniques. Radioactive particles, such as Tc-99m–labeled macroaggregated albumin (20-50 μ in diameter), are injected intravenously; the number of particles impacted in the pulmonary, renal, and cerebral circulations is then measured. Since a small number of particulates (20,000-100,000) is injected, no side effects have been reported. The equation is:

% Right-to-left shunt

$$= \frac{\text{counts (total body} - \text{lung)}}{\text{counts (total body)}} \times 100\%$$

Alternatively, the time-activity curve (relationship between time and the quantity of a radioactive tracer in an organ or region of an organ as measured by an external detector) can be analyzed as the bolus passes over the left ventricle:

% Right-to-left shunt

$$= \frac{\begin{array}{c}\text{Early portion of time-activity curve} \\ \text{(extrapolated shunted flow)}\end{array}}{\text{Total curve (total flow)}}$$

For left-to-right shunts (Figure 9), a time-activity curve is generated over the lung fields and is mathematically processed to obtain a curve representing the pulmonary circulation and a second curve representing pulmonary recirculation. The difference between these two curves is proportionate to systemic flow. The shunt is then calculated as a pulmonary to systemic (Q_p:Q_s) flow ratio; ratios greater than 1.2:1 are abnormal.

Bibliography

Blood DK, McCarthy DM, Sciacca RR, et al: Comparison of single dose and double dose thallium-201 myocardial perfusion scintigraphy for the detection of coronary artery disease and prior myocardial infarction. *Circulation* 58:777, 1978.

Bonow RO, Leon MB, Rosing DR, et al: Effects of verapamil and propranolol on left ventricular systolic function and diastolic filling in patients with coronary artery disease. Radionuclide angiographic studies at rest and during exercise. *Circulation* 65:1337, 1980.

Borer JS, Bacharach SL, Green MV, et al: Real time radionuclide cineangiography in the noninvasive evaluation of global and regional left ventricular function at rest and during exercise in patients with coronary artery disease. *N Engl J Med* 296:839, 1977.

Botvinick EH, Taradash MR, Shames DM, et al: Thallium-201 myocardial perfusion scintigraphy for the clinical clarification of normal, abnormal, and equivocal electrocardiographic stress tests. *Am J Cardiol* 41:43, 1978.

Boucher CA, Zir LM, Beller GA, et al: Increased lung uptake of thallium-201 during exercise myocardial imaging: Clinical, hemodynamic and angiographic implications in patients with coronary artery disease. *Am J Cardiol* 46:189, 1980.

Bough EW, Gandsman EJ, North DL, Shulman RS: Gated radionuclide angiographic evaluation of valve regurgitation. *Am J Cardiol* 46:423, 1980.

Brunken R, Schwaiger M, Grover-McKay M, et al: Positron emission tomography detects tissue metabolic activity in myocardial segments with persistent thallium perfusion defects. *J Am Coll Cardiol* 10:557, 1987.

Buja LM, Tofe AJ, Kulkarni PV, et al: Sites and mechanisms of localization of technetium-99m phosphorus radiopharmaceuticals in acute myocardial infarcts and other tissues. *J Clin Invest* 60:724, 1977.

Bulkley BH, Hutchins GM, Bailey I, et al: Thallium-201 imaging and gated cardiac blood pool scans in patients with ischemic and idiopathic congestive cardiomyopathy: A clinical and pathologic study. *Circulation* 55:753, 1977.

Caldwell JH, Hamilton GW, Sorensen SG, et al: The detection of coronary artery disease with radionuclide techniques: A comparison of rest-exercise thallium imaging and ejection fraction response. *Circulation* 61:610, 1980.

Corbett JR, Lewis M, Willerson JT, et al: ^{99m}Tc-pyrophosphate imaging in patients with acute myocardial infarction: Comparison of planar images with single-photon tomography with and without blood pool overlay. *Circulation* 69:1120, 1984.

Cowley MJ, Mantle JA, Rogers WJ, et al: Technetium-99, stannous pyrophosphate myocardial scintigraphy: Reliability and limitations in assessment of acute myocardial infarction. *Circulation* 51:192, 1977.

DePasquale EE, Nody AC, DePuey EG, et al: Quantitative rotational thallium-201 tomography for identifying and localizing coronary artery disease. *Circulation* 77:316, 1988.

DePuey EG, Guerlter-Krawczynska E, Robbins WL: Thallium-201 SPECT in coronary artery disease patients with left bundle branch block. *J Nucl Med* 29:1479, 1988.

Fintel DJ, Links JM, Brinker JA, et al: Improved diagnostic performance of exercise thallium-201 single photon emission computed tomography over planar imaging in the diagnosis of coronary artery disease: A receiver operating characteristic analysis. *J Am Coll Cardiol* 13:600, 1989.

Fishman AJ, Moore RH, Gill JB, Strauss HW: Gated blood pool tomography: A technology whose time has come. *Semin Nucl Med* 19:13, 1989.

Go RT, MacIntyre WJ, Houser TS, et al: Clinical evaluation of 360° and 180° data sampling techniques for transaxial SPECT thallium-201 myocardial perfusion imaging. *J Nucl Med* 26:695, 1985.

Hansen CL, Corbett JR, Pippin JJ: Iodine-123 phenylpentadecanoic acid and single photon emission computed tomography in identifying left ventricular regional metabolic abnormalities in patients with coronary artery disease: Comparison with thallium-201 myocardial tomography. *J Am Coll Cardiol* 12:78, 1988.

Hellman C, Schmidt DH, Kamath ML, et al: Bypass graft surgery in severe left ventricular dysfunction. *Circulation* 62(Suppl 1):103, 1980.

Hirsowitz GS, Lakier JB, Goldstein S: Right ventricular function evaluated by radionuclide angiography in acute myocardial infarction. *Am Heart J* 108:949, 1984.

Holman BL, Wynne J: Infarct avid (hot spot) myocardial scintigraphy. *Radiol Clin North Am* 18:487, 1980.

Holman BL, Lesch M, Alpert JS: Myocardial scintigraphy with technetium-99m pyrophosphate during the early phase of acute infarction. *Am J Cardiol* 41:39, 1978.

Inouye I, Massie B, Loge D, et al: Abnormal left ventricular filling: An early finding in mild to moderate systemic hypertension. *Am J Cardiol* 53:120, 1984.

Jengo JA, Freeman R, Brizendine M, et al: Detection of coronary artery disease: Comparison of exercise stress radionuclide angiocardiography and thallium stress perfusion scanning. *Am J Cardiol* 45:535, 1980.

Johnson LL, Seldin DW, Becker LC, et al: Antimyosin imaging in acute transmural myocardial infarctions: Results of a multicenter clinical trial. *J Am Coll Cardiol* 13:27, 1989.

Jones RH, McEwan P, Newman GE, et al: Accuracy of diagnosis of coronary artery disease by radionuclide measurement of left ventricular function during rest and exercise. *Circulation* 64:586, 1981.

Kaaja F, Alah M, Goldstein S, et al: Diagnostic value of visualization of the right ventricle using thallium-201 myocardial imaging. *Circulation* 59:182, 1979.

Kolibash AJ, Call TD, Bush CA, et al: Myocardial perfusion as an indicator of graft patency after coronary bypass surgery. *Circulation* 61:882, 1980.

Maddahi J, Garcia EV, Berman DS, et al: Improved noninvasive assessment of coronary artery disease by quantitative analysis of regional stress myocardial distribution and washout of thallium-201. *Circulation* 64:924, 1981.

Massie BM, Botvinick EH, Werner JA, et al: Myocardial scintigraphy with technetium-99m stannous pyrophosphate: An insensitive test for nontransmural myocardial infarction. *Am J Cardiol* 43:186, 1979.

McCarthy DM, Blood DK, Sciacca RR, et al: Single dose myocardial perfusion imaging with thallium-201: Application in patients with nondiagnostic electrocardiographic stress tests. *Am J Cardiol* 43:899, 1979.

Pavel DG, Zimmer AM, Patterson VN: In vivo labeling of red blood cells with Tc: A new approach to blood pool visualization. *J Nucl Med* 18:305, 1977.

Pohost GM, Zir LM, Moore RH, et al: Differentiation of transiently ischemic from infarcted myocardium by serial imaging after a single dose of thallium-201. *Circulation* 55:294, 1977.

Polak JF, Kemper AJ, Bianco JA, et al: Resting early peak diastolic filling rate: A sensitive index of myocardial dysfunction in patients with coronary artery disease. *J Nucl Med* 23:471, 1982.

Reduto LA, Berger HJ, Cohen LS, et al: Sequential radionuclide assessment of left and right ventricular performance after acute transmural myocardial infarction. *Ann Intern Med* 89:441, 1978.

Rigo P, Alderson PO, Robertson RM, et al: Measurement of aortic and mitral regurgitation by gated cardiac blood pool scans. *Circulation* 60:306, 1979.

Ritchie JL, Zaret BL, Strauss WH, et al: Myocardial imaging with thallium-201: A multicenter study in patients with angina pectoris or acute myocardial infarction. *Am J Cardiol* 42:345, 1978.

Rozanski A, Diamond GA, Berman D, et al: The declining specificity of exercise radionuclide ventriculography. *N Engl J Med* 309:518, 1983.

Sharpe DN, Botvinick EH, Shames DM, et al: The noninvasive diagnosis of right ventricular infarction. *Circulation* 57:483, 1978.

Staniloff HM, Forrester JS, Berman DS, Swan HJC: Prediction of death, myocardial infarction, and worsening chest pain using thallium scintigraphy and exercise electrocardiography. *J Nucl Med* 27:1842, 1986.

Strauss HW, McKusick KA, Boucher CA, et al: Of linens and laces: The eighth anniversary of the gated blood pool scan. *Semin Nucl Med* 9:296, 1979.

Strauss HW, Harrison K, Langan JK, et al: Thallium-201 for myocardial imaging: Relation of thallium-201 to regional myocardial perfusion. *Circulation* 51:641, 1975.

Taillefer R, Lette J, Phaneuf DC, et al: Thallium-201 myocardial imaging during pharmacologic coronary vasodilation: Comparison of oral and intravenous administration of dipyridamole. *J Am Coll Cardiol* 8:76, 1986.

Treves S, Fogle R, Lang P: Radionuclide angiography in congenital heart disease. *Am J Cardiol* 46:1247, 1980.

Wackers FJT, Lie KI, Lien KL, et al: Potential value of thallium-201 scintigraphy as a means of selecting patients for the coronary care unit. *Br Heart J* 41:111, 1979.

Wackers FJT, Fetterman RC, Mattera JA, Clements JP: Quantitative planar thallium-201 stress scintigraphy: A critical evaluation of the method. *Semin Nucl Med* 15:46, 1985.

Wackers FJT, Stein R, Pytlik L, et al: Gold-195m for serial first pass radionuclide angiocardiography during upright exercise in patients with coronary artery disease. *J Am Coll Cardiol* 2:497, 1983.

Weich HF, Strauss HW, Pitt B: The extraction of thallium-201 by the myocardium. *Circulation* 56:188, 1977.

Zannad F, Laurens MH, Worms AM, et al: Detection and quantification of left-to-right intracardiac shunts by angiocardioscintigraphy. *Arch Mal Coeur* 75:917, 1982.

Zaret BL, DiCola VC, Donabedian RK, et al: Dual radionuclide study of myocardial infarction: Relationships between myocardial uptake of potassium-43, technetium-99m stannous pyrophosphate, regional myocardial blood flow and creatine phosphokinase depletion. *Circulation* 53:422, 1976.

CHAPTER 6

Exercise Testing and Ambulatory Electrocardiographic Monitoring

LeRoy E. Rabbani
Elliott M. Antman

Although careful scrutiny of the routine resting 12-lead electrocardiogram (ECG) can provide a wealth of information about cardiac disease, it has well-recognized limitations. Even in patients with advanced coronary artery disease, myocardial oxygen supply at rest may not be reduced sufficiently for ischemia to be reflected on the routine supine ECG. Furthermore, since the standard ECG provides, at best, 1 minute of continuous recording of the ECG signal, it is a low-yield procedure for evaluating cardiac arrhythmias. To circumvent these difficulties, exercise testing and ambulatory monitoring are widely applied in clinical practice.

EXERCISE TESTING

METHODS

The standards for adult exercise testing laboratories are shown in Table 1, which summarizes a report of the American Heart Association's Subcommittee on Rehabilitation, Target Activity Group. The proposed standards delineate optimal laboratory conditions and minimum requirements for testing and resuscitative equipment. The usual contraindications to exercise testing are summarized in Table 2. A careful history and physical examination are essential before administering an exercise test so as to exclude the presence of these conditions.

Table 3 lists the recommended procedures for electrocardiographic recording, choice of exercise load, end points for termination of the exercise test, and evaluation of the patient during the recovery period. Controversy exists regarding the number of ECG leads that should be used during exercise testing. Some investigators favor only a single bipolar lead with the active electrode at V_5; others believe that some isch-emic-type ECG responses will be missed if only a single lead is recorded. Although several orthogonal lead systems have been proposed, based on current evidence, the recommended choice of exercise ECG leads is the conventional 12-lead set using the torso (Mason-Likar) locations for limb leads. This enables the physician to use a standard three-channel ECG recorder with the same set of leads for control exer-

---

Table 1. Standards for Adult Exercise Testing Laboratories

Laboratory
  Temperature: 68–75°F, or 20–23°C
  Humidity: 60%
Staff
  Supervised by at least one physician
  At least two staff members present
    during test
Testing equipment
  Motorized treadmill or bicycle ergometer
    for graded exercise testing
  ECG recording instruments
    Conform to AHA standards
    Multiple lead systems: 3, 6, 12
    Continuous oscilloscopic monitoring of
      at least one lead
  Blood pressure: calibrated aneroid or
    mercury manometer
Emergency equipment
  Defibrillator: output through 50 ohm load
    of at least 250 watt-second
  Drugs: atropine, morphine,
    epinephrine, lidocaine, sodium
    bicarbonate, nitroglycerin tablets

AHA = American Heart Association

Table 2. Usual Contraindications to Exercise Testing

Acute myocardial infarction
Unstable angina pectoris
Acute myocarditis
Acute pericarditis
Congestive heart failure
Left main coronary stenosis
Rapid atrial and/or ventricular arrhythmias
Advanced atrioventricular block
Severe aortic stenosis
Uncontrolled hypertension

Table 3. Testing Procedures

ECG recording
  Ensure adequate signal by skin preparation
  Small silver-silver chloride disc electrodes
    mounted in plastic cups with adhesive
    rings
  Obtain 12-lead electrocardiogram and BP
    supine, standing, and after hyperventila-
    tion for 30-45 seconds

Work loads: see Table 4

End points
  Achievement of target level
  85% predicted HR for submaximal test
  Peak performance for maximal test

Indications for termination of test before
  achievement of target level
    Evidence of hypoperfusion and/or dimin-
      ishing cardiac reserve (vasoconstriction,
      abnormal cerebral function, dyspnea, un-
      due fatigue)
    Evidence of progressive myocardial is-
      chemia (worsening ST-segment devia-
      tions or chest discomfort, drop in BP/HR
      as exercise continues, electrical alter-
      nans, progressive widening of QRS com-
      plex)
    Cardiac arrhythmias, unless test specifi-
      cally being performed for assessment of
      arrhythmias (sustained supraventricular
      arrhythmias, increasing VPD frequency,
      ventricular tachycardia of 3 or more con-
      secutive beats)

Recovery
  Monitor HR, BP, and ECG changes
  Confirm that control levels of all patient
    functions have been reestablished

BP = blood pressure; ECG = electrocardiographic; HR = heart rate; VPD = ventricular
premature depolarization.

cise and recovery tracings. Additional considerations include the skin-electrode interface and frequency response of the electrocardiograph machine. The usual skin resistance of 50,000-100,000 ohms may be reduced to 5,000 ohms by rubbing, and as low as 1,000 ohms by application of an intermediate-speed dental burr. The ECG recording instrument should be able to reproduce repolarization events, best accomplished by a low-frequency cut-off of 0.05 Hz. To eliminate "noise" on the ECG signal, a number of exercise testing laboratories use computed signal-averaging techniques to provide a high-fidelity QRS complex and ST segment.

Exercise tests may be maximal or submaximal in design. Maximal tests are limited by symptoms or predetermined signs; they attempt to approximate the physiologic maximal performance, in which oxygen uptake fails to increase further with increasing work. Submaximal exercise tests are usually guided by a specific target heart rate (HR), often representing 85% of maximal predicted HR for the patient's age and sex.

Stress testing protocols may consist of a single level of exercise but usually involve graded or progressive increases in work load. The exercise modes suitable for graded exercise testing include the variable step, treadmill, and bicycle ergometer. The oxygen requirements for these widely used modes are summarized in Table 4. These protocols are oriented to load increments in terms of METs, based on the physician's assessment of the patient's exercise tolerance. (A MET is the energy expenditure at rest equivalent to approximately 3.5 ml of O_2/min/kg body weight.) The most widely used treadmill protocol for routine diagnostic purposes is that described by Bruce. DeBusk developed a reduced-work-load, graded exercise test suitable for evaluation of postinfarction patients and those with a known limited exercise capacity.

Table 4. Oxygen Requirements for Step, Treadmill, and Bicycle Ergometer*

Functional Class	METS	O₂ Requirements (ml O₂/kg/min)	Step Test — Nagle Balke Naughton (2-min stages, 30 steps/min)	Bruce (3-min stages)		Kattus (3-min stages)		Balke % grade at 3–4 mph	Balke % grade at 3 mph	DeBusk (3-min stages)		Bicycle Ergometer (For 70 kg body weight, kgm/min)
				mph	% gr	mph	% gr			mph	% gr	
Normal and I	16	56.0	(Step height increased 4 cm q 2 min)					26				
	15	52.5				mph	% gr	24				
	14	49.0		mph	% gr	4	22	22				1500
	13	45.5	Height (cm)	4.2	16			20		mph	% gr	
	12	42.0	40			4	18	18	22.5			1350
	11	38.5	36					16	20.0			1200
	10	35.0	32	3.4	14	4	14	14	17.5	3	17.5	1050
	9	31.5	28					12	15.0	3	15	900
	8	28.0	24			4	10	10	12.5	3	12.5	750
	7	24.5	20	2.5	12	3	10	8	10.0	2	17.5	
II	6	21.0	16					6	7.5	2	14	600
	5	17.5	12	1.7	10	2	10	4	5.0	2	10.5	450
III	4	14.0	8					2	2.5	2	7	300
	3	10.5	4						0.0	2	3.5	150
	2	7.0								2	0	
IV	1	3.5										

Modified from Ellestad et al., 1979. With permission of the American Heart Association. See Bibliography.
*Oxygen requirements increase with work loads from bottom of chart to top in various exercise tests of the step, treadmill, and bicycle ergometer types.

INTERPRETATION OF EXERCISE TESTS

Table 5 lists the five major components of interpretation of an exercise test.

The establishment of ECG criteria for a positive ischemic response has been the subject of much investigation. The original criterion developed by Masters for the two-step exercise test was 0.5 mm of horizontal or downsloping ST-segment depression in the postexercise recording. Sheffield summarized more recent experience with exercise electrocardiography. Exertionally induced ST-segment displacement can be classified into three types. The first and most common type consists of J-point depression with an ST segment that is entirely flat for the first 80 msec of its duration. The optimal balance between sensitivity and specificity for detection of myocardial ischemia appears to be served by requiring 0.1 mV (1 mm) of flat ST-segment displacement in a standard ECG lead. Other types of ECG leads have sensitivities different from those of the standard leads and warrant different criteria: for bipolar leads, ST-segment displacement of 0.2 mV (2 mm) is often used, and for Frank leads, 0.05 mV to 0.10 mV (0.5 mm to 1 mm) have been proposed.

The type I ischemic ST-segment response is characteristically seen at peak exercise and improves rapidly during recovery (Figure 1). By contrast, the type II ischemic ST-segment response shows progressive negative displacement of the ST segment, which may

Table 5. Interpretation of Test

ECG response
    ST-segment depression
    ST-segment elevation
    Evolution of T-wave inversion
    U-wave inversion
    R-wave-amplitude changes
Symptoms
    Character and distribution of chest discomfort
    Response to rest, NTG, CSP maneuver
Hemodynamic response
Arrhythmias
Quantitation of exercise tolerance
    Functional aerobic capacity
    Functional aerobic impairment

CSP = carotid sinus pressure; NTG = nitroglycerin.

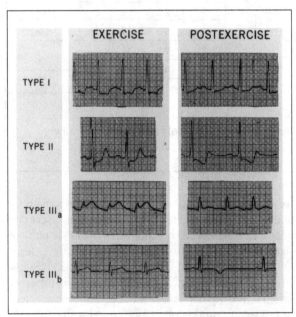

Figure 1. *Types of exertional ST-segment displacement. I: Transient depression during exercise that has almost disappeared 1 minute after exercise. II: Depression during exercise that becomes more pronounced after exercise before belatedly returning to normal. IIIa: ST elevation characteristic of Prinzmetal's angina. IIIb: ST elevation of modest degree usually caused by dyskinesis or scarring of the left ventricle. Reprinted from Sheffield. With permission.*

even become downsloping and be associated with an inverted T wave in the immediate postexercise period. Five to 20 minutes may be required for repolarization changes to resolve. The type III response, ST-segment elevation, is the least common ST-segment response. Once reciprocal changes are accounted for, ST elevation may be due to profound transmural ischemia or, in other cases, may be related to scarring and dyskinesis from previous infarction.

To determine whether patterns of exercise-induced ST depression or elevation provide specific information about the location of an underlying coronary lesion, Mark and co-workers studied 452 consecutive patients with one-vessel disease who underwent exercise testing. ST depression usually occurred in leads V_5-V_6 regardless of the underlying coronary artery involved, demonstrating that ST depression during exercise is not a reliable guide to the underlying pathologic anatomy. However, anterior ST elevation indicated left anterior descending (LAD) coronary artery disease in 93% of cases, and inferior ST elevation indicated a lesion in or proximal to the posterior descending artery in 86% of cases.

More complex ST-segment criteria have been proposed in an attempt to improve the diagnostic accuracy of exercise electrocardiography. For example, the ST-segment index is the algebraic sum of J-point depression (mm) and the ST slope (mV/sec). A negative index is considered abnormal, assuming that the magnitude of ST-segment depression is at least 1 mm and that the index is applied only during exercise or in the immediate recovery period. Another modification, introduced by Kligfield et al., is the ST-segment/heart rate (HR) slope, which normalizes the amount of ST-segment depression occurring during exercise for corresponding changes in HR, using linear regression analysis of these variables. The ST-segment/HR slope more accurately reflects the balance of myocardial oxygen supply and demand because alterations in HR are closely related to changes in myocardial oxygen demand during higher exercise work loads.

McHenry emphasized the need to analyze the ECG for inverted or negative U waves during or after exercise. This may occur in the absence of diagnostic ST-segment shifts and, when present on a V_5 lead, usually indicates significant stenosis of the LAD. Several investigations indicate that a normal ECG response to exercise consists of a decrease in R-wave amplitude. The R-wave amplitude actually increases in many patients with coronary artery disease, partic-

Table 6. Drugs that May Affect Electrocardiographic Exercise Results

Digitalis preparations
Sympathetic nervous system blocking agents:
  propranolol, guanethidine, methyldopa
Diuretics
Nitroglycerin
Nifedipine
Quinidine
Procainamide
Atropine
Tricyclics and other antidepressants
Lithium

ularly those with significant two- or three-vessel obstructions. When used in combination with ST-segment criteria, R-wave amplitude may reduce the number of false-positive and false-negative exercise tests.

Although coronary artery stenoses are the most common cause of the ST-segment shifts described above, abnormal pressure overload of the left ventricle due to either arterial hypertension or obstruction to ventricular outflow may produce profound subendocardial ischemia and an abnormal exercise ECG response. In addition, altered patterns of conduction result in an abnormal activation sequence of the ventricle, with secondary repolarization changes. Thus, as noted by Sheffield, left bundle branch block and the Wolff-Parkinson-White syndrome hamper interpretation of ST-segment changes. Sheffield also noted that hypokalemia can induce equivocal changes in the exercise test response and confound interpretation, as can mitral valve prolapse (through a poorly understood mechanism). Some drugs can modify the significance of an exercise test response, the most common being digitalis, which may cause abnormalities of the ST segment at rest and during exercise. Table 6 lists other drugs that may affect the exercise test response and produce a false-positive result.

Additional information that can be obtained during the exercise test includes the presence or absence of angina pectoris in association with abnormal ST-segment responses. The physician should carefully question the patient and assess the response to interventions. Multivariate analysis has been used to improve predictive capacity of stress testing. Important clinical variables that have emerged as markers for underlying severe coronary artery disease include an inappropriate HR response (failure of HR to increase to >120

beats/min), an inappropriate blood pressure response (drop in BP or failure of the systolic BP to increase to ≥140 mm Hg), and complex ventricular arrhythmias emerging at low exercise work loads.

Maximal oxygen uptake refers to the highest level of oxygen uptake that an ambulatory person can achieve by dynamic exercise of a large fraction of the total body muscle mass. Functional capacity may be expressed as the peak estimated oxygen uptake in ml/min/kg or equivalent MET units during a symptom-limited maximal test. By reference to a nomogram and knowledge of the patient's age, daily activity status, and duration of exercise, the physician can estimate functional aerobic impairment. This represents the percent deviation between observed and predicted values for maximal oxygen consumption, assuming that oxygen consumption can be estimated from exercise duration.

APPLICATIONS OF EXERCISE TESTING

Since the static resting ECG provides only a sample of information limited in time and limited in scope to a single, minimally demanding physiologic state, exercise testing has been developed to increase the myocardial oxygen requirements and unmask a reduced, relatively fixed coronary blood flow. In addition, the controlled atmosphere of the exercise testing laboratory proves an excellent opportunity to quantitate cardiovascular performance and detect stress-induced abnormalities such as cardiac arrhythmias.

The major applications of exercise testing are shown in Table 7. Ellestad et al. (1974) reported that mortality rates of exercise testing established by a survey of multiple centers vary from 1/10,000 to 1/20,000 tests. The infarction rate is approximately 3.6/10,000 tests. Thus, the risks appear to be acceptable and are far outweighed by the benefits of the information obtained during a carefully performed procedure.

INTERPRETATION IN DIFFERENT POPULATIONS

When performing an exercise test for evaluation of coronary artery disease, the physician should be aware of certain important statistical factors. As emphasized by Redwood et al., most symptomatic patients with significant coronary artery obstructions can be diagnosed on clinical grounds alone. In addition, according to Bayes' theorem, the predictive value of a test (the degree of likelihood that a positive result is true)

Table 7. Applications of Exercise Testing

Evaluation of coronary artery disease
 Confirmation of diagnosis of coronary artery disease
 Detection of asymptomatic or subclinical coronary artery disease
 Evaluation of therapy and longitudinal follow-up
 Planning coronary arteriography
 Assessing prognosis in patients with coronary artery disease
 Assessing prognosis in patients post-myocardial infarction
 Diagnosis of silent ischemia in selected patients
Evaluation of arrhythmias
Evaluation of other effort-related symptoms, such as dyspnea, palpitations, and syncope
Functional evaluation of patients with non-coronary cardiovascular disease
Cardiopulmonary exercise testing in congestive heart failure patients

is influenced not only by the sensitivity of the test, but, most especially, by the "prior probability" that an individual has the disease being tested for (i.e., the prevalence of the disease in the population being tested). Thus, if one assumes that an exercise test has a sensitivity for ischemic heart disease of 80% and specificity of 90%, then in a population where the prevalence of ischemic heart disease is 50%, it can be estimated that a patient with a positive exercise test would have an 89% probability of having ischemic heart disease. On the other hand, with a disease prevalence of only 3%, the probability that an individual with a positive test has ischemic heart disease falls to 20%.

Rifkin and Hood used a Bayesian analysis of the ECG response to exercise stress testing and cautioned that terms such as positive and negative may be misleading. Results should be interpreted in terms of a continuum of risk based on a number of variables examined during the exercise test, including peak HR, changes in BP, ST-segment shifts, arrhythmias or conduction disturbances provoked, and symptoms. Hlatky and co-workers used multivariate logistic regression analysis in patients with coronary artery disease who had both an exercise test and cardiac

catheterization, in order to identify factors affecting the sensitivity and specificity of the exercise test. Five factors have significant independent effects on exercise test sensitivity: maximal exercise HR, number of diseased coronary arteries, type of angina, age, and sex. However, the only factor with a significant independent effect on specificity is maximal exercise HR.

Therefore, with these caveats in mind, the clinician who conducts an exercise test to confirm the clinical diagnosis of coronary artery disease hopes to observe the patient during an attack of chest discomfort, determine the degree of stress required to provoke an attack, and record an ECG during an episode of chest discomfort.

ASYMPTOMATIC PATIENTS

Exercise testing is a powerful tool for detecting asymptomatic or subclinical coronary artery disease. Although the chance of recording a false-positive exercise test is increased in the population of asymptomatic patients who have a limited number of cardiovascular risk factors, exercise testing can elicit the presence of underlying coronary artery disease in the asymptomatic patient who possesses a combination of risk factors such as hypertension, diabetes, cigarette smoking, positive family history, or hyperlipidemia. Indeed, a positive exercise test has emerged as an additional independent risk factor for coronary events, as evidenced by a prospective matched study by Giagnoni et al. of 135 asymptomatic subjects. Rautaharju et al. examined the prognostic value of the exercise test in 6,438 asymptomatic middle-aged men with conventional risk factors in the Multiple Risk Factor Intervention Trial, finding that the exercise ST-depression integral was a strong independent predictor of future coronary death. Men with an abnormal ECG at rest, consisting of mainly high-amplitude R waves, and with an abnormal ST response to exercise, had more than a sixfold relative risk for coronary death compared with men with an abnormal ECG at rest and a normal ST response to exercise.

Finally, Gordon et al. described the experience with 3,600 men in the Lipid Research Clinics Mortality Follow-Up Study, which indicated that a positive exercise test was a stronger predictor of cardiovascular death than were high plasma levels of low-density lipoprotein, low plasma levels of high-density lipoprotein, smoking, hyperglycemia, or hypertension. The positive test's impact on risk of cardiovascular death was equivalent to that of a 17.4-year increment in age.

PATIENTS WITH MEDICALLY TREATED DISEASE

Another important aspect in evaluation of patients with coronary artery disease is assessment of medical or surgical therapy. Analysis of data from the Coronary Artery Surgery Study registry by Weiner and colleagues underscores the prognostic importance of the exercise test in medically treated patients with symptomatic coronary artery disease. One independent predictor of survival was ≥1 mm of ST-segment depression and final exercise stage 1 or less, which yielded an annual mortality rate of more than 5%. In a subgroup of 572 patients with three-vessel disease and preserved left ventricular function, four-year survival ranged from 53% for patients only able to achieve stage 1 or 2 of exercise to 100% for patients able to exercise into stage 5. In addition, periodic exercise testing in patients with an established diagnosis of coronary artery disease affords the opportunity to screen for a change in the pattern of myocardial ischemia, as suggested by the emergence of exercise-induced hypotension or ventricular arrhythmias. Furthermore, exercise testing is useful in planning coronary arteriography in patients with coronary artery disease. Thus, persons suspected of having left main coronary obstructions based on the constellation of findings of profound global ST-segment depression and systolic hypotension should be approached more cautiously in the catheterization laboratory. The patient who has a chest pain syndrome typical of angina pectoris but occurring at minimal levels of exertion and who has an equivocal or negative exercise test may be suffering from coronary artery spasm and should be considered for provocative testing with a substance such as ergonovine during coronary arteriography.

POSTINFARCTION RISK STRATIFICATION

Exercise testing is also used to determine risk stratification in the postinfarction patient. As noted by DeBusk et al., submaximal exercise testing performed seven to 14 days after uncomplicated MI is a safe and effective means of assessing prognosis. Approximately 10% of post-MI patients have severe exercise-induced myocardial ischemia, conferring a 15% first-year mortality. These patients should be further evaluated with early cardiac catheterization to deter-

mine whether they should undergo percutaneous transluminal coronary angioplasty (PTCA) or coronary artery bypass grafting (CABG). Preliminary studies by Schaer et al. revealed that the predischarge submaximal exercise test identifies post-thrombolysis patients with a patent infarct artery and jeopardized myocardium. According to DeBusk et al., in the post-MI patients discharged from the hospital with a negative submaximal predischarge exercise test, an additional outpatient symptom-limited, full exercise test conducted six weeks after MI identifies another 10% of patients with severe exercise-induced ischemia. The six-week test is more sensitive than catheterization for prediction of subsequent reinfarction and death. Among the 50% of post-MI patients in whom the symptom-limited exercise test does not manifest severe ischemia, the first-year mortality rate is less than 2%.

A recent Canadian study questions the value of performing both a low-level predischarge exercise test and the post-discharge (six weeks) symptom-limited exercise test in post-MI patients. Senaratne et al. compared the relative values of both tests with respect to predicting the occurrence of subsequent coronary events in 518 consecutive post-MI patients. In terms of assessing prognosis one year after MI, the additional information gleaned from the six-week test was of little importance relative to the predischarge test. The predictive accuracy for coronary events during the first year was 72% using data from the predischarge test and 71% using data from the six-week test. Combining the data from the two exercise tests raised the overall predictive accuracy to only 75%. The investigators recommend that the six-week test not be performed routinely in patients who have already had a negative low-level predischarge test and remain asymptomatic; rather, it should be limited to patients who have new symptoms since discharge or in whom there is a specific indication such as commencement of a physical conditioning program.

Stone et al. examined the prognostic significance of a maximal exercise test performed six months after MI in the MILIS Study Group. Mortality was greater in patients who exhibited any of the following: inability to perform the test because of cardiac limitations, ≥1 mm of ST-segment elevation, inadequate BP response, ventricular premature depolarizations (VPDs) during exercise or recovery, and inability to exercise beyond stage 1 of the modified Bruce protocol. By combining four high-risk prognostic features from the exercise test, patients could be stratified in terms of risk of mortality: 1% if none of these features was present, to 17% if three or four were present.

DEMONSTRATING CARDIAC ARRHYTHMIAS

Although the arrhythmogenicity of exercise has been acknowledged for many years, only recently has exercise been specifically used to reveal cardiac arrhythmias and assess antiarrhythmic drug efficacy. By increasing sympathetic nervous activity, including a marked increase in circulating catecholamines and decreasing parasympathetic nervous activity in association with the development of myocardial ischemia, exercise testing often provokes ventricular ectopic activity. The development of transient left ventricular dysfunction may result in left atrial hypertension and atrial arrhythmias as well.

In a large review of exercise testing for provocation of cardiac arrhythmias, Jelinek and Lown demonstrated that the arrhythmogenicity of isometric (static) exercise is less than that of isotonic (dynamic) exercise. Ventricular arrhythmias during exercise testing can be increased by using maximal symptom-limited protocols and using a continuous recording system, which allows identification of all arrhythmias or conduction disturbances. Although patients who exhibit single VPDs during exercise testing do so with limited reproducibility, patients who exhibit frequent complex repetitive forms may be expected to do so with less variability than those who exhibit only rare, isolated ectopic beats. Since VPDs usually emerge at peak exercise and within the initial 3 minutes of recovery, the patient must be monitored carefully during these periods. In some patients, exercise-induced arrhythmias may show overdrive suppression as exercise continues and heart rate accelerates (Figure 2).

Podrid et al. recently reviewed the changing role of exercise testing in the evaluation of arrhythmias. In 10% of patients with a history of serious arrhythmia, exercise is the sole method for eliciting arrhythmia. Moreover, exercise testing is efficacious in evaluating the effect of antiarrhythmic drugs that work by decreasing membrane automaticity, prolonging myocardial impulse conduction, and increasing membrane refractoriness. Exercise-induced catecholamine secretion exerts the opposite effect. Therefore, exercise may negate the major effects of the antiarrhythmic agents. Furthermore, exercise testing may expose adverse drug reactions that may not be evident at rest, such as conduction abnormalities, negative

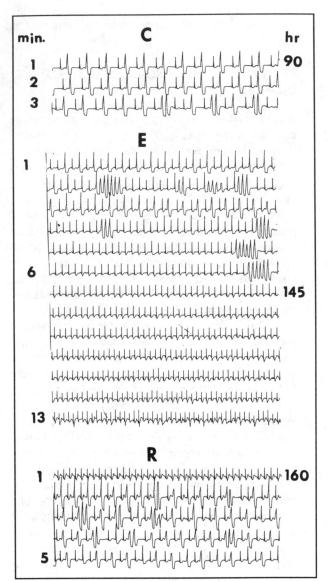

Figure 2. *Slow-speed continuous ECG recording, or trendscription, can be used to record the control (C), exercise (E), and recovery (R) phases of the stress test. In this case, ventricular bigeminy and ventricular couplets occurred during control; salvos of ventricular tachycardia emerged beginning in the second minute of exercise, followed by overdrive suppression as heart rate accelerated.*

inotropy, congestive heart failure, and aggravation of arrhythmia. If arrhythmia is reproducibly elicited by exercise testing, this technique can be used to determine drug efficacy. In summary, exercise testing is a useful method for eliciting arrhythmia, evaluating drug efficacy, and identifying adverse drug effects.

Henry et al. maintain that predischarge exercise-induced ventricular ectopy is a much better predictor of cardiac death in the post-MI patient than that detected by ambulatory monitoring.

OTHER APPLICATIONS

Additional applications of exercise testing include evaluation of other effort-related symptoms such as dyspnea or palpitations and functional evaluation of patients with noncoronary cardiovascular disease. By referring to established nomograms, the physician may quantitate the degree of effort tolerance and use this as a guide to management. As noted by Sheffield, infrequent but still valuable indications for exercise testing include evaluating functional capacity to dictate timing of surgical replacement of diseased valves; assessing the efficacy of surgical treatment; and determining in the catheterization lab the effects of exercise on hemodynamic conditions in disease states such as cardiac shunts or stenotic valves. Finally, PF Cohn asserts that exercise testing is useful for detecting silent myocardial ischemia in asymptomatic patients after MI and in patients at high risk for developing coronary artery disease because of two or more risk factors, particularly diabetes.

McElroy and co-workers applied cardiopulmonary exercise testing to patients with congestive heart failure. This technique entails monitoring of respiratory gases and airflow to determine oxygen uptake, carbon dioxide production, respiratory rate, tidal volume, and minute ventilation during a graded maximal exercise test. The maximal oxygen uptake, which correlates with the maximal exercise cardiac output, can be used to grade the severity of heart failure. The anaerobic threshold, which occurs at 60-70% of the maximal oxygen uptake, is another index of the severity of heart failure and indicates that the patient is close to performing a maximal test. Both maximal oxygen uptake and anaerobic threshold serve as objective measures of the efficacy of therapy for congestive heart failure. In addition, a pulmonary limitation to exercise can be revealed by failure to attain the anaerobic threshold or the maximal oxygen uptake, as well as by exhaustion of the ventilatory reserve (estimated by the maximal voluntary ventilation). In this regard, Cohn and Rector identified peak oxygen consumption during a progressive maximal exercise test, LV ejection fraction, and resting plasma norepinephrine concentration as being the strongest univariate predictors of prognosis in patients with severe congestive heart failure.

RADIONUCLIDE STRESS TESTING AND OTHER EXERCISE PROCEDURES

Recently, radionuclide stress testing, particularly thallium-201 scintigraphy and exercise radionuclide angiography, has emerged as a technique that improves the sensitivity and specificity of the exercise stress testing procedure (see also Chapter 5). As noted by Beller and Gibson, radionuclide techniques provide important physiological and functional information with respect to the presence and extent of ischemia that cannot be derived from cardiac catheterization. Such radionuclide studies are particularly helpful when the standard ECG is confounded by the presence of ventricular hypertrophy, conduction defects, the pre-excitation syndrome, and drugs such as those listed in Table 6.

As delineated by Beller and Gibson, thallium-201, a radiopharmaceutical potassium analogue, is employed in exercise myocardial scintigraphy. After intravenous injection, the initial myocardial uptake of thallium-201 is related to regional myocardial blood flow and the 85% extraction fraction of thallium-201 by the heart. In contrast to normal myocardial tissue, damaged myocardial tissue is incapable of concentrating thallium-201 intracellularly. After IV injection, thallium-201 continuously washes out of the heart and is exchanged for recirculating tracer in a process of *redistribution*. Thallium-201 redistribution is evident after transient regional myocardial hypoperfusion or chronic diminution in regional flow. Redistribution is the total or partial resolution of initial defects over time after thallium-201 injection, defined by obtaining delayed views 2-4 hours after initial injection. When thallium-201 is injected during peak exercise, there is a heterogeneity of flow between normal and relatively underperfused myocardium in the presence of a significant coronary lesion. With termination of exercise and resumption of relatively homogeneous flow to normal myocardium and to the hypoperfused region, normalization of the defect occurs as thallium-201 washes out of normal myocardium, thereby revealing the delayed accumulation or flat *washout* from the hypoperfused region. When thallium-201 is injected intravenously during exercise or at rest into a totally occluded coronary artery or in the presence of a myocardial scar, a persistent defect is evident in the irreversibly damaged region. If this region is fibrotic, then views obtained 2–4 hours after thallium-201 injection will fail to show delayed redistribution. Partial redistribution occurs if there is physiologically significant collateral flow to viable myocardium in the distribution of the occluded vessel. Gill et al. identified increased thallium uptake by the lungs during exercise, a marker of left ventricular dysfunction during exercise, as a powerful harbinger of a subsequent cardiac event.

Beller and Gibson maintain that the overall sensitivity and specificity of thallium-201 exercise scintigraphy by visual analysis for coronary artery disease detection is 83% and 90% respectively, compared to 58% and 82% respectively for values ≥1.0 mm of ST-segment depression on exercise. The sensitivity of thallium-201 exercise scintigraphy is decreased by the presence of circumflex, diagonal, or distal vessel stenosis; single-vessel disease; lesser stenosis severity; nonjeopardized coronary collaterals; and a low level of exercise. In contrast, its sensitivity is increased by advanced age, prior myocardial infarction, left main disease, and associated ST depression or angina. Decreased specificity may be due to breast tissue attenuation, marked obesity, right ventricular dilatation, apical thinning, upper septal thinning, noncoronary heart disease, and, possibly, propranolol therapy.

Beller and Gibson note that IV infusion of dipyridamole is an alternative to exercise thallium-201 imaging. The coronary vasodilating property of dipyridamole augments blood flow in regions perfused by normal coronary vessels, but not in areas supplied by diseased arteries, creating inhomogeneity of flow that is demonstrated by abnormal thallium-201 uptake at peak vasodilatory effect. Delayed redistribution is manifest 2–4 hours later if the patient has coronary artery disease without infarction or scar. The sensitivity and specificity of dipyridamole thallium-201 imaging for coronary artery disease detection is approximately 90%. This technique should be considered in patients who attain suboptimal work loads on exercise testing or who have orthopedic or peripheral vascular disease conditions which make it difficult to adequately assess exercise performance.

Exercise radionuclide angiography determines left and right ventricular performance during exercise by utilizing either equilibrium-gated or first-pass techniques. Beller and Gibson define the normal ventricular response to exercise as an absolute increase of at least 5% in the right ventricular EF and left ventricular EF without the concomitant development of new regional wall motion defects, or >5% increase in end-systolic volume during exercise. In the postinfarction patient, an abnormal response consistent with ischemia will cause the left ventricular EF to fall more than 5%. The clinical indications for exercise radionuclide angiography are similar to those described for thallium-201 scintigraphy: determining the functional significance of known coronary artery disease; helping in the differential diagnosis of chest pain; prognostic applications, particularly, identifying high- and low-risk groups after myocardial infarction; and evaluating efficacy of thrombolytic therapy, PTCA, and CABG. When a new regional wall motion abnormality is combined with failure to increase ejection fraction by ≥5%, the exercise radionuclide angiogram has an overall sensitivity of 86% and specificity of 91% in detecting coronary artery disease.

Finally, it should be noted that Armstrong et al. have reported preliminary results combining two-dimensional exercise echocardiography with routine treadmill exercise testing in the diagnosis of coronary artery disease. Exercise-induced regional wall motion abnormalities on echo appears to be an accurate means of making or excluding a diagnosis of coronary artery disease.

AMBULATORY MONITORING

Ambulatory monitoring, also called ambulatory electrocardiography, ambulatory recording, Holter monitoring, Holter recording, or long-term ECG recording, is designed to record the ECG signal over an extended period for later playback and analysis. It differs from continuous monitoring (as is found in coronary care units or exercise stress testing laboratories), which provides on-line ECG printouts for immediate analysis. The principle and techniques used in current ambulatory monitoring procedures were originally devised by Norman J. Holter more than 20 years ago. Improvements since the original models were introduced consist of miniaturization of the recording apparatus, greater fidelity of the recorded signal, and improved playback and scanning devices.

The optimal duration of monitoring has been the subject of much investigation. As summarized by Winkle (1980), ambulatory monitoring for more than a 6-12-hour period not only improves the total yield of VPDs, but greatly enhances the chance of finding complex or high-grade VPDs (ventricular couplets and salvos of ventricular tachycardia). Thus, recording over a 24-hour period enables the physician to cor-

Table 8. Components of an Ambulatory Monitoring System
Recording apparatus
Scanner
Data analysis
Quality control

Table 9. Lown Grading System	
Grade	Characteristics
0	No ventricular beats
1a	Occasional, isolated VPDs, <30/hr: <1/min
1b	Occasional, isolated VPDs, <30/hr: >1/min
2	Frequent VPDs: >30/hr
3	Multiform VPDs
4a	Repetitive VPDs: couplets
4b	Repetitive VPDs: salvos, or ventricular tachycardia
5	Early VPDs: abutting or interrupting the T wave

relate a patient's complaint of palpitations or lightheadedness with disturbances of cardiac rhythm. In addition, one can catalog the frequency and complexity of VPDs, which many investigators feel are a marker for sudden cardiac death.

SYSTEM COMPONENTS

The components of an ambulatory monitoring system are shown in Table 8. As with exercise electrocardiography, skin impedance must be reduced by rubbing. Pre-gelled adhesive electrodes are applied to the torso to provide either single- or dual-channel recording. The leads monitored correspond most closely to standard precordial lead V_5 for single-channel recordings and leads V_5 and V_1 for dual-channel recordings. The recording apparatus consists of a lightweight (2 lb) tape recorder, which may be worn on the belt. The ECG signal may be recorded on a standard cassette or reel-to-reel system. The most widely used apparatus is the continuous recorder, which provides a complete recording of all ECG activity. Less widely used is the event recorder. These are of two types. The first may be activated by the patient in response to symptoms such as palpitations or lightheadedness. In the event that such a non-full-disclosure event recorder system is used, the accuracy of the algorithm must be confirmed. The second type of event recorder continuously monitors the ECG signal, but will only record rhythm disturbances outside a previously programmed range.

Playback scanners operate at 60 or 120 times real time and provide the technician with a superimposed image of QRS complexes. This is coupled to an audio signal. Changes in HR or rhythm are manifested as a shift in the visual image or audio signal, and a direct ECG printout may be obtained of selected portions of the tape recording. Since a typical 24-hour recording may contain over 100,000 QRS complexes, a method of data analysis is required. A simple approach is to provide a count of all the VPDs that

occurred during a 24-hour period. Since it appears that the risk of sudden cardiac death is related to the frequency of complex VPDs, Lown and Wolf introduced a grading system for VPDs (Table 9). Michelson and Sami criticized this system for not providing a quantitative assessment of ventricular ectopic activity or reflecting the density of VPDs during a given portion of the tape. Nevertheless, it is the most popular and clinically useful system at present.

Semiautomated scanning systems are available that report an overall error rate, compared with real time of 5-10% in detection of ectopic beat frequency. Fully automated, computer-based systems are being developed that may reduce the error rate to less than 1%. Introduction of technician editing capabilities improves the accuracy of semiautomated recordings, but at the expense of speed of interpretation.

CLINICAL APPLICATIONS OF AMBULATORY MONITORING

DIAGNOSIS OF CARDIAC ARRHYTHMIAS

Winkle (1980) summarized the results of 11 studies examining the incidence of ventricular arrhythmias during ambulatory recordings on normal subjects. Infrequent VPDs are common but complex ventricular arrythmias are unusual, particularly in younger patients. A number of epidemiologic studies suggest an association between frequent and high-grade ventricular arrhythmias in patients with coronary artery disease and risk of sudden cardiac death.

Cardiac arrhythmias are often sporadic events resulting in variability in arrhythmia frequency over a 24-hour period or when two 24-hour periods are com-

Table 10. Major Clinical Indications for Ambulatory Monitoring

Diagnosis of suspected cardiac arrhythmias
Diagnosis of suspected myocardial ischemia
Diagnosis of silent ischemia
Evaluation of therapy
   Antiarrhythmic drugs
   Pacemaker function
   Post-myocardial infarction

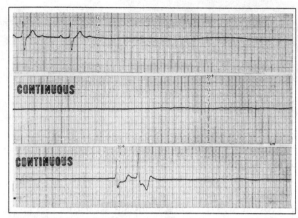

Figure 3. *This elderly patient's complaints of light-headedness were documented on ambulatory monitoring to be caused by profound sinus arrest and ventricular standstill.*

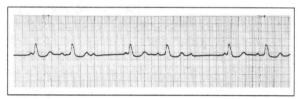

Figure 4. *Classic Wenckebach-type second-degree atrioventricular block was found to be the etiology of this patient's "irregular pulse" and complaints of "palpitations."*

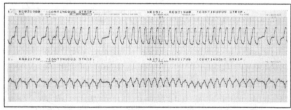

Figure 5. *This 16-year-old with familial hypertrophic cardiomyopathy had episodic lightheadedness related to paroxysms of supraventricular tachycardia with a rapid ventricular response. Sinus rhythm is seen at the left, with a wide QRS complex, representing an intraventricular conduction delay and/or conduction over an accessory tract (two-channel recording).*

pared. Recent sophisticated statistical analyses of the variability of arrhythmia frequency and complexity on serial ambulatory recordings propose stringent criteria for the diagnosis of antiarrhythmic drug efficacy. These statistically oriented studies have several shortcomings. The number of subjects analyzed were small and the subjects who underwent repeated ambulatory recordings were from selected groups with widely disparate cardiac diagnoses. It is not clear that information gained from such a selected group of patients can be extrapolated to people with a different clinical profile. Patients exhibiting marked variability of ectopic beat frequency often have minimal structural heart disease and may not require antiarrhythmic therapy. However, patients with malignant ventricular arrhythmias and recurrent cardiac arrests show considerably less variability in ventricular arrhythmias and probably should not be subjected to such rigorous statistical standards. It may be necessary to establish for each subject the degree of arrhythmia variability, using control recordings, before initiating drug therapy.

The major clinical indications for obtaining ambulatory recordings are listed in Table 10. Cardiac arrhythmias are usually suspected when patients complain of lightheadedness, palpitations, dizziness, or syncope. The symptoms may be due to bradyarrhythmias, such as profound sinus bradycardia or sinus arrest (Figure 3) or disturbances of atrioventricular conduction leading to pauses in ventricular activity (Figure 4). Alternatively, supraventricular arrhythmias with a poorly controlled ventricular response (Figure 5) or bursts of rapid ventricular tachycardia or ventricular flutter can cause diminished cerebral perfusion and alterations of consciousness (Figure 6). Widespread application of ambulatory monitoring has yielded dramatic examples of accelerating ventricular tachyarrhythmias in patients out of the CCU setting

(Figure 7). Patients suffering sudden cardiac death during ambulatory recordings have been described.

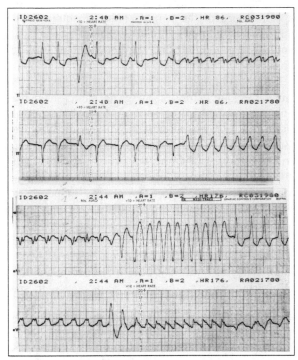

Figure 6. *This middle-aged man with severe biventricular failure had repetitive paroxysms of ventricular tachycardia (VT). In this continuous two-channel recording, VT is initiated at the right end of the top strip; an R-on-T beat occurs in the middle of the third strip, causing a shift in axis and acceleration of the rate of VT, which later slows and terminates spontaneously.*

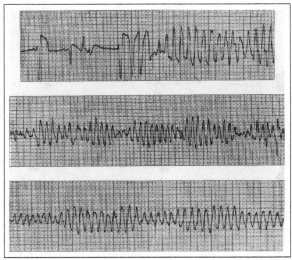

Figure 7. *In this continuous recording, rapid repetitive early-cycle VPDs in the middle of the top strip are seen initiating a run of coarse ventricular flutter/fibrillation, with oscillation of the amplitude of QRS complexes.*

Most had ventricular fibrillation initiated by early-cycle ventricular complexes.

DIAGNOSIS OF SUSPECTED ISCHEMIA

Myocardial ischemia is usually suspected when patients complain of effort-related substernal chest discomfort. Ambulatory recordings in such patients give the clinician an opportunity to perform repeated "exercise tests" on patients with coronary disease as they engage in daily activities. Slow-speed ECG recordings by Maseri et al. revealed an unexpected high frequency of transient ST-T-wave shifts in patients with coronary disease. Occasionally, patients reveal spontaneous ST-segment elevation during ambulatory recordings, which may or may not occur in association with chest discomfort. One should be cautious when interpreting ST-T-wave shifts on ambulatory recordings because of some peculiarities of the ECG pattern obtained by such techniques compared with the standard ECG leads. These peculiarities include deeper S waves, notches, or dips before the following T waves; shifts in ST-segment position; and T-wave lability, probably due to a combination of physiologic changes in the patient as well as alterations of patient position during the recording (e.g., from the supine to standard position). More recently, as reviewed by PF Cohn, Holter monitoring has emerged as a potent vehicle for detecting silent myocardial ischemia, a frequent manifestation of coronary artery disease.

EVALUATION OF ANTIARRHYTHMIC THERAPY

Another major indication for ambulatory recording is evaluation of therapy. The efficacy of antiarrhythmic drugs during acute drug testing or more chronic therapy is easily evaluated by ambulatory monitoring. In this regard, Morganroth examined the evaluation of antiarrhythmic therapy using Holter monitoring. Holter monitoring is the principal method for detecting and evaluating the presence of potentially lethal ventricular arrhythmias. These arrhythmias undergo a high degree of spontaneous variability. In order to define a therapeutic drug effect, a reduction in the frequency

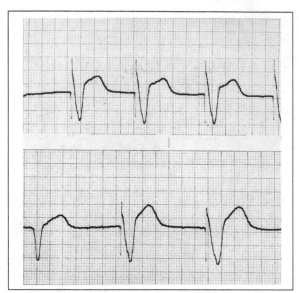

Figure 8. *Two isolated segments of 24-hour ambulatory monitoring session of a patient with a permanent ventricular demand pacemaker. An apparent inappropriate decrease in pacing rate is seen when one compares the intervals between pacing spikes in the top and bottom strips. This was due in this case to variation in the tape drive speed of the monitoring device—note the difference in QRS width and QT interval in the two strips—rather than pacemaker generator malfunction or sensing of isoelectric VPDs in the lead being recorded.*

of VPDs of at least 75% and a reduction in the frequency of nonsustained ventricular tachycardia by at least 90% are required to eliminate the likelihood of spontaneous variability as the cause of this change in the frequency of arrhythmia. In defining proarrhythmia, a different algorithm must be applied. When using antiarrhythmic drugs, Morganroth notes that a quantitative ventricular arrhythmia baseline for both frequency and type of arrhythmia must be established, thereby enabling repeat Holter monitoring after therapeutic intervention to determine whether efficacy, inefficacy, or proarrhythmia has occurred. Holter monitoring clearly reveals differential antiarrhythmic response rates among classes of antiarrhythmic drugs in patients with benign or potentially lethal arrhythmias. Transtelephonic monitoring and full 24-hour recordings may be used to evaluate characteristic forms of pacemaker malfunction: failure to sense, failure to capture the myocardium, or inappropriate alterations in pacing rate (Figure 8). Since pacemaker therapy

has become an extraordinarily complex field, the specifications of the particular device implanted in any patient should be reviewed before basing a diagnosis of pacemaker malfunction on ambulatory recordings.

Holter monitoring may also be used to detect ventricular ectopy before discharge in patients recuperating from acute MI as well as at varying intervals during the first year after acute MI. As delineated by Bigger et al. (1984), several studies suggest that ventricular arrhythmias in postinfarction patients are associated with increased mortality within one to four years of follow-up. Indeed, Bigger et al. reported the results of a large multicenter study concluding that ventricular arrhythmias and LV dysfunction are independently related to mortality risk in the post-MI patient. Mukharji et al. found that patients in the MILIS study with ≥10 VPDs/hr after infarction had a mortality rate nearly four times that of patients with <10 VPDs/hr after readjusting for LVEF. The NIH-sponsored Cardiac Arrhythmia Pilot Study (CAPS), published in 1988, was a study of 502 postinfarction patients in a multicenter, double-blind, randomized trial. All patients had ≥10 VPDs/hr on a 24-hour Holter monitor and an LVEF >20%. Enrolled six to 60 days after acute MI, the patients were randomly assigned to one of five antiarrhythmic drug therapy tracks: flecainide, encainide, moricizine, imipramine, or placebo. During a double-blind drug and dose selection phase, investigators could switch patients to the next drug in their assigned track or change dosage to attain 70% or greater VPD frequency suppression and more than 90% suppression of runs of VPDs except for patients assigned to placebo. Patients were followed for one year. As first drugs, encainide and flecainide had higher efficacy rates (79% and 83%, respectively) than imipramine (52%), moricizine (66%), or placebo (37%). Encainide and flecainide also had high efficacy rates, 68% and 69%, in patients in whom therapy with imipramine or moricizine failed.

The CAPS results paved the way for the Cardiac Arrhythmia Suppression Trial (CAST), a large, multicenter, randomized, placebo-controlled trial designed to examine the effect of antiarrhythmic treatment (encainide, flecainide, or moricizine) on mortality in post-MI patients with asymptomatic or mildly symptomatic ventricular arrhythmia (defined as ≥ 6 VPDs/hr). The surprising preliminary results were recently published. As of March 30, 1989, 2,309 patients had been enrolled in the initial drug-titration phase of

CAST; 1,727 patients (75%) had Holter monitor-documented initial suppression of their arrhythmia by one of the three study drugs and were randomly assigned to placebo or study drug. During an average follow-up period of 10 months, patients receiving study drugs had a *higher* mortality from arrhythmia than patients receiving placebo. Indeed, encainide and flecainide were responsible for the excess fatalities from arrhythmia and nonfatal cardiac arrests, as well as higher total mortality. As a result, the CAST phase employing encainide and flecainide was discontinued. The CAST investigators concluded that, even though encainide and flecainide may be initially efficacious in suppressing ventricular arrhythmias, these two class IC antiarrhythmic agents should not be utilized in the treatment of post-MI patients with asymptomatic or mildly symptomatic ventricular arrhythmias. It should be noted that it would be premature to extrapolate the CAST results to other patient groups or other antiarrhythmic drugs.

Ambulatory recordings appear to be superior to the standard exercise test for detection of ventricular arrhythmias in patients with coronary heart disease, the mitral valve prolapse syndrome, and hypertrophic cardiomyopathy. However, about 10% of patients have ventricular arrhythmias only on exercise testing; therefore, the two techniques should be considered complementary. Recent attention has been devoted to the comparison of Holter monitoring and electrophysiologic study (EPS) in patients with ventricular arrhythmias. Swerdlow and Peterson conducted a prospective comparison of the two techniques in 43 consecutive patients with coronary artery disease and sustained ventricular tachyarrhythmias. Overall, Holter monitoring detected arrhythmias suitable for antiarrhythmic drug assessment in 50% of the patients, whereas sustained monomorphic ventricular tachycardia suitable for electropharmacologic testing was induced at EPS in 82%. Drug efficacy could be assessed in 70% of patients evaluated by Holter monitoring, compared with 96% evaluated by EPS. Kim et al. studied the value of EPS in assessing the efficacy of antiarrhythmic agents in 52 patients with sustained ventricular tachycardia. They concluded that demonstration of antiarrhythmic efficacy by EPS predicts a good clinical outcome and that inefficacy as manifest by the EPS protocol may not preclude a good outcome if there is a marked reduction of spontaneous VPDs on Holter monitoring. Mitchell et al. performed a randomized clinical trial of noninvasive methods (Holter monitoring and exercise testing) versus an invasive approach (EPS) to drug therapy in 57 patients with symptomatic and demonstrable ventricular tachyarrhythmias. The noninvasive approach required fewer drug trials and fewer hospital days and identified a therapy predicted to be effective for more patients than did the invasive approach. However, patients randomly assigned to the noninvasive approach had more symptomatic recurrences of tachyarrhythmia than those treated by the invasive approach.

Kim recently reviewed the values and limitations of EPS and Holter monitoring in the management of ventricular tachycardia. Kim maintains that EPS is sensitive but not specific, while Holter monitoring is specific but not sensitive for evaluating the efficacy of antiarrhythmic drugs in patients with recurrent ventricular tachycardia. Failure to suppress VPDs on Holter monitoring during drug therapy predicts poor outcome. Suppression of VPDs by drug therapy, however, does not preclude a poor outcome. If ventricular tachycardia is no longer induced by EPS during drug therapy, the patient will have a good outcome. However, a persistent induction of ventricular tachycardia during drug therapy does not preclude good outcomes. Thus, some investigators suggest alternative EPS efficacy criteria such as changes in the rate of induced ventricular tachycardia during therapy. Kim contends that further studies should be conducted to confirm the latter suggestions. Because both EPS and Holter monitoring have values and limitations, Kim recommends using a combination of the two methods to enhance the clinician's ability to predict the outcome of antiarrhythmic therapy. Studies designed to prove that one of the two methods is superior to the other may prove futile.

FUTURE DIRECTIONS

New therapies are actively being investigated for treatment of angina pectoris and the reduction of infarct size. The impact of these therapies on ventricular function and long-term patient survival requires careful scrutiny. Techniques such as exercise testing and ambulatory monitoring are excellent tools for both epidemiologic studies and individual patient considerations. Computer-assisted electrocardiographic diagnosis of ischemic ST-segment shifts and cardiac arrhythmias holds great promise for the busy clinician but should be viewed as complementary to the judgment and experience of a skilled observer. On the horizon is signal-averaged electrocardiography, a noninvasive test for identifying patients at risk for ventricular arrhythmias. As noted by Vatterott et al., this computerized method of analyzing standard ECGs averages multiple QRS complexes. Signal averaging minimizes the level of noise that contaminates the periodic ECG signal and thereby exposes particular microvolt-level signals called late potentials, which are normally hidden with noise. Low-level late potentials that are contiguous with the terminal QRS complexes have been described. Late potentials, representing delayed depolarizations from damaged myocardial tissue and the substrate for reentrant ventricular tachycardia, have been correlated with clinical ventricular tachycardia, and are predictive of ventricular tachycardia inducibility at the time of EPS, and of post-MI arrhythmias.

Another concept that has recently generated interest is decreased HR variability and its association with increased mortality after acute MI. Kleiger et al. note that a high degree of HR variability is found in the compensated heart with good function, while HR variability can be decreased with severe coronary artery disease, congestive heart failure, aging, and diabetic neuropathy. To test the hypothesis that HR variability is a predictor of long-term survival after acute MI, Kleiger et al. analyzed the Holter tapes of 808 post-MI patients. Heart rate variability was defined as the standard deviation of all normal RR intervals in a 24-hour Holter mode 11 ±3 days after MI. Mean follow-up time was 31 months. Of all Holter variables measured, HR variability had the strongest univariate correlation with mortality. The relative risk of mortality was 5.3 times higher in the group with HR variability of <50 msec than the group with HR variability of >100 msec. Heart rate variability remained a significant predictor of mortality after adjusting for clinical factors, demographics, other Holter features, and EF. Kleiger et al. raise the hypothesis that decreased HR variability correlates with increased sympathetic or decreased vagal tone, which may predispose to ventricular fibrillation.

Finally, as noted by Antman et al., transtelephonic ECG transmission has emerged as a valuable addition to the cardiologist's diagnostic armamentarium. Clinical indications for routine transtelephonic ECG transmission include 12-lead ECG, pacemaker surveillance (bradycardia), antiarrhythmic drug surveillance, complex pacemaker function in the presence of coexistent tachyarrhythmias, monitoring an exercise/rehabilitation program, and possibly detection of silent ischemia. Emergency transmission indications consist of evaluation of infrequent, episodic symptoms; emergency triage; and evaluation of chest pain.

Bibliography

Antman EM, Ludmer PL, Friedman PL: Clinical applications of transtelephonic ECG transmission. *Clin Prog Electrophysiology and Pacing* 4:168, 1986.

Armstrong WF, O'Donnell J, Dillon JC, et al: Complementary value of two-dimensional exercise echocardiography to routine treadmill exercise testing. *Ann Intern Med* 105:829, 1986.

Beller GA, Gibson RS: Sensitivity, specificity, and prognostic significance of noninvasive testing for occult or known coronary disease. *Prog Cardiovasc Dis* 29:241, 1987.

Bigger JT, Fleiss JL, Kleiger R, et al: The relationships among ventricular arrhythmias, left ventricular dysfunction, and mortality in the 2 years after myocardial infarction. *Circulation* 69:250, 1984.

Bigger JT, Wenger TL, Heissenbuttel RH: Limitations of the Lown grading system for the study of human ventricular arrhythmias. *Am Heart J* 93:727, 1977.

Bruce RA: Progress in exercise cardiology. In: Yu PN and Goodwin JF, eds. *Progress in Cardiology*. Philadelphia: Lea and Febiger; 1974, p. 113.

Bruce RA, Hornsten TR: Exercise stress testing in evaluation of patients with ischemic heart disease. *Prog Cardiovasc Dis* 11:371, 1969.

The CAPS Investigators: Effects of encainide, flecainide, imipramine, and moricizine on ventricular arrhythmias during the year after acute myocardial infarction: The CAPS. *Am J Cardiol* 61:501, 1988.

The CAST Investigators: Preliminary report: Effect of encainide and flecainide on mortality in a randomized trial of arrhythmia suppresson after myocardial infarction. *N Engl J Med* 321:406, 1989.

Clarke LJ, Bruce RA: Exercise testing. In: Cohn PF, ed. *Diagnosis and Therapy of Coronary Artery Disease*. Boston: Little, Brown; 1979, p. 81.

Cohn JN, Rector TS: Prognosis of congestive heart failure and predictors of mortality. *Am J Cardiol* 62:25A, 1988.

Cohn PF: Silent myocardial ischemia. *Ann Intern Med* 109:312, 1988.

Davidson DM, DeBusk RF: Prognostic value of a single exercise test 3 weeks after uncomplicated myocardial infarction. *Circulation* 61:236, 1980.

DeBusk R: The value of exercise stress testing. *JAMA* 232:956, 1975.

DeBusk RF, Blomqvist CG, Kouchoukos NT, et al: Identification and treatment of low-risk patients after acute myocardial infarction and coronary artery bypass graft surgery. *N Engl J Med* 314:161, 1986.

Ellestad MH, Blomqvist CG, Naughton JP: Standards for adult exercise testing laboratories. American Heart Association Subcommittee on Rehabilitation, Target Activity Group. *Circulation* 59:241A, 1979.

Ellestad MH, Cooke BM, Greenberg PS: Stress testing: Clinical application and predictive capacity. *Prog Cardiovasc Dis* 16:479, 1974.

Faris JV, McHenry PL, Morris SN: Concepts and applications of treadmill exercise testing and the exercise electrocardiogram. *Am Heart J* 95:102, 1978.

Force T, Graboys TB: Exercise testing and ambulatory monitoring in patients with preexcitation syndrome. *Arch Intern Med* 141:88, 1981.

Froelicher VF, McKirnan MD: Rehabilitation and exercise early after acute myocardial infarction. In: Karliner JS and Gregoratos G, eds. *Coronary Care.* New York: Churchill Livingstone; 1981, p. 897.

Giagnoni E, Secchi MB, Wu SC, et al: Prognostic value of exercise EKG testing in asymptomatic normotensive subjects: A prospective matched study. *N Engl J Med* 309:1085, 1983.

Gill JB, Ruddy TD, Newell JB, et al: Prognostic importance of thallium uptake by the lungs during exercise in coronary artery disease. *N Engl J Med* 317:1485, 1987.

Gordon DJ, Lars-Goran E, Karun JM, et al: Predictive value of the exercise tolerance test for mortality in North American men: The Lipid Research Clinics Mortality Follow-up Study. *Circulation* 74:252, 1986.

Graboys TB: Detection of cardiac arrhythmias and conduction abnormalities in coronary artery disease. In Cohn PF, ed. *Diagnosis and Therapy of Coronary Artery Disease.* Boston: Little Brown; 1979, p. 63.

Graboys TB, Wright RF: Provocation of supraventricular tachycardia during exercise stress testing. *Cardiovasc Rev and Reports* 1:57, 1980.

Henry RL, Kennedy GT, Crawford MH: Prognostic value of exercise-induced ventricular ectopic activity for mortality after acute myocardial infarction. *Am J Cardiol* 59:1251, 1987.

Hlatky MA, Pryor DB, Harrell FE, et al: Factors affecting sensitivity and specificity of exercise electrocardiography: Multivariable analysis. *Am J Med* 77:64, 1984.

Holter NJ: Radioelectrocardiography: A new technique for cardiovascular studies. *Ann NY Acad Sci* 65:913, 1957.

Jelinek MV, Lown B: Exercise stress testing for exposure of cardiac arrhythmia. *Prog Cardiovasc Dis* 16:497, 1974.

Kennedy HL, Caralis DG: Ambulatory electrocardiography: A clinical perspective. *Ann Int Med* 87:729, 1977.

Kim SG: Values and limitations of programmed stimulation and ambulatory monitoring in the management of ventricular tachycardia. *Am J Cardiol* 62:71, 1988.

Kim SG, Seiden SW, Felder SD, et al: Is programmed stimulation of value in predicting the long-term success of antiarrhythmic therapy for ventricular tachycardias? *N Engl J Med* 315:356, 1986.

Kleiger RE, Miller JP, Bigger JT, et al: Decreased heart rate variability and its association with increased mortality after acute myocardial infarction. *Am J Cardiol* 59:256, 1987.

Kligfield P, Okin PM, Ameisen O, et al: Evaluation of coronary artery disease by an improved method of exercise electrocardiography: The ST segment/heart rate slope. *Am Heart J* 112:589, 1986.

Lown B, Matta RJ, Besser HW: Programmed trendscription: A new approach to electrocardiographic monitoring. *JAMA* 232:39, 1975.

Lown B, Podrid PJ, DeSilva RA, et al: Sudden cardiac death: Management of the patient at risk. *Curr Prob Cardiol* 4:7, 1980.

Lown B, Wolf M: Approaches to sudden death from coronary heart disease. *Circulation* 44:130, 1971.

Mark DB, Hlatky MA, Lee KL, et al: Localizing coronary artery obstructions with the exercise treadmill test. *Ann Intern Med* 106:53, 1987.

Maseri A, Severi S, Nes MD, et al: "Variant" angina: One aspect of a continuous spectrum of vasospastic myocardial ischemia: Pathogenic mechanisms, estimated incidence and clinical and coronary arteriographic findings in 138 patients. *Am J Cardiol* 42:1019, 1978.

Master AM: The master two-step test. *Am Heart J* 75:810, 1968.

McElroy PA, Janicki JS, Weber KT: Cardiopulmonary exercise testing in congestive heart failure. *Am J Cardiol* 62:35A, 1988.

McHenry PL: The actual prevalence of false positive ST-segment responses to exercise in clinically normal subjects remains undefined. *Circulation* 55:63, 1977.

Michelson EL, Morganroth J: Spontaneous variability of complex ventricular arrhythmias detected by long-term electrocardiographic recording. *Circulation* 61:690, 1980.

Mitchell LB, Duff HJ, Manyari DE, et al: A randomized clinical trial of the noninvasive and invasive approaches to drug therapy of ventricular tachycardia. *N Engl J Med* 317:1681, 1987.

Morganroth J: Evaluation of antiarrhythmic therapy using Holter monitoring. *Am J Cardiol* 62:18H, 1988.

Morganroth J, Michelson EL, Horowitz LN, et al.: Limitations of routine long-term electrocardiographic monitoring to assess ventricular ectopic frequency. *Circulation* 58:408, 1978.

Moss AJ, Davis JH, DeCamilla J: Ventricular ectopic beats and their relation to sudden and nonsudden cardiac death after myocardial infarction. *Circulation* 60:998, 1979.

Mukharji I, Rude RE, Poole WK, et al: The MILIS Study Group. Risk factors for sudden death after acute myocardial infarction: two-year follow-up. *Am J Cardiol* 54:31, 1984.

Podrid PJ, Venditti FJ, Levine PA, et al: The role of exercise testing in evaluation of arrhythmias. *Am J Cardiol* 62:24H, 1988.

Rautaharju PM, Prineas RJ, Eifler WJ, et al. Prognostic value of exercise electrocardiogram in men at high risk of future coronary heart disease: Multiple Risk Factor Intervention Trial. *J Am Coll Cardiol* 8:1, 1986.

Redwood DR, Borer JS, Epstein ST: Whither the ST segment during exercise? *Circulation* 54:703, 1976.

Rifkin RD, Hood WB: Bayesian analysis of electrocardiographic exercise stress testing. *N Engl J Med* 297:681, 1977.

Ruberman W, Weinblatt E, Goldberg JD, et al: Ventricular premature beats and mortality after myocardial infarction. *N Engl J Med* 297:750, 1977.

Ruberman W, Weinblatt E, Goldberg JD, et al: Sudden death after myocardial infarction: Runs of ventricular premature beats and R on T as high risk factors. *Am J Cardiol* 45:444, 1980.

Sami M, Kraemer H, Harrison DC, et al: A new method for evaluating antiarrhythmic drug efficacy. *Circulation* 62:1172, 1980.

Schaer DH, Leiboff RH, Wasserman AG, et al: Exercise testing after infarction/thrombolysis identifies patent vessels and residually ischemic myocardium. *Circulation* 72(Suppl III):462, 1985.

Schultze RA, Strauss WH, Pitt B: Sudden death in the year following myocardial infarction: Relation to ventricular premature contractions in the late hospital phase and left ventricular ejection fraction. *Am J Med* 62:192, 1977.

Senaratne MPJ, Hsu L, Rossall RE, et al: Exercise testing after myocardial infarction: Relative values of the low level predischarge and postdischarge exercise test. *J Am Coll Cardiol* 12:1416, 1988.

Sheffield LT: Exercise stress testing. In: Braunwald E, ed. *Heart Disease: A Textbook of Cardiovascular Medicine.* Philadelphia: Saunders; 1988, p. 223.

Sheffield LT, Reeves TJ, Blackburn H, et al: The exercise test in perspective. *Circulation* 55:681, 1977.

Sheffield LT, Rottman D: Stress testing methodology. *Prog Cardiovasc Dis* 19:33, 1976.

Stone PH, Turi ZG, Muller JE, et al: Prognostic significance of the treadmill exercise test performance 6 months after myocardial infarction. *J Am Coll Cardiol* 8:1007, 1986.

Swerdlow CD, Peterson J: Prospective comparison of Holter monitoring and electrophysiologic study in patients with cor-

onary artery disease and sustained ventricular tachyarrhythmias. *Am J Cardiol* 56:577, 1985.

Vatterott PJ, Hammill SC, Bailey KR, et al: Signal-averaged electrocardiography: A new noninvasive test to identify patients at risk for ventricular arrhythmias. *Mayo Clin Proc* 63:931, 1988.

Weiner DA, Ryan TJ, McCabe CH, et al: Prognostic importance of a clinical profile and exercise test in medically treated patients with coronary artery disease. *J Am Coll Cardiol* 3:772, 1984.

Winkle RA: Antiarrhythmic drug effect mimicked by spontaneous variability of ventricular ectopy. *Circulation* 57:116, 1978.

Winkle RA: Ambulatory electrocardiography and the diagnosis, evaluation and treatment of chronic ventricular arrhythmias. *Prog Cardiovasc Dis* 23:99, 1980.

Echocardiography; Jugular and Arterial Pulse Recordings

Joshua Wynne
Priscilla Peters

Echocardiography is the most widely used noninvasive cardiac diagnostic method available (aside from the chest x-ray and electrocardiogram), and it may provide definitive information in a wide variety of valvular, pericardial, myocardial, and congenital diseases. It uses short pulses (1-2 μsec duration) of high-frequency (1.9-5 million cycles/sec or MHz) sound waves, repeated many times each second (typically, 1,000 Hz). Because of the short duration of the ultrasound pulses, no deleterious effects occur with echocardiography. The sound waves are generated by a piezoelectric crystal, which has the unique property of transforming electrical energy into mechanical energy (i.e., sound) and vice versa. A transducer containing the crystal is placed on the chest wall and acts as both a transmitter and receiver of the short pulses of ultrasound that reflect off surfaces of the heart and return to the crystal. Ultrasound waves are reflected when they strike an interface composed of two tissues of differing acoustic impedance (which is related to tissue density).

In the traditional M-mode (or "motion") study, the sound waves are transmitted and received along a single line; the resulting image has been called an "ice-pick" view of the heart (Figure 1). Identification of cardiac structures requires careful, and sometimes tedious, positioning of the transducer on the patient's chest by the operator, who must change the orientation and position of the transducer in order to see different parts of the heart. All current echocardiographic machines provide a cross-sectional or two-dimensional (2D) view by steering the echocardiographic beam through an arc of up to 90°, producing a tomographic image of excellent spatial resolution (Figure 2). If many such images are obtained each second (typically, 30–60 images/sec), the motion of the heart can be viewed in real time. In

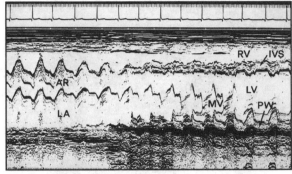

Figure 1. *M-mode echocardiographic sweep from a normal subject, obtained by rotating the transducer so that various cardiac structures come into view. AR = aortic root; IVS = interventricular septum; LA = left atrium; LV = left ventricle; MV = mitral valve; PW = posterior wall; RV = right ventricle.*

current clinical practice, M-mode studies are done only as an adjunct to the two-dimensional study, as the two-dimensional technique typically provides more definitive and anatomically specific information.

CLINICAL APPLICATIONS

Echocardiography is probably the best method currently available, invasive or noninvasive, for evaluating structural cardiac abnormalities larger than 1–2 mm. Because the air within the lungs disperses echocardiographic signals, adequate images may be difficult or impossible to obtain in about 10% of patients in whom an optimal transducer position cannot be found, particularly those with obstructive lung disease. All four cardiac valves and chambers usually can be seen, as well as the interventricular septum and interatrial septum. The main pulmonary artery, the base of the aorta and proximal aortic root, and

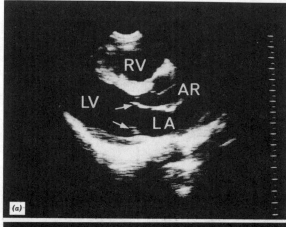

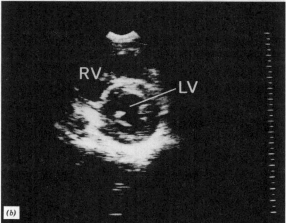

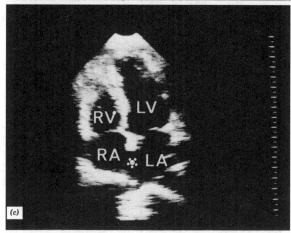

Figure 2. *Two-dimensional echocardiographic views from a normal subject. (a) Long-axis parasternal view, demonstrating the coaptation in diastole of two of the aortic valve leaflets in the center of the aorta. (b) Short-axis parasternal view at the level of the papillary muscles, which are the indentations within the LV at 3 and 8 o'clock. (c) Apical four-chamber view, showing the normal dropout of echo signal from the region of the septum primum (·). AR = aortic root; LA = left atrium; LV = left ventricle; RA = right atrium; RV = right ventricle. The arrows indicate the anterior and posterior mitral valve leaflets.*

the inferior vena cava can be imaged easily. Direct visualization of the ostia of both the right and left coronary arteries is also possible. However, because the ultrasound beam can typically evaluate only the proximal portions of the vessels, consistently reliable and reproducible assessment of coronary artery stenosis is not yet practical. The left ventricular wall motion abnormalities seen with myocardial infarction or ischemia can be readily imaged and are valuable for initial assessment and follow-up.

VALVULAR HEART DISEASE

Echocardiography permits evaluation of the site, cause, and severity of a variety of forms of valvular heart disease. Differentiation of subvalvular, valvular, and supravalvular involvement is usually determined easily (although this is usually a consideration only with the aortic valve). The cause of the valvular disease can often be ascertained or at least suggested by echocardiographic findings, since the echocardiogram can identify thickening and calcification of the valve (e.g., rheumatic disease) or its supporting structures (e.g., calcified mitral annulus); disruption of the valve (e.g., ruptured chordae tendineae); abnormal motion of the valve (e.g., mitral valve prolapse); or other disease processes (e.g., vegetations of infective endocarditis). The severity of valvular disease is determined by both direct imaging of the valve and by evaluation of the secondary functional and structural abnormalities produced by the valve lesion, such as left atrial and left ventricular enlargement and volume overload from left-sided regurgitant lesions.

In addition to evaluating suspected diseases, echocardiography is useful in excluding significant valvular involvement. Although there are exceptions, the presence of an apparently normal valve and supporting apparatus in a technically adequate 2D echocardiogram essentially excludes hemodynamically significant involvement in most forms of valvular heart disease. A normal Doppler study can confirm the absence of significant functional valve abnormality (see Chapter 8).

MITRAL VALVE

The normal mitral valve appears as two thin mobile leaflets with the anterior leaflet demonstrating the larger excursion (Figure 1). The motion of the posterior leaflet is a mirror image of the anterior leaflet, although its excursion is substantially less. The pattern of mo-

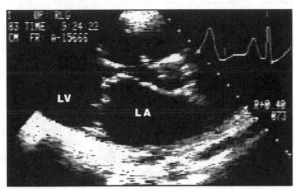

Figure 3. *Long-axis two-dimensional echocardiogram from a patient with mitral stenosis, demonstrating diastolic doming of the anterior leaflet. LA = left atrium; LV = left ventricle.*

tion of the leaflets is one of rapid opening in diastole (during the period of rapid ventricular filling), with anterior and posterior leaflets moving in opposite directions. At the end of the rapid filling phase and the start of the slow filling phase, the leaflets float toward each other, assuming a more neutral position. With left atrial systole, transmitral flow again increases, and the leaflets are driven further apart, only to coapt completely upon ventricular systole.

Mitral Stenosis

In mitral stenosis there is thickening of the leaflets, fusion of the commissures, and shortening, fusion, and thickening of the chordae tendineae. It is characterized on the 2D echocardiogram by diastolic doming of the anterior leaflet (secondary to commissural fusion) and restricted excursion and diminished separation of the leaflet tips (Figure 3). Thickening and fibrosis of the leaflets, as well as shortening and fusion of the chordal apparatus, typically occurs and ranges from mild (rheumatic deformity without significant stenosis) to severe (densely thickened, relatively immobile leaflets with calcific extension into the subvalvular apparatus).

Diminished compliance (increased stiffness) of the left ventricle, usually as a consequence of left ventricular hypertrophy, may result in prolongation of the period of rapid filling, and the M-mode echocardiographic appearance may superficially mimic that of mitral stenosis. In such cases of diminished compliance, the mitral leaflets continue to move independently, rather than concordantly as in mitral stenosis,

and the mitral valve is morphologically normal on the 2D echocardiogram. Other less common causes of pulmonary venous hypertension can usually be distinguished by echocardiography, including a left atrial myxoma, supravalvular ring, cor triatriatum, and congenital mitral stenosis ("parachute" valve).

The noninvasive evaluation of isolated mitral stenosis is particularly useful in distinguishing those patients for whom balloon valvuloplasty is appropriate from those with marked subvalvular fusion or heavily calcified valves who require surgical intervention. Cardiac catheterization in *isolated* straightforward mitral stenosis is rarely indicated. A normal echocardiogram (including Doppler flow studies) *excludes* valvular mitral stenosis.

Mitral Regurgitation

It is unusual to be able to directly identify mitral regurgitation on the echocardiogram. Only when gross disruption of the valve is found (as in rupture of chordae tendineae or papillary muscle) can one be certain of mitral regurgitation. In most other forms of mitral regurgitation, indirect signs must be studied, including an enlarged left ventricle (often with preserved systolic function), a dilated left atrium, and systolic left atrial expansion.

Doppler echocardiography is particularly useful in assessing the presence and severity of mitral regurgitation. By positioning the sample volume at the level of the leaflet tips, the regurgitant jet can be identified; using the pulsed mode, it is possible to map the extent of the left atrial jet, and thus gauge the severity of the regurgitation.

Mitral valve prolapse may or may not be associated with mitral regurgitation. The absence of a reliable "gold standard" has hindered the identification of firm echocardiographic criteria for the diagnosis of prolapse, and equivocal cases occur. Echocardiography may be useful in identifying prolapse of the tricuspid or aortic valves, since some patients have multiple valve involvement. (This syndrome has been called the "multiple floppy valve syndrome.")

Mitral regurgitation may result from either structural deformity of the valve and/or its supporting apparatus, or from functional abnormalities of the valve apparatus and papillary muscles (termed papillary muscle dysfunction). The functional abnormalities typically are associated with normal appearing mitral valve leaflets, although left ventricular wall motion abnormalities can often be identified. Pathologic de-

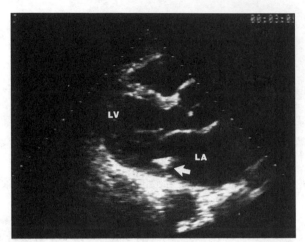

Figure 4. *Long-axis two-dimensional echocardiogram from a patient with severe calcification of the mitral annulus (arrow). LA = left atrium; LV = left ventricle.*

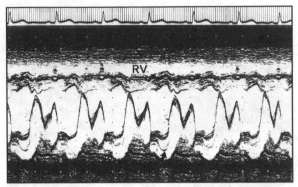

Figure 5. *M-mode echocardiogram from a patient with marked mitral valve prolapse. Note the striking mid- and late-systolic posterior motion of the mitral valve (arrow). RV = right ventricle.*

formity of the valve itself may be due to a variety of causes, principally, rheumatic disease, rupture of chordae tendineae, infective endocarditis, hypertrophic obstructive cardiomyopathy, calcified mitral annulus, and mitral valve prolapse. Thickening of the valve is found in rheumatic disease, while calcification of the annulus presents a distinctive echocardiographic appearance, with a shelf of calcium behind the posterior mitral valve leaflet (Figure 4). In ruptured chordae tendineae, hypermobile and flail components can be identified. In mitral valve prolapse, one or both leaflets bow posteriorly and cephalad into the left atrium, often commencing in midsystole but sometimes occurring throughout systole (Figure 5).

The major use of echocardiography is in identifying the presence or absence of structural abnormalities of the mitral valve. It is less useful in assessing the severity of regurgitation. Doppler techniques typically provide reasonably reliable information to aid in the assessment of the severity of the lesion, although in complex mixed valvular disease, cardiac catheterization is often necessary. On echocardiography, the magnitude of enlargement of the left atrium and especially the left ventricle is a further general guide to the severity of regurgitation. Since the development of LV dysfunction is a dreaded outcome in this condition, echocardiography is often used to monitor LV function over time. Screening for mitral valve prolapse is one of the major reasons echocardiograms in general are ordered; however, careful cardiac auscultation by an experienced physician is

probably as reliable as echocardiography for the diagnosis of clinically significant mitral valve prolapse. It has been suggested that mitral valve prolapse occurs more frequently than usual in young patients with focal cerebral ischemic events, and that the two may be etiologically related. It probably is reasonable to obtain echocardiograms in this group of patients, although the best management strategy remains unclear.

AORTIC VALVE

The aortic valve cusps are normally thin, symmetrical, and mobile. In diastole, they meet in the center of the aorta, and during systole they open until they are adjacent to the aortic wall (Figures 2 and 6).

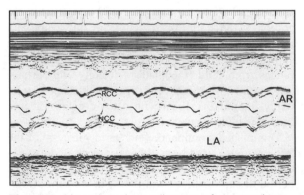

Figure 6. *M-mode echocardiogram of a normal aortic valve. Note the movement of the right coronary cusp (RCC) and noncoronary cusp (NCC). AR = aortic root; LA = left atrium.*

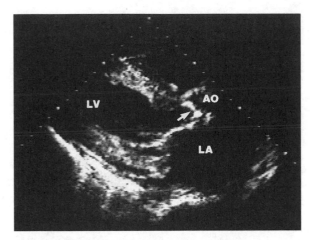

Figure 7. *Long-axis two-dimensional echocardiogram from a patient with calcific aortic stenosis. This panel is taken in midsystole, and there is markedly reduced opening of the cusps (arrow). There is also increased left ventricular wall thickness indicative of left ventricular hypertrophy. AO = aorta; LA = left atrium; LV = left ventricle.*

Aortic Stenosis

In younger adults, a bicuspid aortic valve may not be thickened or calcified, but these changes are the rule in older patients with bicuspid or acquired aortic stenosis (Figure 7). The typical 2D echocardiographic findings of a bicuspid aortic valve are systolic doming into the aorta, as imaged in the parasternal long-axis view, and demonstration of two leaflets and two commissures from the short-axis view (Figure 8). Commissures may be oriented right-left, with the leaflets opening anteroposteriorly, or the commissures may be inserted anteroposteriorly with the leaflets then opening right-left.

Determination of the site of left ventricular outflow tract obstruction usually is determined easily by echocardiography. Subvalvular stenosis may be either fixed or dynamic. The fixed variety may be caused by a fibrous or muscular membrane or channel, while the dynamic is caused by systolic anterior movement (SAM) of the mitral valve toward the septum. Two-dimensional echocardiography also permits determination of the extent, location, and type of supravalvular stenosis.

The determination of normal cuspal appearance and motion on 2D echocardiography essentially excludes valvular aortic stenosis. While 2D echocardiography can identify patients with severe aortic stenosis based

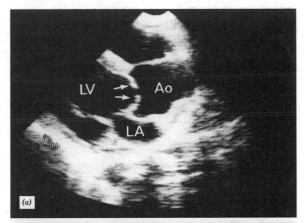

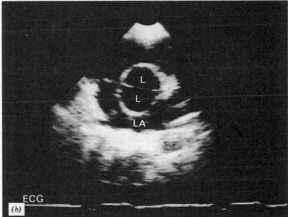

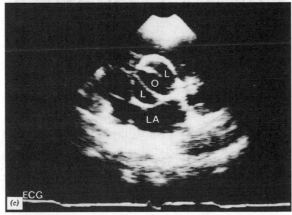

Figure 8. *Two-dimensional echocardiographic studies of a bicuspid aortic valve. (a) Recorded during systole with the transducer in the long-axis parasternal position; demonstrates leaflet doming and thickening (arrows). The ascending aortic root is mildly dilated. Panels b and c were recorded using a short-axis parasternal transducer position. (b) During diastole, the leaflet (L) closure line is seen to be somewhat eccentric. (c) During systole, there is compromise of valve leaflet opening with a stenotic orifice (O). Ao = aorta; LA = left atrium; LV = left ventricle. (Reproduced from Borow KM: Congenital aortic stenosis in the adult. J Cardiovasc Med 8:1163, 1983. With permission.)*

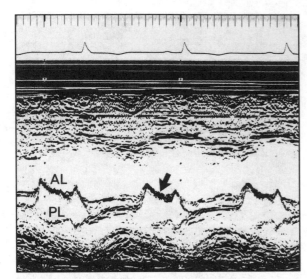

Figure 9. *M-mode echocardiogram of the mitral valve in a patient with aortic regurgitation. High-frequency diastolic vibration (arrow) of the anterior leaflet (AL) of the mitral valve is found. PL = posterior leaflet.*

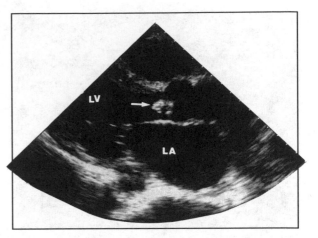

Figure 10. *Long-axis two-dimensional echocardiogram from a patient with a large vegetation of the aortic valve (arrow). LA = left atrium; LV = left ventricle.*

on markedly reduced cuspal excursion, it has not been completely reliable in determining the severity of obstruction. In aortic stenosis (in contrast to mitral stenosis) the planimetered aortic valve area correlates poorly with catheterization findings, as does the degree of cuspal separation. The echocardiogram tends to overestimate the severity of stenosis, particularly in patients with left ventricular dysfunction and reduced cardiac output. While adults without stenosis can be reliably distinguished from those with severe stenosis, the separation of patients with moderate from severe stenosis is more equivocal. The evaluation of Doppler flow velocities across the stenotic aortic valve (using the modified Bernoulli equation) is particularly useful in determining the severity of aortic stenosis.

Aortic Regurgitation

Although Doppler echocardiography is now probably the most reliable means of detecting even the most trivial of aortic regurgitant jets, there are several M-mode echocardiographic findings that help to establish the diagnosis. High-frequency diastolic vibration of the anterior leaflet of the mitral valve is commonly noted (Figure 9); diastolic fluttering of the septum can be seen as well. Occasionally diastolic flutter of the aortic valve itself can be seen, typically when

there is cuspal rupture, with or without a vegetation. Mitral valve and septal vibration reflect only the direction of the regurgitant jet, not the severity of the aortic regurgitation.

The echocardiogram usually is able to distinguish between the two principal causes of aortic regurgitation: disease of the aortic cusps (typically due to rheumatic or calcific disease or to infective endocarditis) (Figure 10); and enlargement of the aortic root (due to hypertension, aortic aneurysm, or anuloaortic ectasia) without direct involvement of the cusps themselves. Acute severe aortic regurgitation with markedly elevated left ventricular end-diastolic pressure, occurring as a consequence of endocarditis, may result in premature closure of the mitral valve or premature opening of the aortic valve. Patients with these findings are typically in severe congestive heart failure and usually require immediate aortic valve replacement.

The echocardiogram is quite reliable in distinguishing the various causes of aortic regurgitation. It is less useful in estimating the *severity* of chronic aortic regurgitation, although, as in mitral regurgitation, the degree of LV enlargement is a general guide and Doppler provides additional information. It has been suggested that asymptomatic patients with aortic regurgitation undergo serial echocardiographic evaluation, and those developing evidence of LV dysfunction (manifested by an end-systolic dimension >55 mm) be considered for valve replacement. The echocardiographic appearance of acute severe aortic re-

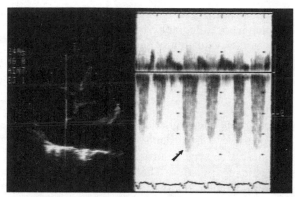

Figure 11. *Modified apical four-chamber echocardiographic and Doppler study demonstrating a systolic signal in the right atrium (arrow), indicative of tricuspid regurgitation.*

gurgitation with an aortic vegetation due to endocarditis, resulting in early closure of the mitral valve, is sufficiently diagnostic that aortic valve replacement can usually be undertaken without diagnostic cardiac catheterization.

TRICUSPID VALVE

The normal tricuspid valve is similar in echocardiographic appearance to the mitral valve. The M-mode technique usually achieves only partial imaging of the valve, which is best seen in systole. Two-dimensional echocardiography affords a more complete evaluation of the valve and is the preferred method of examination.

Tricuspid Valve Disease

Tricuspid stenosis, typically due to rheumatic valve disease, has an echocardiographic appearance similar to that of rheumatic mitral stenosis. Associated right-heart enlargement and abnormal systolic motion of the interventricular septum suggest significant tricuspid regurgitation. Doppler echocardiography can reliably confirm and evaluate the presence and severity of tricuspid regurgitation, and can provide a useful estimate of pulmonary artery pressure (Figure 11).

There are three important causes of structural tricuspid valve disease: rheumatic stenosis; involvement by vegetative endocarditis (typically in drug addicts or patients with central intravenous catheters); and Ebsteins's anomaly of the tricuspid valve. Thickening of the valve with rheumatic involvement is sim-

ilar to that seen in rheumatic mitral stenosis. A vegetation appears distinctively as a shaggy mass attached to the valve. Ebstein's anomaly is best appreciated on 2D echocardiography, in which the tricuspid valve appears situated more apically than usual in the right ventricle.

The most common cause of tricuspid regurgitation, however, is right-heart dilatation and failure, often due to mitral or pulmonary disease; the tricuspid valve is normal in appearance.

Doppler echocardiography is the most reliable method available for diagnosing tricuspid regurgitation. Two-dimensional echocardiography is also reliable in identifying tricuspid stenosis, and it provides an approximate qualitative estimation of its severity. However, the lack of a quantitative estimate of stenosis is usually not an important limitation, since rheumatic tricuspid stenosis virtually never occurs in the absence of rheumatic mitral stenosis. Thus, echocardiographic demonstration of tricuspid stenosis demands exploration of the tricuspid valve at the time of mitral valve surgery.

PULMONARY VALVE

The pulmonary valve is the most difficult of all the cardiac valves to image and the least likely to be structurally abnormal in an adult patient. If the valve could be seen in its entirety, it would resemble the aortic valve. M-mode echocardiographic imaging is usually limited to the cuspal closure line in diastole and the movement of the posterior cusp in systole; the 2D exam typically allows for visualization of two of the three cusps of the valve as they open and close in the pulmonary artery (Figure 12).

Pulmonary Valve Disease

Structural abnormalities of the pulmonary valve are unusual except for mild thickening with congenital pulmonic stenosis. Rarely, they may occur from a vegetation involving the cusps or with the carcinoid syndrome. Abnormalities of motion of the valve are more common. Doming of the valve on the 2D study (or an abnormally prominent movement of the valve on M-mode echocardiography as a consequence of forceful right atrial contraction) indicates the presence of congenital pulmonic stenosis. Enhanced imaging of the valve, with systolic fluttering of the valve cusps, and ablation of the movement of the valve after right atrial systole often indicate pulmonary hypertension.

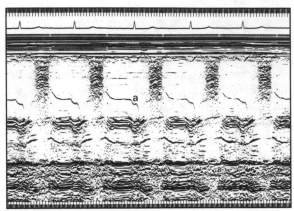

Figure 12. *M-mode echocardiogram of a normal pulmonary valve. Atrial systole (a) partially opens the valve before the vigorous posterior movement of the cusp as a consequence of ventricular systole.*

While the echocardiogram can determine the presence and location of right ventricular outflow tract obstruction, the echocardiographic estimation of the severity of valvular pulmonic stenosis is only a rough semiquantitative guide. The addition of the Doppler technique can provide further information about the site and degree of obstruction. Cardiac catheterization may be required in the adult patient in order to be confident about the degree of obstruction and to look for associated lesions. Significant valvular pulmonic stenosis can be excluded by a normal 2D study of good technical quality.

PROSTHETIC VALVES

Two principal forms of prosthetic valves are used: an entirely mechanical one, with a rigid ball or disc occluder; and a bioprosthetic type, with a rigid or semi-rigid prosthetic base and cusps composed of human or animal tissue (most commonly the cusps from the aortic valve of a pig). Because of the large difference in density between the mechanical occluder and human tissue, the occluder typically is easy to image. Consequently, the function of the mechanical valve is easy to evaluate echocardiographically, particularly in view of the precise timing of cardiac events made possible by M-mode echocardiography. Movement of the occluder within its cage or supporting base is easily evaluated. Conversely, it may be difficult on occasion to image adequately the normally thin cusps of bioprostheses—although, when visualized, the cusps

move in a pattern quite similar to that of native valves. Doppler echocardiography has been shown to be reliable in the evaluation of prosthetic valve function.

Prosthetic Dysfunction

Stenosis and/or regurgitation may be seen with each type of valve. Partial dehiscence of the sewing ring of either valve type from its annulus leads to paraprosthetic regurgitation. There are usually no specific echocardiographic findings to indicate this abnormality, aside from secondary changes that may occur (such as ventricular enlargement). If the valve prosthesis is sufficiently detached, abnormal rocking of the valve may be demonstrable echocardiographically.

Dysfunction of a mechanical prosthesis may be caused by thrombosis, ingrowth of fibrous tissue, or vegetations. If motion of the occluder is disturbed as a result, echocardiography will identify such abnormalities of motion, especially sticking. Mobile vegetations or pedunculated clots are typically easier to identify than laminated thrombus or fibrous ingrowth.

Acquired bioprosthetic dysfunction is usually heralded by thickening and, at times, calcification of the cusps. Diminished or abnormal motion of the leaflets may be identified when stenosis is present. Spontaneous tearing of a leaflet (or dysfunction as a consequence of endocarditis) usually results in a dramatic and virtually diagnostic echocardiographic appearance, with the flail portion of the valve vibrating violently and chaotically in the associated regurgitant jet of blood.

When the echocardiogram demonstrates major prosthetic dysfunction (such as sticking of the occluder or disruption of a bioprosthetic leaflet), further evaluation (including cardiac catheterization) may not be required. Conversely, the failure to identify an abnormality may be misleading, and substantial prosthetic dysfunction may occur on occasion despite the lack of diagnostic echocardiographic abnormalities. An echocardiographic evaluation should be routine in cases of suspected prosthetic valve dysfunction, although simply fluoroscoping a mechanical valve may reveal definitive evidence of dysfunction in some cases. The echocardiogram is often critical in identifying other causes of symptoms in patients with suspected prosthetic valve dysfunction, including unappreciated left ventricular dysfunction, progression of disease in other native valves, and postoperative pericardial effusion or constriction.

AORTA

The proximal few centimeters of the ascending aorta above the aortic valve can usually be imaged echocardiographically; by placing the transducer in other locations, portions of the aortic arch and descending aorta often can be visualized.

AORTIC ANEURYSM

Enlargement of a visualized portion of the aorta can be determined by echocardiography; assessment of the size of a dilated aorta has shown excellent agreement with catheterization findings. It is possible to image the false lumen of a dissecting aortic aneurysm as an extra channel located adjacent to the true lumen. Portions of the intimal flap itself may be identified in some patients with dissections. As tangential imaging with the M-mode method may simulate a dissection when none is present, two-dimensional echocardiography with its wide field of view (supplemented as necessary by transesophageal imaging) is required for optimal evaluation of the aorta.

Since failure to demonstrate an aneurysm of the aorta echocardiographically may be due to failure to image the involved segment, an aneurysm, particularly a localized one, cannot be excluded by echocardiography. Conversely, demonstration of aortic root enlargement by echocardiography is quite accurate. In patients with echocardiographically demonstrated aortic aneurysm, the distinction between a saccular aneurysm and a dissection may be difficult. The extent of the aneurysm may be difficult to determine if technical considerations limit imaging portals. Cardiac Doppler is useful in determining the presence of associated aortic regurgitation, typically present if the base of the aorta is involved. Most patients with suspected aortic aneurysms who require more definitive evaluation, especially the assessment of involvement of the coronary arteries, will need to undergo computed tomography and/or aortography.

INTRACARDIAC MASSES

Echocardiography is the procedure of choice for the evaluation of suspected intracardiac masses, includ-

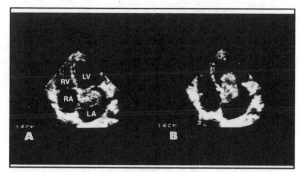

Figure 13. *Apical four-chamber two-dimensional echocardiogram from a patient with a large atrial myxoma attached to the interatrial septum. (A) Systole. (B) Diastole, during which the myxoma prolapses through the mitral orifice into the left ventricle. LA = left atrium; LV = left ventricle; RA = right atrium; RV = right ventricle.*

ing intracavitary tumors, atrial and ventricular thrombi, and valvular vegetations.

TUMORS

The most common intracavitary cardiac tumor by far is the myxoma, which typically is found in the left atrium but occasionally is seen in the right atrium and rarely in other locations. It may grow quite large and virtually fill the left atrium. The myxoma appears as a mass, often somewhat heterogeneous in appearance, that usually is pedunculated and attaches to the interatrial septum in the region of the septum primum (fossa ovalis) (Figure 13). Frondlike protuberances from the mass are common.

Other tumors beside myxomas may be found within a cardiac chamber; hypernephromas may extend up the inferior vena cava and fill the right atrium in a manner reminiscent of a myxoma. Left atrial thrombi may also simulate a myxoma; they are seen in patients with rheumatic mitral valve disease, and may be pedunculated.

The echocardiographic identification of a suspected left atrial myxoma is almost always definitive; the next step is removal of the tumor at cardiac surgery. Cardiac catheterization is rarely necessary and, in fact, is probably contraindicated in most patients, for fear of dislodging a portion of the tumor and resultant embolization. While the symptoms of a myxoma may be protean (fever, malaise, etc.), an echocardiogram ordinarily should not be ordered unless there are specific factors suggesting a myxoma (diastolic murmur, embolization, etc.), or unless more common clinical entities have been excluded.

VEGETATIONS

Vegetations are identified echocardiographically on the basis of morphologic as well as functional features. They appear as masses that typically are attached to the valve leaflets and usually are mobile (Figure 10). M-mode echocardiography often shows them vibrating violently as a consequence of the attendant valve destruction and regurgitation.

It may not be possible to differentiate a vegetation from an avulsed or disrupted portion of valve leaflet that is hypermobile. Except for rupture of mitral chordae tendineae, however, most disrupted valves result from endocarditis. The redundant and thickened valve seen in the mitral valve prolapse syndrome without endocarditis may simulate involvement by a vegetation; one should be cautious about diagnosing a vegetation in this setting unless there are unequivocal findings, or a change in the echocardiographic appearance is noted.

Most patients with typical endocarditis will have echocardiographic evidence of vegetations. Although the presence of a vegetation is not an absolute predictor of clinical outcome, patients with vegetations tend to have a higher incidence of complications leading to valve replacement or death. Patients without visible vegetations less frequently develop complications, require surgery, or die. One should not, however, use the mere presence of a vegetation to decide about surgery; the usual clinical criteria (congestive heart failure, embolization, uncontrolled sepsis) remain operant. Vegetations may persist despite apparent bacteriologic cure, and there is only a loose correlation between the size or appearance of the vegetation and the risk of embolization and other complications.

THROMBI

Thrombi may be encountered within all four cardiac chambers, as well as within the pulmonary artery; they are most commonly seen in the left ventricle. Left ventricular thrombi usually are located at the cardiac apex, and usually are seen following a myocardial infarction (Figure 14). Thrombi are found overlying dyskinetic or "paradoxically" moving left

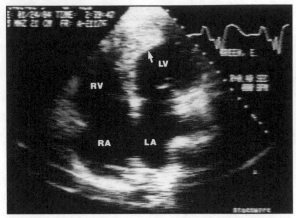

Figure 14. *Apical four-chamber two-dimensional echocardiographic study from a patient with a large laminated apical thrombus (arrow) in an enlarged LV. LA = left atrium; LV = left ventricle; RA = right atrium; RV = right ventricle.*

ventricular segments; except in extremely rare instances, a left ventricular thrombus is not found when normal wall motion is present in all left ventricular regions. Left atrial thrombi are seen on occasion but usually only when mitral stenosis is present; even then, a visualized thrombus is unusual.

Although it is a frequently cited reason for ordering echocardiograms, the attempt to identify an intracardiac thrombus ultrasonically is often not worth the effort. Patients with manifestly normal left ventricular function and without mitral stenosis are at exceedingly low risk of harboring a thrombus in the heart. Similarly, visible ventricular thrombi after a myocardial infarction usually are limited to patients with anterior infarcts, and even then are found in fewer than half.

LEFT VENTRICLE

Left ventricular cavity size, contour, orientation, and thickness are easily evaluated with echocardiography. A variety of indices of function may be calculated with M-mode echocardiography, including the ejection fraction, mean velocity of circumferential fiber shortening (Vcf), and percent fractional shortening (%$\triangle$D). Because the M-mode echocardiogram images a limited portion of the ventricle, assessment of left ventricular performance with this technique requires that function be uniform throughout the ventricle. The regional variations in left ventricular wall motion seen with coronary artery disease are reliably evaluated with 2D echocardiography. Because the 2D echocardiogram provides a tomographic image of the ventricle, it is necessary to obtain at least two orthogonal views so that the proper three-dimensional contour of the ventricle can be estimated.

A major use of echocardiography is in evaluating a patient with an enlarged cardiac silhouette on chest roentgenography; the principal issue is whether the cardiac chambers are dilated, or if there is a pericardial effusion. Echocardiography is unparalleled in this role (Figure 14). When the heart itself is enlarged, the left ventricle is commonly the most dilated chamber (although patients with mitral stenosis or an atrial septal defect may present with a dramatically increased cardiac silhouette due to right ventricular enlargement, despite a small left ventricle).

LEFT VENTRICULAR ENLARGEMENT

Left ventricular enlargement is usually due to one of three principal causes: volume overload (due to aortic or mitral regurgitation); coronary artery disease with myocardial infarction; or primary myocardial disease (dilated or congestive cardiomyopathy). Volume overload is characterized by an enlarged ventricle with preserved or increased systolic function; the stroke volume is thus increased. Evidence of valvular disease may be found. This distinctive pattern may become less clear once LV dysfunction supervenes, and the pattern then approximates that of dilated cardiomyopathy, characterized by a dilated, hypokinetic ventricle.

The unique feature of LV dysfunction due to coronary artery disease and myocardial infarction is its focal and regional nature, although an end-stage patient with multiple myocardial infarctions may have diffuse abnormalities of wall motion that are indistinguishable from a cardiomyopathy or volume overload with dysfunction.

CORONARY ARTERY DISEASE

It has long been known that a severe reduction in coronary perfusion results in cessation of systolic motion of the ischemic myocardium. However, most patients with coronary artery disease have near-normal coronary blood flow at rest, and these patients demonstrate normal left ventricular wall motion. With

stress, such as exercise, the limited coronary reserve cannot keep pace with the increased demand for nutrients, and ischemia results. Increasing success has been reported with imaging patients with 2D echocardiography during and after exercise; the technique is limited principally by the difficulty in maintaining an adequate imaging portal. When imaging is successful, however, the development of a regional wall motion abnormality is strong evidence of ischemia.

Most echocardiographic studies are performed at rest, usually after a myocardial infarction. There are a number of off-line analysis systems available for the quantification of left ventricular wall motion. Currently, no system used in the evaluation of wall motion abnormalities has been universally accepted. Recent extensive evaluation of off-line analysis packages has shown that no system is without sources of error. There is no question, however, that LV function can be accurately categorized by visual assessment into clinically useful groups (e.g., good versus poor, regional versus diffuse). Patients in whom severe LV dysfunction is demonstrated echocardiographically probably can be spared further invasive evaluation.

Two-dimensional echocardiography (along with Doppler techniques) is also quite useful in evaluating the complications of myocardial infarction, both acute and chronic. Acute complications that can be detected include ventricular septal rupture, papillary muscle rupture, and pericardial effusion. Chronic complications that can be evaluated include left ventricular aneurysms (true versus false), papillary muscle dysfunction, and left ventricular thrombi.

CARDIOMYOPATHY

It is often useful to divide the cardiomyopathies into groups with similar echocardiographic, hemodynamic, and clinical findings, rather than grouping them by cause. Echocardiography permits definitive evaluation of some of these cases, although the precise causal factor rarely is apparent from the echocardiogram.

The three principal functional groups are *dilated* (formerly called congestive), *restrictive,* and *hypertrophic* (Table 1). The primary feature of the dilated form is left ventricular dilatation and dysfunction; of the restrictive type, increased wall stiffness producing elevated filling pressures; and of the hypertrophic form, inappropriate myocardial hypertrophy. The distinc-

Table 1. Echocardiographic Features of the Cardiomyopathies

	Dilated	Restrictive	Hypertrophic
LV size	↑	N	N or ↓
LV systolic function	↓	N (or ↓)	N or ↑
LV wall thickness	N	↑	↑
Other features		PE	ASH ` SAM

ASH = asymmetric septal hypertrophy; PE = pericardial effusion; LV = left ventricular; N = normal; SAM = systolic anterior motion of the mitral valve; ↑, increased; ↓, decreased.

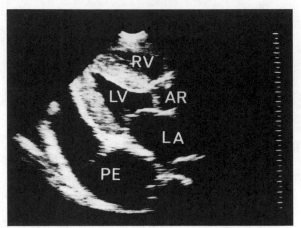

Figure 15. *Long-axis parasternal two-dimensional echocardiogram from a patient with cardiac amyloidosis. Note the marked increase in thickness of the left ventricular (LV) walls, and the unusually echodense appearance. There is also a large pleural effusion (PE). AR = aortic root; LA = left atrium.*

tions are not absolute, and a given disease may have features from two of the functional groups.

Dilated Cardiomyopathy

Although caused by a variety of toxic substances (alcohol, drugs such as Adriamycin, etc.), this cardiomyopathy is most frequently of unknown cause. Although four-chamber cardiac enlargement is the rule, the left ventricle typically is most involved, demonstrating enlargement and hypokinesis. The asynergy commonly is diffuse and involves all LV segments, which in many cases distinguishes dilated cardiomyopathy from coronary artery disease. However, end-stage LV damage due to multiple infarctions also may appear diffusely hypokinetic. Wall thickness is typically normal, and left ventricular thrombi may be found. No intrinsic valvular pathology is seen.

Restrictive Cardiomyopathy

Grouped in this category are primary restrictive processes and secondary diseases, most frequently infiltrative diseases of the myocardium (e.g., amyloid, sarcoid, iron overload, etc.). The typical echocardiographic feature is a normal-sized left ventricle with increased wall thickness. While the rigorous classification of the restrictive cardiomyopathies excludes secondary types (i.e., infiltrative diseases), these in fact are the most commonly encountered form of restrictive disease in clinical practice. Although systolic function is normal in idiopathic restrictive cardiomyopathy, it often is depressed in the infiltrative diseases. One striking feature of these diseases (particularly with amyloid involvement of the myocardium) is an unusual sparkling, echo-dense appearance (Figure 15).

Hypertrophic Cardiomyopathy

The characteristic feature in this category is inappropriate left ventricular hypertrophy. In many cases, there is asymmetric involvement of the septum (asymmetric septal hypertrophy, ASH), with the septum at least 1½ times the thickness of the posterior wall. The septum can reach dramatic widths; we have seen patients whose septa were 25 mm thick or more (normal is 11 mm or less). In rare cases, other LV locations are preferentially involved, including the anterolateral wall and apex. In a minority of cases, symmetric hypertrophy is noted. Wall motion typically is normal or increased, and the LV cavity size is small. (See also Chapter 18.)

When dynamic obstruction is present, systolic anterior motion (SAM) of the anterior leaflet of the mitral valve is found. The subaortic pressure gradient produces turbulent blood flow, which causes the aortic valve to vibrate violently. The severity of SAM and aortic valve fluttering bear a good relationship to the degree of outflow gradient. The M-mode technique on occasion may suggest ASH when the septum

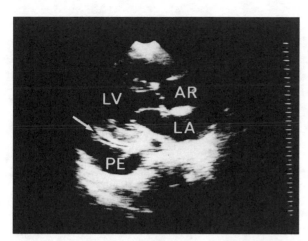

Figure 16. *Long-axis parasternal two-dimensional echocardiogram from a patient with a large pleural effusion (PE). The arrow indicates minimal amount of pericardial fluid between the posterior left ventricular (LV) wall and the pericardium. AR = aortic root; LA = left atrium.*

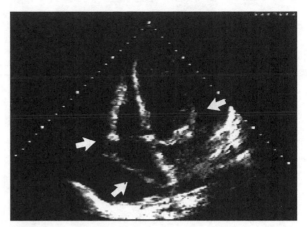

Figure 17. *Apical four-chamber two-dimensional echocardiographic study demonstrating large pericardial effusion (arrows) surrounding the heart.*

is imaged tangentially, but the two-dimensional technique usually removes any doubt. Cardiac Doppler, with the sample volume placed in the LV outflow tract below the aortic valve, provides useful information about the presence and degree of pressure gradient. Since the magnitude of the pressure gradient usually is of little clinical importance except when surgery is being considered, we do not ordinarily perform catheterization, unless there are other unanswered questions (such as whether coronary artery disease is contributing to the patient's symptoms).

PERICARDIUM

The posterior pericardium generates a strong echocardiographic signal and usually is easily identified. A minimal separation may normally be found between the epicardial and pericardial surfaces, and represents less than 15 ml of pericardial fluid (Figure 16).

PERICARDIAL EFFUSION

More than a minimal separation of epicardium and pericardium identifies a pericardial effusion. Free-flowing fluid will move to dependent locations within the pericardial space, so the apparent size of an effusion depends upon the position of the patient during

imaging. Precise estimation of the size of a pericardial effusion is probably both unnecessary and unreliable, but semiquantitative distinctions (trivial, small, medium, large) are clinically meaningful; these estimates are based on the degree of epicardial/pericardial separation (Figure 17). Both M-mode and two-dimensional techniques are useful for detecting and sizing effusions, although loculated effusions are best evaluated with the 2D technique. Pericardial thickening is suggested by an unusually broad and prominent pericardial signal, and is often associated with concordant movement of the epicardium and pericardium, suggesting symphysis of these structures as a consequence of fibrosis.

In large pericardial effusions, fibrous strands and masses can be imaged within the pericardial fluid, as can tumor masses with neoplastic involvement of the pericardium.

There are numerous technical pitfalls in the evaluation of the pericardium, but strict adherence to proper techniques eliminates most spurious impressions. The differentiation of a left pleural effusion from a pericardial effusion may be difficult on occasion with the M-mode technique; two-dimensional echocardiography is almost always definitive in forming this distinction (Figure 16).

While echocardiography is highly reliable in detecting pericardial effusions, it is less useful in establishing the hemodynamic burden caused by the fluid. Specific echocardiographic signs (such as gross cardiac oscillation, and respirophasic right atrial and ventricular diastolic collapse) suggest hemodynamic compromise, but the diagnosis of tamponade still rests more solidly on clinical and invasively determined information.

CONGENITAL HEART DISEASE

The development of 2D echocardiography had its earliest and perhaps its most profound influence in the evaluation of congenital cardiac anomalies. Because of its wide field of view, 2D echocardiography permits analysis of the often complex spatial relationships and orientations. Atrial, ventricular, and great vessel anatomy, orientation, and connections can be evaluated with a high degree of accuracy and reliability. Cardiac catheterizations have become more stylized since the introduction of 2D echocardiography, since now the anatomical features often are known prior to catheterization and only specific questions (such as pressures, flows, and resistances) remain to be determined. In selected patients with certain lesions—such as secundum-type atrial septal defect (ASD) and coarctation of the aorta—catheterization is no longer required or routine before surgery but rather is performed only when there are unresolved issues following echocardiography.

Since a review of all the congenital cardiac anomalies is beyond the scope of this chapter, the discussion will be limited to the most common nonvalvular congenital defect found in the adult patient—the atrial septal defect.

ATRIAL SEPTAL DEFECT

The most reliable echocardiographic feature of an ASD is right ventricular enlargement, a consequence of the increased blood flow through the right side of the heart. A normal-sized right ventricle essentially excludes a hemodynamically significant ASD. On the other hand, the degree of right ventricular enlargement is not a precise guide to the actual size of the left-to-right shunt. The interventricular septum demonstrates normal thickening, but often moves "paradoxically" anteriorly during systole, in contrast to its normal posterior motion. This is the result of posterior displacement of the septum during diastole as a consequence of the right ventricular volume overload.

Direct visualization of the atrial septum is possible with 2D echocardiography. Low-lying defects in the septum in the region of the atrioventricular valves are seen with a primum-type ASD (endocardial cushion defect). Associated abnormalities of the atrioventricular valves and ventricular septum may also be seen. Secundum-type ASDs are found in the region of the fossa ovalis, which is so thin normally that it may not be visualized even in a patient without a defect, thus simulating an ASD. Orienting the echocardiographic beam more perpendicularly to the atrial septum (using subcostal portals) increases the reliability of direct visualization of the defect, but ordinarily, apparent holes in the atrial septum near the fossa ovalis should be diagnosed with caution because of the normal "drop out" of echocardiographic signals in this region (Figure 2c). Mitral valve prolapse is frequently seen with a secundum ASD.

The Doppler technique is a useful adjunct to the echocardiographic evaluation of atrial septal defects, particularly when the clinical suspicion is high but the defect cannot be visualized directly. The recording of a continuous, low-velocity Doppler signal in the region of the atrial septum strongly suggests a shunt. Visualization of flow from left atrium to right atrium by color Doppler is definitive. (See Chapter 8 and p. *xix*.)

Right ventricular volume overload (right ventricular enlargement and abnormal interventricular septal motion) may be found in a variety of conditions besides ASD, including tricuspid regurgitation; the echocardiographic findings must be interpreted in the clinical setting. Doppler echocardiography may be of benefit in equivocal cases.

The echocardiographic findings form an important decision-point in managing a patient with a suspected atrial septal defect. A normal study without right ventricular enlargement essentially excludes a hemodynamically significant ASD. Further evaluation is rarely fruitful or indicated. Should there be unusual features that suggest an ASD despite a negative echocardiogram (including Doppler echocardiography), a radionuclide angiocardiogram should be obtained. If no shunt is detected, an ASD of significance is excluded (although a "probe patent" foramen ovale is not).

The distinction between a primum and secundum ASD is usually an easy one to make. Associated defects are often apparent. Some patients with an uncomplicated secundum ASD may be sent directly to surgery without cardiac catheterization.

TRANSESOPHAGEAL ECHOCARDIOGRAPHY

The transesophageal echocardiographic (TEE) technique is emerging as a useful adjunct to the standard precordial two-dimensional examination, frequently providing more specific pathologic and anatomic information with better resolution of intracardiac structures than the precordial technique allows.

The transesophageal technique is often used in the conscious patient. Occasionally, premedication is indicated if the patient appears anxious. Topical anesthetic such as lidocaine spray is administered to the oropharynx to suppress the gag reflex, and a bite guard is typically used to prevent damage to the probe. The patient may be in the left lateral decubitus position, which aids in the elimination of salivary secretions, or in a sitting position, depending on imaging needs and physician and patient interaction. The probe is lubricated with surgical jelly and introduced in the same fashion as a standard gastroscope. In addition to the physician performing the procedure, an assistant should be present to aid in monitoring the patient's vital signs, and to adjust machine controls to ensure adequate image quality. A routine examination can usually be accomplished within 10 minutes.

The transesophageal exam involves several standard imaging planes, including a basal short-axis scan, a four-chamber view, and a transgastric short-axis view. As the transducer is withdrawn back through the esophagus, the thoracic aorta can be evaluated.

Transesophageal echocardiography is particularly useful in the evaluation of prosthetic valve dysfunction, mitral regurgitation, thoracic aortic dissection, detection of intracardiac and paracardiac masses, and for the evaluation of congenital heart disease, especially when the standard precordial study is inadequate and/or additional detailed information is required. Transesophageal echocardiography is also of use in the operating room to evaluate the success of valve repair and to monitor left ventricular function.

PULSE RECORDINGS

By placing an ultrasound transducer over the carotid artery, internal jugular vein, and cardiac apex impulse, a tracing may be obtained that displays in graphic form the pressure and volume fluxes of the underlying structures. Although the resulting external recordings

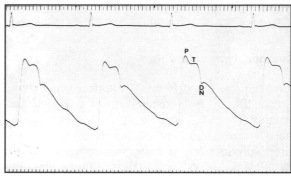

Figure 18. *Normal carotid pulse tracing. The percussion wave (P) is more prominent than the subsequent tidal wave (T). DN = dicrotic notch.*

are not direct measurements of intraluminal pressure, the morphology of the carotid, jugular, and apex pulse tracings closely mirrors the intracavitary pressure recordings obtained from within the aorta, right atrium, and left ventricle, respectively. In specific pathologic conditions, tracings may be obtained from other locations, such as recording the right ventricular impulse with pressure overload of the right ventricle, or the hepatic pulse with tricuspid regurgitation. The use of pulse recordings as clinical tools has largely been replaced by the echo/Doppler technique, but pulse recordings remain invaluable as teaching aids.

CAROTID PULSE

The normal carotid pulse tracing is composed of a rapid upstroke (anacrotic limb) terminating in an initial peak or percussion wave (Figure 18). The percussion wave is followed by a less prominent, somewhat more rounded tidal wave. The percussion wave appears to be related primarily to the peak aortic flow rate, while the tidal wave is related to peak aortic pressure. Thus the tidal wave often becomes more prominent with systemic hypertension, following the infusion of a vasoconstrictor, and in elderly patients. The descending limb of the carotid pulse tracing, which normally is less steep than the ascending limb, is interrupted by the incisura or dicrotic notch. The notch is due to aortic valve closure. Although the morphology of the carotid pulse tracing resembles that of an intra-aortic pressure recording, it is delayed by approximately 20–50 milliseconds, which is the time it takes the pulse wave to travel from the chest to the neck.

Systolic Time Intervals

Although interesting from an historical perspective, systolic time intervals are rarely used today in clinical practice. They are measurements derived from simultaneous recording of the electrocardiogram, the indirect carotid pulse, and the phonocardiogram; the systolic time intervals consist of *total systole*, the *pre-ejection period*, and the *left ventricular ejection time*. Total systole is measured from the onset of the Q wave of the electrocardiogram to the first high-frequency component of the second heart sound. The left ventricular ejection time is measured from the initial carotid upstroke to the dicrotic notch of the externally recorded carotid pulse tracing, while the pre-ejection period is derived by subtracting the left ventricular ejection time from total systole.

Used in the past to aid in the noninvasive evaluation of valvular heart disease and ventricular performance, STIs have been largely supplanted by 2D echocardiographic and Doppler techniques.

Carotid Pulse Abnormalities

Atherosclerosis of the carotid artery may produce abnormalities of the carotid pulse tracing. In the absence of local carotid disease, abnormalities of the pulse may be generally categorized as hyperkinetic or hypokinetic (Table 2). In a variety of disease states, specific abnormalities of the carotid pulse often can be identified. Aortic stenosis typically shows a small hypokinetic pulse with a delayed systolic peak (Figure 19). An anacrotic shoulder, occurring in the early to mid-portion of the ascending limb of the carotid pulse tracing, reflects decreased aortic flow secondary to obstruction to left ventricular emptying, as well as turbulent flow. A "shudder" is often noted, also a consequence of turbulent blood flow.

In contrast to the findings in fixed orifice left ventricular outflow obstruction, in the dynamic obstruction seen with hypertrophic cardiomyopathy there is a hyperkinetic pulse of large amplitude with a rapid upstroke (Figure 20). As left ventricular volume decreases during systole, the anterior leaflet of the mitral valve moves towards the septum and narrows the outflow tract. Consequently, there is a sudden decrease in the carotid pulse amplitude, reflecting a sudden fall in ejection rate. A secondary wave is generated

Table 2. General Causes of Abnormalities of the Carotid Pulse Tracing
Hyperkinetic pulse
Increased cardiac output states, such as anxiety, fever, exercise, pregnancy, and anemia
Widened pulse pressure, as with aortic regurgitation, persistent ductus arteriosus, and Paget's disease of the bone
Decreased arterial distensibility
Hypokinetic pulse
Fixed left ventricular outflow tract obstruction, as with aortic stenosis and discrete subaortic stenosis
Reduced forward stroke volume as with myocardial infarction, cardiomyopathy, and severe mitral regurgitation
Narrow pulse pressure, as with cardiac tamponade, constrictive pericarditis

until the end of systole, resulting in the characteristic "spike and dome" pulse curve configuration.

JUGULAR VENOUS PULSE

The normal jugular venous pulse recording consists of two major peaks (*a* and *v*) and two major descents (*x* and *y*) (Figure 21). The a-wave is the result of the displacement of blood into the jugular vein by right atrial systole; it is the most prominent positive wave and is absent when effective atrial systole is lacking. Atrial relaxation is associated with the x descent, which continues to the x trough, the most negative wave of the normal jugular pulse recording. The x descent usually is interrupted by the c-wave, a small wave resulting from closure of the tricuspid valve. Further accumulation of blood behind the still-closed tricuspid valve results in the v-wave, due to passive filling of the right atrium. The *y* descent is generated by the opening tricuspid valve and flow of blood from the right atrium into the right ventricle.

Jugular Venous Pulse Abnormalities

A prominent a-wave is found when right atrial systole is unusually forceful as a consequence of an impediment to right atrial emptying. This is usually the result of increased stiffness (diminished compliance)

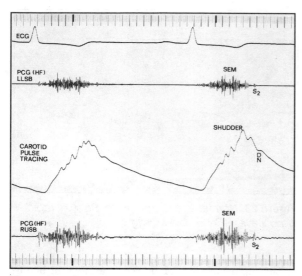

Figure 19. *Carotid pulse tracing from a patient with severe valvular aortic stenosis, showing a low anacrotic shoulder and systolic shudder. The phonocardiogram (PCG) demonstrates a mid- to late-peaking systolic ejection murmur (SEM) with soft aortic component of the second heart sound (S₂). DN = dicrotic notch; HF = high frequency; LLSB = left lower sternal border; RUSB = right upper sternal border. (Reproduced from Borow KM, Wynne J: External pulse recordings, systolic time intervals, apexcardiography, and phonocardiography. In: Cohn PF, Wynne J, eds. Diagnostic Methods in Clinical Cardiology. Boston: Little Brown; 1982, 144. With permission.)*

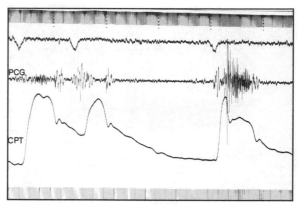

Figure 20. *Carotid pulse tracing (CPT), phonocardiogram (PCG), recorded at the left lower sternal border, and electrocardiogram in a patient with provocable dynamic subaortic obstruction due to hypertrophic cardiomyopathy. Recordings made after an atrial premature beat demonstrate precipitation of a spike and dome configuration on CPT and accentuation of the systolic ejection murmur, indicating that dynamic obstruction was provoked. (Reproduced from Borow KM, Wynne J: External pulse recordings, systolic time intervals, apexcardiography, and phonocardiography. In: Cohn PF, Wynne J, eds. Diagnostic Methods in Clinical Cardiology. Boston: Little, Brown; 1982, 148. With permission.)*

of the right ventricle as a consequence of right ventricular hypertrophy of any etiology (chronic obstructive lung disease, mitral valve disease, pulmonary artery hypertension, pulmonic stenosis, etc.).

The x descent is reduced in atrial fibrillation, since atrial relaxation is absent. It is shallow or obliterated in tricuspid insufficiency, since there is active regurgitation of blood into the right atrium. A positive systolic wave (or c-v wave) replaces the x trough in severe tricuspid regurgitation. With severe tricuspid regurgitation, a similar systolic pulsation may often be recorded from over the liver (Figure 22). In cardiac tamponade, a prominent x descent is noted. Conversely, the x descent is reduced with constrictive pericarditis; a prominent x descent in this setting strongly suggests effusoconstrictive disease.

The v-wave is more prominent with enhanced passive refilling of the atrium, as seen in an atrial septal defect. As noted above, an early and large systolic regurgitant wave is seen in tricuspid regurgitation.

Although by common usage regurgitant waves have been referred to as v waves, strictly speaking a v-wave is solely the result of passive atrial filling, while

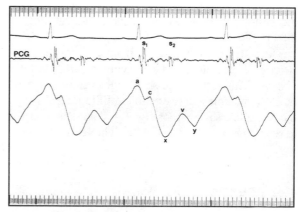

Figure 21. *Jugular venous pulse recording from a normal subject. The a-wave is the largest positive wave, while the x trough is the more prominent negative wave. The phonocardiogram (PCG) is a low-frequency recording at the lower left sternal border, showing first (S₁) and second (S₂) heart sounds.*

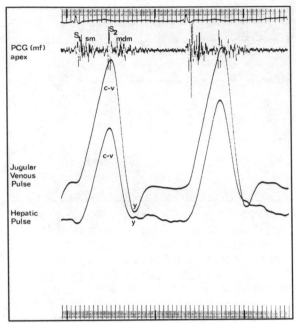

Figure 22. *Jugular venous and hepatic pulse tracings from a patient with Ebstein's anomaly and tricuspid regurgitation. A giant c-v systolic wave is noted, with an abrupt y descent. The hepatic pulse recording is similar to the jugular pulse tracing. PCG = phonocardiogram; sm = systolic murmur, mf = mid-frequency; mdm = mid-diastolic murmur. (Reproduced from Borow KM, Wynne J: External pulse recordings, systolic time intervals, apexcardiography, and phonocardiography. In: Cohn PF, Wynne J, eds. Diagnostic Methods in Clinical Cardiology. Boston: Little, Brown; 1982, 131. With permission.)*

the systolic wave is due to active systolic filling of the atrium.

The y descent is unusually rapid and brief in constrictive pericarditis, and ends with an early diastolic plateau. This reflects the small right ventricular end-diastolic volume and restriction to filling, resulting in the so-called square root sign. A deep and sharp y descent may also be found with right ventricular failure.

THE APEXCARDIOGRAM

The movement of the heart against the chest wall throughout the cardiac cycle results in motion of the left precordial surface, which can be recorded on the apexcardiogram. This closely resembles the left ventricular pressure pulse in morphology (Figure 23).

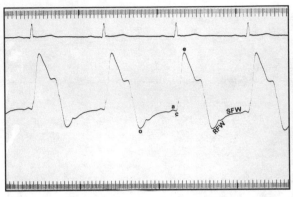

Figure 23. *Normal apexcardiogram. RFW = rapid filling wave; SFW = slow filling wave.*

The rapid upstroke of the apexcardiogram begins with left ventricular isovolumic systole (*c* point). The upstroke terminates at the *e* point, which coincides with the onset of left ventricular ejection. During the second half of LV systole, the curve usually undergoes a gentle decline. At approximately the time of aortic valve closure, the curve begins a sharp decline, correlating with the onset of the ventricular isovolumic relaxation period. This downward deflection terminates near the end of mitral valve opening (end of isovolumic relaxation period), an event that is approximated by the 0 point of the apexcardiogram. Vigorous ventricular filling in early diastole produces the rapid filling wave (RFW), which is followed by the less vigorous slow filling wave (SFW). The a-wave is the final diastolic wave, and corresponds to the distention of the left ventricle as a consequence of left atrial contraction.

APEXCARDIOGRAPHIC ABNORMALITIES

The a-wave is absent in patients with atrial fibrillation, and is increased (greater than 15% of the overall height of the apical pulse tracing) in cases of diminished left ventricular compliance (Figure 24).

The systolic bulge of the apexcardiogram may be unusually forceful, although typically not sustained, in volume overload of a compensated left ventricle (increased stroke volume). This may be found in mitral or aortic regurgitation, anemia, anxiety, thyrotoxicosis, and so forth. A sustained apical impulse, on the other hand, is found with left ventricular pressure overload (aortic stenosis or systemic hypertension), and with left ventricular dysfunction

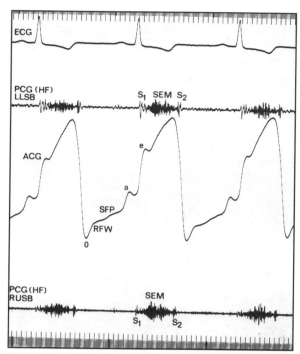

Figure 24. *Apexcardiogram (ACG) in a patient with severe valvular aortic stenosis. The systolic wave is sustained, with a continued rise throughout ventricular ejection. The a-wave is exaggerated. HF = high frequency; LLSB = left lower sternal border; PCG = phonocardiogram; RFW = rapid filling wave; RUSB = right upper sternal border; SEM = systolic ejection murmur; SFP = slow filling phase. (Reproduced from Borow KM, Wynne J: External pulse recordings, systolic time intervals, apexcardiography, and phonocardiography. In: Cohn PF, Wynne J, eds. Diagnostic Methods in Clinical Cardiology. Boston: Little, Brown; 1982, 145. With permission.)*

(cardiomyopathy, left ventriuclar failure, left ventricular aneurysm) (Figure 24).

An unusual double or bifid apical impulse may be seen with hypertrophic cardiomyopathy with obstruction. Since diminished LV compliance is also often found, the a wave may be quite prominent as well, resulting in a characteristic triple apical impulse.

A prominent rapid filling wave is found in patients with augmented early diastolic filling, often as a result of LV volume overload (mitral regurgitation being the most commonly encountered example). The rapid filling wave is reduced with diminished left ventricular compliance, since the increased stiffness of the ventricle limits its ability to expand in early diastole. The rapid filling wave is blunted and shortened in duration with mitral stenosis.

The apexcardiogram is particularly useful in clarifying the timing of auscultatory events. An ejection sound occurs in relationship to the e point. A mitral valve opening snap is found near the 0 point, while a third heart sound is found later, at the peak of the rapid filling wave. The fourth heart sound is found at the time of the a-wave.

Bibliography

Alam M, Rosman HS, Lakier JB, et al: Doppler and echocardiographic features of normal and dysfunctioning bioprosthetic valves. *J Am Coll Cardiol* 10:851, 1987.

Armstrong WF: Exercise echocardiography: Ready, willing and able. *J Am Coll Cardiol* 11:1359, 1988.

Chan P, Ogilby JD, Segal B: Tricuspid valve endocarditis. *Am Heart J* 117:1140, 1989.

Douglas PS, Fiolkoski J, Berko B, et al: Echocardiographic visualization of coronary artery anatomy in the adult. *J Am Coll Cardiol* 11:565, 1988.

Jaffe WM, Roche AHG, Coverdale HA, et al: Clinical evaluation versus Doppler echocardiography in the quantitative assessment of valvular heart disease. *Circulation* 78:267, 1988.

Khandheria BK, Tajik AJ, Taylor CL, et al: Aortic dissection: Review of value and limitations of two-dimensional echocardiography in a six year experience. *J Am Soc Echo* 2:17, 1989.

Labovitz AJ, Pearson AC, McCluskey MT, et al: Clinical significance of the echocardiographic degree of mitral valve prolapse. *Am Heart J* 115:842, 1988.

Lipshultz SE, Sanders SP, Mayer JE, et al: Are routine preoperative cardiac catheterization and angiography necessary before repair of ostium primum atrial septal defect? *J Am Coll Cardiol* 11:373, 1988.

O'Rourke RA: Value of Doppler echocardiography for quantifying valvular stenosis or regurgitation. *Circulation* 78:483, 1988.

Pinamonti B, Alberti E, Cigalotto A, et al: Echocardiographic findings in myocarditis. *Am J Cardiol* 62:285, 1988.

Ryan T, Armstrong WF, O'Donnell JA, et al: Risk stratification after acute myocardial infarction by means of exercise two-dimensional echocardiography. *Am Heart J* 114:1305, 1987.

Vargas-Barron J, Attie F, Skronme D, et al: Two-dimensional echocardiography and color Doppler imaging in patients with systolic-diastolic murmurs. *Am Heart J* 114:1461, 1987.

CHAPTER 8

Doppler Echocardiography

Sherif B. Labib
Steven L. Schwartz
Natesa G. Pandian

Echocardiography is the most useful diagnostic technique for evaluation of most cardiac disorders. Two-dimensional echocardiography provides detailed information on the morphology of the valves, the myocardium and pericardium, the function of the valves, and the size of the cardiac chambers. The last decade has established Doppler echocardiography as an important tool for studying cardiac flow dynamics. Based on the ability of Doppler to determine the direction and velocity of blood flow, an enormous amount of hemodynamic information can be deduced noninvasively. In obstructive valvular lesions, transvalvular pressure gradients and an estimate of the valve areas can be obtained. Regurgitant and shunt flows are readily detected and evaluated. Doppler is also very useful in the assessment of ischemic heart disease, constrictive and restrictive disorders, and cardiac tamponade. The combination of hemodynamic information gained from the various Doppler modalities and the anatomic information provided by two-dimensional echocardiographic imaging makes ultrasound a powerful diagnostic tool.

PRINCIPLES AND TECHNICAL ASPECTS

The basis of Doppler ultrasound is relatively simple. A high-frequency sound signal, ultrasound, is generated by a crystal within a transducer and is aimed at various regions within the cardiovascular system where red blood cells reflect the ultrasound signals back to the transducer (Kremkau; McDicken; Wells). The frequency of the reflected ultrasound waves is altered according to the relative motion of the reflective surface encountered. The difference between the emitted and the reflected frequency is termed the *Doppler shift*. If the reflected surface is stationary, the emitted and reflected signals will have identical frequencies and no Doppler shift is observed. If the reflective surface is moving toward or away from the ultrasound source, the reflected signal will be "shifted" to a higher or lower frequency, respectively. A higher-frequency shift will be displayed as a positive deflection on the spectral display screen and a lower-frequency shift as a negative deflection. The magnitude of the frequency shift is proportional to the velocity at which the reflective surface is moving towards or receding away from the ultrasound source. Thus, application of these Doppler principles allows for the determination of flow direction and flow velocity.

The precise mathematical relationship between flow velocity and the Doppler shift is represented by the Doppler equation:

$$F(d) = \frac{2f}{c} V \cos \theta$$

where F(d) is the frequency or Doppler shift; f is the frequency of the ultrasound generated by the transducer; c is the velocity of ultrasound in tissues (1,540 m/sec); V is the velocity of the blood column that is being interrogated; and θ, or the Doppler angle, is the angle between the ultrasound beam and the long axis of the column of blood. Inspection of the Doppler equation reveals that the shift in frequency is not only related to blood flow velocity but also to the Doppler angle. The larger the angle, the lesser the magnitude of the frequency shift detected. Only the velocity of the vector component in the direction of the ultrasound beam will be measured. A large Doppler angle will thus underestimate the blood velocity. It is therefore desirable for the ultrasound beam to be as parallel as possible to the column of blood being interrogated. Generally, when the Doppler angle is

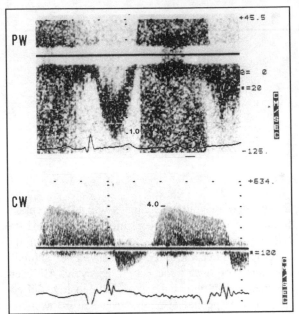

Figure 1. *Pulsed and continuous-wave Doppler. The transducer is placed at the apex in these recordings. The top tracing is a PW recording where the sample volume is placed in the left ventricular outflow tract. The negative deflection that follows the QRS complex represents systolic ejection. Note the normal laminar appearance (hollow center). The curtain-like signals seen in diastole represent the turbulent flow of aortic regurgitation, which aliases, making the true direction and velocity difficult to determine. The CW Doppler tracing at the bottom clearly characterizes the aortic regurgitation flow as directed toward the transducer (positive deflection and a peak velocity of 4 m/sec).*

20° or less, underestimation of true velocity is negligible.

Two forms of Doppler are commonly used: continuous wave (CW) and pulsed wave (PW). They are used in a complementary fashion. The differences between them are illustrated in Figure 1.

In CW Doppler, the transducer is continuously emitting and receiving ultrasound data, and the CW display depicts Doppler shift information reflected from every red blood cell along the path of the ultrasound beam. The advantage of such a system is that high-velocity flows can be accurately measured.

In PW Doppler, the transducer alternates between transmission and reception of ultrasound waves, making depth discrimination possible. The pulsing of the ultrasound waves allows the selective sampling of an operator-defined region along the path of the ultra-

sound beam, known as the *sample volume*. The PW Doppler examination is frequently performed with the guidance of two-dimensional echocardiography (Griffith and Henry) or color flow Doppler, where the sample volume is moved to varying depths and positioned in the regions of interest by the examiner. The number of transmitted pulses per second, or the sampling rate, is limited by their total travel time to and from the target distance (depth of the sample volume). When high-velocity flows are encountered, the sampling rate in the pulsed Doppler mode is too slow to accurately measure their velocity, and an artifact known as *aliasing* occurs. Aliasing on the spectral display is depicted as a cutoff of a given flow-velocity envelope and the placement of the cut portion on the other side of the reference (zero velocity) baseline. When the blood velocity is high enough, signals on both sides of the baseline merge and a curtain-like pattern is seen (Figure 1). In this situation, it becomes difficult to discern the direction and velocity of blood flow with certainty. The maximum velocity that can be recorded without aliasing (generally 1.5-2.0 m/sec) is termed the Nyquist limit, which varies according to the transducer frequency, depth of the sample volume, and the position of the reference baseline.

Color flow Doppler imaging allows direct, two-dimensional, real-time visualization of flow velocity as a color-coded pattern superimposed on a two-dimensional echo image (Miyatake et al. 1984; Pandian et al. 1987; Pandian et al. 1989). It is essentially a form of PW Dopper, whereby hundreds of sampling sites within a given sector are analyzed simultaneously and assigned a color according to blood flow direction and velocity relative to the transducer. There are several algorithms and color maps that may be used for expression of the processed data. The most commonly used method assigns a red or blue color to blood flow moving toward or away from the transducer, respectively (Figure 2, p. *xviii*). High velocities are represented by brighter hues of these colors. Since color flow Doppler is a form of PW Doppler, it is subject to aliasing; if the Nyquist limit is exceeded, color reversal will occur. Important color flow controls include gain-setting and sector size and location. Their proper adjustment is essential for obtaining optimum results. When the gain is set too high, for example, excessive bright color signals obscure the image. If set too low, color flow signals will appear weak, flow jets will appear small, and the sensitivity of the technique for the detection of abnormal flow will be decreased. The gain-setting should be care-

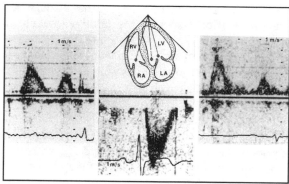

Figure 3. *PW Doppler recording of normal flow as imaged from the cardiac apex. The sample volume is positioned within the flow of interest. The tracing on the left represents diastolic tricuspid flow. In the center tracing, flow in the left ventricular outflow tract is seen during systole. Diastolic mitral flow is recorded in the right tracing. Note the biphasic appearance of flow across the atrioventricular valves.*

fully adjusted, in as standardized a manner as possible. This may be achieved by initially turning the setting down completely, then gradually increasing it until background noise begins to appear faintly. Sector size and location can also be selected. Use of large sector sizes, however, will result in a slower sampling rate, thus compromising the spatial and temporal resolution.

NORMAL AND ABNORMAL FLOW

When a normally functioning valve opens, full communication between the two chambers, or chamber and great vessel, is established. Only a minimal pressure difference exists (1-2 mm Hg) to drive the blood flow forward. Therefore, normal blood flow across the cardiac valves is low in velocity. It is also laminar because most of the red blood cells are moving at about the same velocity. The direction of the flow velocity envelope on the spectral display depends on the location of the transducer relative to the direction of blood flow. When the transducer is placed at the cardiac apex and the sample volume is placed in the left ventricular outflow tract (Figure 3) or in the aorta just beyond the aortic valve, blood ejected by the left ventricle into the aorta is moving away from the transducer and is depicted as a negative or downward deflection following the QRS complex. The same flow will have a positive deflection when interrogated from the suprasternal notch. The hollow center of a PW

Doppler tracing, surrounded by a dark grey narrow band, reflects normal laminar flow with uniform red blood cell acceleration and deceleration. Normal aortic flow is also characterized by a rapid rise in velocity that reaches its peak value of <1.5 m/sec usually during the first half of systole.

From the apex, the sample volume may be placed in the left ventricle beneath the mitral valve; there, the direction of mitral flow is oriented towards the transducer, and will be depicted by a positive or upward deflection. Normal mitral flow, as seen in Figure 3, is also laminar and low in velocity (usually under 1 m/sec), and is biphasic in individuals with an intact sinus mechanism. Most left ventricular filling takes place in early diastole (E wave), followed by diastasis and then by a smaller A wave representing late diastolic filling (which occurs as a result of atrial contraction).

Flows within the right-sided chambers and vessels are interrogated in a manner similar to that of left-sided flows—by placing the sample volume of the PW Doppler or directing the CW beam to intercept the flow in question. Generally, when comparing right- and left-sided flows across their respective atrioventricular and semilunar valves, right-sided flow profiles tend to have similar morphology to, but lower velocity than, their left-sided counterparts (Figure 3).

Several features characterize abnormal flows. They have increased velocity, reflecting the pressure gradient driving the flow. Red blood cells passing through a narrowed or deformed orifice create a turbulent jet consisting of red blood cells with varying direction and velocity; the jet is depicted on the PW spectral display as a broad spectral pattern. In the case of regurgitant lesions, the abnormal flow will travel in a retrograde direction relative to the valve.

HEMODYNAMICS

Traditionally, hemodynamic assessment of cardiovascular disorders has been done primarily in the catheterization laboratory. The advent of flow-directed, balloon-tipped catheters brought hemodynamic monitoring to the bedside in the intensive care unit. These methods are invasive, however. Doppler echocardiography allows noninvasive assessment of intracardiac hemodynamics.

The key to the noninvasive hemodynamic assessment is the Bernoulli equation, which describes the relationship between the pressure gradient and flow velocity across a restrictive orifice. In most clinical situations, pressure gradients can be determined using the modified Bernoulli equation:

$$P_2 - P_1 = 4 (V_2^2 - V_1^2)$$

where $P_2 - P_1$ equals the pressure gradient; V_1 is the flow velocity proximal to the stenosis; and V_2 is the maximum velocity of the stenotic jet. Usually, V_1^2 is much less than V_2^2 and is therefore assumed to equal zero. The modified Bernoulli equation can be even further simplified as:

$$P_2 - P_1 = 4 V^2$$

where V represents the maximum post-stenotic flow velocity. This equation has been applied to jets across stenotic valves (Stamm and Martin) as well as regurgitant valves (Nishimura and Tajik; Yock and Popp; Currie et al.).

Knowing the maximum velocity across a stenotic valve, we can calculate the gradient across that valve, as in aortic stenosis. Likewise, with knowledge of the maximum velocity of a regurgitant jet, we may determine the pressure on one side of the regurgitant valve if we know the pressure on the other side. This principle can be applied to examination of right ventricular systolic pressures in patients with tricuspid regurgitation. As will be discussed later, the changes in velocity, time intervals, and slopes of spectral tracings can give important hemodynamic information as well.

When using this method to calculate pressure gradients, the following points must be adhered to in order to insure accuracy: (1) The Doppler beam must be as parallel as possible to the jet in order to record maximal velocity; and (2) the proximal velocity (V_1) should be much less than V_2.

Another hemodynamic variable that can be assessed noninvasively is cardiac output. Flow across an orifice can be determined by

$$Q = A \times V$$

where Q equals flow, A equals orifice area, and V is the integral of the velocity curve over time, or time-velocity integral. Using this equation, stroke volume can be determined by measuring the area of any valve orifice and obtaining the velocity across that valve. Cardiac output can be calculated by simply multiplying the stroke volume by the heart rate. Usually, aortic flows and dimensions are used in such calculations because the velocity across a normal aortic valve is easily obtainable, the aortic orifice is relatively circular so the area can be calculated from its diameter, and the orifice size remains relatively constant throughout systole.

Determination of stroke volume in this manner can be applied to other situations as well. Comparing flow across the pulmonic valve to that across the aortic valve in patients with an intracardiac shunt gives the shunt ratio, or Qp:Qs. The continuity equation is another application of stroke volume measurement. This equation states that flow on one side of an orifice must equal that on the other side of the orifice, and is expressed as follows:

$$A_1 \times V_1 = A_2 \times V_2$$

where V_1 and V_2 are flow velocities proximal and distal to the orifice, and A_1 and A_2 are the areas at the site where velocity is measured. By rearranging this equation, one can calculate a stenotic valve area by knowing the area and velocity proximal to the valve and the maximal flow velocity through the valve. This equation has proven very useful for noninvasive assessment of aortic stenosis.

VALVULAR HEART DISEASE

AORTIC STENOSIS

The two-dimensional echocardiographic study is useful in delineating the aortic valve morphology. While valvular thickening and limited aortic cusp separation readily identify patients with abnormal aortic valves, these features are unreliable in determining the degree of aortic valvular narrowing (DeMaria et al.; Godley et al.). It is not uncommon to note marked valvular restriction on the 2D echo examination and ultimately find no transvalvular pressure gradient. Use of Doppler provides the necessary information to assess the hemodynamic significance of the stenotic valve. Significant aortic valvular obstruction creates turbulent flow, and the pressure drop across the valve during systole results in increased flow velocity (Figure 4); peak velocity is reached later in systole. Although PW Doppler may be used for the detection and localization of such turbulent flows, it has little value in estimating severity because of its inability to measure high-flow velocities. Such flows are accurately measured with CW Doppler, and with use of the modified Bernoulli equation the pressure gradient across the aortic valve can be readily derived (Stamm and

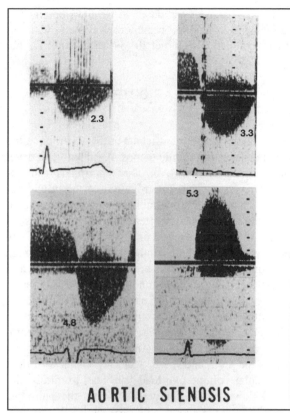

AORTIC STENOSIS

Figure 4. *CW Doppler recordings from four patients with aortic stenosis of varying severity. The peak velocity of the tracing on top left is 2.3 m/sec, which corresponds to a maximum instantaneous gradient (MIG) of 21 mm Hg, consistent with mild aortic stenosis. The tracing on top right is from a patient with moderate aortic stenosis; the MIG is 44 mm Hg. The recording on bottom left, from a patient with critical aortic stenosis, has a peak velocity of 4.8 m/sec and an MIG of 92 mm Hg. The tracing on bottom right was recorded from the suprasternal position in a patient with critical aortic stenosis; the flow is toward the transducer and recorded as positive. The MIG is 110 mm Hg.*

Martin; Berger et al. 1984; Oh et al.). When the maximum velocity is used in the calculation, the maximum instantaneous gradient or "peak gradient" is obtained; this reflects the largest systolic pressure difference between the left ventricle and aorta. This maximum instantaneous gradient is usually higher than the customary "peak to peak" gradient obtained in the catheterization laboratory. One may also average multiple instantaneous gradient measurements to obtain a mean gradient.

Accurate estimation of pressure gradients depends on precise measurement of blood flow velocity through the stenotic orifice. In order to record the true maximum velocity, it is imperative that the ultrasound beam be aligned as parallel as possible to the long axis of the stenotic jet flow. Otherwise, the flow velocity and the calculated pressure gradient may be significantly underestimated. Since the direction of stenotic jets is often eccentric and unpredictable in a given patient, the examiner must use multiple sampling sites for CW Doppler interrogation of the ascending aorta, and use the highest value obtained in the calculation of pressure gradients. Doppler sampling sites in patients with aortic stenosis should include the apical, subcostal, right parasternal, and suprasternal views. Occasionally, color flow Doppler is helpful in aligning the CW beam with the stenotic jet orientation. Acquisition of the highest possible flow velocity requires a compulsive, systematic examination by an experienced operator.

It is important to note that pressure gradients, whether obtained by Doppler or by catheterization, are related not only to valve area but to cardiac output as well. Therefore, in states of abnormal cardiac output, the use of velocity and pressure gradients alone to assess the severity of valvular stenosis may lead to erroneous conclusions. Flow velocity is increased in high cardiac output states, such as are encountered with a hyperdynamic left ventricle or in aortic regurgitation, and will therefore lead to overestimation of the severity of aortic stenosis. Conversely, velocity is decreased in low output states, such as in ischemic cardiomyopathy or end-stage aortic stenosis, and will lead to underestimation of true severity. Doppler validation studies with cardiac catheterization, however, show that peak aortic flow velocity of >3 m/sec, or a ratio of left ventricular outflow velocity to aortic velocity of <0.25, are highly sensitive indicators for detecting significant AS. Their absence can therefore be used reliably to exclude AS (Oh et al.). Flow velocity >4.5 m/sec is highly specific for critical aortic stenosis, but not sensitive (Oh et al.). Values in between have less diagnostic value. A velocity of only 3.5 m/sec, for example, may represent the maximum velocity obtained in critical AS patients with coexisting depressed left ventricular function. In such settings of abnormal cardiac output, the noninvasive calculation of aortic valve area using the continuity equation, rather than the use of pressure gradients alone, more accurately reflects aortic stenosis severity. The previously discussed continuity equation is based on the principle that flow volume proximal to, distal to, and at the site of obstruction is identical. The equation may be rearranged in the following manner to solve for the stenotic aortic valve area:

$$A_2 = \frac{A_1 \times V_1}{V_2}$$

The diameter of the left ventricular outflow tract is measured in the parasternal long-axis view, and its cross-sectional area (A_1), which is assumed to have a circular configuration, is calculated with the simple algebraic formula Area $= \pi r^2$. Flow velocity in the LV outflow tract (V_1) is obtained with PW Doppler from the apical views, where the sample volume is positioned immediately beneath the aortic valve. V_2 is the maximum flow velocity obtained at or beyond the valve by CW Doppler examination from multiple transducer orientations. In using the continuity equation, V_1 and V_2 may be expressed as peak velocities, mean velocities, or time-velocity integrals. In the presence of atrial fibrillation, the average of multiple consecutive beats is used in the calculation. Because velocity information from the LV outflow tract proximal to the obstruction (which is directly influenced by cardiac output) is incorporated into the continuity equation, this method is especially useful in estimating aortic stenosis severity in the setting of abnormal cardiac output.

Some caution should be advised in the use of the continuity equation to derive aortic valve area. Derivation of the left ventricular outflow tract area (A_1) assumes a circular configuration. The LV outflow tract, bounded by the interventricular septum and the anterior mitral valve leaflet, is dynamic throughout the cardiac cycle and may not have a perfectly circular cross-section. Furthermore, the diameter of the LV outflow tract may be difficult to accurately measure in patients with stenotic valves, which are occasionally surrounded by echo-bright calcifications. Flow velocity in the LV outflow tract (V_1) may vary with minor alterations in the position of the sample volume, especially in the region where pre-stenotic acceleration of flow occurs. Finally, obtaining the maximum velocity across the stenotic valve (V_2) via proper alignment of the CW beam with the stenotic jet is time-consuming and requires a considerable amount of operator expertise. Despite these difficulties, however, the noninvasive calculation of aortic

valve area has been validated with values obtained at cardiac catheterization in numerous centers, with excellent correlations (Otto et al.; Skjaerpe et al.; Zoghbi et al. 1986).

RIGHT VENTRICULAR OUTFLOW OBSTRUCTION

Obstruction to right ventricular outflow can be at the valvular level (pulmonic stenosis), subvalvular level (infundibular stenosis), or at the periphery (pulmonary artery stenosis). Interrogation of the infundibulum, pulmonic valve, pulmonary trunk, and proximal right and left pulmonary arteries can be accomplished from either the parasternal or subcostal window. Flow profiles seen in valvular pulmonic stenosis and main pulmonary artery stenosis are similar to those seen in aortic stenosis, while infundibular stenosis gives a profile similar to that of subaortic obstruction. As with other valvular lesions, gradients calculated from CW Doppler recordings correlate well with hemodynamic data (Hatle and Angelsen). Increased flow across the pulmonic valve, seen in patients with right ventricular volume overload, can lead to mildly elevated flow velocities recorded across the pulmonic valve. These patients can be differentiated from others with stenotic lesions by noting increased flow in the right ventricle as well as the pulmonary artery, without a localized increase in flow velocity (Hatle and Angelsen).

MITRAL STENOSIS

Two-dimensional echocardiography plays an important role in the evaluation of mitral valve stenosis. It is used to survey the various cardiac chamber sizes and to provide detailed morphologic information pertaining to the mitral and submitral structures. Estimation of mitral valve area is possible by direct planimetry of the valve orifice in those patients with technically satisfactory parasternal short-axis images. Doppler is used to provide important hemodynamic information to supplement and confirm the 2D echo findings (Hatle et al. 1978, 1979; Holen et al.).

When a normally functioning mitral valve opens, early diastolic filling occurs and the left atrium and left ventricular diastolic pressures rapidly equalize, as depicted by the normal swift diastolic descent of the Doppler flow velocity profile. In mitral stenosis, the transmitral pressure gradient is initially elevated and

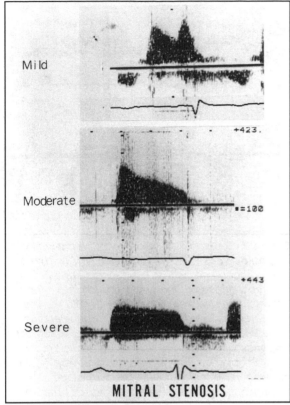

Figure 5. *CW Doppler recordings from the apex in mitral stenosis. The top tracing is from a patient with mild mitral stenosis; valve area was calculated as 2.2 cm². The middle tracing is from a patient with moderate mitral stenosis. The tracing on the bottom was recorded from a patient with critical mitral stenosis; mitral valve area was 0.5 cm². Notice that the deceleration slope is flatter as mitral stenosis becomes more severe.*

persists longer into diastole, resulting in a high peak velocity at the onset of left ventricular filling and a slow decline of the diastolic velocity profile. The rate of decline corresponds to the degree of obstruction and is used to gauge its severity (Figure 5). The best mitral flow velocity profile is obtained when the transducer is placed at the cardiac apex. Since the Doppler flow velocity does not usually exceed the Nyquist limit even in severe MS, either PW or CW Doppler may be used. Color Doppler may serve as a guide to orient the Doppler ultrasound beam as parallel as possible to the stenotic jet. The mean transmitral pressure gradient is derived by measuring multiple instantaneous velocities at short time inter-

vals throughout diastole and employing the modified Bernoulli equation.

Doppler may also be used for the noninvasive estimation of mitral valve area using the principle of pressure half-time. This is especially pertinent in situations where factors other than the degree of valvular stenosis may influence the mean gradient—such as increased flow across the mitral valve from significant coexistent mitral regurgitation, or changes in diastolic filling times from variations in heart rate. Pressure half-time ($t_{1/2}$) is defined as the time (in milliseconds) it takes for the transvalvular diastolic gradient to decay to half its initial peak value. Since the spectral display reflects velocity measurements and the relationship between pressure and velocity is quadratic ($\Delta P = 4 \times V^2$), $t_{1/2}$ may be expressed in terms of velocity rather than pressure, i.e., the time required for the velocity to fall to a value corresponding to the initial velocity divided by $\sqrt{2}$ (or simply multiplied by 0.7). The $t_{1/2}$ in normal individuals ranges between 20 msec and 60 msec. The narrower the mitral orifice, the flatter the diastolic slope of the velocity profile and the more prolonged the $t_{1/2}$ will be. Hatle and co-workers have shown that a mitral valve area of 1 cm² corresponds to a $t_{1/2}$ of 220 msec. Accordingly, mitral valve area (MVA) may be estimated by dividing 220 by the $t_{1/2}$:

$$MVA = \frac{220 \text{ msec}}{t_{(1/2)}}$$

The pressure half-time derivation of mitral valve area is independent of heart rate, stroke volume, mitral regurgitation, aortic regurgitation, and the presence of atrial fibrillation. The effects of left atrial compliance, as seen following balloon valvuloplasty, and of abnormal left ventricular compliance with coexistent aortic stenosis, systemic hypertension, and coronary artery disease on $t_{1/2}$, have not been fully resolved. To ensure diagnostic accuracy, both modalities for estimating mitral valve area (Doppler-derived $t_{1/2}$ and planimetry of the mitral orifice in the 2D echo examination) should be used whenever possible and their results compared.

TRICUSPID STENOSIS

Tricuspid valve stenosis (TS) should be carefully searched for in all patients with rheumatic heart disease. Like MS, the hallmark of TS is the demonstration of valve thickening and diastolic doming on the 2D echo study. Direct planimetry of the tricuspid orifice, however, is not possible. Doppler evaluation of tricuspid flow in TS is performed similarly to that of mitral flow in MS, but because of the relatively uncommon occurrence of TS, it is less well studied. With increasing severity of TS, the peak tricuspid flow is increased and the diastolic descent of the flow velocity is prolonged (Parris et al.). The mean diastolic gradient and pressure half-time are calculated in the same manner as in MS, but the latter is less useful, as the mathematical relationship required to estimate tricuspid valve area has not yet been fully elucidated.

AORTIC REGURGITATION

Doppler echocardiography has proven to be a highly sensitive method for the diagnosis of aortic insufficiency. The presence of aortic regurgitation detected by Doppler echocardiography, even if very mild, indicates at least a minor abnormality of the aortic valve (Berger et al. 1989). Both pulsed and continuous-wave Doppler recordings of aortic regurgitation are seen as a high velocity, holodiastolic flow, as shown in Figure 1. The appearance of aortic insufficiency on PW tracings is that of a curtain-like holodiastolic flow pattern, due to aliasing. Continuous-wave Doppler recorded from the apex (Figures 1 and 6) reveals a characteristic profile with a decrescendo pattern in which the peak velocity, at least 3 m/sec, occurs immediately after aortic valve closure. The timing of onset of flow is an important point differentiation from mitral flow, which commences after the isovolumic relaxation phase. Spectral recordings of the flow in the proximal descending aorta with the transducer in the suprasternal position may exhibit a retrograde diastolic flow signal. In the presence of severe regurgitation, these tracings may resemble a "sine wave" pattern (Figure 6). Color Doppler is useful for the identification of aortic insufficiency. As shown in Figure 7 (p. *xviii*), a bright, mosaic, retrograde jet emanating from the aortic valve and persisting throughout diastole is seen in the left ventricular outflow tract in the parasternal long-axis, short-axis, or apical views. The color of the jet depends upon transducer location and jet orientation. From the apical views, the jet is predominantly red; however, from the parasternal views the color is variable. If the jet is directed toward the anterior mitral leaflet, as in the majority of cases, it will be a shade of blue. However,

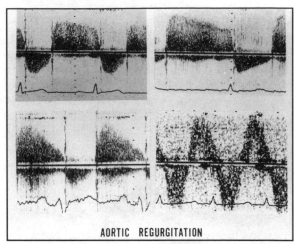

AORTIC REGURGITATION

Figure 6. *Doppler recordings from four patients with varying degrees of aortic insufficiency (AI). The top left, top right, and bottom left tracings are CW Doppler recordings from the apex. The tracing in the top left was recorded from a patient with mild AI. The deceleration slope is 1.8 m/sec. The deceleration slope seen on the top right is 3.2 m/sec, which corresponds with moderate AI. The bottom left recording was obtained from a patient with severe AI who required valve replacement. The downslope of the tracing in this patient is steep, 6.9 m/sec. The tracing on bottom right is a PW Doppler recording with the transducer at the suprasternal position and the sample volume in the descending aorta. The retrograde flow seen in diastole is almost equal to the forward flow in systole, consistent with severe AI.*

if the jet is directed toward the septum, a reddish hue will be seen.

Pulsed Doppler, CW Doppler, and color flow imaging can be used to grade the severity of aortic insufficiency. Pulsed Doppler sampling of the left ventricular outflow tract may be employed to "map" the jet. The farther from the aortic valve the jet is detected, the more severe the regurgitation. Grading systems have employed intracardiac landmarks for determination of severity; just beneath the valve is grade I; up to the tip of the anterior mitral leaflet is grade II; up to the papillary muscles is grade III; and beyond the papillary muscle level is grade IV. The problems with this method are that the technique may be time-consuming and tedious to perform accurately and the depth at which regurgitant flow is detected can vary with different sized ventricles. Additionally, antegrade mitral flow, especially in the presence of mitral stenosis or a mitral prosthesis, may contaminate the aortic regurgitation flow signal. For these reasons, other Doppler echocardiographic methods are preferable.

The ability to measure instantaneous gradients with CW Doppler has proven useful in assessing the severity of aortic insufficiency (Figure 6). Severe regurgitation tends to result in a rapid decrease in diastolic transvalvular pressure gradient. This relationship forms the basis for analysis of CW tracings. A steeper deceleration slope and shorter pressure half-time, both indicative of a more rapidly diminishing gradient between the aorta and left ventricle, are observed with increasing severity of aortic insufficiency (Masuyama et al.; Teague et al.; Labovitz et al.). It has been suggested that a slope of >2 m/sec and a pressure half-time of <400 m/sec indicate at least moderate aortic insufficiency, and a pressure half-time of <180 m/sec may represent very severe regurgitation. A drawback to quantification of aortic regurgitation in this manner is that properties of the ventricle may also affect the aortic-ventricular gradient and the flow velocity profile. Patients with elevated ventricular diastolic pressures for reasons other than aortic insufficiency, e.g., aortic stenosis, may have relatively steeper deceleration slopes and shorter pressure half-times; therefore, the gradient measurement method may overestimate the severity of regurgitation in these patients (Beyer et al.).

Color flow mapping, with the ability to visualize regurgitation jets, is an attractive method for gauging the severity of valvular insufficiency. Attempts to use the length and area of the jet in the ventricle, as recorded from the apical views, have proved less than satisfactory (Perry et al.; Smith et al.). Examination of the regurgitant jets in the parasternal views is useful. By comparing the height of the jet in the left ventricular outflow tract, as seen in the parasternal long-axis view, to the height of the outflow tract, one can accurately assess the severity of aortic insufficiency (Perry et al.). Likewise, the ratio between the area of the jet as visualized from the parasternal short-axis view and the area of the outflow tract also correlates well with the severity of regurgitation (Perry et al.; Baumgartner et al.). Though the grading system has yet to be precisely defined, data from one report support the following scheme: for the parasternal long-axis, a jet height/outflow-tract height ratio of $<25\%$ would signify grade I insufficiency, 25-46% grade II, 47-64% grade III, and $\geq65\%$ grade IV (Perry et al.). These cutoff points, while useful, have yet to be validated.

PULMONIC REGURGITATION

Mild regurgitation across the pulmonic valve is a common finding in healthy adults. It can be detected by pulsed or CW Doppler, as with aortic insufficiency, a holodiastolic flow is recorded. The flow profile recorded using CW Doppler is similar to that of aortic insufficiency, except that the accentuated decrease in velocity following atrial contraction is seen in patients in normal sinus rhythm. The peak velocities are lower than those recorded with aortic regurgitation, an expected finding because the gradient between the pulmonary artery and right ventricle in diastole is lower than that between the aorta and left ventricle. In healthy individuals, the peak diastolic velocity is <2 m/sec, although it is higher in patients with pulmonary hypertension. Pulmonic regurgitation is seen on color Doppler display as a red, candle flame-shaped jet emanating from the valve cusps. It can be visualized in the right ventricular outflow view and the parasternal short-axis view.

No system has been devised yet for grading pulmonic insufficiency, although regurgitant jets seen by PW Doppler or color Doppler that are restricted to 1 or 2 cm proximal to the pulmonic valve are considered within normal limits, and can be detected in the majority of healthy individuals (Yoshida et al.; Takao et al.). In patients with pathologic pulmonic regurgitation, the jets are wider and extend deeper into the right ventricle.

MITRAL REGURGITATION

All Doppler modalities have demonstrated excellent sensitivity and specificity for detecting mitral regurgitation (Quinones et al.; Abbasi et al.; Miyatake et al. 1986). With PW Doppler, only diastolic mitral flow is recorded when the sample volume is placed in the left atrium just above a normally functioning mitral valve; there is no systolic flow. In the presence of MR, a retrograde turbulent signal that aliases will be detected during systole. The full flow profile may be obtained with CW Doppler. As shown in Figure 8, it is characterized by a high peak velocity reaching 4-6 m/sec, reflecting the systolic pressure gradient across the mitral valve. The flow profile also appears symmetric and broad based, spanning both the isovolumic contraction and relaxation phases of the cardiac cycle. This serves as a useful feature to distinguish MR flow from aortic flow. With color flow Doppler, MR is readily identified as a bright systolic jet (be-

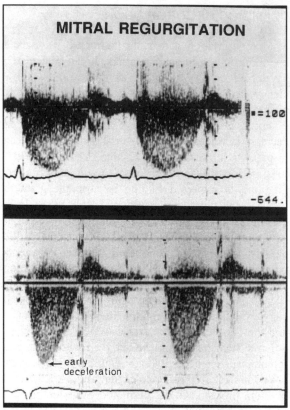

Figure 8. *Tracings obtained from two patients with mitral regurgitation. Note the symmetric contour of the top tracing. In contrast, the bottom tracing shows early deceleration, signifying a rapid decline in pressure gradient between the left ventricle and left atrium during systole that results from the precipitous rise in left atrial pressure. This is the correlate of the hemodynamic V wave.*

cause of its high velocity) spurting out from the mitral valve orifice and filling varying portions of the left atrial cavity. When the transducer is placed at the cardiac apex, the jet is blue (flow is oriented away from the transducer) and usually displays a mosaic pattern, reflecting the velocity spectrum variance within turbulent flow (Figure 9, p. *xix*).

There are several approaches for gauging MR severity. Quantitation of regurgitant volume is possible (Karen et al.) by subtracting forward systolic aortic flow from total mitral diastolic flow (flow estimates are the product of the flow velocity integral and the respective valvular cross-sectional areas, as previously discussed). The signal intensity and the deceleration rate of the CW-derived flow profile may also yield useful information. The most widely used ap-

proach, however, is a semiquantitative grading system using PW or color flow Doppler. With PW Doppler, the sample volume is systematically moved to explore various regions within the left atrial cavity to map out the size of the flow disturbance (Abbasi et al.). Grading is based on the maximum depth at which flow disturbance is detected within the left atrium. Although this approach has shown acceptable correlation with angiographic grading of MR, the technique requires the point-by-point mapping of the entire left atrium in multiple views; this can be time-consuming and may underestimate severity, especially when the jet is eccentric or clinging to an atrial wall, or overestimate severity when a narrow jet extends far into the left atrium.

Color flow Doppler allows direct observation of the dynamic features and orientation of a regurgitant jet and thus permits rapid and more precise evaluation of MR severity (Miytake et al. 1986; Helmcke et al.; Spain et al.). From multiple orthogonal views, the three-dimensional characteristics of the jet may be mentally reconstructed (Figure 9, p. *xix*). The best correlation with angiographic grading of MR is achieved when jet area, rather than length, is considered from multiple views, or when the ratio of jet area to cross-sectional left atrial area is utilized. A maximum jet area from multiple views measuring ≥ 8 cm^2 or a jet area-to-left atrial area ratio of $\geq 40\%$ indicates severe MR. A jet area measuring ≤ 4 cm^2 or a jet area-to-left atrial area ratio of $\leq 20\%$ indicates mild MR (Helmcke et al.; Spain et al.).

Several points should be considered when using the color Doppler approach to gauge MR severity. Factors other than regurgitation volume may influence jet area. Jets visualized with color Doppler are composed not only of regurgitant flows but also atrial blood displaced by the regurgitant flow, making it difficult to define the jet's precise boundaries. In addition, the effect of the interaction between incoming pulmonary venous flow and the regurgitant jet's velocity is not well known. Jet areas may also vary from one ultrasound machine to another depending on the respective converter algorithm and resolution (Bolger et al.). Other technical factors that influence jet area are sector size and gain-settings. These should be employed in as standardized a manner as possible by an experienced operator. Also, since the area of flow disturbance represents velocity data, it is subject to underestimation if the Doppler angle is large. This is not likely to represent a significant confounding factor, however, because multiple views are used and

MR flow velocity is high. Further, the precise measurement of the jet is less relevant than its mere detection in a given area. Despite these potential influences, the technique yields good correlations with angiography and serves as a very useful noninvasive means of detecting MR, gauging its severity, and following its progression over time.

TRICUSPID REGURGITATION

Tricuspid regurgitation may be diagnosed by the presence of a retrograde holosystolic flow disturbance proximal to the tricuspid valve. The spectral tracings observed are similar to those seen in mitral regurgitation, except the peak velocity recorded from tricuspid regurgitation is lower due to the lower pressure gradient between the right atrium and right ventricle in systole. Color Doppler images of tricuspid regurgitant jets also appear similar to images of mitral regurgitant jets, although the lower flow velocity of tricuspid insufficiency leads to less aliasing. Many views can be employed to detect tricuspid regurgitation, including the right ventricular inflow view, the parasternal short-axis view at the aortic valve level, the apical four- and five-chamber views, subcostally via the four-chamber or the short-axis view, and the right parasternal view. Flow is away from the transducer and is therefore depicted as "negative" on spectral tracings and blue on color imaging, although, when imaging subcostally or from the right thorax, this is not always the case.

When assessing the severity of triscuspid regurgitation, it should be kept in mind that, depending on age, from 15% to 80% of otherwise healthy individuals have tricuspid regurgitation detectable by Doppler (Yoshida et al.; Akasaka et al.). In general, tricuspid regurgitant flows detectable only in the vicinity of the tricuspid valve and with flow velocities in the range of 2.0-2.6 m/sec in the presence of a normal-sized right atrium are considered physiologic. Patients with more severe tricuspid regurgitation are identifiable by a regurgitant jet detected in a larger portion of the right atrium or by retrograde systolic flow in the hepatic vein (Figure 10). A regurgitant jet seen by color Doppler in greater than one third of the area of the right atrium is judged to necessitate tricuspid annuloplasty. As illustrated in Figure 10, in the presence of severe valvular pathology such as Ebstein's anomaly, carcinoid, or endocarditis, the profile of the regurgitant triscuspid jet may be of relatively low velocity (<3 m/sec) and may appear laminar in

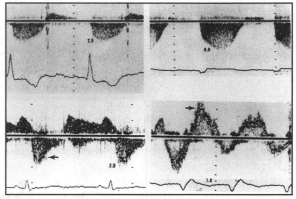

Figure 10. *Doppler recordings of tricuspid regurgitation. The tracing on top left was recorded from a patient with mild tricuspid regurgitation and normal right ventricular pressures. Peak velocity is 2.5 m/sec. The recording on top right is from a patient with tricuspid regurgitation. Peak velocity is 4 m/sec, corresponding to a 64 mm Hg systolic pressure gradient between the right ventricle and right atrium and indicating the presence of pulmonary hypertension. The bottom two tracings are recorded from a patient with severe tricuspid regurgitation secondary to carcinoid heart disease. The regurgitant orifice is large and right atrial pressure is markedly elevated, but right ventricular systolic pressure is only mildly elevated so the peak velocity is only 2 m/sec. Right atrial pressure rises rapidly, causing the flow velocity to decelerate rapidly (arrow). The bottom right tracing is a pulsed Doppler recording from the hepatic vein in the same patient. Severe tricuspid regurgitation causes retrograde systolic flow in the systemic veins (arrow).*

PW tracings. These findings signify a very large regurgitant orifice that blood can flow through without turbulence; in extreme cases, a functionally common right-sided chamber may be present (Hatle and Angelsen).

PROSTHETIC VALVES

The basic principles described for Doppler assessment of native valves apply to prosthetic valves as well. The normally functioning prosthetic valve differs from the native valve in that higher flow velocities are recorded across prosthetic valves in the absence of pathology. Transvalvular flow velocities of up to 4 m/sec have been recorded across normal prosthetic valves in the aortic position (Ramirez et al.; Sagar et al.; Panidis et al.). Despite high flow velocities, Doppler recordings of prosthetic valves differ from stenotic native valves in that peak velocity occurs earlier and the acceleration slope is steeper. There is a weak inverse correlation between peak velocity and valve size. In general, velocities and gradients are higher and observed valve areas lower for ball-in-cage valves, followed by bioprosthetic valves and disc valves. Gradients calculated by the Bernoulli equation and mitral valve areas calculated by the pressure half-time method correlate well with those obtained by catheterization (Cooper et al.; Alam et al.).

Regurgitation across prosthetic valves is common and is detectable by Doppler across many normally functioning valves. However, it is usually trivial or mild and limited to the vicinity of the prosthesis. Color Doppler has proven useful in the detection of pathologic prosthetic valve insufficiency, in that it is able to differentiate between transvalvular and paravalvular regurgitation. However, assessment of regurgitation by standard transthoracic echocardiography may be difficult in some patients because of reverberation artifact. While precordial Doppler examination has been shown to correctly diagnose prosthetic valvular regurgitation (Panidis et al.; Williams and Labovitz; Dittrich et al.), recent studies have shown transesophageal color Doppler echocardiography to be superior in this setting (Nellessen et al.; Taams et al.). Not only is the diagnosis and assessment of the severity of regurgitation more precise, but the differentiation between transvalvular and paravalvular regurgitation is made more accurately, especially when the prosthesis is in the mitral position. Transesophageal echocardiography is thus a useful adjunct to transthoracic echocardiography in the evaluation of prosthetic valve dysfunction.

INTRACARDIAC SHUNTS

Doppler plays a major role in the evaluation of acquired and congenital shunt flows (Stevenson). The detection of shunt flows has been greatly facilitated by the advent of the color flow Doppler. Figures 11 and 12 (pp. *xix–xx*) are examples of intracardiac shunt flows, which appear as jets originating on the one side of the interatrial or interventricular septum (where prestenotic acceleration of flow begins) and crossing the septum to reach the receiving chamber. Usually the direction of shunt flow is from left to right, except in cases where the normal left-to-right-sided pressure gradient is reversed. Although interatrial shunting may be seen in several views, the subcostal and modified

right-parasternal views, which allow parallel alignment of the ultrasound beam with shunt flow, are particularly useful (Figure 11). A PW Doppler recording of interatrial shunt flow may be obtained, with or without the guidance of color flow Doppler, by placing the sample volume within the shunt flow. Because the pressure difference between the right and left atria is relatively small, the interatrial shunt flow is low in velocity and thus must be differentiated from physiologic venous flows. The inferior vena caval, superior vena caval, and coronary sinus flow dynamics within the right atrium often may make the diagnosis of atrial-septal defect flows difficult. The latter, depicted in Figure 11, is characteristically continuous throughout the cardiac cycle, showing only minor variation with respiration when compared with caval flows.

Shunt flows across ventricular septal defects are evaluated in a similar manner. Membranous ventricular septal defects are easily seen in the parasternal long- and short-axis views. These lesions are characterized by systolic flow jets with a high velocity commensurate with the systolic pressure gradient across the interventricular septum. Shunt flow occurring between the aortic right sinus of Valsalva and the right ventricle is also high in velocity but occurs during both systole and diastole (Yokoi et al.). Shunt flow across a ductus arteriosus is best evaluated from the parasternal view, although visualization from the suprasternal window is also possible. This is a high-velocity flow occurring during systole and diastole.

All flows described thus far occur initially in a left-to-right direction. With progression over time, the elevation of right-sided pressures results in the reversal of shunt flow direction. The quantitative assessment of shunt size is based on the comparison of pulmonary and systemic flow rates (Qp:Qs). Right ventricular and left ventricular stroke volumes can be estimated noninvasively by calculating the product of the flow velocity integral obtained by PW Doppler and the cross-sectional areas of the right ventricular and left ventricular outflow tracts (Goldberg et al.; Sanders et al.)

Doppler-derived shunt flow ratio correlates well with calculations by other modalities but is subject to limitations due primarily to defining the precise borders of the right ventricular and left ventricular outflow tracts, and to a lesser extent, the recording of their flow measurements. It is important to note that the pulmonary-to-systemic ratio as calculated by any technique, whether invasive or noninvasive, is unreliable in the presence of significant valvular regurgitation.

The Doppler technique is useful not only for the detection of shunt flows and estimation of pulmonary-to-systemic flow ratio, but also for the detection and evaluation of concomitant congenital lesions, as well as the estimation of pulmonary artery systolic pressure using tricuspid regurgitant flow velocity. The hemodynamic information gained by the Doppler examination and the anatomic information gathered by the two-dimensional echo examination are complementary and provide a comprehensive evaluation of most patients with abnormal shunt flows.

ESTIMATION OF INTRACARDIAC PRESSURES

RIGHT VENTRICULAR AND PULMONARY ARTERIAL PRESSURE

An important use of Doppler is the hemodynamic analysis of the right heart. One way this can be done is by evaluating the characteristics of flow velocity in the pulmonary artery. There is an inverse correlation between acceleration time, defined as the interval between onset of flow and peak velocity, and pulmonary artery pressure. Patients with pulmonary hypertension, who have a mean pulmonary artery pressure >22 mm Hg, have acceleration times of <100 m/sec. The downslope of the velocity profile is also altered, with a small period of reacceleration sometimes evident. Other Doppler indices that have been shown to correlate well with pulmonary artery pressure are the interval between pulmonic valve closure and tricuspid valve opening and the ratio of the pre-ejection period to ejection time (Kitabatake et al.).

The most widely used method for estimation of right ventricular or pulmonary artery systolic pressure is analysis of the tricuspid regurgitation flow profile. As demonstrated in Figure 10, by measuring the peak velocity, pressure gradient can be calculated according to the Bernoulli equation (Yock and Popp; Currie et al.). Pulmonary artery systolic pressure can then be determined by adding an estimate of the right atrial pressure to the pressure gradient. The advantage to this method is the ease with which pulmonary arterial systolic pressure can be estimated from a spectral tracing. The tricuspid regurgitant profile can be enhanced by intravenous injection of agitated saline (Himelman et al.). Estimation of right atrial pressure

may lead to some error, but several methods have been proposed to minimize this problem (Yock and Popp; Currie et al.; Simonson and Schiller). In our laboratory, we estimate right atrial pressure as follows: if right atrial size is normal, right atrial pressure is estimated to be 5 mm Hg; if the right atrium is enlarged, 10 mm Hg; if the inferior vena cava is dilated as well, 15 mm Hg; and if inspiratory collapse is not evident in a dilated inferior vena cava, 20 mm Hg. Using the peak velocity of the tricuspid regurgitant profile to estimate pulmonary artery pressure allows for the acquisition of accurate, clinically relevant information without the need for invasive monitoring.

VENTRICULAR DIASTOLIC PRESSURE

Analysis of the pulmonary insufficiency profile also gives hemodynamic information. Peak diastolic velocity correlates well with mean pulmonary artery pressure; values >2 m/sec indicate pulmonary hypertension. End-diastolic velocity measured by Doppler correlates well with hemodynamic measurements of end-diastolic gradient between the pulmonary artery and right ventricle as well as the right ventricular end-diastolic pressure. Although the correlation is excellent, predicted values are consistently underestimated by this technique (Masuyama et al.). Nevertheless, a pulmonary regurgitant profile that exhibits a steep deceleration slope or premature cessation of flow is a reliable sign of elevated right ventricular end-diastolic pressure. Similarly, an aortic regurgitant profile with a steep deceleration slope or premature cessation of flow indicates elevated left ventricular end-diastolic pressure.

ASSESSMENT OF LEFT VENTRICULAR FUNCTION

SYSTOLIC FUNCTION

The aortic flow velocity curve can be used to assess left ventricular systolic function as well as stroke volume and cardiac output. In patients with left heart failure, decreases in peak velocity and acceleration have been described. The aortic tracing exhibits a more rounded form, with the peak velocity occurring later in systole (Hatle and Angelsen). A normal flow pattern, however, does not exclude the presence of a myopathic ventricle, and overlap between groups has been noted (Pandian et al. 1988; Gardin et al.). Continuous-wave Doppler tracings of mitral regurgitant jets can also supply information about left ventricular performance. The rate of rise in systolic pressure, or *dp/dt*, is reflected in the upslope of the mitral regurgitation tracing. Those patients with impaired systolic function, therefore, would have a more gradual upslope (Hatle and Angelsen).

DIASTOLIC FUNCTION

With increasing realization that left ventricular diastolic dysfunction can lead to symptoms of congestive heart failure, recent work has focused on mitral flow patterns to gain insight into this phenomenon. Several abnormalities in mitral flow patterns have been described, including alterations in the early filling velocity (E wave), atrial filling velocity (A wave) and the ratio of the former to the latter (E/A ratio). Other useful parameters are the isovolumic relaxation time, the period between aortic closure and mitral opening, and the deceleration time, or the interval between peak early velocity and cessation of flow. If the A wave commences before cessation of flow, the deceleration slope is extrapolated to baseline.

Figure 13 depicts the two basic patterns that have been described. The first pattern is seen in patients with ischemic heart disease, left ventricular hypertrophy, hypertrophic cardiomyopathy, and aortic stenosis, and is characterized by a lower peak E velocity,

increased atrial filling velocity, E/A ratio <1, a prolonged deceleration time, and a prolonged isovolumic relaxation time (Nishimura et al.). These changes have been attributed to impaired relaxation of the left ventricle, since patients with coronary disease who exhibit this pattern also have prolonged time constants of relaxation (Stoddard et al.). The other pattern results from restriction to filling, and consists of an elevated early velocity, decreased atrial filling velocity, a high E/A ratio, and shortened isovolumic relaxation and deceleration times (Nishimura et al.). This pattern is usually seen in patients with restrictive cardiomyopathy and constrictive pericarditis.

The precise diastolic abnormality cannot always be determined from the mitral flow velocity tracing, however. Progressive increases in left atrial pressure in patients with ischemic or dilated cardiomyopathy cause the mitral valve to open earlier, and the resulting higher early diastolic gradient leads to a higher E velocity. Therefore, despite prolonged relaxation as determined by hemodynamic recordings, the isovolumic relaxation time shortens, and the E/A ratio increases. The mitral flow tracing observed in this situation may change from the abnormal relaxation pattern to the restrictive pattern (Appleton et al. 1988b). There is an intermediate stage in this process during which the mitral flow profile may appear normal. This finding has been described in patients with chronic ischemic disease and also those with aortic stenosis and elevated end-diastolic pressures (Appleton et al.

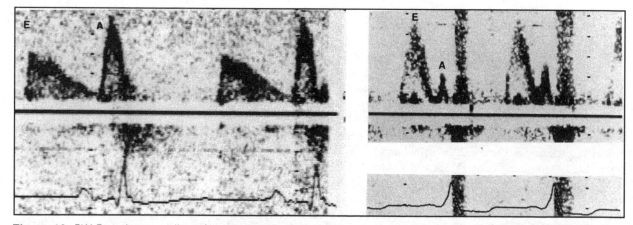

Figure 13. *PW Doppler recordings from two patients, with the sample volume placed at the tips of the mitral valve leaflets. The tracing on the left, from a patient with coronary artery disease, represents the abnormal isovolumic relaxation pattern, with a slow deceleration time of the E wave and an E/A ratio of <1. The recording on the right is from a patient with restrictive cardiomyopathy. Note the rapid downslope of the E wave and an E/A ratio of approximately 2:1.*

1988b; Gallino et al.). Prominent reversal of pulmonary venous flow during atrial systole may aid in recognizing such pseudo-normalization. Changes in mitral flow velocity that occur with elevation of diastolic pressures may be due to either intrinsic changes in ventricular compliance or a rightward shift along the pressure-volume curve induced by higher filling pressures. The mitral flow velocity profile has also been shown to change with age, heart rate, and loading conditions. Therefore, when evaluating mitral flow for evidence of diastolic dysfunction, the fact that diastole is a complex, multifactorial event should be considered.

ISCHEMIC HEART DISEASE

DETECTION OF ISCHEMIC HEART DISEASE

As mentioned, measurements of global left ventricular systolic function such as cardiac output and stroke volume can be measured by Doppler. Exercise-induced changes in the aortic flow velocity profile have been examined in the hope that changes in global LV function resulting from ischemia could be detected. While initial work suggested that aortic flow velocity falls during exercise in patients with coronary artery disease (Bryg et al.), later reports show that it may not. The increases in peak velocity and peak acceleration in patients with coronary disease, however, are often less than the increases seen in healthy individuals (Pandian et al. 1988; Harrison et al.). Aortic flow velocity is influenced by a number of other factors, such as changes in loading conditions and heart rate, and thus is not a useful parameter to detect ischemia.

The effects of ischemia on diastolic function have been discussed (Figure 13). Diminution of the E/A ratio occurs frequently during ischemia and is often noted in patients with myocardial infarction. Changes in the mitral flow pattern, however, cannot be used to reliably detect ischemic heart disease.

COMPLICATIONS OF ACUTE MYOCARDIAL INFARCTION

Doppler is extremely useful in the diagnosis of complications of acute myocardial infarction, namely, ventricular septal defect and acute mitral regurgitation. Prompt, accurate diagnosis is important, as these complications are life-threatening. The details of Doppler flow patterns in ventricular septal defect and mitral regurgitation have been discussed, but some differences may exist when these conditions complicate an acute myocardial infarction. Both are heralded by new murmurs. Early deceleration of the mitral regurgitant jet profile, indicative of a noncompliant left atrium, is highly suggestive of an acute increase in left atrial pressures (and a prominent v-wave) and may give a clue about the acuteness of the regurgitation (Hatle and Angelsen). Patients with acute, acquired, ventricular septal defects may have a low-velocity diastolic flow across the septum due to elevated left ventricular diastolic pressure, although the predominant flow is systolic (Hatle and Angelsen). Triphasic flow, consisting of a low-velocity mid-diastolic flow, a pre-systolic wave, and high-velocity systolic flow, has also been described (Bhatia et al.). Color flow Doppler is also useful for detection and localization of acquired ventricular septal defects and is especially useful in patients with serpiginous tracts through the interventricular septum (Amico et al.). Preliminary work also suggests that the area of the color jet correlates with the pulmonary-to-systemic flow ratio.

HYPERTROPHIC OBSTRUCTIVE CARDIOMYOPATHY

The presence of a subaortic obstruction can be detected by a high-velocity systolic jet directed away from the apex. This jet can be differentiated from that seen with aortic stenosis by the contour and relative time of the peak velocity. The typical tracing, as in Figure 14, is described as "dagger shaped," with a gradual early systolic upslope and a late systolic peak. The maximal instantaneous gradient derived from the peak systolic velocity indicates the severity of the intraventricular obstruction (Sasson et al. 1988). The peak velocity also occurs simultaneously with maximum septal contact of the anterior mitral leaflet in patients with systolic anterior motion of the mitral valve (Yock et al.).

The site of obstruction can be localized with pulsed Doppler by moving the sample volume within the left ventricle and noting the location of flow acceleration. Cessation of flow can be observed during mid-systole in patients with mid-ventricular obstruction when the pulse sample is placed at the point of cavity obliteration. Color flow mapping can locate the site as well. A narrow, mosaic flow pattern can be seen at the site of obstruction. These methods can be used to deter-

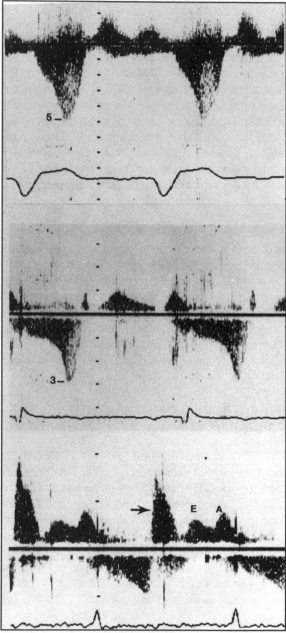

Figure 14. *CW Doppler recordings from the apex, illustrating altered flows in patients with hypertrophic or hyperdynamic ventricles. The top recording is from a patient with hypertrophic obstructive cardiomyopathy. The recording, with the Doppler beam aimed at the left ventricular outflow tract, exhibits the typical dagger-shaped appearance. Peak flow velocity is 5 m/sec. The patient from whom the middle tracing was recorded had a hyperdynamic ventricle without obstruction or hypertrophy. The increased flow velocity late in systole is presumably caused by obliteration of the outflow tract due to markedly in-*

mine if the obstruction is subaortic, mid-ventricular, or apical.

Diastolic flow abnormalities are also seen in the majority of patients with hypertrophic cardiomyopathy. The mitral flow pattern typically resembles the abnormal relaxation pattern, with an E/A ratio <1 and a prolonged deceleration time. An additional flow during the isovolumic relaxation period can be recorded. As shown in Figure 14, this flow is typically directed toward the apex and is believed to be due to an interventricular gradient caused by asynchronous relaxation (Sasson et al. 1987). Flow from apex to base during isovolumic relaxation has been described in patients with mid-cavity obstruction and is believed to be secondary to a residual post-systolic gradient between the apex and the basal portion of the ventricle (Zoghbi et al. 1988). It should be noted that the systolic and diastolic flow abnormalities described are not specific, and may be observed in the presence of a hyperdynamic ventricle or left ventricular hypertrophy with partial cavity obliteration in systole (Figure 14). Hypertrophic cardiomyopathy can be nonobstructive, so the absence of a systolic gradient does not exclude the diagnosis.

RESTRICTIVE CARDIOMYOPATHY

The hallmarks of restrictive cardiomyopathy are abnormal ventricular diastolic function, elevation of ventricular and atrial pressures, and a "dip and plateau" appearance to the ventricular pressure tracings. These findings are reflected in mitral and tricuspid recordings as a shortened isovolumic relaxation time, increased E velocity and E/A ratio, and decreased deceleration time (Figure 13). For tricuspid flows, inspiration is associated with an exaggeration of these abnormalities, but mitral flows are essentially unchanged throughout the respiratory cycle (Appleton et al. 1988a; Hatle et al. 1989). Diastolic mitral and tricuspid regurgitation, due to markedly elevated ventricular pressures, may be present. Marked elevations

creased systolic function. Note that the peak velocity occurs later in systole than it did in the example above. The bottom tracing illustrates exaggerated flow velocity during the isovolumic relaxation period (arrow). This can be observed in patients with hypertrophic cardiomyopathy or in the setting of a hyperdynamic ventricle with cavity obliteration. E=E wave; A=A wave.

in right ventricular end-diastolic pressure can be identified by the presence of antegrade flow across the pulmonic valve at end-diastole.

Examination of venous flow patterns may also be useful. Normally, the flow pattern recorded from systemic veins consists of a systolic and diastolic phase, with the systolic velocity slightly higher. In the presence of restrictive cardiomyopathy, systemic and pulmonary venous flow patterns exhibit higher flow velocities in diastole. Diastolic velocities in systemic veins increase with inspiration but are relatively constant in the pulmonary veins (Appleton et al. 1988a; Klein et al.). Systolic flow reversal is seen in the presence of severe tricuspid regurgitation. Additionally, atrial systole is accompanied by an exaggerated flow reversal in the pulmonary veins (Klein et al.). It should be noted that the above mentioned signs are seen in patients with symptomatic restrictive cardiomyopathy or those with advanced disease; early in the course of amyloidosis the mitral flow pattern may show an abnormal relaxation pattern (Klein et al.). Also, other disorders, namely, constrictive pericarditis, may be accompanied by similar Doppler findings. Thus, when evaluating for the presence of restrictive cardiomyopathy, clinical as well as two-dimensional echocardiographic and other findings play an important role.

CONSTRICTIVE PERICARDITIS

Constrictive pericarditis is associated with preserved systolic function and impairment of ventricular filling. The clinical, hemodynamic and Doppler findings of constrictive pericarditis and restrictive pericarditis may be similar, but differentiation is possible. Normally, intrathoracic and intracardiac pressures are altered to a similar degree throughout the respiratory cycle. In constrictive pericarditis, the abnormal pericardium acts as a buffer to changes in pressure, hence there is a dissociation between intrathoracic and intracardiac pressures with respiration. This dissociation is detected by variations in flow velocities with respiration, as illustrated in Figure 15 (Nishimura et al.). With inspiration, intrathoracic and pulmonary capillary wedge pressures decrease, yet ventricular pressures are unchanged. This leads to a decreased gradient between the pulmonary circulation and the left ventricle, so mitral flow velocity decreases. The reverse happens with expiration. Right-sided flow velocities vary in the opposite direction; tricuspid flow increases with inspiration and decreases with expi-

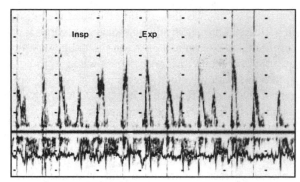

Figure 15. *PW Doppler recording of mitral inflow in a patient with calcific constrictive pericarditis. The flow velocity during inspiration (Insp) is at least 35% higher than during expiration (Exp). Similar changes with respiration, often to a greater degree, are seen in patients with tamponade.*

ration. While the typical atrioventricular flow pattern, high E velocity, rapid deceleration time, and increased E/A ratio are seen in both restrictive cardiomyopathy and constrictive pericarditis, these respiratory variations are seen only in the latter and are thus useful in differentiating the two (Hatle et al. 1989).

Evaluation of venous flow patterns is also useful. In constrictive pericarditis, the systolic component of systemic venous flow is greater than the diastolic component. An early, rapid deceleration with late systolic retrograde flow may be seen in this condition (Von Bibra et al.). Pulmonary venous flows in constrictive pericarditis exhibit predominant systolic flow during inspiration with equalization of systolic and diastolic flows during expiration, while a predominant diastolic flow occurs throughout the respiratory cycle in restrictive cardiomyopathy (Schiavone et al.). Other abnormalities, such as diastolic mitral and tricuspid regurgitation and end-diastolic antegrade flow across the pulmonic valve, can be seen in constrictive pericarditis, although they are more common in restrictive cardiomyopathy. Thus, the hemodynamic and physiologic differences between restrictive cardiomyopathy and constrictive pericarditis can be used to help differentiate the two.

CARDIAC TAMPONADE

The hemodynamic alterations seen in cardiac tamponade are caused by the pericardium exerting positive pressure on the cardiac chambers, resulting in impairment to ventricular filling. As in constrictive pericarditis, there is dissociation between alterations in pericardial pressures and pulmonary pressures with respiration. The gradient between the pulmonary circulation and the left heart decreases with inspiration, so the mitral flow velocity decreases as well. Respiratory changes in flow velocities, or "flow velocity paradoxus," has been observed across all four valves (Figure 15). Flow velocity decreases with inspiration and increases with expiration across the mitral and aortic valves; changes in the opposite direction are observed across the tricuspid and pulmonic valves (Leeman et al.; Appleton et al. 1988; King et al.). These changes are also detectable by color Doppler. The antegrade flow jet across the tricuspid valve appears larger with inspiration, and the mitral jet smaller. The magnitude as well as the presence of these respiratory variations in flow velocities are of diagnostic importance. In tamponade, respiratory changes in mitral velocity are at least 40%, with even greater changes seen in tricuspid velocities. Patients who have effusion without tamponade have lesser degrees of respiratory changes in flow velocity (Appleton et al. 1988). In addition to transvalvular flows, respiration affects flow velocities recorded from the superior vena cava. With expiration, there is a marked decrease or reversal in diastolic flow that is sometimes associated with decreased systolic flow (Appleton et al. 1988). The presence of these Doppler findings, in association with right ventricular diastolic collapse and right atrial collapse seen on 2D echocardiography, strongly indicates cardiac tamponade.

PROBLEMS AND PITFALLS

Doppler, like two-dimensional echocardiography, is very operator- and patient-dependent. Locating a jet, delineating it, determining its peak velocity, and correctly interpreting its importance require patience and skill. Several sites should be interrogated, often with the patient in different positions. Failure to be compulsive may result in inadequate or incorrect information. The Doppler beam must be as parallel to the flow jet interrogated as possible in order to obtain the maximal velocity. Image-guided transducers using color Doppler facilitate beam orientation. The location of the transducer and the timing of the flow in relation to the cardiac cycle should always be considered when interpreting a tracing. Also, when performing a study, it is important to know which modality of Doppler to use to get the information desired. Finally, as with other techniques, findings observed with Doppler must be interpreted in light of the entire clinical picture.

We thank our cardiac sonographers, Marjory E. Caldeira RDMS, Janet Simonetti BS, Brenda S. Kusay BS, and Teresa Murphy BS, for their valuable help with Doppler recordings. We are grateful to Mrs. Linda Wing for her excellent secretarial assistance.

Bibliography

Abbasi AS, Allen MW, DeCristofaro D, Ungar I: Detection and estimation of the degree of mitral regurgitation by range-gated pulsed Doppler echocardiography. *Circulation* 61:143, 1980.

Akasaka T, Yoshikawa J, Yoshida K, et al: Age-related valvular regurgitation: A study by pulsed Doppler echocardiography. *Circulation* 76:262, 1987.

Alam M, Rosman HS, Lakier JB, et al: Doppler and echocardiographic features of normal and dysfunctioning bioprosthetic valves. *J Am Coll Cardiol* 10:851, 1987.

Amico A, Iliceto S, Rizzo A, Cascella V, Rizzon P: Color Doppler findings in ventricular septal dissection following myocardial infarction. *Am Heart J* 117:195, 1989.

Appleton CP, Hatle LK, Popp RL: Cardiac tamponade and pericardial effusion: Respiratory variation in transvalvular flow velocities studied by Doppler echocardiography. *J Am Coll Cardiol* 11:1020, 1988.

Appleton CP, Hatle LK, Popp RL: Demonstration of restrictive ventricular physiology by Doppler echocardiography. *J Am Coll Cardiol* 11:757, 1988a.

Appleton CP, Hatle LK, Popp RL: Relation of transmitral flow velocity patterns to left ventricular diastolic function: New insights from a combined hemodynamic and Doppler echocardiographic study. *J Am Coll Cardiol* 12:426, 1988b.

Baumgartner H, Kratzer H, Helmreich G, Kuhn P: Quantitation of aortic regurgitation by colour coded cross-sectional Doppler echocardiography. *European Heart J* 9:380, 1988.

Berger M, Berdoff RL, Gallerstein PE, Goldberg E: Evaluation of aortic stenosis by continuous wave ultrasound. *J Am Coll Cardiol* 3:150, 1984.

Berger M, Hecht SR, Van Tosh A, Lingam U: Pulsed and continuous wave Doppler echocardiographic assessment of valvular regurgitation in normal subjects. *J Am Coll Cardiol* 13:1540, 1989.

Beyer RW, Ramirez M, Josephson MA, Shah PM: Correlation of continuous-wave Doppler assessment of chronic aortic regurgitation with hemodynamics and angiography. *Am J Cardiol* 60:852, 1987.

Bhatia SJS, Plappert T, Theard MA, St. John Sutton M: Transseptal Doppler flow velocity profile in acquired ventricular septal defect in acute myocardial infarction. *Am J Cardiol* 60:372, 1987.

Bolger A, Eigler N, Pfaff JM, Resser K, Maurer G: Computer analysis of Doppler color flow mapping images for quantitative assessment of in vitro fluid jets. *J Am Coll Cardiol* 12:450, 1988.

Bryg RJ, Labovitz AJ, Mehdirad AA, Williams GA, Chaitman BR: Effect of coronary artery disease on Doppler-derived parameters of aortic flow during upright exercise. *Am J Cardiol* 58:14, 1986.

Cooper DM, Stewart WJ, Schiavone WA, et al: Evaluation of normal prosthetic valve function by Doppler echocardiography. *Am Heart J* 114:576, 1987.

Currie PJ, Seward JB, Chan KL, et al: Continuous wave Doppler determination of right ventricular pressure: A simultaneous Doppler-catheterization study in 127 patients. *J Am Coll Cardiol* 6:750, 1985.

DeMaria AN, Bommer W, Joye J, et al: Value and limitations of cross-sectional echocardiography of the aortic valve in the diagnosis and quantification of valvular aortic stenosis. *Circulation* 62:304, 1980.

Dittrich H, Nicod P, Hoit B, Dalton N, Sahn D: Evaluation of Bjork-Shiley prosthetic valves by real-time two-dimensional Doppler echocardiographic flow mapping. *Am Heart J* 115:133, 1988.

Gallino RA, Milner MR, Goldstein SA, et al: Left ventricular filling patterns in aortic stenosis in patients older than 65 years of age. *Am J Cardiol* 63:1103, 1989.

Gardin JM, Iseri LT, Elkayam U, et al: Evaluation of dilated cardiomyopathy by pulsed Doppler echocardiography. *Am Heart J* 106:1057, 1983.

Godley RW, Green D, Dillon JC, et al: Reliability of two-dimensional echocardiography in assessing the severity of valvular aortic stenosis. *Chest* 79:657, 1981.

Goldberg SJ, Sahn DJ, Allen HD, et al: Evaluation of pulmonary and systemic blood flow by two-dimensional Doppler echocardiography using fast Fourier transform spectral analysis. *Am J Cardiol* 50:1394, 1982.

Griffith JM, Henry WL: An ultrasound system for combined cardiac imaging and Doppler blood flow measurement in man. *Circulation* 57:925, 1978.

Harrison MR, Smith MD, Friedman BJ, DeMaria AN: Uses and limitations of exercise Doppler echocardiography in the diagnosis of ischemic heart disease. *J Am Coll Cardiol* 10:809, 1987.

Hatle L, Angelsen B, Tromsdal A: Noninvasive assessment of atrioventricular pressure half-time by Doppler ultrasound. *Circulation* 60:1096, 1979.

Hatle L, Angelsen B: *Doppler Ultrasound in Cardiology: Physical Principles and Clinical Applications*. Philadelphia: Lea & Febiger; 1985.

Hatle L, Brubakk A, Tromsdal A, Angelsen B: Noninvasive assessment of pressure drop in mitral stenosis by Doppler ultrasound. *Br Heart J* 40:131, 1978.

Hatle LK, Appleton CP, Popp RL: Differentiation of constrictive pericarditis and restrictive cardiomyopathy by Doppler echocardiography. *Circulation* 79:357, 1989.

Helmcke F, Nanda NC, Hsiung MC, et al: Color Doppler assessment of mitral regurgitation with orthogonal planes. *Circulation* 75:175, 1987.

Himelman RB, Stulbarg M, Kircher B, et al: Noninvasive evaluation of pulmonary artery pressure during exercise by saline-enhanced Doppler echocardiography in chronic pulmonary disease. *Circulation* 79:863, 1989.

Holen J, Aaslid R, Landmark K, Simonsen S: Determination of pressure gradient in mitral stenosis with a noninvasive ultrasound Doppler technique. *Acta Med Scand* 199:455, 1976.

Karen G, Katz S, Strom J, Sonnenblick EH, LeJemtel TH: Non-invasive quantification of mitral regurgitation in dilated cardiomyopathy: Correlation of two Doppler echocardiographic methods. *Am Heart J* 116:758, 1988.

King SW, Pandian NG, Gardin JM: Doppler echocardiographic findings in pericardial tamponade and constriction. *Echocardiography* 5:361, 1988.

Kitabatake A, Inoue M, Masao M, et al: Noninvasive evaluation of pulmonary hypertension by a pulsed Doppler technique. *Circulation* 68:302, 1983.

Klein AL, Hatle LK, Burstow DJ, et al: Doppler characterization of left ventricular diastolic function in cardiac amyloidosis. *J Am Coll Cardiol* 13:1017, 1989.

Kremkau FW: Transducers and sound beams. In: *Diagnostic Ultrasound—Physical Principles and Exercises*. New York: Grune & Stratton; 1980, pp. 54–78.

Labovitz AJ, Ferrera RP, Kern MJ, et al: Quantitative evaluation of aortic insufficiency by continuous wave Doppler echocardiography. *J Am Coll Cardiol* 8:1341, 1986.

Leeman DE, Levine MJ, Come PC: Doppler echocardiography in cardiac tamponade: Exaggerated respiratory variation in transvalvular blood flow velocity integrals. *J Am Coll Cardiol* 11:572, 1988.

Masuyama T, Kodama K, Kitabatake A, et al: Continuous-wave Doppler echocardiographic detection of pulmonary regurgitation and its application to non-invasive estimation of pulmonary artery pressure. *Circulation* 74:484, 1986.

Masuyama T, Kodama K, Kitabatake A, et al: Noninvasive evaluation of aortic regurgitation by continuous-wave Doppler echocardiography. *Circulation* 73:460, 1986.

McDicken WN: Detection of motion by the Doppler effect. In: *Diagnostic Ultrasonics—Principles and Use of Instruments*. New York: Wiley; 1976, pp. 219–35.

Miyatake K, Izumi S, Okamoto M, et al: Semiquantitative grading of severity of mitral regurgitation by real-time two-dimensional Doppler flow imaging technique. *J Am Coll Cardiol* 7:82, 1986.

Miyatake K, Okamoto M, Kinoshita N, et al: Clinical application of a new type of real-time two-dimensional Doppler flow imaging system. *Am J Cardiol* 54:857, 1984.

Nellessen U, Schnittger I, Appleton CP, et al: Transesophageal two-dimensional echocardiography and color Doppler flow velocity mapping in the evaluation of cardiac valve prostheses. *Circulation* 78:848, 1988.

Nishimura RA, Abel MD, Hatle LK, Tajik AJ: Assessment of diastolic function of the heart: Background and current applications of Doppler echocardiography. Part II. Clinical studies. *Mayo Clin Proc* 64:181, 1989.

Nishimura RA, Tajik AJ: Determination of left-sided pressure gradients by utilizing Doppler aortic and mitral regurgitant signals: Validation by simultaneous dual catheter and Doppler studies. *J Am Coll Cardiol* 11:317, 1988.

Oh JK, Taliercia CP, Holmes DR Jr., et al: Prediction of the severity of aortic stenosis by Doppler aortic valve area determination: Prospective Doppler-catheterization correlation in 100 patients. *J Am Coll Cardiol* 11:1227, 1988.

Otto CM, Pearlman AS, Comess KA, et al: Determination of stenotic aortic valve area in adults using Doppler echocardiography. *J Am Coll Cardiol* 7:509, 1986.

Pandian NG, Kusay BS, Caldeira M, et al: Color Doppler flow imaging in cardiac diagnosis. *Echocardiography* 6:99, 1989.

Pandian NG, Thanikachalam S, Elangovan D, Caldeira ME, Salem DN: Color Doppler flow imaging in valvular stenosis. *Echocardiography* 4:515, 1987.

Pandian NG, Wang SS, Thanikachalam S: Role of Doppler echocardiography in ischemic heart disease. In: Kerber RE, ed. *Echocardiography in Coronary Artery Disease*. Mount Kisco: Futura; 1988, p. 259–80.

Panidis IP, Ross J, Mintz GS: Normal and abnormal prosthetic valve function as assessed by Doppler echocardiography. *J Am Coll Cardiol* 8:317, 1986.

Parris TM, Panidis IP, Ross J, Mintz GS: Doppler echocardiographic findings in rheumatic tricuspid stenosis. *Am J Cardiol* 60:1414, 1987.

Perry GJ, Helmcke F, Nanda NC, Byard C, Soto B: Evaluation of aortic insufficiency by Doppler color flow mapping. *J Am Coll Cardiol* 9:952, 1987.

Quinones MA, Young JB, et al: Assessment of pulsed Doppler echocardiography in detection and quantification of aortic and mitral regurgitation. *Br Heart J* 44:612, 1980.

Ramirez ML, Wong M, Sadler N, Shah PM: Doppler evaluation of bioprosthetic and mechanical aortic valves: Data from four models in 107 stable, ambulatory patients. *Am Heart J* 115:418, 1988.

Sagar KB, Wann LS, Paulsen WHJ, Romhilt DW: Doppler echocardiographic evaluation of Hancock and Bjork-Shiley prosthetic valves. *J Am Coll Cardiol* 7:681, 1986.

Sanders SP, Yeager S, Williams R: Measurement of sytemic and pulmonary blood flow and Qp:Qs ratio using Doppler and two-dimensional echocardiography. *Am J Cardiol* 51:952, 1983.

Sasson Z, Hatle L, Appleton CP, et al: Intraventricular flow during isovolumic relaxation: Description and characterization by Doppler echocardiography. *J Am Coll Cardiol* 10:539, 1987.

Sasson Z, Yock PG, Hatle LK, Alderman EL, Popp RL: Doppler echocardiographic determination of the pressure gradient in hypertrophic cardiomyopathy. *J Am Coll Cardiol* 11:752, 1988.

Schiavone WA, Calafiore PA, Salcedo EE: Transesophageal Doppler echocardiographic demonstration of pulmonary venous flow velocity in restrictive cardiomyopathy and constrictive pericarditis. *Am J Cardiol* 63:1286, 1989.

Simonson JS, Schiller NB: Sonospirometry: A new method for noninvasive estimation of mean right atrial pressure based on two-dimensional echographic measurements of the inferior vena cava during measured inspiration. *J Am Coll Cardiol* 11:557, 1988.

Skjaerpe T, Hegrenaes L, Hatle L: Noninvasive estimation of valve area in patients with aortic stenosis by Doppler ultrasound and two-dimensional echocardiography. *Circulation* 72:810, 1985.

Smith MD, Grayburn PA, Spain MG, et al: Observer variability in the quantitation of Doppler color flow jet areas for mitral and aortic regurgitation. *J Am Coll Cardiol* 11:579, 1988.

Spain MG, Smith MD, Grayburn PA, Harlamert EA, DeMaria AN: Quantitative assessment of mitral regurgitation by Doppler color flow imaging: Angiographic and hemodynamic correlations. *J Am Coll Cardiol* 13:585, 1989.

Stamm RB, Martin RP: Quantification of pressure gradients across stenotic valves by Doppler ultrasound. *J Am Coll Cardiol* 2:707, 1983.

Stevenson JG: Echo Doppler analysis of septal defects. In: Peronneau P, Diebold B, ed. *Cardiovascular Application of Doppler Echocardiography*. Paris: Inserm; 1983, p. 515.

Stoddard MF, Pearson AC, Kern MJ, et al: Left ventricular diastolic function: Comparison of pulsed Doppler echocardiographic and hemodynamic indexes in subjects with and without coronary artery disease. *J Am Coll Cardiol* 13:327, 1989.

Taams MA, Gussenhoven EJ, Cahalan MK, et al: Transesophageal Doppler color flow imaging in the detection of native and Bjork-Shiley mitral valve regurgitation. *J Am Coll Cardiol* 13:95, 1989.

Takao S, Miyatake K, Izumi JS, et al: Clinical implications of pulmonary regurgitation in healthy individuals: Detection by cross-sectional pulsed Doppler echocardiography. *Br Heart J* 59:542, 1988.

Teague SM, Heinsimer JA, Anderson JL, et al: Quantification of aortic regurgitation utilizing continuous wave Doppler ultrasound. *J Am Coll Cardiol* 8:592, 1986.

von Bibra H, Schober K, Jenni R, et al: Diagnosis of constrictive pericarditis by pulsed Doppler echocardiography of the hepatic vein. *Am J Cardiol* 63:483, 1989.

Wells PNT: Fundamental physics. In: *Physical Principles of Ultrasonic Diagnosis*. London: Academic Press; 1969, pp. 1–27.

Williams GA, Labovitz AJ: Doppler hemodynamic evaluation of prosthetic (Starr-Edwards and Bjork-Shiley) and bioprosthetic (Hancock and Carpentier-Edwards) cardiac valves. *Am J Cardiol* 56:325, 1985.

Yock PG, Hatle L, Popp RL: Patterns and timing of Doppler-detected intracavitary and aortic flow in hypertrophic cardiomyopathy. *J Am Coll Cardiol* 8:1047, 1986.

Yock PG, Popp RL: Noninvasive estimation of right ventricular systolic pressure by Doppler ultrasound in patients with tricuspid regurgitation. *Circulation* 70:657, 1984.

Yokoi K, Kambe T, Ichimiya S, et al: Ruptured aneurysm of the right sinus of Valsalva: Two pulsed Doppler echocardiographic studies. *J Clin Ultrasound* 9:505, 1981.

Yoshida K, Yoshikawa J, Shakudo M, et al: Color Doppler evaluation of valvular regurgitation in normal subjects. *Circulation* 78:840, 1988.

Zoghbi WA, Farmer KL, Soto JG, Nelson JG, Quinones MA: Accurate noninvasive quantification of stenotic aortic valve area by Doppler echocardiography. *Circulation* 73:452, 1986.

Zoghbi WA, Haichin RN, Quinones MA: Mid-cavity obstruction in apical hypertrophy: Doppler evidence of diastolic intraventricular gradient with higher apical pressure. *Am Heart J* 116:1469, 1988.

CHAPTER 9

Cardiac Catheterization

L. David Hillis
Richard A. Lange
Ricardo G. Cigarroa

Since its inception in the 1940s, cardiac catheterization has played an important role in the understanding of cardiac and circulatory physiology and pathophysiology and in the diagnosis of assorted cardiac abnormalities. More recently, it has been used with increasing frequency as a therapeutic procedure in patients with valvular abnormalities and atherosclerotic coronary artery disease (CAD). During its early years, catheterization was performed sparingly and with substantial risk. Over time, however, it has become established throughout the world, and the associated morbidity and mortality have fallen drastically. Today, diagnostic cardiac catheterization is performed with only minimal risk, and therapeutic catheterization (i.e., coronary angioplasty and valvuloplasty) is performed without incident in the vast majority of patients. Therefore, cardiac catheterization now plays a vital role in the *diagnostic* evaluation of the patient with suspected cardiac disease; at the same time, it offers increasingly sophisticated *therapeutic* possibilities in these individuals.

INDICATIONS AND CONTRAINDICATIONS

Diagnostic cardiac catheterization is appropriate in several clinical circumstances. First, it is indicated to confirm or exclude the presence of a condition already suspected because of findings on physical examination or noninvasive evaluation. In such a circumstance, it allows the establishment of the presence of cardiac disease as well as its severity. Second, catheterization is indicated to clarify a confusing or obscure clinical problem, that is, to arrive at a diagnosis in a patient whose clinical presentation and noninvasive evaluation are inconclusive. Third, with only rare exceptions, catheterization should be performed in all patients for whom corrective cardiac surgery is contemplated, in order to confirm the suspected abnormality and to exclude associated defects that might require the surgeon's attention. Fourth, cardiac catheterization is occasionally performed purely as a research procedure.

Therapeutic cardiac catheterization is indicated in the patient with symptomatic CAD (in the case of coronary angioplasty) whose coronary anatomy is believed to be suitable for the procedure. Aortic or mitral valvuloplasty is indicated in the individual with symptomatic aortic or mitral stenosis in whom corrective surgery may offer an unfavorable risk:benefit ratio, due, for example, to advanced age or concomitant disease (such as chronic pulmonary, hepatic, or renal disease or an underlying malignancy).

Catheterization is absolutely contraindicated if a mentally competent individual does not consent. It is relatively contraindicated if an intercurrent condition exists which, if corrected, would improve the safety of the procedure. Examples of such conditions include ventricular irritability, uncontrolled cardiac failure, digitalis toxicity, electrolyte imbalance, high fever, severe anemia, hypovolemia, uncontrolled systemic arterial hypertension, and an uncontrolled bleeding diathesis.

TECHNIQUES OF CARDIAC CATHETERIZATION

Catheterization of the right and left sides of the heart can be accomplished by the introduction of catheters either by direct vision (into the brachial vein and artery) or by percutaneous puncture (of the femoral vein and artery). In the brachial approach, local anesthetic is introduced into an area 3–4 cm in diameter 1–2 cm above the flexor crease of the arm, after which a transverse cutdown is performed. If both right- and left-heart catheterization is planned, the incision should be wide (2–3 cm in length) and located over the brachial artery; if only right-heart catheterization is contemplated, a small incision can be made directly over a medial vein. Once the skin incision is made, the subcutaneous tissues are separated by blunt dissection with a curved hemostat, and the vein and artery are isolated, separated from adjacent tissues, and tagged. The catheters are introduced under direct vision and are advanced into the great vessels and heart.

Following catheterization by the brachial approach, the catheters are removed, and the vein used for right-heart catheterization is ligated. The artery used for left-heart catheterization is cleaned and rendered free of thrombi, and the arteriotomy is repaired. After the arteriotomy is closed and blood flow restored to the distal arm, the wound is flushed with saline, the incision is sutured, and the site of the cutdown is dressed.

To use the percutaneous femoral approach, local anesthetic is introduced into an area 3–4 cm in diameter 1–2 cm below the inguinal crease. A small incision (about 0.5 cm long) is made over the vessels to be used for catheter introduction and passage, after which a "tunnel" is constructed with a straight hemostat from the skin incision to the desired femoral vessel. An 18-gauge needle (Seldinger needle) is introduced through the skin incision and tunneled at a 30–45° angle into the lumen of the femoral artery or vein. Once there is free blood flow through the needle, a guide wire is advanced into the lumen of the punctured vessel. The wire is held firmly in place as the needle is removed. Then, with the wire in the vessel, a catheter is threaded onto it and into the vessel lumen, and the wire is removed.

Following catheterization by this approach, the catheters are removed, and hemostasis is achieved by hand pressure over the puncture site until bleeding stops; this is usually achieved after pressure has been placed on the femoral vein for 5–10 minutes and on the femoral artery for 15–20 minutes. Subsequently, the patient must remain in bed with the involved leg immobilized for 12–24 hours.

The choice of approach (brachial or femoral) for both venous and arterial catheterization is determined by the preference and experience of the cardiologist and by the anatomic and pathophysiologic abnormalities of the patient. In general, right-heart catheterization is easier via the brachial approach in the patient with right ventricular and right atrial dilatation. In contrast, right-heart catheterization is performed preferentially via the femoral approach in the patient with a suspected secundum atrial septal defect. Thus, in choosing the route for right-heart catheterization, it is necessary to know anatomic abnormalities and specific disease entities. In most patients, left-heart catheterization can be performed by either the brachial or femoral approach. Certain conditions make it difficult to perform left-heart catheterization by the femoral approach, such as extensive peripheral vascular disease, severe obesity, severe systemic arterial hypertension, bleeding diatheses, and any disorder that causes a markedly augmented arterial pulse pressure (e.g., severe aortic regurgitation). In turn, the brachial approach for left-heart catheterization is relatively contraindicated if there is evidence of severe brachiocephalic arterial disease.

In most catheterization laboratories, the brachial or femoral approach is used in almost all procedures. Occasionally, catheterization of one or more cardiac chambers is necessary via another route. For example, a rare patient with severe left-sided valvular disease may require a direct puncture of the left ventricle to measure left ventricular pressure and to perform a ventriculogram.

HEMODYNAMIC MEASUREMENTS

CARDIAC OUTPUT

The role of the heart is to deliver an adequate quantity of blood to the body. This flow of blood is known as the cardiac output (CO) and is expressed in liters per minute. Since the magnitude of CO is proportional to body surface area, one person may be compared to another by means of the cardiac index (CI), the CO adjusted for body surface area. The normal CI is 2.6 L/min/m^2 of body surface (Table 1).

There are two major methods of measuring CO: the Fick method and the indicator dilution technique. The latter can be performed by the injection of indocyanine green or by the thermodilution technique.

Fick Method

The measurement of CO by the Fick method is based on the hypothesis that the uptake or release of a substance by an organ is the product of the blood flow to that organ and the regional arteriovenous (AV) concentration difference of the particular substance.

Table 1. Normal Hemodynamic Values

Flows	
Cardiac index (L/min/m²)	2.6–4.2
Stroke volume index (ml/m²)	30–65
Pressures (mm Hg)	
Systemic arterial	
Peak systolic/end-diastolic	100-140/60-90
Mean	70–105
Left ventricle	
Peak systolic/end-diastolic	100-140/3-12
Left atrium (PCW)	
Mean	1–10
a-wave	3–15
v-wave	3–15
Pulmonary artery	
Peak systolic/end-diastolic	16-30/0-8
Mean	10–16
Right ventricle	
Peak systolic/end-diastolic	16-30/0-8
Right atrium	
Mean	0–8
a-wave	2–10
v-wave	2–10
Resistances	
Systemic vascular resistance	
Dynes-sec-cm⁻⁵	770–1500
Resistance units	10–20
Pulmonary vascular resistance	
Dynes-sec-cm⁻⁵	20–120
Resistance units	0.25–1.5
Oxygen consumption (ml/min/m²)	110–150
AV O₂ difference (ml/100 ml)	3.0–4.5

PCW = pulmonary capillary wedge; AV = arteriovenous.

volume of this collection is measured, and the difference in O_2 content between inspired and expired air is calculated. From these data, the person's O_2 consumption (in ml/min) is determined. Determining the AV O_2 difference across the lungs requires that blood from the vessels adjacent to the lungs (i.e., the pulmonary artery and vein) be analyzed for O_2 content. Since the saturation of pulmonary venous blood is similar to that of systemic arterial blood, pulmonary arterial and systemic arterial samples are usually obtained for the Fick determination of CO. The O_2 content of pulmonary and systemic arterial blood may be measured directly or calculated from the O_2 saturation of the blood: O_2 content = Hgb (in g/100 ml) $\times$ 1.39 $\times$ saturation, where 1.39 ml is the maximum O_2-carrying capacity of 1 g of Hgb.

The normal O_2 consumption index (O_2 consumption/m² of body surface) is 110–150 ml/min/m² (Table 1). In general, the O_2 consumption is slightly higher in young people than in the elderly. It increases with hyperthyroidism, hyperthermia, and exercise and decreases with hypothyroidism and hypothermia. The normal AV O_2 difference is 3.0–4.5 volumes percent (ml O_2/100 ml of blood).

The following is an example of the Fick calculation of CO: (1) O_2 consumption = 250 ml/min; (2) Hgb = 15 g/100 ml; (3) systemic arterial O_2 saturation = 0.95 (95%); (4) pulmonary arterial O_2 saturation = 0.70 (70%); (5) 10 = dl/L.

$$CO = \frac{250}{(15)(1.39)(10)(0.95) - (15)(1.39)(10)(0.70)}$$
$$= \frac{250}{198.1 - 145.9} = 4.78 \text{ L/min}$$

The Fick method has several potential sources of error: (1) An incomplete collection of expired air causes an underestimation of O_2 consumption, leading to a falsely low figure for CO. This is the most common source of error. (2) Incorrect timing of the expired air collection leads to a faulty estimate of O_2 consumption. (3) The Douglas bag analysis should be performed soon after its collection, since air diffuses in and out of the bag if there is a substantial delay. (4) The spectrophotometric determination of O_2 saturations in the blood samples may be inaccurate if certain substances, such as indocyanine green, have been introduced into the blood. (5) The mixed venous blood sample (pulmonary arterial) must, indeed, be *mixed venous*. It must be obtained from the pulmonary artery, not from a systemic vein, right atrium, or right

To measure CO in humans, this principle is applied to the lungs, and the substance measured is oxygen. By measuring the amount of O_2 extracted from inspired air by the lungs and the AV O_2 difference across the lungs, pulmonary blood flow may be calculated. Since pulmonary blood flow equals systemic blood flow in most people, the Fick method allows one to measure systemic blood flow.

The Fick formula for the calculation of CO is:

$$CO \text{ (L/min)} = \frac{O_2 \text{ consumption (ml/min)}}{AV \text{ } O_2 \text{ difference across the lungs}}$$

The O_2 consumption is determined directly by collecting a timed sample (usually 3–4 min) of expired air in a special receptacle called a Douglas bag. The ventricle; and it must not be partially contaminated by pulmonary capillary wedge blood.

The average error in determining O_2 consumption is about 6%, and the error in AV O_2 difference is 5%. When the AV O_2 difference is small, errors in measurement are particularly likely to occur. Therefore, the Fick method is most accurate in the patient with a low CO and least accurate in one with a high CO.

Indicator Dilution Technique

This technique is based on the principle that the volume of fluid within a container can be measured if one adds a known quantity of indicator to the fluid and then measures the concentration of the indicator after it has been completely mixed with the fluid. The indicator most often used is indocyanine green, an easily detectable, water-soluble, nontoxic substance. To measure CO using indocyanine green, a known concentration of indicator must be injected, and there must be complete mixing of the indocyanine green between the sites of injection and sampling. In most catheterization laboratories, CO is measured by injecting indocyanine green into the pulmonary artery while blood is withdrawn at a constant rate from a systemic artery through an optical densitometer. The lungs, left atrium, and left ventricle act as adequate mixing sites, and there is no degradation of indocyanine green between the pulmonary and systemic arteries.

More recently, cold saline or 5% dextrose-in-water have been used as indicators to measure CO. The catheter used for this measurement is a balloon-tipped, flow-directed, polyvinylchloride catheter with two openings, one at the tip and the other 25–30 cm proximal to the tip. In addition, a small thermistor is located 2–5 cm from the tip. This catheter is inserted into a vein and advanced to the pulmonary artery. Thus, the distal opening is in a large pulmonary artery, and the proximal opening is in the right atrium. Iced fluid is injected into the right atrial opening, and the temporary change in temperature at the thermistor is recorded.

The calculation of CO by the indicator dilution technique is usually done by a minicomputer, which establishes that the downslope of the inscribed curve is exponential and then computes the area under the curve, while excluding the recirculation peak. These calculations can be done manually but require a clear mathematical separation of the initial circulation peak from that of normal recirculation.

With both indocyanine green and cold saline or dextrose, therefore, CO can be determined by assessing the concentration of an indicator after adequate mixing with blood has occurred. To insure an accurate assessment of CO, great care must be taken, first, to inject an exact amount of indicator; second, to inject the indicator as rapidly as possible (so that it is actually delivered as a bolus); third, to calibrate the densitometer and recorder systems precisely; and fourth, to insure that the withdrawal of blood (in the case of indocyanine green) at the sampling site is uniform and not accompanied by air bubbles. If care is taken to eliminate these sources of error, the indicator dilution technique is a reliable method of measuring CO. This technique is most accurate for individuals with a high CO. It is least accurate in those with a low CO and in those with valvular regurgitation between the sites of indicator injection and sampling (i.e., tricuspid or pulmonic regurgitation with thermodilution, aortic or mitral regurgitation with indocyanine green).

PRESSURE MEASUREMENTS

One of the most important functions of cardiac catheterization is the accurate measurement and recording of intracardiac pressures. Once a catheter has been positioned in the desired cardiac chamber, it is connected either directly or through stiff, fluid-filled tubing to a pressure transducer, which transforms a pressure signal into an electrical signal. The accurate measurement of pressures requires close attention to the details of the catheter-transducer system, including proper transducer balancing as well as removing air bubbles from the catheters and connections. Errors in pressure measurement may occur in several ways. An accurate zero reference is essential. All manometers must be referenced to the same zero level, which must be changed if the patient's position is altered. Pressure transducers must be calibrated frequently, preferably before each pressure recording.

During most catheterizations, pressures are measured directly from each of the cardiac chambers except the left atrium. A direct pressure measurement is obtained with a catheter in the right atrium, right ventricle, pulmonary artery, ascending aorta, and left ventricle. In contrast, the left atrium is seldom entered unless a transseptal catheterization is performed (passage of a catheter from the right atrium across

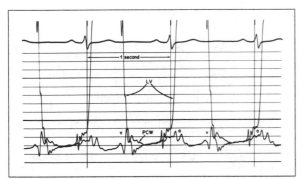

Figure 1. *Simultaneous recording of left ventricular (LV) and pulmonary capillary wedge (PCW) pressures in a patient without mitral valve disease. The distance between each horizontal line above the baseline represents 4 mm Hg, and the distance between each vertical line represents 1 sec. The PCW a-wave occurs in conjunction with the a-wave of the LV pressure trace, and the PCW v-wave occurs with the downslope of the LV trace. Note that during diastole the LV and PCW pressures are superimposed; that is, there is no pressure gradient between the PCW and LV.*

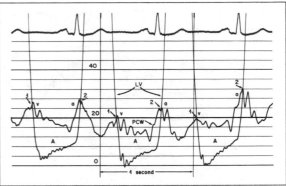

Figure 2. *Simultaneous recording of LV and PCW pressures in a patient with mitral stenosis. Throughout diastole, from points 1 to 2, there is a pressure gradient between the PCW and LV pressures. The patient, a 28-year-old woman, had a cardiac output of 3,740 ml/min, measured simultaneously with this pressure tracing. The heart rate was 68 beats/min, the mean diastolic filling period was 0.49 sec/beat, and the mean pressure gradient, derived by dividing A by the average gradient duration, was 12.7 mm Hg. Using the Gorlin formula, the mitral valve area was*

$$\frac{3740/(68)(0.49)}{(38)(\sqrt{12.7})} = 0.82 \ cm^2$$

the interatrial septum into the left atrium). The left atrial pressure is generally recorded "indirectly," that is, as the pulmonary capillary wedge pressure. To accomplish this, an end-hole catheter is placed in the pulmonary artery and advanced into the pulmonary arterial tree until it is effectively wedged. If the catheter is wedged adequately, the resulting pressure is left atrial in origin, and the blood withdrawn from it is fully saturated. The demonstration that fully saturated blood can be withdrawn from the catheter confirms that the pressure is indeed left atrial.

In addition to the recording of pressures from each of the cardiac chambers, it is important that the pressures from certain chambers be examined simultaneously to confirm or exclude the presence of valvular lesions. Thus, left ventricular and pulmonary capillary wedge pressures should be recorded simultaneously to ascertain if mitral stenosis is present (Figures 1 and 2). Likewise, the left ventricular and systemic arterial pressures should be displayed concurrently to evaluate the presence or absence of left ventricular outflow tract obstruction (Figures 3–5).

Recording intracardiac and peripheral vascular pressures can demonstrate hemodynamic evidence of valvular regurgitation. For instance, large regurgitant waves in the pulmonary capillary wedge tracing may

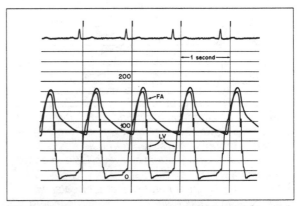

Figure 3. *Simultaneous recording of LV and femoral arterial (FA) pressures in a patient without LV outflow tract obstruction. Pressures are indicated in mm Hg on the vertical scale. Note that there is no pressure gradient during systole between LV and FA; in fact, the peak systolic FA pressure is about 5 mm Hg higher than LV. See Figure 4 for an explanation of this phenomenon.*

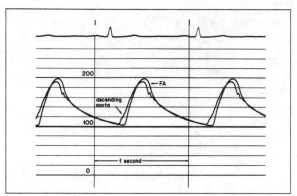

Figure 4. *Simultaneous recording of ascending aortic and FA pressures in a normal individual. The peak systolic FA pressure is slightly higher than the peak systolic ascending aortic pressure, due to peripheral amplification of pressure, a normal phenomenon.*

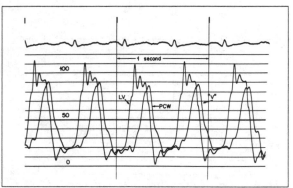

Figure 6. *Simultaneous recording of LV and PCW pressures from a patient with severe, acute mitral regurgitation due to an inferior myocardial infarction with resulting papillary muscle rupture. Note that there is no gradient between LV and PCW during diastole. However, the PCW tracing demonstrates large regurgitant v-waves as high as 90 mm Hg.*

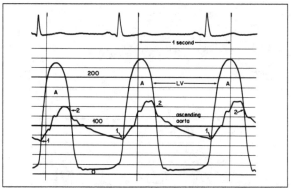

Figure 5. *Simultaneous recording of LV and ascending aortic pressures in a patient with severe aortic stenosis. Throughout systole, from points 1 to 2, there is a pressure gradient between LV and aorta. The patient, a 50-year-old man, had a cardiac output of 3,350 ml/min, a heart rate of 62 beats/min, a mean systolic ejection time of 0.36 sec/beat, and a mean pressure gradient throughout systole of 83 mm Hg, determined by dividing A by the average duration of the gradient. Thus, the aortic valve area equals*

$$\frac{3350/(62)(0.36)}{(44.5)(\sqrt{83})} = 0.37 \text{ cm}^2$$

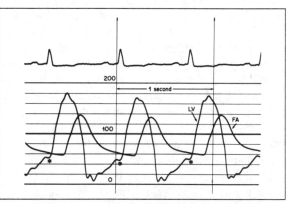

Figure 7. *Simultaneous recording of LV and FA pressures from a patient with mixed aortic stenosis and regurgitation. The FA upstroke occurs later than that of the LV, due to the time required for pulse wave transmission from the LV to the FA. There is a systolic gradient between LV and FA of about 40 mm Hg peak to peak. The FA pulse pressure is only minimally widened. During diastole, the LV pressure demonstrates a gradual and steady rise, so that the LV pressure at end-diastole (*) is about 50 mm Hg.*

indicate severe mitral regurgitation (Figure 6). Conversely, a wide peripheral arterial pulse pressure in conjunction with a greatly elevated left ventricular end-diastolic pressure suggests aortic regurgitation (Figure 7). In short, both the absolute level and the qualitative configuration of the intracardiac and peripheral vascular pressures are important in the diagnosis and quantitation of valvular heart disease.

The normal intracardiac and peripheral vascular flows, pressures, and resistances are listed in Table 1.

RESISTANCES

The resistance of a vascular bed can be calculated by dividing the pressure gradient across the bed by the flow through it. Thus,

systemic vascular resistance =

$$\frac{\text{mean systemic arterial pressure} - \text{mean right atrial pressure}}{\text{systemic blood flow}}$$

and

pulmonary vascular resistance =

$$\frac{\text{mean pulmonary arterial pressure} - \text{mean pulmonary venous pressure}}{\text{pulmonary blood flow}}$$

Resistances are expressed in either resistance units (mm Hg/L/min) or dynes-sec-cm^{-5} (resistance unit determination × 80). The normal values for vascular resistances are displayed in Table 1.

An increased systemic vascular resistance is usually present in patients with systemic arterial hypertension. It may also be seen in the patient with a reduced forward CO and compensatory arteriolar vasoconstriction. In turn, a reduced systemic vascular resistance may be present in the patient with an inappropriately increased CO, the causes of which include AV fistula, severe anemia, high fever, and thyrotoxicosis. An elevated pulmonary vascular resistance may be present because of primary lung disease, Eisenmenger's syndrome (alterations in the pulmonary vasculature in response to increased pulmonary blood flow), and a greatly elevated pulmonary venous pressure due to left-sided myocardial or valvular dysfunction.

VALVE AREAS

Through the application of standard fluid dynamic principles, the resistance to blood flow through a stenosed valve can be expressed as a valve orifice area. The data required for the calculation of a valve area may be obtained during cardiac catheterization. Specifically, the pressures on either side of a stenotic valve and the flow across it must be known. The Gorlin equation is then used to calculate the valve area.

$$\text{Valve area} = \frac{\text{CO/(DFP or SEP)(heart rate)}}{\text{(constant)}(\sqrt{\text{mean pressure gradient}})}$$

where DFP = diastolic filling period, and SEP = systolic ejection period. If an atrioventricular valve (mitral or tricuspid) is in question, the diastolic filling period is employed; if the aortic or pulmonic valve is involved, the systolic ejection period is used. The constant used is 38 for the mitral valve and 44.5 for the other valves. The mean pressure gradient is the average gradient throughout systole (for aortic and pulmonic valves) or diastole (for mitral or tricuspid valves). Note that the square root of the mean pressure gradient is used in the calculation.

The normal mitral valve orifice is 3-5 cm^2. Substantial stenosis can develop before a pressure gradient appears. A mitral valve with an area of 0–1.0 cm^2 is considered severely stenotic (Figure 2); 1.0–1.5 cm^2, moderately stenotic; and 1.5–2.0 cm^2, mildly stenotic. A valve area >2.0 cm^2 is not necessarily normal but does not usually represent a hemodynamically significant obstruction to blood flow. The normal aortic valve has a cross-sectional area of 3–4 cm^2, but hemodynamically important aortic stenosis does not develop until the valve area becomes <1.1–1.2 cm^2. Specifically, an aortic valve with an area of <0.7 cm^2 is severely stenotic (Figure 5); 0.7–1.0 cm^2, moderately stenotic; and 1.0–1.2 cm^2, mildly stenotic.

It is essential that all the variables used to calculate a valve area (CO, systolic ejection period or diastolic filling period, heart rate, and pressure gradient) are measured in close temporal proximity to one another and with the patient hemodynamically stable. Great care must be exercised in acquiring these data, since the decision for surgical intervention is based on the calculated valve area.

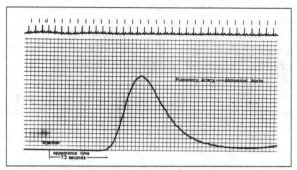

Figure 8. *A normal curve following the injection of 5 mg of indocyanine green into the pulmonary artery, with simultaneous withdrawal of blood from the abdominal aorta. The time between injection and first appearance of the indicator is 7.3 sec.*

SHUNT DETECTION AND MEASUREMENT

The detection and quantitation of an intracardiac shunt can be accomplished by several techniques. First, the measurement of O_2 content within the cardiac chambers and the peripheral vessels allows one to locate the site of intracardiac shunting and determine its magnitude. Once the site of intracardiac shunting is determined, the blood flow to the pulmonary and systemic circulations can be calculated. The oximetric determination of intracardiac shunting is highly specific but relatively insensitive; that is, an oximetric assessment reliably demonstrates the presence of a large shunt but usually fails to detect a small one.

Second, the presence and magnitude of an intracardiac shunt can be demonstrated and quantitated by indicator dilution injections. By performing the injection of indocyanine green and the simultaneous withdrawal of blood from several sites within the heart and great vessels, one can determine the site and size of the intracardiac shunt (Figures 8–10). Indocyanine green injections are more sensitive than oximetry for detecting and quantitating small intracardiac shunts. The intravenous injection of hydrogen (dissolved in saline), with simultaneous sensing with a platinum-tipped electrode in the aorta, can be used to detect very small right-to-left shunts. This technique is the most sensitive method available for the detection of right-to-left shunts. Similarly, the inhalation of hydrogen with simultaneous sensing with a platinum-tipped electrode in the pulmonary artery can be used to detect very small left-to-right shunts.

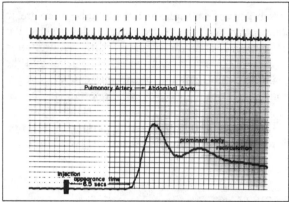

Figure 9. *A curve following the injection of 5 mg of indocyanine green into the pulmonary artery, with blood withdrawal from the abdominal aorta, in a patient with a large left-to-right intracardiac shunt (in this case an atrial septal defect). In comparison to a normal curve (Figure 8), there is a very prominent early recirculation peak. The appearance time is normal, thus excluding a right-to-left shunt distal to the site of injection.*

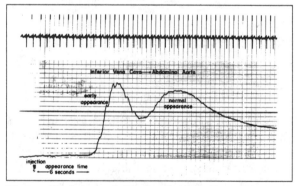

Figure 10. *A curve following the injection of 5 mg of indocyanine green into the inferior vena cava, with blood withdrawal from the abdominal aorta, in a patient with a large right-to-left intracardiac shunt (a large ventricular septal defect with pulmonary infundibular stenosis, or tetralogy of Fallot). The initial peak represents early appearance of indocyanine green in the abdominal aorta, reflecting the right-to-left shunt through the VSD. The second peak represents normal appearance of indocyanine green.*

Third, angiography can be used to demonstrate an intracardiac shunt, but this technique does not allow quantitation of the shunt. For example, a ventricular septal defect with shunting from the left to the right ventricle can be demonstrated with a left ventriculogram in a 30–40° left anterior oblique projection. Alternatively, a patent ductus arteriosus with shunting from the aorta to the pulmonary artery can be detected via a proximal aortogram.

BALLOON-TIPPED, FLOW-DIRECTED (SWAN-GANZ) CATHETERS

In 1970, the balloon-tipped, flow-directed catheter was introduced for right-heart catheterization at the bedside, without the need for fluoroscopy. At present, it is widely used to monitor pulmonary arterial and pulmonary capillary wedge pressures in the critically ill patient in an intensive care unit. The catheter, which has an inflatable balloon at its tip, is made of polyvinylchloride and is extremely soft. The standard balloon-tipped catheter has two lumina—the smaller lumen allows inflation of the balloon, the larger lumen allows measurement of pressures and collection of blood specimens.

Before using the balloon-tipped catheter, the balloon should be inflated in a bowl of saline to exclude an air leak, and the catheter lumen should be flushed with saline. The catheter may be inserted at the bedside either percutaneously (via the femoral, internal jugular, or subclavian vein) or by direct exposure of the brachial vein. When it is introduced without the use of fluoroscopy, it should be passed into the vasculature for 10–30 cm (depending on the site of introduction) before the balloon is inflated. The catheter is marked at 10-cm intervals to facilitate this procedure. Before advancing the catheter, blood should be aspirated through it to insure that it is intravascular. Then the balloon is inflated gently with up to 1 ml of air. If there is resistance to balloon inflation, the catheter should be advanced or withdrawn carefully until the balloon can be inflated freely. The catheter is then connected to a pressure transducer to record right atrial pressure. It is also valuable to obtain a blood sample for oximetric analysis in each right-heart chamber or vessel where pressures are recorded, to exclude left-to-right intracardiac shunting.

Once a blood sample and pressure have been obtained from the right atrium, the catheter is advanced gently with the balloon inflated, while pressure and the electrocardiogram are observed. Particular care must be exercised while traversing the right ventricle; if more than two or three consecutive ventricular premature beats are provoked, the catheter should be withdrawn quickly. If the catheter does not pass eas-

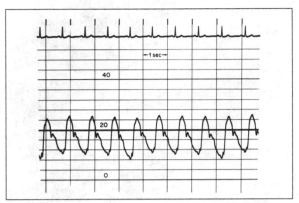

Figure 11. *A recording of pulmonary arterial pressure with a Swan-Ganz catheter; the pressure averages about 25/10 mm Hg.*

ily from the right ventricle to the pulmonary artery, it should be withdrawn to the right atrium and the procedure repeated. Once it has passed to the pulmonary artery and the pressure has been recorded (Figure 11), it is advanced gently (with the balloon still inflated) until the waveform changes to that of a pulmonary capillary wedge pressure (Figure 12). A fully oxygenated blood specimen from this site confirms that the catheter is truly in a wedged position. When the balloon is deflated, the waveform should change to that of pulmonary arterial pressure.

It is occasionally impossible to pass the balloon-tipped catheter without the use of fluoroscopic control, particularly in the patient with a large right atrium, right ventricle, or pulmonary hypertension. It may be

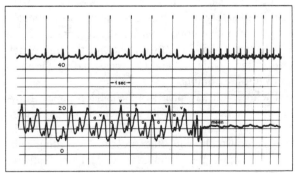

Figure 12. *A recording of PCW pressure from the same patient as in Figure 11. For each QRS complex, there are two pressure waves: a and v. The mean PCW pressure is 13 mm Hg.*

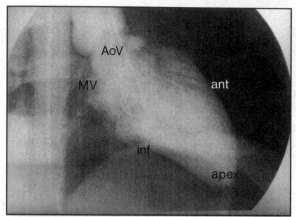

Figure 13. *The end-diastolic image from a right anterior oblique (RAO) left ventriculogram in a patient with normal wall motion. AoV = aortic valve; MV = mitral valve; inf = inferior wall; ant = anterior wall; apex = apex of the left ventricle.*

necessary to use a guide wire to stiffen the catheter while it is passed under fluoroscopic visualization. It is generally easier to pass the catheter without the use of fluoroscopy when the site of vascular entry is central (i.e., internal jugular or subclavian vein) rather than peripheral.

The balloon-tipped, flow-directed catheter offers several advantages over the more traditional stiff catheter used for right-heart catheterization; at the same time, it has certain drawbacks. Since it is unusually soft, perforation of the major vessels and heart is virtually impossible, whereas perforation occasionally occurs with a stiff catheter. As indicated, the flow-directed catheter can be inserted and advanced without fluoroscopic control, although catheter manipulation is easier with fluoroscopic assistance. Apart from its safety, the balloon-tipped, flow-directed catheter can be equipped with a distal thermistor and a third lumen 25–30 cm from the tip, through which iced saline is injected and CO measured by the thermodilution technique.

The major disadvantages of the balloon-tipped, flow-directed catheter stem from the same features that are responsible for its advantages. First, because the catheter is unusually soft, the pressure recordings obtained through it contain a good deal of "catheter whip," that is, artifact introduced by the movement of the catheter itself within the heart. Second, since the catheter is no larger than 7 French in size and yet contains two or (in the case of a thermodilution catheter) three lumina, the distal lumen is small, making

blood sampling difficult. Third, since this catheter is advanced in the direction of blood flow, its placement in the pulmonary artery may be impossible if flow within the right-heart chambers is bidirectional. For example, advancing a balloon-tipped, flow-directed catheter to the pulmonary artery in a patient with severe tricuspid regurgitation may be impossible, since the regurgitant jet directs the catheter from the right ventricle back into the right atrium. Despite these limitations, this catheter allows one to measure right- and left-sided filling pressures and make appropriate therapeutic decisions regarding fluid and drug administration.

The risks and complications of the balloon-tipped, flow-directed catheter are similar to those of any catheter used for right-heart catheterization: ventricular irritability during passage through the right ventricle, and local inflammation or infection at the site of entrance. In addition, because of its softness, the balloon-tipped catheter is easily knotted. Improper inflation and deflation of the balloon can lead to rupture of a small pulmonary artery or to subsegmental pulmonary infarction. By and large, however, the balloon-tipped, flow-directed catheter is extremely safe. Once it is positioned in the pulmonary artery, it may be left in place for 48–72 hours.

ANGIOGRAPHIC MEASUREMENTS

LEFT VENTRICULOGRAPHY

The opacification and simultaneous cineangiocardiography of the left ventricle allows one to assess global and segmental left ventricular function, left ventricular volumes and ejection fraction, and the presence and severity of mitral regurgitation. To achieve adequate opacification, a large bolus of radiographic contrast material must be delivered to the LV over a short period of time. In the normal adult, 55–60 ml of contrast material is injected over 3–4 seconds; thus, approximately 13–20 ml are injected per second. As the contrast material is injected into the LV, cineangiocardiography is performed. The filming of the LV may be performed in one projection (single plane) or two (biplane). Single-plane left ventriculography is usually performed in a 30° right anterior oblique projection (Figures 13 and 14). If biplane angiography is available, a 60° left anterior oblique projection (thus, two projections 90° apart in obliquity) is also performed.

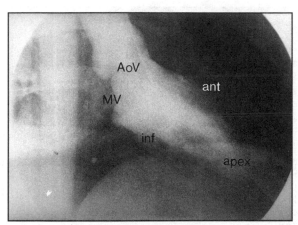

Figure 14. *The end-systolic images from an RAO left ventriculogram in the same patient as shown in Figure 13. Abbreviations are also similar. In comparison to Figure 13, all segments of the left ventricular wall have contracted normally.*

A number of different catheters may be used for left ventriculography, but all should have certain features. (1) The catheter should be of sufficient size so that a high-pressure injection of contrast material does not cause it to recoil and cause ventricular irritability. (2) The catheter should be designed so that the jet of injected contrast material exits through a series of side-holes rather than through an end-hole; the chance of a high-pressure jet of contrast material being injected into the endocardium (so-called endocardial staining) is thus minimized. (3) Although the angiographic catheter should have multiple side-holes for the injection of contrast material, these should be confined to the distal 2–3 cm of the catheter, or else the contrast material will be injected into both the LV and the proximal ascending aorta.

From the left ventriculogram, left ventricular volumes and ejection fraction may be calculated using a standard area-length formula. End-diastolic and end-systolic volumes are both measured; from these, left ventricular stroke volume is derived (end-diastolic volume minus end-systolic volume), and ejection fraction is calculated (stroke volume divided by end-diastolic volume). The normal values for left ventricular volumes and ejection fraction are displayed in Table 2. In addition to the calculation of left ventricular volumes, segmental wall motion may be assessed. A segment of the LV wall with reduced systolic motion is said to be hypokinetic; a segment that does not move at all during ventricular contraction is akinetic; and one that moves paradoxically during ven-

Table 2. Normal Angiographic Values	
LV end-diastolic volume index	50–100 ml/m²
LV end-systolic volume index	15–35 ml/m²
LV stroke volume index	30–65 ml/m²
LV ejection fraction	0.55–0.80
LV = left ventricular.	

tricular systole is dyskinetic (Figures 15 and 16). Finally, the presence and severity of mitral regurgitation may be evaluated and quantitated in rough terms (Figure 17).

AORTOGRAPHY

Aortography is the rapid injection of a large amount of contrast material into the aorta. A proximal aortogram is performed to assess the competency of the aortic valve and to evaluate the anatomy of the proximal aorta and large vessels that supply the head and neck. In turn, a distal aortogram is performed to assess the presence of vascular abnormalities (e.g., aneurysm, intraluminal thrombus). The catheters employed for aortography are similar to those used for left ventriculography. For proximal aortography, 50–60 ml of contrast material is injected over 2–2.5 seconds and filmed either by cineangiography or rapid cut-film angiography. The standard proximal aorto-

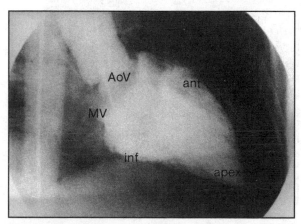

Figure 15. *The end-diastolic image from an RAO left ventriculogram in a patient with a previous inferior myocardial infarction. Abbreviations are those used in Figure 13.*

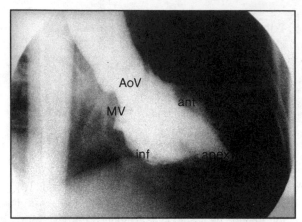

Figure 16. *The end-systolic image from an RAO left ventriculogram in the same patient as shown in Figure 15. Note that the anterior wall (ant) and apex move normally during systole but that the inferior wall (inf) is akinetic; that is, it does not move during systole.*

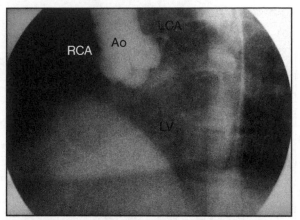

Figure 18. *A selected frame from an LAO supravalvular aortogram in a patient without aortic regurgitation. Ao = proximal aorta; RCA = proximal right coronary artery; LCA = proximal left coronary artery; LV = left ventricle. The three aortic valve cusps are easily discernible.*

gram is filmed in a 45–60° left anterior oblique projection (Figure 18).

PULMONARY ANGIOGRAPHY

Pulmonary angiography is performed primarily to confirm or exclude the presence of pulmonary emboli. A large-bore angiographic catheter is advanced from a systemic vein to the main pulmonary artery

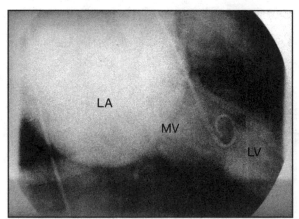

Figure 17. *A selected frame from an RAO left ventriculogram in a patient with severe, long-standing mitral regurgitation. Note that the LA is larger than the LV and that it is more densely opacified with contrast material. MV = mitral valve.*

and is positioned so that catheter recoil during contrast injection does not cause the catheter tip to fall back into the right ventricle, with resulting ventricular irritability. A large injection of contrast material (55–60 ml) is performed over 2–2.5 seconds. During the injection, rapid cut-filming is performed.

If the mainstream injection of the pulmonary artery does not allow a definitive diagnosis, several subselective injections are made into those segments of lung where the suspicion of pulmonary emboli is highest. These injections can be made with either a small power injection through the same angiographic catheter or a hand injection through a balloon-tipped catheter, with simultaneous cut-film angiography.

Once the films have been obtained, they must be interpreted meticulously. Several radiographic signs are diagnostic of pulmonary embolism, including a large intraluminal filling defect or an abrupt pulmonary arterial cutoff. Other radiographic signs, such as localized oligemia and asymmetry of pulmonary blood flow, are suggestive but not strictly diagnostic of embolism.

SELECTIVE CORONARY ARTERIOGRAPHY

Selective coronary arteriography is usually performed to determine the presence and severity of fixed, atherosclerotic coronary artery disease. It is occasionally performed to evaluate the presence of dynamic alterations of coronary arterial tone, that is, coronary ar-

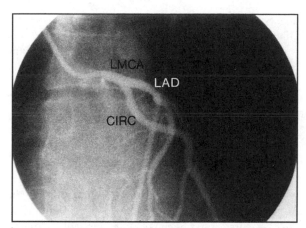

Figure 19. *An anteroposterior view of a normal left coronary artery. LMCA = left main coronary artery; LAD = left anterior descending; CIRC = left circumflex.*

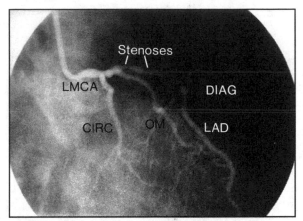

Figure 21. *An RAO projection of the left coronary artery in a patient with two stenoses of the proximal LAD. LMCA = left main coronary artery; CIRC = left circumflex coronary artery; OM = obtuse marginal branch of circumflex coronary artery; LAD = left anterior descending coronary artery; DIAG = diagonal branch of the LAD.*

terial spasm. Each coronary arterial ostium is selectively engaged with a catheter, after which injections of contrast material are made by hand. Since CAD is often eccentric within the coronary arterial lumen, injections of each of the two coronary arteries are performed and filmed in several different obliquities (Figures 19–24).

Several important features about selective coronary arteriography deserve emphasis. Systemic arterial pressure and heart rate should be observed closely during arteriography, since the procedure can induce transient hypotension or bradycardia. The latter can

be treated with intravenous atropine and, if necessary, placement of a temporary transvenous ventricular pacemaker. Cineangiography of the coronary arteries should be performed with as much image magnification and, at the same time, as little image distortion as possible. With very few exceptions, coronary arteriography should not be performed during an episode of angina. Rather, the patient should receive sublingual nitroglycerin, and sufficient time should

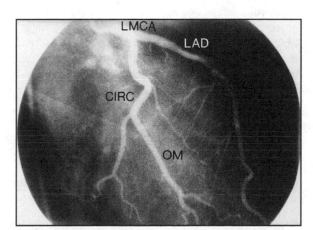

Figure 20. *An RAO projection of a normal left coronary artery. Abbreviations are similar to those used in Figure 19. OM = obtuse marginal branch of the circumflex.*

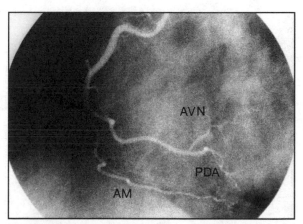

Figure 22. *A left anterior oblique (LAO) projection of a normal right coronary artery. AM = acute marginal branch; PDA = posterior descending artery; AVN = atrioventricular nodal artery.*

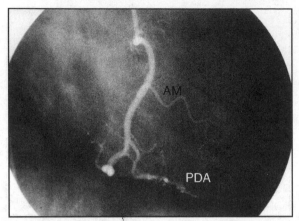

Figure 23. *An RAO projection of a normal right coronary artery. AM = acute marginal branch; PDA = posterior descending artery.*

be allowed for pain to resolve. Then, arteriography may proceed.

CORONARY ANGIOPLASTY

Coronary angioplasty involves the inflation of a distensible balloon within a significant coronary stenosis, with subsequent compression or disruption of the atheromatous lesion (see Chapter 16). After baseline coronary arteriography, a large-bore guiding catheter is advanced to the appropriate coronary ostium, through which a smaller-sized balloon dilatation catheter is advanced over a soft guide wire. Once the guide wire

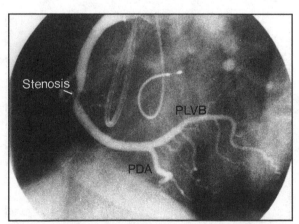

Figure 24. *An LAO projection of a right coronary artery with a severe stenosis in its midportion. PDA = posterior descending artery; PLVB = posterior left ventricular branch.*

has been advanced beyond the stenosis that is to be dilated, the balloon dilatation catheter is gently advanced over it. Once within the stenosis, the balloon is fully inflated for 30–120 seconds with 6–12 atmospheres of pressure, after which it is deflated. The brief inflation of the balloon may be repeated several times within a period of several minutes. The balloon initially is seen to expand at both ends, with a central indentation due to the profile of the coronary stenosis. This central indentation typically resolves as the stenosis is successfully dilated.

Coronary angioplasty has been used successfully in patients with several manifestations of ischemic heart disease. First, it has been widely employed in patients with stable angina of effort who continue to have limiting symptoms despite appropriate medical therapy. Second, angioplasty has been performed safely and effectively in patients with unstable angina pectoris. In these individuals, the risk of death or myocardial infarction does not appear to be substantially higher than that reported for patients with stable angina. Third, angioplasty has been used in patients with acute myocardial infarction, either alone or in close temporal proximity to thrombolytic therapy. When used alone, the procedure is often successful in reestablishing antegrade flow through a totally occluded infarct artery. When used 2–48 hours after thrombolytic therapy, angioplasty allows the operator to dilate the high-grade residual coronary stenosis that presumably was the site of thrombus formation.

Fourth, angioplasty has been employed with modest success in patients with stable angina and a totally occluded coronary artery not in the setting of acute myocardial infarction. In these individuals, the chance of reestablishing antegrade flow is related to the elapsed time from total occlusion to attempted angioplasty. If the procedure is performed within 12 weeks of total occlusion, the chance of success is good (65–70%); if it is performed later than 12 weeks after occlusion, the chance of success falls to below 20%. Finally, angioplasty has been used successfully in patients with saphenous vein or internal mammary grafts who have developed angina and have angiographic evidence of a discrete graft stenosis. In these individuals, angioplasty is most likely to yield a good result when the stenosis is located in the body or distal end of the graft.

In experienced hands, coronary angioplasty is an effective therapeutic modality in patients with limiting angina who would otherwise require coronary artery bypass grafting for symptomatic relief. Its overall success rate depends on patient selection, but in most series it averages 85–90%. Although complications are reported in 5–10% of patients undergoing angioplasty, most are correctable by emergency coronary bypass surgery, so that the overall mortality for the procedure is less than 1%. During the four to six months after successful angioplasty, 25–35% of stenoses recur, but these are usually amenable to repeat angioplasty.

BALLOON VALVULOPLASTY

Over the past two to three years, percutaneous balloon valvuloplasty has been used with some success in patients with aortic or mitral stenosis as an alternative to surgical commissurotomy or valve replacement. During this procedure, two large balloon catheters are positioned across the valve to be dilated and are inflated with 3–5 atmospheres of pressure for 15–30 seconds. Balloon inflations are usually repeated several times (see Chapter 16).

Preliminary data suggest that balloon valvuloplasty is modestly successful in most patients with aortic stenosis, but a recurrence of stenosis occurs in the majority within 6–12 months of dilatation. As a result, aortic balloon valvuloplasty is recommended only for those individuals in whom an aortic valve replacement is thought to carry a prohibitive risk (i.e., the patient with severe chronic lung disease). Mitral balloon valvuloplasty appears to yield successful results in selected patients, especially those without extensive valvular calcification or concomitant regurgitation. The likelihood of recurrence following mitral balloon valvuloplasty appears to be low, but long-term follow-up data are not yet available.

RISKS AND COMPLICATIONS

As cardiac catheterization has become performed more frequently, the incidence of complications has diminished; however, even in the most skilled hands, the procedure is not without risk. The overall incidence of a major complication—death, myocardial infarction, or cerebrovascular accident—during or within 24 hours of catheterization is 0.2–0.4%. Of these major complications, death in the catheterization laboratory or within 24 hours of catheterization occurs in 0.1–0.2% of patients, the majority of whom have extensive cardiac disease. Such deaths may be caused by perforation of the heart or great vessels, cardiac arrhythmias, or acute myocardial infarction, with re-

sulting left ventricular dysfunction. Myocardial infarction during or immediately following catheterization occurs in 0.3% of patients, but most infarctions are small and uncomplicated. Cerebrovascular accidents in the peri-catheterization period are either embolic (from the arterial catheter or thrombus in the left ventricle or atrium) or thrombotic (i.e., existence of previous extensive cerebrovascular disease that, in association with the hemodynamic alterations induced by arteriography, leads to inadequate cerebral perfusion).

Numerous minor complications may cause morbidity but have no effect on mortality. Following arterial catheterization by the brachial approach, restoration of blood flow to the arm can be imperfect and the patient may require a thrombectomy after catheterization. Hemorrhage or hematoma formation can occur at the site of the femoral arterial puncture and, if severe, may require limited surgical exploration. Occasionally, a femoral arterial thrombectomy is required following a percutaneous puncture, and the very rare patient may require a lower limb partial amputation. Local infection may occur at the site of catheter entry and manipulation, but this can usually be treated with meticulous wound care and a short course of antibiotic therapy. The injection of contrast material commonly causes nausea and vomiting as well as a transient fall in systemic arterial pressure. Occasionally, the injections are associated with allergic reactions of varying severity, and an occasional individual develops anaphylaxis due to contrast material. In addition, the endocardial injection of contrast material during ventriculography can cause ventricular irritability.

POSTCATHETERIZATION CONCERNS

During the 24 hours after catheterization, there are several important considerations. The patient should remain at complete bedrest for 8–12 hours if the arterial catheterization was performed by the brachial approach and for 24 hours if it was performed via the femoral approach. The patient should be observed closely after catheterization to insure that heart rate and blood pressure are stable and that the arterial and venous entry sites do not show evidence of bleeding. Radiographic contrast material is extremely hyperosmolar and, as a result, causes an osmotic diuresis during the 12–24 hours after catheterization. Therefore, sufficient oral and intravenous fluids should be administered to insure that such a diuresis does not induce intravascular volume depletion.

Bibliography

Adams DF, Fraser DB, Abrams HL: The complications of coronary arteriography. *Circulation* 48:609, 1973.

Branthwaite MA, Bradley RD: Measurement of cardiac output by thermal dilution in man. *J Appl Physiol* 24:434, 1968.

Croft CH, Lipscomb K, Mathis K, et al: Limitations of qualitative angiographic grading in aortic or mitral regurgitation. *Am J Cardiol* 53:1593, 1984.

Dalen JE, Brooks HL, Johnson LW, et al: Pulmonary angiography in acute pulmonary embolism: Indications, techniques, and results in 367 patients. *Am Heart J* 81:175, 1971.

Dehmer GJ, Firth BG, Hillis LD: Oxygen consumption in adult patients during cardiac catheterization. *Clin Cardiol* 5:436, 1982.

Forrester JS, Ganz W, Diamond G, et al: Thermodilution cardiac output determination with a single flow-directed catheter. *Am Heart J* 83:306, 1972.

Gorlin R, Gorlin SG: Hydraulic formula for calculation of area of stenotic mitral valve, other cardiac valves, and central circulatory shunts. *Am Heart J* 41:1, 1951.

Hamilton WF, Riley RL, Attyah AM, et al: Comparison of the Fick and dye injection methods of measuring the cardiac output in man. *Am J Physiol* 153:309, 1948.

Hillis LD: Percutaneous transluminal coronary angioplasty. *Am J Med Sci* 288:89, 1984.

Hillis LD, Firth BG, Winniford MD: Analysis of factors affecting the variability of Fick versus indicator dilution measurements of cardiac output. *Am J Cardiol* 56:764, 1985.

Hillis LD, Firth BG, Winniford MD: Variability of right-sided cardiac oxygen saturations in adults with and without left-to-right intracardiac shunting. *Am J Cardiol* 58:129, 1986.

Hillis LD, Winniford MD, Dehmer GJ, Firth BG: Left ventricular volumes by single plane cineangiography: In vivo validation of the Kennedy regression equation. *Am J Cardiol* 53:1159, 1984.

Hillis LD, Winniford MD, Jackson JA, Firth BG: Measurements of left-to-right intracardiac shunting in adults: Oximetric versus indicator dilution techniques. *Cathet Cardiovasc Diagn* 11:467, 1985.

Judkins MP: Percutaneous transfemoral selective coronary arteriography. *Radiol Clin N Amer* 6:467, 1968.

McBride W, Lange RA, Hillis LD: Restenosis after successful coronary angioplasty. Pathophysiology and prevention. *N Engl J Med* 318:1734, 1988.

Niggemann EH, Ma PTS, Sunnergren KP, et al: Detection of intracardiac left-to-right shunting in adults: A prospective analysis of the variability of the standard indocyanine green technique in patients without shunting. *Am J Cardiol* 60:355, 1987.

Rackley CE, Dear HD, Baxley WA, et al: Left ventricular chamber volume, mass, and function in severe coronary artery disease. *Circulation* 41:605, 1970.

Sasahara AA, Stein M, Simon M, et al: Pulmonary angiography in the diagnosis of thromboembolic disease. *N Engl J Med* 270:1075, 1964.

Seldinger SI: Catheter replacement of the needle in percutaneous arteriography, a new technique. *Acta Radiol* 39:368, 1953.

Sones FM, Shirey EK: Cine coronary arteriography. *Mod Concepts Cardiovasc Dis* 31:735, 1962.

Swan HJC, Ganz W, Forrester J, et al: Catheterization of the heart in man with use of a flow-directed balloon-tipped catheter. *N Engl J Med* 283:447, 1970.

10 Electrophysiologic Testing

Joseph P. Ilvento

Clinical electrophysiologic testing of the heart began in 1968, when Damato and coworkers measured signals from the Bundle of His with a transvenously placed electrode catheter. Initially, further progress was limited by the available technology; however, with the advent of sophisticated recording and analysis equipment, the technique of electrophysiologic study (EPS) has become a useful tool not only for the assessment of atrioventricular block, but also for the diagnosis of sinus node dysfunction, supraventricular and ventricular tachyarrhythmias, and complex, reflex-mediated cardiac rhythm disturbances. Selection and guidance of therapy, be it pharmacologic, bradycardia or antitachycardia pacemakers, automatic defibrillators, or surgical or catheter ablation, have been greatly aided (indeed, spawned in some instances) by electrophysiologic testing. The technique is still evolving and indications for its use are being refined as our understanding of mechanisms of arrhythmias increases and as technological advances allow for more effective treatment. What follows is a guide for the appropriate use of EPS for diagnostic and therapeutic purposes.

TECHNIQUES OF ELECTROPHYSIOLOGIC STUDY

Electrophysiologic studies should be performed with sterile technique in a laboratory equipped with defibrillation equipment, fluoroscopy, all cardioactive drugs and solutions necessary for safe resuscitation, and archival data storage equipment which permits rapid analysis of acquired data. Much of the direction of the EP study depends upon data acquired in the laboratory during the case, making efficiently gathered and easily interpretable signals of paramount importance. Ideally, 16 channels of simultaneous data acquisition are desirable with the ability to record all 12 leads of the electrocardiogram simultaneously. A critical care nurse should be present to administer medications and document the case. A technician certified in fluoroscopy should also be present for operation of the imaging equipment. Single-plane fluoroscopy is adequate for most applications; however, for mapping procedures, biplane is valuable.

The study is performed with the patient sedated with drugs that have minimal effects on sympathetic and parasympathetic tone. This is particularly important when supraventricular arrhythmias or syncope are to be evaluated, because changes in autonomic tone may alter the ability to induce arrhythmia. Accordingly, midazolam and diazepam are preferable over meperidine and morphine. However, for programmed ventricular stimulation in patients whose sinus node and AV node function have been already assessed, the latter two drugs can be useful adjuncts, particularly for patients with back pain. After instrumentation, heparin should be administered (2,500 units IV bolus and 500 units/hr thereafter) unless contraindicated, as the risk of deep vein thrombosis may be as high as 2% in patients who undergo serial EPS. Heparin should probably not be given in cases of catheter ablation or right atrial mapping with stiff mapping catheters that may perforate the atrium. Full anticoagulation should be administered in all cases in which catheters are placed in the left heart.

Access is attained most commonly via the right femoral vein for right atrial, His bundle (Figure 1), and right ventricular recordings. The left subclavian vein is particularly useful for accessing the coronary sinus because the lateral right atrium deflects the catheter toward the ostium of the coronary sinus, located posteromedially above the tricuspid annulus. The right internal jugular vein is also useful for this purpose and particularly for catheters that are to remain in place after the study for right ventricular apical pacing. Although temporary pacing catheters may remain

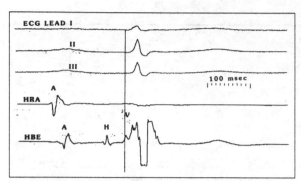

Figure 1. *Endocavitary measurements made during sinus rhythm from electrode catheters positioned in the high right atrium (HRA) and across the tricuspid valve for recording the His potential (HBE). Upper three tracings are surface electrocardiogram leads I, II, and III. The His potential occurs 45 msec before the onset of the surface QRS in this case. The normal HV interval ranges from 35-60 msec. Note the earlier appearance of the atrial signal in the HRA recording, indicating a wave front of activation moving from the high to low right atrium, consistent with a sinus node mechanism.*

in place via the right femoral vein, the internal jugular approach is preferable to assure both sterility and patient comfort. In situations that require left ventricular access for stimulation or mapping, the right femoral and right or left brachial arteries are useful entry points. A wide variety of catheters are available for particular applications and will not be specifically discussed here.

STIMULATION PROTOCOLS

Stated most succinctly, EPS is a form of perturbation analysis. The conduction system is disturbed from equilibrium by a pacing stimulus or other manipulation and the response to the disturbance is recorded and analyzed. There are two general types of stimulation. *Burst* and *incremental pacing* consist of the delivery of a train of impulses at a constant or progressively increasing rate. They are most often used for the assessment of conduction properties of the AV node or bypass tract and for the induction of an arrhythmia. *Programmed stimulation* refers to the delivery of short trains of from one to four extrastimuli in which the coupling intervals between successive impulses are varied in some organized fashion in order to assess refractoriness or to induce an arrhyth-

mia. Programmed stimulation protocols vary widely among laboratories (Akhtar et al.), but are most often characterized by a drive stimulus train of six to eight impulses followed by a programmed set of one to four impulses whose coupling intervals are progressively decreased until refractoriness is attained or an arrhythmia is induced.

Except in the case of atrial fibrillation, studies usually begin with an evaluation of the sinus node, atrium, and AV node. Measurement of the sinus node recovery time or sinoatrial conduction time may provide evidence of sinus node dysfunction in syncope patients, but is often unrevealing. The sinus node recovery time is defined as the time of appearance of the first sinus complex after a fixed period of atrial pacing, generally 30 seconds. Sinoatrial conduction times are measured after single premature extrastimuli are delivered during sinus rhythm (Reiffel et al.). Other techniques useful in the laboratory for the evaluation of syncope include carotid sinus massage and tilt table testing. These are typically performed with continuous arterial pressure monitoring via an arterial catheter.

INDICATIONS FOR ELECTROPHYSIOLOGIC STUDY

GENERAL DIAGNOSTIC CONSIDERATIONS

The decision to perform electrophysiologic study is based on the type and frequency of symptoms, whether an arrhythmia has been documented, and the presence of organic heart disease. Ambulatory or telemetric electrocardiographic monitoring may be useful only in those patients who have frequent episodes of arrhythmia. If physical injury has resulted from a syncopal episode, outpatient monitoring to document a second event may place the patient at an unacceptably high risk of serious injury. Certainly, however, all available electrocardiographic data should be reviewed before EPS is undertaken. Treadmill testing should be performed before EPS in most instances, particularly if the patient's symptoms are exertionally or stress related or if chest pain is a feature of the symptom complex. Likewise, some assessment of cardiac anatomy may be helpful. The likelihood of inducing an arrhythmia during EPS that can be implicated as a cause of the patient's symptoms is significantly increased if organic heart disease is present.

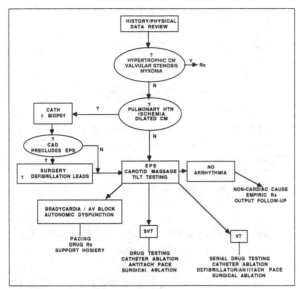

Figure 2. *A decision algorithm for the evaluation of patients with unexplained syncope. See text for discussion. CM = cardiomyopathy; CAD = coronary artery disease; EPS = electrophysiologic study; SVT = supraventricular tachycardia; VT = ventricular tachycardia; Y = yes; N = no.*

Echocardiography is a useful, noninvasive method to assess structural abnormalities prior to EPS.

UNEXPLAINED SYNCOPE

Approximately 50% of patients with syncope never suffer a second episode. However, those patients who have a cardiovascular etiology established for syncope have a 30% mortality rate after one year of untreated follow-up, significantly higher than the 12% mortality rate for noncardiovascular syncope (Kapoor et al.). The distribution of arrhythmic causes of syncope is highly dependent upon the population studied but can be estimated roughly as evenly divided between bradycardia and ventricular tachycardia. Newer protocols have provided greater sensitivity in the diagnosis of reflex mediated or autonomic syncope (Benditt). Because 50% of patients with syncope will have a cardiovascular cause established, it is crucial to rule out organic heart disease carefully before a single episode of syncope is permitted to recur.

The history and physical examination are useful about half the time in predicting a cardiac cause for syncope and they are the most important diagnostic

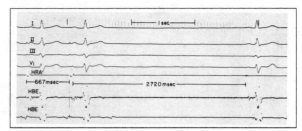

Figure 3. *Measurement of the sinus node recovery time in a patient with syncope. The right atrium was paced for 30 seconds at a cycle length of 667 msec. The last two paced beats are at the left. Upon cessation of pacing, a 2,720-msec interval elapses before the first sinus beat occurs. The corrected sinus node recovery time in this patient was 1,920 msec (2,720 msec − 800 msec, the resting sinus cycle length). The corrected sinus node recovery time should be <550 msec. Pacing is indicated in this case.*

tools in directing the evaluation of a patient with syncope (Figure 2). Neurologic and metabolic causes of syncope should be actively elicited and treated before EPS is considered. Cardiac mechanisms such as atrial myxoma, aortic or mitral stenosis, hypertrophic obstructive cardiomyopathy, right-to-left shunting, and pulmonary hypertension must be excluded with the appropriate diagnostic studies. Indeed, EPS may be dangerous in patients with obstructive forms of heart disease who have syncope. As noted, if coronary artery disease is suspected, treadmill testing should be performed before EPS, particularly if syncopal events are related to exertion.

Typically, EPS for syncope is performed with indwelling arterial pressure monitoring and with electrode catheters placed in the high right atrium, across the tricuspid valve for His potential recording, and in the right ventricle. Atrial pacing is performed for the assessment of sinus and AV node function as well as for induction of supraventricular arrhythmias. Carotid sinus massage should be performed only in those patients without objective evidence of atherosclerotic carotid disease. Tilt table testing with isoproterenol infusion should be performed if no significant coronary disease is present. Patients are monitored for bradycardia and/or hypotension while at an upright angle of 30-60° for approximately 30 minutes, with subsequent infusion of isoproterenol if the initial observation period is not fruitful. Programmed ventricular stimulation should also be undertaken in a standard

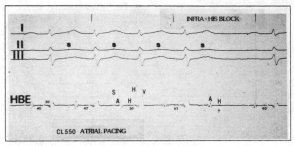

Figure 4. *Infra-Hisian block during atrial pacing in a patient with syncope. The right atrium was paced at a cycle length of 550 msec. S marks the stimulus artifact. Note the progressive prolongation of the HV interval with the occurrence of a non-conducted His potential (at arrow). Permanent pacing is indicated in this case.*

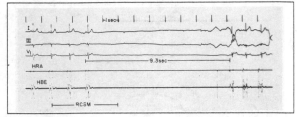

Figure 5. *Recording made during right carotid sinus massage (RCSM) in a patient with syncope. A 9.3-sec sinus pause was elicited with approximately 5 sec of carotid massage. Pauses of greater than 3-3.5 sec are generally considered abnormal. Pacing is indicated in this case.*

syncope study, in addition to the above, in an effort to elicit ventricular tachycardia. A more detailed discussion of EPS as it relates to bradyarrhythmias and tachyarrhythmias follows below.

BRADYARRHYTHMIAS

If electrocardiographic evidence of AV block or sinus bradyarrhythmias is available, and the observed abnormality can be correlated with symptoms, then EPS need not be performed to confirm the need for permanent pacemaker implantation. However, if bi- or trifascicular block is present or bradyarrhythmias have not been documented, EPS can be helpful to elicit evidence of sinus node dysfunction (Figure 3) or infra-Hisian block (Figure 4). Although the presence of either of these abnormalities can confirm the clinical suspicion, their absence at EP study does not exclude them as a cause in a given patient, and clinical considerations must ultimately guide selection of pacing therapy. Current methods of evaluating bradyarrhythmias and AV block lack sufficient sensitivity to have a significant negative predictive value (see Chapter 20). Further refinement of the techniques for provocation of these arrhythmias is needed to provide greater sensitivity.

Carotid sinus hypersensitivity and the relative contributions of the cardioinhibitory and vasodepressor components of this syndrome can be very accurately evaluated by EPS (Figure 5); it is very useful in demonstrating the need for and allowing selection of the appropriate pacemaker or pharmacotherapy (particularly in the instance of a marked vasodepressor component). Tilt table testing with infusion of isoproterenol

can be helpful in provoking bradycardia and hypotension in patients with syncope. Although the mechanism of this reflex has not been defined conclusively, receptors in the posterior left ventricular wall are thought to mediate an abnormal reflex that results in circulatory compromise similar to that observed in carotid sinus hypersensitivity. More importantly, treatment results in resolution of symptoms. Patients being considered for pacemaker implantation should undergo ventricular pacing to evaluate the effects of AV dyssynchrony so that an AV sequential pacemaker can be implanted if significant phasic variations in pressure are documented.

SUPRAVENTRICULAR TACHYARRHYTHMIAS

Electrophysiologic study is perhaps more useful in the provocation of supraventricular and ventricular tachycardias than in the evaluation of bradyarrhythmias. While of no practical use in elucidating the mechanism of atrial fibrillation (except as described below), EPS can help in differentiating the ventricular or supraventricular origin of wide-complex tachycardias. If a His potential is observed before the QRS complex, then aberrant supraventricular conduction can be safely diagnosed, with rare exceptions such as a nodoventricular bypass tract or His-Purkinje reentrant tachycardias. If a prolonged HV interval is observed during atrial fibrillation in a patient with syncope, bradyarrhythmias secondary to AV block should be sought. Syncope may also result from a prolonged sinus pause following the termination of atrial fibrillation or other atrial tachyarrhythmia. This is best evaluated by ambulatory ECG monitoring but can sometimes be observed in the EP laboratory. In any patient with an infarction scar or, more generally, organic heart disease and atrial fibrillation with symptoms suspicious for arrhythmia, programmed ventricular stimulation should be performed to be certain that ventricular tachycardia is not inducible. Atrial fibrillation can be the terminating event in orthodromic reciprocating AV reentrant tachycardia involving an accessory bypass tract or in AV nodal reentrant tachycardia. The atrial fibrillation that occurs as a result of orthodromic or AV nodal reentrant tachycardia is usually of short duration. Careful analysis of Holter data before EPS may provide important clues as to the etiology of the arrhythmia and so guide the electrophysiologist during study. In the patient with an irregular wide-complex tachycardia, the presence of an accessory bypass tract can be accurately evaluated by EPS.

Paroxysmal narrow complex tachycardias are readily diagnosed by electrophysiologic study. Intraatrial reentry, AV nodal reentry, and orthodromic reciprocating tachycardias (Figure 6) can be clearly defined and the results of treatment evaluated by EPS. EPS should be performed in any patient with recurrent, symptomatic narrow-complex tachycardias, particularly as ablative therapies emerge. These techniques, currently under active evaluation, may prove to be a safe method to interrupt or modify conduction through the AV node or an accessory pathway.

VENTRICULAR TACHYARRHYTHMIAS

Any patient with sustained ventricular tachycardia (Figure 7) or aborted sudden cardiac death not associated with myocardial infarction should be considered for electrophysiology study. EPS should not, however, be considered a risk stratification technique in this group of patients, as 20% of patients with a clinical episode of VT/ventricular fibrillation who are not inducible will suffer an arrhythmia recurrence or arrhythmic death (Wilber et al.). Similarly, 20% of patients rendered noninducible by serial drug testing in the EP laboratory will suffer an arrhythmia recurrence. Thus, EPS should more appropriately be considered a diagnostic tool for guiding therapy selection rather than a prognostic tool. Clearly, a patient rendered noninducible by an antiarrhythmic drug has a lower risk of recurrence than one who is treated with an ineffective drug (Mason and Winkle), but the recurrence rate, particularly in patients with poor ventricular function (ejection fraction <30-35%), is unacceptably high. If VF or VT occurs in the periinfarction period (generally considered to be within

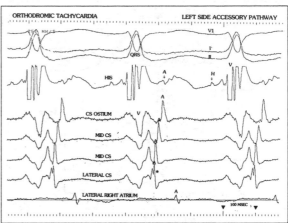

Figure 6. *Recordings made during an episode of orthodromic reciprocating AV reentrant tachycardia in a patient with a left-side accessory bypass tract. Top to bottom: Three surface ECG leads, His bundle electrogram, and four tracings from a catheter positioned within the coronary sinus (CS), with uppermost trace from an electrode positioned at the coronary sinus ostium and each successive trace 1 cm further lateral. Bottom trace is from a Gallagher mapping catheter positioned in the low lateral right atrium. The local atrial (A), His (H), and ventricular (V) signals are labeled. Notice the relatively long AH interval and the short VA time. The activation sequence of the atria begins in the lateral coronary sinus, as opposed to the normal retrograde activation that might occur through the AV node, which would manifest as the His bundle atrial electrogram occurring first. These tracings, recorded simultaneously, show a left lateral bypass tract conducting retrograde with antegrade conduction occurring via the AV node-His bundle. Note the normal QRS duration and morphology.*

10-14 days after infarction), it may be related to the acute infarct and not presage subsequent arrhythmias.

Risk stratification of postinfarction patients with or without peri-infarction arrhythmias is a subject of active investigation. Gomes et al. defined a high-risk subset of patients with depressed ejection fraction, >30 premature ventricular complexes per hour, and late potentials detected by signal-averaged electrocardiography. These patients have a significantly higher risk of ventricular arrhythmias and may be a subgroup who require electrophysiologic testing even though spontaneous sustained arrhythmias have not occurred. Clinical considerations still rule in this case, however, and any patient with the above triad or VT/VF in the peri-infarction period should be carefully re-

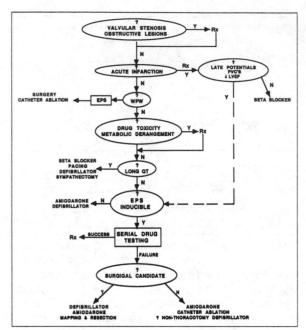

Figure 7. *A decision algorithm for the evaluation of patients with sustained ventricular tachycardia (VT) or ventricular fibrillation (VF). The broken line indicates an approach to the postinfarction patient that is not yet widely accepted but is the subject of active investigation. See text for discussion. PVC = premature ventricular complex; LVEF = left ventricular ejection fraction; EPS = electrophysiologic study; WPW = Wolff-Parkinson-White syndrome.*

viewed before discharge to decide whether further rhythm evaluation is necessary. Empiric pharmacotherapy (except perhaps amiodarone) without an adequate baseline study and evaluation of efficacy by repeat EPS provides little or no added benefit over no therapy at all for the prevention of sudden death (Schaffer and Cobb). While ambulatory ECG monitoring may be useful, evidence supports EPS as a more sensitive and specific indication of drug efficacy in postinfarction patients with monomorphic VT (Platia and Reid).

The usefulness of EPS from diagnostic and therapeutic viewpoints in patients with nonischemic cardiomyopathies is markedly diminished. However, if a patient has suffered aborted sudden death or sustained VT, EPS can help document AV node function and the presence of other tachycardias and therefore guide nonpharmacologic therapy with devices such as an implantable cardioverter-defibrillator. In patients with nonsustained VT and organic heart disease, sustained monomorphic VT is inducible in approxi-

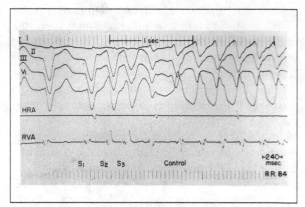

Figure 8. *Induction of ventricular tachycardia by programmed ventricular stimulation. Recordings were made from the right ventricular apex (RVA) and high right atrium (HRA). Four surface ECG leads are also shown. Eight drive stimuli (S_1) were delivered, followed by two extrastimuli (S_2 and S_3). The first abnormal QRS complex is of intermediate morphology followed by a monomorphic sustained VT, cycle length 240 msec.*

mately 30% of patients. In this subgroup with inducible VT, the risk of a clinical arrhythmic event is significantly higher than in the noninducible group.

Programmed stimulation with up to three or sometimes four extrastimuli can be performed at several drive cycle lengths and in several ventricular locations in order to induce VT (Figure 8). In our laboratory, we typically deliver up to three extrastimuli to two right ventricular sites at two basic drive cycle lengths. If this protocol does not result in the induction of an arrhythmia, isoproterenol is administered to elevate the heart rate by approximately 20 beats/min if no significant risk of ischemia is present. If the arrhythmia is still not induced, left ventricular stimulation is undertaken. If a patient with sustained VT or sudden death not associated with acute infarction is not inducible at EPS, a failure of the method is more likely than the absence of risk. If metabolic causes have been excluded, then empiric therapy with amiodarone or implantation of an automatic defibrillator should be considered.

THERAPEUTIC USES OF ELECTROPHYSIOLOGIC TESTING: SELECTION OF DRUG THERAPY

VENTRICULAR TACHYCARDIA AND SUDDEN DEATH

Programmed electrical stimulation was initially employed to evaluate the effectiveness of antiarrhythmic drug therapy and is still most widely used today in the evaluation of drug therapy of ventricular tachycardia. Ventricular tachycardia is inducible in approximately 90% of patients with a prior clinical episode of VT and prior myocardial infarction and approximately 60% of patients who have suffered an episode of aborted sudden death. Baseline testing is therefore required in all patients in these two categories before serial drug testing is undertaken, in order to ascertain inducibility, the number of morphologies, and the rate spectrum in a given patient. If pharmacotherapy renders a patient noninducible, then the two-year likelihood of recurrence of a clinical arrhythmia is approximately 20%.

Implicit in these data is the fact that coronary disease is likely to progress and left ventricular function is likely to worsen in some of these patients. Those with poor left ventricular function, from either ischemic or nonischemic cardiomyopathies, are at high risk of sudden death. Indeed, the worse the ventricular function, the higher the risk of arrhythmia. This evidence indirectly argues that, even though a drug successfully suppresses ventricular tachycardia in the EP laboratory, patients with poor ventricular function may be at a >20% risk of recurrent ventricular arrhythmias. Thus, patients with poor left ventricular function must be rendered completely noninducible before drug therapy is accepted. In those patients with good left ventricular function and inducible VT, there are certain situations in which one can accept a slowing of the rate or a conversion to nonsustained VT as an end point. Measurement of blood pressure during VT in an upright tilt provides further evidence of the level of arrhythmia tolerance. The risk of recurrence in this population of partial responders is intermediate in comparison with complete responders, and only in those patients with minimal additional coronary disease and good left ventricular function should an intermediate end point be accepted.

In general, the likelihood of successful drug therapy decreases nonlinearly with each successive drug failure. In our laboratory, an average of three drugs or combinations of drugs is evaluated serially before nonpharmacologic therapy is considered. If a patient is inducible, procainamide is usually evaluated at the time of the first study. If the left ventricular ejection fraction is >35%, a type 1C antiarrhythmic (most commonly propafenone) alone or in combination with procainamide is evaluated at the second study, and, if indicated, amiodarone at a third study (one week after initiation of therapy at 1200-1600 mg daily).

Because of the slow kinetics of amiodarone, induction of VT at EPS one week after initiation of amiodarone does not necessarily indicate drug failure, and the patient should not be prematurely directed to nonpharmacologic therapy. However, waiting longer before testing (two weeks or six weeks) places the patient at increased and very real risk (approximately 10%) of arrhythmia recurrence or sudden death. If a patient remains inducible to an arrhythmia and is hemodynamically unstable or has poor left ventricular function at the one-week study, then nonpharmacologic approaches should be considered.

SUPRAVENTRICULAR ARRHYTHMIAS

Drug effects on the inducibility of supraventricular arrhythmias can be evaluated by EPS. However, the effects of endogeneous catecholamine release during stressful clinical situations may diminish the effectiveness of a drug that was found to suppress the arrhythmia in the electrophysiology laboratory. Isoproterenol infusion can help mimic this situation and should be employed in order to give a better understanding as to the likelihood of arrhythmia recurrence. Repeat EPS after AV junction modification or accessory pathway ablation is necessary to document success. Perhaps the most important role for EPS pertaining to supraventricular arrhythmias is in cases of atrial fibrillation in Wolff-Parkinson-White syndrome (Klein et al.). Documentation of adequate slowing of accessory pathway conduction is important for risk stratification. Those patients with shortest pre-excited RR intervals during atrial fibrillation of <250 msec should be considered for further intervention, i.e., drugs, catheter ablation, or surgical interruption of the bypass tract.

NONPHARMACOLOGIC THERAPIES FOR ARRHYTHMIAS

Perhaps the most exciting area in clinical electrophysiology today is the development of nonpharmacologic means of arrhythmia control for supraventricular arrhythmias. Quality of life is an increasingly important parameter in nonpharmacologic decision making as the risks of these therapies decrease. Currently, the trend is in the direction of more aggressive treatment for patients who are poorly controlled with drugs, even if they are at low risk for sudden death. Surgical and catheter ablation, defibrillator implantation, and antitachycardia pacing are playing a larger role in the management of arrhythmias in general and are briefly discussed below.

SURGERY FOR SUPRAVENTRICULAR ARRHYTHMIAS

With an experienced surgeon and electrophysiologist, accessory pathways can be successfully ablated with low mortality and a low risk of AV block. The initial EPS is of great importance in planning the surgical approach. Electrophysiologic mapping must also be performed intraoperatively and after the dissection to confirm success. Success rates are better than 98% with a low risk of AV block, most of which is associated with septal accessory pathways (which require dissection close to the region of the His bundle); in these cases, the risk of AV block is technique-dependent but certainly less than 5%. Surgical approaches to correction of atrial fibrillation and flutter are being studied and may provide further information as to the structural etiology and nonpharmacologic cures for these arrhythmias.

CATHETER ABLATION FOR SUPRAVENTRICULAR ARRHYTHMIAS

This promising technique was initially employed for the control of atrial fibrillation refractory to drug therapy. Complete destruction of the His bundle has allowed for rate control and the elimination of antiarrhythmic drug therapy in 80% of patients. Patients also may require fewer drugs for control of congestive heart failure and reactive airway disease after AV junction ablation. After His bundle destruction, patients are pacemaker-dependent. While, on the surface, this remedy appears to be high-risk, adequate data are not yet available to support or refute this possibility. Indeed, the risks of the initial arrhythmia and its drug treatment may be greater than the risks of pacer dependence. A 2% incidence of late sudden death has also been reported with this technique. Organic heart disease has been present in this subgroup and a causal link of ablation to mortality has not been established. In patients with a dilated left ventricle, left ventricular size has been demonstrated to decrease after ablation, presumably due to adequate rate control. More recently, ablative impulses delivered to the floor of the right atrium have allowed for the abolition of AV nodal reentrant tachycardia without AV block, obviating the need for permanent pacing (Haissaguerre et al.). Accessory pathways have been ablated on both the right and left side of the AV ring. The largest experience has been with posterior septal pathways, where 60% have been successfully controlled.

ANTITACHYCARDIA PACING FOR SUPRAVENTRICULAR TACHYCARDIA

Sophisticated pacemakers are available to pace-terminate atrial, AV nodal reentrant, and orthodromic reciprocating tachycardias; however, they have proven to be of limited usefulness. Although they can reliably terminate these arrhythmias, recurrence, most often during exertion or stress, has been a difficult problem. With the advent of ablative therapies, antitachycardia pacing will play an even smaller role for the treatment of supraventricular tachycardias. The experience with these devices has proven useful, however, in developing detection and termination algorithms for ventricular tachycardia.

SURGERY FOR VENTRICULAR ARRHYTHMIAS

Surgical removal of the focus of ventricular tachycardia has its greatest use in patients with frequent or incessant arrhythmias. The best results are obtained in those patients with discrete aneurysms and good left ventricular function. Preoperative and intraoperative EP mapping and postoperative EP study are necessary to guide the surgery and prove efficacy. However, even in patients rendered noninducible by surgery, there is still a 10-30% recurrence rate within the first five years. We implant a defibrillator lead system at the time of surgery in most patients and perform postoperative EPS to aid in the decision to implant the defibrillator itself. Whether all patients who undergo ablative surgery for VT should receive a defibrillator or empiric amiodarone postoperatively is widely debated. However, the significant recurrence rate in noninducible patients argues that this may be the correct approach, particularly in patients with significantly impaired ventricular function. Computer-aided EP mapping techniques may improve accuracy and postoperative recurrence rates, as these techniques allow for faster, more complete mapping.

CATHETER ABLATION FOR VENTRICULAR TACHYCARDIA

Catheter ablative techniques are less useful for ventricular tachycardia than for supraventricular arrhythmias. Catheter ablation should be reserved for patients with poorly controlled or incessant VT who are not surgical candidates. Significant procedure-related morbidity and mortality have been reported. However, this is in part related to the debilitated status of most patients who have undergone the procedure (Evans et al.).

IMPLANTABLE CARDIOVERTER-DEFIBRILLATORS

The advent of the automatic defibrillator in 1978 provided a major breakthrough in the therapy of sudden death. Five-year survival figures are better than 95% in a patient subgroup who, when treated with other therapies, would generally have a 50-70% survival. The device can be safely implanted in patients who might not tolerate ablative surgery; operative mortality and infection rates are low. However, there can be significant psychological problems encountered by patients who receive the device (or their caretakers). Therefore, psychological factors, intercurrent disease, and long-term prognosis independent of the arrhythmia should be taken into account before the decision is made to implant a defibrillator. Currently, VT or VF must be inducible at the time of EPS for Medicare to cover payment for the device. However, it is clear that a significant number of sudden death survivors are noninducible, yet at high risk of recurrence. EPS is necessary before implantation to allow for proper device selection and programming. Newer devices have antitachycardia and bradycardia pacing capabilities, allowing the termination of the arrhythmia in some instances without the unpleasant sensation of a shock, but still providing defibrillator backup should the pacing therapy cause degeneration of the tachycardia (Figure 9). Most patients do not lose consciousness before the defibrillator discharges, so those who are pace-terminable may have fewer psychological difficulties. Currently, energies of 20-30 joules are typically delivered; however, different waveforms

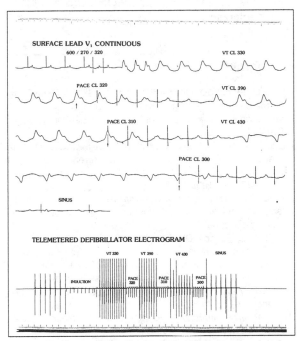

Figure 9. *Composite illustration of the response of an automatic implantable defibrillator with antitachycardia pacing capabilites to the induction of ventricular tachycardia by programmed stimulation. Upper five traces are continuous from surface ECG lead V_1, while the bottom trace is the electrogram recorded from the pacing leads placed epicardially on the left ventricle. Stimulation in the first four lines comes from the defibrillator. The fifth line shows p-triggered ventricular pacing after conversion to sinus rhythm. In the first line, the defibrillator was noninvasively programmed to deliver two extrastimuli after a drive train of eight pulses at 600 msec. VT (cycle length 330 msec) results and the paper speed is increased after the third VT complex. At the arrow in the second line the defibrillator delivers six pacing pulses at a coupling interval of CL 320 msec, which causes the VT to slow to CL 390 msec. At the arrow in the third line, the defibrillator delivers a similar pulse train, now at a 10-msec shorter coupling interval of 310 msec. This results in a slowing of the VT to CL 430 msec. Finally, a third pulse train is delivered at 300 msec, terminating the tachycardia, followed by p-triggered ventricular pacing from the patient's previously implanted AV sequential pacemaker. In the bottom trace, the episode, which lasted approximately 16 sec, was recalled from the memory of the defibrillator. This feature allows verification of the appropriate function of the device as well as assisting in diagnostic and trouble-shooting issues.*

may allow for lower energy requirements and better patient tolerance.

Bibliography

Akhtar M, Fisher JD, Gillette PC, et al: NASPE Ad Hoc Committee on Guidelines for Cardiac Electrophysiological Studies. North American Society of Pacing and Electrophysiology. PACE 8:611, 1985.

Almquist A, Goldenberg IF, Milstein S, et al: Provocation of bradycardia and hypotension by isoproterenol and upright posture in patients with unexplained syncope. *N Engl J Med* 320:346, 1989.

Benditt DG: Provocation of bradycardia and hypotension by isoproterenol and upright posture in patients with unexplained syncope. *N Engl J Med* 320:346, 1989.

Benditt DG, Benson DW, Jr., Klun GJ, et al: Prevention of recurrent sudden cardiac arrest: Role of provocative electrophysiologic testing. *J Am Coll Cardiol* 2:418, 1985.

Cox JL: Patient selection criteria and results of surgery for refractory ischemic ventricular tachycardia. *Circulation* 79 (Suppl I):I-163, 1989.

Denes P: Atrioventricular and intraventricular block. *Circulation* 75 (Suppl III):III-19, 1987.

Denes P, Ezzi MD: The Role of electrophysiologic studies in the management of patients with unexplained syncope. *PACE* 8:424, 1985.

Evans GT Jr., Scheinman MM, Zipes DP, et al: The percutaneous cardiac mapping and ablation registry (Final summary of results). *PACE* 11:1621, 1988.

Gomes JA, Winters SL, Martinson M, et al: The diagnostic significance of quantitative signal averaged variables relative to clinical variables, site of myocardial infarction, ejection fraction and ventricular premature beats. *J Am Coll Cardiol* 13:377, 1989.

Haissaguerre M, Warin JF, Lemetayer P, et al: Closed chest ablation of retrograde conduction in patients with atrioventricular nodal reentrant tachycardia. *N Eng J Med* 320:426, 1989.

Kapoor WN, Karpf M, Wieland S, Peterson JR, Levey GS: A prospective evaluation and follow-up of patients with syncope. *N Eng Med* 309:197, 1983.

Kelly PA, Cannom DS, Garan H, et al: The automatic cardioverter-defibrillator: Efficacy, complications and survival in patients with malignant ventricular arrhythmias. *J Am Coll Cardiol* 11:1278, 1988.

Klein GJ, Bashore TM, Sellers TD, et al: Ventricular fibrillation in the Wolff-Parkinson-White syndrome. *N Eng J Med* 30:1081, 1979.

Kudenchuk PJ, McAnulty JH: Syncope: Evaluation and treatment. *Mod Conc Cardiovasc Dis* 54:25, 1985.

Mason JW, Winkle RA: Electrode catheter arrhythmia induction in the selection and assessment of antiarrhythmic therapy for recurrent ventricular tachycardia. *Circulation* 58: 971, 1978.

Milstein S, Reyes WJ, Benditt DG: Upright body tilt in evaluation of patients with recurrent unexplained syncope. *PACE* 12:117, 1989.

Platia EV, Reid PR: Comparison of programmed electrical stimulation and ambulatory electrocardiographic (Holter) monitoring in the management of ventricular tachycardia and ventricular fibrillation. *J Am Coll Cardiol* 4:493, 1984.

Reiffel JA, Ferrick K, Zimmerman J, Bigger JT Jr.: Electrophysiologic studies of the sinus node and atria. In: Dreifus LS, ed. *Cardiac Arrhythmias: Electrophysiologic Techniques and Management.* Philadelphia: F.A. Davis Co.; 1985, pp. 37–59.

Ritchie JL, Hallsnam AP, Troubaugh GB, Caldwell JH, Cobb LA: Out-of-hospital sudden coronary death: Rest and exercise radionuclide left ventricular function in survivors. *Am J Cardiol* 55:645, 1985.

Ruskin JN, DiMarco JP, Garan H: Out-of-hospital cardiac arrest: Electrophysiologic observation and selection of long-term antiarrhythmic therapy. *N Eng J Med* 303:607, 1980.

Schaffer WA, Cobb LA: Recurrent ventricular fibrillation and modes of death in survivors of out-of-hospital ventricular fibrillation. *N Eng J Med* 293:259, 1975.

Scheinman MM, Morady F, Hess DS, Gonzales R: Catheter induced ablation of the atrioventricular junction to control refractory arrhythmia. *JAMA* 248:851, 1982.

Scherlag BJ, Lau SH, Helfant RH, et al: Catheter technique for recording His bundle activity in man. *Circulation* 39:13, 1969.

Uther JB, Richards DAB, Denniss AR, Ross DL: The prognostic significance of programmed ventricular stimulation after myocardial infarction: A review. *Circulation* 75 (Suppl III):III-161, 1987.

Wilber DJ, Garan H, Finkelstein D, et al: Out-of-hospital cardiac arrest. Use of electrophysiologic testing in the prediction of long-term outcome. *N Engl J Med* 318:19, 1988.

CHAPTER 11

Newer Cardiac Imaging Techniques

Maleah Grover-McKay
David J. Skorton

IMAGING METHODS

The goal of cardiac imaging is to accurately portray a mobile, contracting three-dimensional structure, a particular challenge considering that image acquisition is usually two-dimensional. Current cardiac imaging methods employ a variety of energy forms, including x-rays, ultrasonic waves, gamma rays from radioisotopes, and the combination of magnetic and electrical fields in nuclear magnetic resonance methods. Concepts of planar versus tomographic imaging and considerations of image resolution are common to all techniques.

PLANAR VERSUS TOMOGRAPHIC IMAGING

Medical images may be broadly categorized as planar or tomographic. *Planar* imaging consists of projecting energy through the patient's body at a single orientation (e.g., chest roentgenogram) or by collecting emitted energy at a single orientation (e.g., planar [201]thallium imaging). The transmitted or emitted energy is detected or recorded on a planar surface (e.g., gamma camera crystal). Therefore, in planar imaging a three-dimensional structure is represented in two dimensions with resulting superimposition of structures. *Tomographic* imaging produces cross-sectional images through the body by recording transmitted or emitted energy at each of several orientations, then integrating data from these views by computer to generate a "slice-like" image. These slices can be obtained at several levels, thereby providing information in the third dimension. If images are acquired over time, a four-dimensional representation can be obtained.

IMAGE RESOLUTION

An important concept in evaluation of imaging techniques is resolution, defined as the ability to distinguish detail such as the separation of closely approximated objects. Three types of resolution are important: spatial, temporal, and contrast resolution.

Spatial Resolution

Spatial resolution as applied to medical imaging refers to the ability to visually distinguish two closely spaced objects. A simple, conceptual definition of spatial resolution is a measure of how closely the objects can be approximated while still being resolved as two individual objects. Using this definition, a spatial resolution of 2 mm would indicate that objects could be placed as close together as 2 mm and still be distinguished as individual objects. Other, more complex definitions of spatial resolution are available (Coulam et al.). Modern and evolving cardiac imaging techniques vary considerably in their spatial resolution, from the submillimeter resolution achievable with angiography to resolutions of 5-10 mm in radioisotope imaging.

Temporal Resolution

Temporal resolution refers to the ability to evaluate changes in an image attribute over time. Thus, sampling rate and frame rate are commonly used as measures of image temporal resolution. As was the case with spatial resolution, the temporal resolution of different imaging techniques also varies considerably, from the M-mode echocardiographic technique, which samples greater than 1,000 ultrasound echoes per second, to ultrafast computed tomography which generates approximately 15 cardiac images per second.

Contrast Resolution

Contrast resolution is commonly defined as the ability to distinguish closely adjacent regions of tissue based on image brightness or gray scale. The meaning of brightness or intensity in a given image varies depending on the type of energy used to create the image. Thus, increased brightness in an echocardiogram is due to increased ultrasound "backscatter." Other imaging techniques have regional intensity or brightness attributes based on quite different variables, including electron density and atomic number (radiography and angiography), radioisotope concentration (radioisotope imaging), and regional proton density, nuclear magnetic resonance relaxation behavior, and blood flow (nuclear magnetic resonance imaging).

GOALS OF CARDIAC DIAGNOSIS

The goals of cardiac diagnosis include evaluation of anatomy, function, metabolism, tissue characteristics, and blood flow. The latter includes evaluation of regional myocardial blood flow (perfusion), blood flow across heart valves, and abnormal flow (shunts) between the left and right sides of the circulation. These goals are attainable, in part, using the standard cardiac imaging methods of chest roentgenography, echocardiography, standard radionuclide imaging, and angiography. However, the standard techniques mainly provide insight into cardiac structure and function and, using Doppler methods, intracardiac and great vessel blood flow. Information on myocardial perfusion is currently only qualitative and relative using ^{201}thallium scintigraphy. Recently, several newer methods have evolved, including digital computer-assisted echocardiography, digital angiography, computed tomography using radionuclides or x-rays, and nuclear magnetic resonance methods. In many cases the newer techniques not only provide better spatial, temporal, and contrast resolution but are capable of obtaining quantitative rather than qualitative data on myocardial perfusion, as well as information about metabolism and tissue characteristics. In the remainder of this discussion, we offer an introduction to some of the capabilities and potential of the newer cardiac imaging methods.

DIGITAL ANGIOCARDIOGRAPHY

Depiction of cardiac structure and function using angiographic techniques has long involved storage of images on cine film or large format "cut" film. The storage of angiographic images in these forms has the advantages of very high spatial resolution and reasonably high contrast resolution. Several disadvantages accrue to these methods, however, including the high cost of film, massive storage requirements for cineangiograms and cut film, and the fact that analog images, such as those stored on cine or cut film, cannot be manipulated by computer unless they are digitized using optical methods. In the last decade, affordable systems have become available which permit direct acquisition and storage of angiographic data in digital form on high-speed digital disks (Heintzen). These systems have permitted such common methods of angiographic image acquisition as digital subtraction angiography. In this method, used in the vascular system throughout the body, an initial, preliminary "scout" image is first obtained, followed by an image recorded after the introduction of radiopaque contrast material into the vascular system. The scout image is then subtracted from the post-infusion image, and the differences in brightness between the images represent the distribution of radiopaque contrast in the vascular system. A substantial amplification of contrast resolution is produced by the subtraction process. The improved contrast resolution is sufficient to permit, for example, high-quality left ventriculography after intravenous injection of contrast material (Mancini and Vogel). One of the ultimate goals of digital angiography when it was initially developed was the ability to visualize the coronary arterial system after intravenous injection. Unfortunately, this has not yet come to fruition. Nonetheless, exciting new types of information have been gleaned from digital analysis of selective left-heart and coronary artery injections. Two basic types of analysis have been used in investigations employing digital techniques to evaluate selective coronary angiograms: static and dynamic methods of assessing the significance of individual coronary stenoses.

STATIC ANALYSES OF CORONARY STENOSES

Digital analysis of single angiographic frames can be used to extract improved anatomical and functional information compared to that available from standard visual analyses of these images. For example, the well-known large inter- and intraobserver variability in visual assessment of coronary angiograms (De-Rouen et al.; Zir et al.) may be reduced by digital analysis. Further, particularly in patients with multivessel coronary disease, visual estimation of percent diameter stenosis on angiograms may correlate poorly with the lesion's functional significance (White et al.). Quantitative computer analyses of single or orthogonal angiographic frames have improved our ability to assess the functional significance of individual coronary stenoses. Automated methods of coronary contour detection (Fleagle et al.), three-dimensional reconstruction techniques (Brown et al.), and video-densitometric measurements (Johnson MR et al.) have been used to approximate the actual minimal luminal area within the atheromatous portion of the coronary artery. All of these approaches offer benefits compared to the simple, visual estimation of percent diameter stenosis (Marcus et al.).

DYNAMIC ANALYSES

Techniques of digital subtraction angiography have been used to assess the kinetics of radiographic contrast entry into and washout from the myocardium for the purposes of estimating myocardial perfusion or, more frequently, coronary flow reserve (Hodgson et al.). Gray scale (Cusma et al.) and color encoding methods (Vogel et al.) have been used to produce parametric images in which regional gray tone or color indicates regional coronary flow reserve. The information on coronary flow reserve may prove to be a useful adjunct to the standard coronary angiogram.

DIGITAL COMPUTER-ASSISTED ECHOCARDIOGRAPHY

Although ultrasound of the heart must be considered a mature technology with well-established methods of data acquisition and interpretation, several lines of active investigation promise to further expand the uses of this energy form for cardiovascular diagnosis.

DIGITAL CONTRAST ECHOCARDIOGRAPHY

Echocardiographic contrast agents include a variety of solutions, usually containing "microbubbles," that can be injected safely into the vascular system and used to increase echo reflectance from the blood in the heart chambers and great vessels (Gramiak et al.).

Ultrasound contrast agents may be safely injected intravenously, causing opacification of right-heart blood, or directly into the aortic root or coronary arteries, providing visualization of the distribution of myocardial blood flow (Feinstein et al; Armstrong). Newer ultrasound contrast agents appear to have the capability of passing through the pulmonary vasculature after intravenous injection and producing some enhancement of echo reflectance from blood on the left side of the heart without the necessity of a left-heart catheterization (Keller et al.). Even if the use of contrast echocardiography for analysis of myocardial blood flow always required left-heart catheterization, this technique might still be very useful as an adjunct to the cardiac catheterization procedure to yield some assessment of the presence and degree of regional hypoperfusion of the myocardium due to coronary artery disease. Although it is too early to assess its eventual clinical relevance, digital contrast echocardiography is beginning to show promise for the assessment of myocardial perfusion.

ULTRASOUND TISSUE CHARACTERIZATION

Echocardiographers have long been aware that certain abnormalities of myocardial structure (such as calcification or deposition of collagen as scar after infarction) will increase regional tissue brightness by increasing the amount of ultrasound energy reflected from cardiac tissue. Recently, investigators have attempted to identify and characterize abnormalities of cardiac tissue structure or physiologic state by quantitatively assessing the amount and pattern of ultrasound reflections from tissue—so called "ultrasound tissue characterization" (Skorton; Miller et al.). Measurements of the overall amplitude of ultrasound reflected from a region of myocardium (referred to as ultrasound backscatter) and computerized analysis of the pattern of echo reflections (referred to as tissue texture) have been two methods used to identify several abnormalities of myocardial structure or perfusion. Acute ischemia (Mimbs et al. 1981; McPherson et al. 1986), acute infarction (Haendchen et al.; Fitzgerald et al.; Skorton et al.), chronic infarction (Mimbs et al. 1980; Vered et al. 1989), and cardiomyopathy (Chandrasekaran et al.; Vered et al. 1987) have all been identified using quantitative ultrasound tissue characterization methods. Currently available technology does not permit the clinical use of ultrasound tissue characterization to assess myocardial composition on a routine basis, but intensive ongoing research makes this a potential additional use of echocardiography in the near future.

THREE-DIMENSIONAL RECONSTRUCTION

Computer technology is often used to construct three-dimensional models of complex-shaped structures for industrial applications such as computer-aided design and computer-aided engineering (Ranky). Techniques of combining several tomographic images to produce a 3D picture of the structure of interest arc being increasingly applied in clinical and investigative medical applications. Three-dimensional reconstructions have found widest use to date in computed tomographic scanning, where available software permits routine 3D reconstruction and display of bony structures (Hemmy et al.). Echocardiography (Geiser et al.) and other tomographic imaging techniques may also be used to produce 3D reconstructions of the heart throughout its cycle. These reconstructions permit assessment of cardiac chamber volume (Moritz et al.; Ariet et al.), calculation of functional indices, and calculation of complex parameters of myocardial performance including stress/strain relationships of the myocardium (McPherson et al. 1987). These computer-generated 3D reconstructions may prove particularly useful in evaluating complex 3D cardiac geometry such as that of the right ventricle and in congenital heart disease. Once again, the area of 3D reconstruction from ultrasound (or other) imaging must currently be considered investigational, but this promising technique may become clinically applicable in the next few years.

COMPUTED TOMOGRAPHY

As mentioned earlier, computed tomography consists of generating slice-like images by computerized reconstruction of image data acquired at many orientations with respect to the heart. Computed tomography can be performed using conventional radioisotopes, positron-emitting isotopes, and x-rays.

RADIOISOTOPE COMPUTED TOMOGRAPHY

Single-Photon Emission Computed Tomography (SPECT)

The radioisotopes used in conventional, planar radioisotope imaging (^{201}thallium and ^{99m}technetium)

emit photons at discrete energy levels. In radioisotope tomography, these photons are detected by a gamma camera that rotates around the patient, yielding data used to create tomographic images. This technique is called single photon emission computed tomography (SPECT) (Croft). Single photon emission computed tomography is being applied to assessment of myocardial perfusion, cardiac function, identification of injury, and metabolic imaging.

New myocardial perfusion tracers. Although ^{201}thallium scanning has proven of clinical value, the suboptimal characteristics of thallium as an imaging agent have motivated research into the development of perfusion tracers based on ^{99m}technetium. ^{99m}Technetium-labeled myocardial perfusion tracers are currently investigational (Sia and Holman; Heo et al.). Many of the advantages of the ^{99m}technetium-labeled myocardial perfusion tracers are related to the higher energy of ^{99m}technetium (140 keV) as compared with the photopeak with the highest relative abundance for ^{201}thallium (80 keV). The resulting advantages of ^{99m}technetium-labeled tracers include higher spatial resolution, more favorable radiation dosimetry, and the possibility that attenuation correction can be performed (discussed further below).

Quantitation. Methods have been developed to quantitate tomographic images of relative regional myocardial perfusion by using circumferential profile analysis. One approach employs a "bullseye" display, presenting the short-axis slices as concentric circles (Figure 1) (Caldwell et al.; Garcia et al.; dePasquale et al.).

Technical considerations. Increased anatomic information and the lack of superimposition of counts from different myocardial regions are two advantages of SPECT. However, the technique is more complex than planar imaging. Some of the factors that influence measurement of radioactivity and, therefore, might affect image interpretation, include scattered photons, attenuation, uniformity of detector response, and patient motion. Correction of images for scattered photons is still investigational but can be performed by determination of a "scatter mask" either from the tomograms (Axelsson et al.) or from radioactivity measured at a photopeak below that of the radioisotope being imaged (Jaszczak et al.). Initial attempts at attenuation correction require acquisition of a transmission image, yielding information about attenuation coefficients of the different tissues surrounding the heart (Manglos et al.). Quantitative estimation of regional radioisotope concentration may be improved

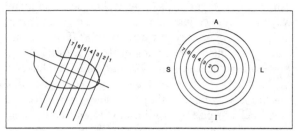

Figure 1. *Illustration of "bullseye" display of data from SPECT ²⁰¹thallium images. At left is a schematic of the left ventricle, indicating the location of short-axis images from the apex (slice 1) to the base (slice 7). At right, data on ²⁰¹thallium uptake in these slices are displayed concentrically with the apex at the center. Data for the apex can be obtained either from the short-axis image as shown or from the vertical, long-axis image. A = anterior left ventricle; I = inferior left ventricle; L = lateral left ventricle; S = interventricular septum. (From Brundage B: Correlative Cardiac Imaging. Aspen; 1990. With permission of Aspen Publishers, Inc.)*

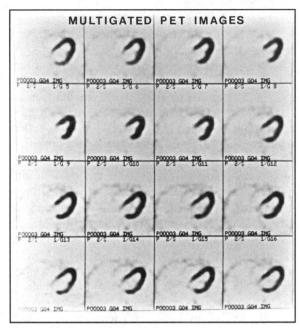

Figure 2. *Gated ¹⁸F-deoxyglucose PET images of the left ventricle are shown, with end-diastole at the upper left corner, going through systole, to end-diastole again at the lower right. In each frame, the interventricular septum is at the upper left, the anterior wall and apex at the upper right and the lateral wall at the lower right. The changes in wall thickness and ventricular cavity size with contraction can be seen.*

after attenuation correction. Attempting to correct for the uniformity of response to a photon for all detectors is extremely important for SPECT imaging. Finally, as little as 3-mm motion by the patient has been shown to create ²⁰¹thallium image artifacts that can mimic perfusion defects (Eisner et al.; Friedman et al.).

Positron Emission Tomography (PET)

The radioisotopes used in positron emission tomography (PET) emit a positive electron, or positron, that travels a short distance before it combines with an electron. The combined mass of the positron and electron is converted to two gamma rays, an event called annihilation. The two gamma rays leave the site of interaction at approximately 180°. A ring of detectors is placed around the heart to detect the annihilation events. Measurement and correction for scattered photons and for attenuation are possible. Gated PET images of the heart of excellent clarity can be acquired (Figure 2). The main radioisotopes that have been used in PET include tracers of myocardial blood flow (¹³N ammonia, ⁸²rubidium and ¹⁵O water), a tracer of exogenous glucose utilization (¹⁸F 2-deoxyglucose), a tracer of fatty acid metabolism (¹¹C palmitic acid), and a tracer of the tricarboxylic acid cycle (¹¹C acetate). Tracers of myocardial receptors are still

under investigation (Syrota). Quantitation of regional myocardial blood flow and metabolism are possible using a tracer kinetic model for a given radiotracer (Huang and Phelps).

X-RAY COMPUTED TOMOGRAPHY

X-ray computed tomography (CT) has several advantages compared with conventional x-ray imaging. On x-ray CT images, superimposition of structures inherent to conventional, planar x-ray imaging techniques does not occur. The x-ray CT technique is able to record x-ray intensity differences of less than 0.1% and to determine the attenuation coefficient of a given structure to within 0.5%. Determination of attenuation coefficients is possible in part because of more exact mathematical methods for correction of problems related to "beam hardening." This term refers to changes in the x-ray spectrum that occur due to x-ray/tissue interactions when the x-ray source is polyenergetic (Robb and Morin). Finally, less scattered radiation is detected in x-ray CT because the beam is collimated.

However, conventional x-ray CT has several limitations in cardiac imaging. Spatial resolution is limited by the fact that objects that are smaller than the resolution of the machine may not be accurately measured; this is called the "partial volume" effect (Hoffman and Ritman). Resolution is also limited by the blurring due to cardiac and respiratory motion. More x-ray photons are detected with longer imaging times; however, greater patient motion will also be detected. After image acquisition using conventional x-ray CT, the gantry must rotate back to its original position. In addition, other mechanical and electrical events limit the time for scan acquisition to approximately 2 seconds and for the interscan delay to approximately 3 seconds. In response to these problems, two methods of rapid CT scanning have been recently developed to permit dynamic CT imaging of the heart.

Dynamic computed tomography was initially performed using the Dynamic Spatial Reconstructor (DSR) at Mayo Clinic (Ritman et al.). Simultaneous acquisition of up to 240 adjacent, 1-mm thick image planes at rates of up to 60/sec is possible with the DSR.

Ultrafast Computed Tomography

This method differs from conventional x-ray CT because acquisition of rapid images is made possible by using an electron beam rather than an x-ray tube (Boyd et al.). The electron beam is deflected onto four stationary 210° tungsten target rings, producing an x-ray beam that is transmitted through the patient. Up to eight image levels are generated, since the radiation is detected by two banks of solid-state detectors above the patient. Depending on whether single- or multiple-slice imaging is being performed, image acquisition time may be as short as 50 msec. Image acquisition can be gated to the cardiac cycle.

CLINICAL APPLICATIONS OF EMISSION COMPUTED TOMOGRAPHY

Single Photon Emission Computed Tomography (SPECT)

The major advantages of SPECT are that the radiotracers employed are used in conventional cardiac nuclear imaging studies, and that the tomographic gamma cameras and other details of the technique are in many ways similar to conventional gamma camera imaging. To date the major uses of cardiac SPECT studies include assessment of (1) regional myocardial blood flow with [201]thallium- and [99m]technetium-labeled perfusion tracers; (2) global and regional myocardial function and volumes using [99m]technetium-labeled red blood cells to perform radioisotope ventriculograms; and (3) myocardial damage with [99m]technetium pyrophosphate, antimyosin antibodies, or [201]thallium. In addition, metabolic studies have been performed using iodinated fatty acids.

Evaluation of regional myocardial blood flow. Studies have demonstrated that, for the diagnosis of coronary artery disease, [201]thallium SPECT imaging results in improved diagnostic performance when compared with planar imaging (Tamaki et al.; Fintel et al.). This is particularly true for the left anterior descending and circumflex coronary arteries in men. The addition of quantitative analysis improves detection of circumflex disease (Port et al.). Applying the bullseye analysis method to 210 patients, 179 with and 31 without coronary disease, resulted in a sensitivity of 95%, a specificity of 74%, and accuracy of 92% for prediction of the presence or absence of coronary disease (Garcia). Although not all initial studies using [99m]technetium-labeled perfusion tracers were performed using SPECT, the preliminary data suggest that imaging with the technetium-labeled tracers provides information comparable to [201]thallium imaging (Kiat et al.; Seldin et al.). In addition, using [99m]technetium-labeled perfusion tracers, simultaneous measurement of ventricular function can be performed in conjunction with evaluation of myocardial perfusion (Sporn et al.).

Evaluation of global and regional myocardial function and volume. Several studies have demonstrated that tomographic radioisotope ventriculograms detect regional wall motion abnormalities and estimate ventricular volumes with reasonable accuracy (Corbett et al. 1985; Underwood et al.; Faber et al.).

Evaluation of myocardial damage. Detection of nontransmural acute myocardial infarction is improved using SPECT rather than planar ^{99m}Tc pyrophosphate imaging (Corbett et al. 1984), and estimation of infarct size is possible (Holman et al.; Lewis et al.; Jansen et al.). Infarcted myocardium can also be imaged with antimyosin antibody. The area delineated by pyrophosphate is larger than the area identified by antimyosin antibody, possibly because pyrophosphate is seen in both infarcted and ischemic myocardium whereas antimyosin antibody is only seen in infarcted myocardium (Khaw et al.; Johnson LL et al.). [201]Thallium SPECT imaging has also been used to quantitate infarct size (Caldwell et al.; Johnson LL et al.; Mahmarian et al.).

Evaluation of myocardial fatty acid metabolism.
Radioiodinated fatty acid tracers have been synthesized and used to evaluate myocardial fatty acid metabolism, hence viability, in normal, ischemic, and reperfused myocardium, and in cardiomyopathy (Rellas et al.; Vyska et al.; Miller et al.). The large iodine molecule attached to the fatty acid raises the question of whether the tracers are transported and metabolized in an identical manner to non-iodinated fatty acids.

Positron Emission Tomography (PET)

Cardiac PET has been used to evaluate myocardial blood flow and metabolism, and initial investigations of receptors have been performed. The ability to investigate myocardial metabolism has provided unique information regarding myocardial viability and biochemistry. The dietary state of the patient (e.g., fasted or fed) can influence metabolic images. In the fasted state, arterial fatty acids are increased, and normal myocytes preferentially utilize fatty acids; whereas after a glucose load, normal myocytes increase glucose utilization (Neely et al.). However, when oxygen delivery is decreased, for example, during ischemia, fatty acid metabolism is impaired because oxygen is necessary to perform beta-oxidation. Energy can still be obtained by anaerobic glycolysis, and therefore, glucose utilization increases in myocytes with insufficient oxygen delivery (Liedtke).

Detection of coronary artery disease. Several studies have demonstrated the ability to accurately detect coronary artery stenoses with the positron-emitting tracers of myocardial blood flow, ^{13}N ammonia (Schelbert et al. 1981; Yonekura et al.), [82]rubidium (Gould et al.; Demer et al.), and [15]O water (Bergmann et al. 1984). Sensitivities for the detection of coronary disease ranged from 94% to 98% and specificities from 95% to 100%, compared with visual analysis of coronary angiograms. Regional myocardial blood flow can be quantitated by applying a tracer kinetic model to data obtained from serial images (Figure 3).

Myocardial fatty acid metabolism. Evaluation of myocardial fatty acid metabolism is possible using ^{11}C palmitate (Schon et al.). Ischemic and infarcted myocardium can be detected (Sobel et al. 1977; Lerch

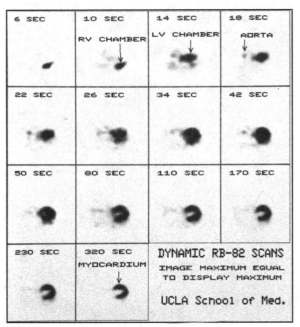

Figure 3. *Dynamic [82]rubidium PET images of the heart. The blood flow tracer, [82]rubidium, is seen initially in the right ventricular (RV) chamber, subsequently in the left ventricular (LV) chamber, and finally in the left ventricular myocardium.*

et al.; Geltman et al. 1982) as can the effect of different workloads (Schelbert et al. 1983; Grover-McKay et al.). Myocardial fatty acid metabolism can improve after coronary thrombolysis, and this improvement can be evaluated with ^{11}C palmitate (Bergmann et al. 1982; Sobel et al. 1984; Knabb et al.). Altered regional myocardial metabolism has been detected in congestive cardiomyopathy (Geltman et al. 1983).

Detection of infarcted and viable myocardium.
Detection of infarcted and viable myocardium is also possible using both a tracer of myocardial blood flow and a tracer of metabolism, such as a tracer of exogenous glucose utilization, [18]F 2-deoxyglucose. Infarcted myocardium demonstrates a concordant decrease in the uptake of both tracers (Figure 4). In ischemic but viable myocardium, which cannot utilize fatty acids in a normal manner, exogenous glucose utilization is increased, presumably because of increased anaerobic glycolysis. Therefore, regional myocardial [18]F 2-deoxyglucose uptake is increased relative to blood flow, a pattern which has been called "mismatch" (Figure 5). This pattern has been observed in several clinical situations including after myocardial infarction, and in patients with coronary

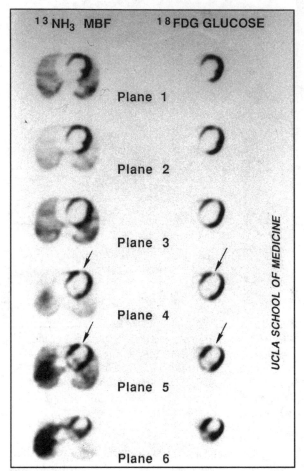

Figure 4. *Positron emission tomographic (PET) images of myocardial blood flow (MBF) obtained using ^{13}N-ammonia are seen on the left at six myocardial levels from the base (at top) to the apex (at bottom). Myocardial images of exogenous glucose utilization (^{18}F-deoxyglucose, FDG) are seen on the right. Concordant decrease in blood flow and glucose utilization is seen in the anteroseptal region from the midventricle towards the apex, as demonstrated by the arrows. This finding is consistent with prior myocardial infarction. (From Schelbert H and Buxton D: Insights into coronary artery disease gained from metabolic imaging. Circulation 78:496, 1988. Published with permission of the American Heart Association.)*

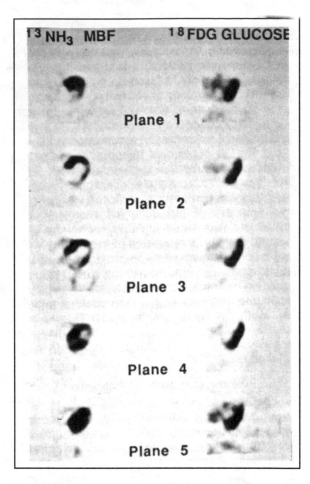

Figure 5. *Images of myocardial blood flow (MBF) obtained with ^{13}N-ammonia are seen on the left and of exogenous glucose utilization obtained with ^{18}F-deoxyglucose (FDG) on the right. The base of the heart is at the top and the apex is at the bottom. Myocardial blood flow is decreased in the lateral wall. Glucose utilization is increased in the lateral wall compared with the septum. This pattern has been called a "mismatch" (of perfusion vs. substrate uptake) and is believed to represent an increase in anaerobic glycolysis in the ischemic lateral wall. (From Schelbert H and Buxton D.: Insights into coronary artery disease gained from metabolic imaging. Circulation 78:496, 1988. Published with permission of the American Heart Association.)*

artery disease studied at rest and also after exercise (Marshall et al; Schwaiger et al.; Camici et al.). Abnormal wall motion has been shown to improve in myocardium with this pattern following successful coronary artery bypass grafting (Tillisch et al.). This

pattern has been demonstrated in myocardium represented by Q waves on the electrocardiogram (Brunken et al. 1986) and by persistent thallium defects (Brunken et al. 1987). Detection of viable but jeopardized myocardium may enable improved identifi-

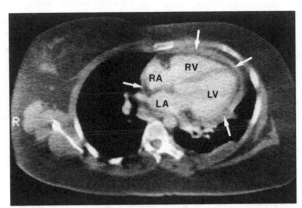

Figure 6. *Ultrafast computed tomography (CT) image of the heart. The right atrium (RA) and right ventricle (RV) are at the top and the left atrium (LA) and left ventricle (LV) are at the bottom. A thickened pericardium can be seen (arrows). (Courtesy of William Stanford, M.D., The University of Iowa Department of Radiology.)*

cation of patients who will benefit from acute interventions such as coronary thrombolysis and angioplasty.

CLINICAL APPLICATIONS OF DYNAMIC X-RAY COMPUTED TOMOGRAPHY

Anatomy and function. Assessment of cardiac geometry with dynamic CT methods permits remarkably precise measurements of several clinically important parameters. Myocardial mass (Feiring et al.; Iwasaki et al.), chamber volumes (Reiter et al. 1986), cardiac output (Garrett et al.) and regurgitant volumes (Reiter et al. 1987) can be calculated extraordinarily accurately using rapid CT methods. Detection of pericardial thickening and fluid (Figure 6), cardiac tumors (Figure 7), aortic aneurysm/dissection, and thrombus is possible with a high degree of success. High-resolution, dynamic CT methods may even potentially permit coronary artery visualization (Block et al.). Global function and regional function have been accurately evaluated at rest and during exercise, ischemia, and pharmacologic and hemodynamic interventions (Farmer et al.; Lanzer et al.; Feiring et al. 1988).

Coronary artery bypass grafts. A particular strength of ultrafast CT is in the assessment of coronary artery bypass graft patency. Experience at several centers supports the use of CT to evaluate grafts in the clin-

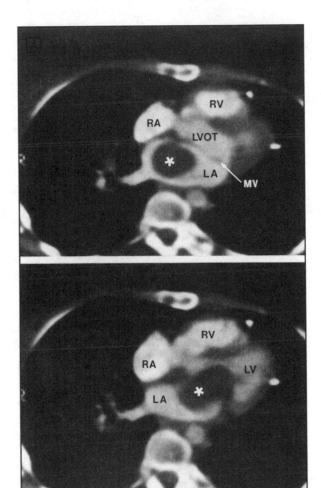

Figure 7. *Ultrafast CT image of left atrial myxoma. A. Images obtained during systole demonstrate the left atrial myxoma (*) surrounded by the contrast material in the left atrium (LA). B. During diastole the left atrial myxoma is seen to cross the mitral valve (MV) into the left ventricle (LV). The right atrium (RA), right ventricle (RV), and left ventricular outflow tract (LVOT) are also filled with contrast material. (Courtesy of William Stanford, M.D., The University of Iowa Department of Radiology.)*

ical setting (Figure 8) (Bateman et al.; Stanford et al.). This appears to be the most accurate noninvasive method available at present for directly identifying graft patency.

Myocardial perfusion. Initial attempts at quantitation of myocardial blood flow (Rumberger et al.; Wolfkiel et al.) demonstrated that CT-based methods were promising. Ongoing investigations suggest that evaluation of endocardial versus epicardial myocardial blood flow may be possible with ultrafast CT.

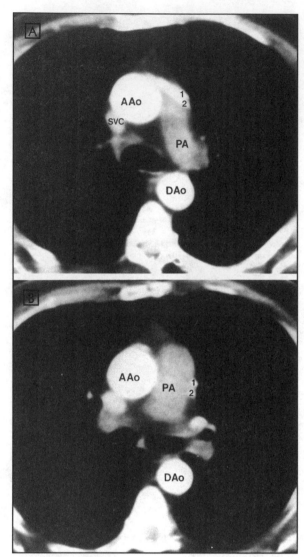

Figure 8. *Ultrafast CT images demonstrating coronary artery bypass graft patency. A. The ascending aorta (AAo) and descending aorta (DAo) are filled with contrast material. The two linear structures which are filled with contrast material and are attached to the ascending aorta represent two venous bypass grafts (1,2). B. The two grafts are seen in cross-section after they have traversed the pulmonary artery (PA). SVC = superior vena cava. (Courtesy of William Stanford, M.D., The University of Iowa Department of Radiology.)*

MAGNETIC RESONANCE IMAGING AND SPECTROSCOPY

The nuclear magnetic resonance (NMR) phenomenon is based on the fact that nuclei with an odd number of protons, neutrons, or both, have the property of angular momentum, or "spin." These spinning, charged particles produce local magnetic fields. Because the magnetic fields are normally randomly distributed, the *net* magnetic field of an object, such as a patient, is zero. However, when the patient is placed in a strong external magnetic field, enough of the local magnetic fields (such as those produced by spinning hydrogen nuclei or protons) align with the external field to produce a small, net magnetic moment. By quantum theory, the spinning nuclei can exist in two states: aligned with or against the external magnetic field. The protons aligned with the magnetic field are in a lower energy state than those aligned against the field. When an additional magnetic field in the form of a radiofrequency pulse is delivered, some of the protons "flip" into the higher energy state, but slowly return, or relax, back to the equilibrium state. It is the energy emitted as protons relax back to the lower energy state that is used to produce magnetic resonance (MR) images. The brightness of a region in an MR image depends upon several factors, including the concentration of protons (essentially, water content), the rate of relaxation, and blood flow (Pohost and Canby).

In addition to the ability to obtain images, the magnetic resonance imaging technique enables tissue characterization both by evaluation of relaxation times and by spectroscopy. The relaxation times, T1 and T2, represent in part the time required for the protons to return to equilibrium. T1 is called the spin-lattice relaxation time because it denotes relaxation due to energy exchange between the nucleus (spin) and its surrounding environment (lattice). T2 is called the spin-spin relaxation time because this relaxation phenomenon is due in part to exchange of energy between neighboring spins. Differences in relaxation times are present in different types of tissue and different states of the same tissue (e.g., infarcted vs. normal).

Nuclear magnetic resonance spectroscopy yields noninvasive information about the chemical composition of tissue. This information results from evaluating the unique magnetic fields created by the chemical environment of the nucleus under study (Gadian).

CLINICAL APPLICATIONS OF MAGNETIC RESONANCE IMAGING

Anatomy and function. Magnetic resonance images are high-resolution tomograms yielding excellent depiction of the details of cardiac anatomy, including the demonstration of pericardial disease, aortic aneurysm/dissection (Kersting-Sommerhoff et al.), and cardiac masses (Freedberg et al.). Such geometric variables as left ventricular mass can be quite accurately determined by MR imaging (Keller et al.; Florentine et al.). Similarly, alterations in regional wall thickness due to scar or aneurysm can be readily visualized with MR imaging techniques (Higgins et al.). Particularly with the improvement in temporal resolution offered by cine MR techniques, global and regional left ventricular function can also be analyzed (Sechtem et al. 1987; van Rossum et al.). Alterations in blood pool appearance related to changes in blood flow velocity (Kaufman et al.) and turbulence (discussed further below) can also be exploited to visualize "jets" of blood moving through regurgitant valves (Utz et al.; Sechtem et al. 1988) (Figure 9) and intracardiac defects.

Tissue characterization by MR relaxometry. The T1 and T2 MR relaxation times can give substantial information concerning the molecular environment of protons in normal and abnormal tissue. Thus, relaxation times have been found to be significantly altered by myocardial ischemia (Johnston et al.; Pflugfelder et al.) and infarction (McNamara et al.; Wisenberg et al.1988; Been et al.). Since relaxation times are important determinants of regional tissue brightness in MR images, the altered relaxation behavior of infarcted myocardium can sometimes be directly visualized as increased tissue brightness on T2-weighted images (Figure 10). Although the tissue determinants of alterations in myocardial relaxation times have not been fully explored, image-based assessment of relaxation times appears to be one noninvasive approach to tissue characterization of the myocardium. Acute and chronic injury attendant to myocardial ischemia has been the most carefully studied myocardial abnormality utilizing magnetic resonance imaging or relaxometry. Infarct-related alterations in magnetic resonance T1 and T2 and in image intensity are related in greater part to changes in tissue water content. Cardiac transplant rejection is another process that may be potentially detected using MR methods (Aherne et al.; Wisenberg et al. 1987).

Vascular imaging. The appearance of blood in magnetic resonance images is greatly dependent on the rate of blood flow with respect to the imaging plane. For spin-echo MR pulse sequences, an inverse relationship exists between the rate of blood flow and image intensity, with more rapid blood flow causing

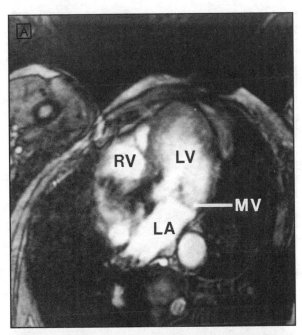

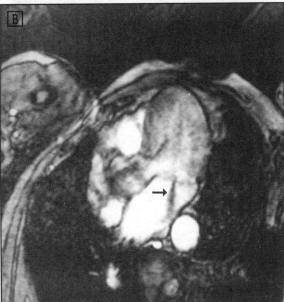

Figure 9. *Cine-magnetic resonance images from a patient with mitral regurgitation. A. Diastolic image depicting right ventricle (RV), left ventricle (LV), left atrium (LA), and the mitral valve (MV). B. Systolic image demonstrating a jet of mitral regurgitation (arrow). (Courtesy of William Stanford, M.D., The University of Iowa Department of Radiology.)*

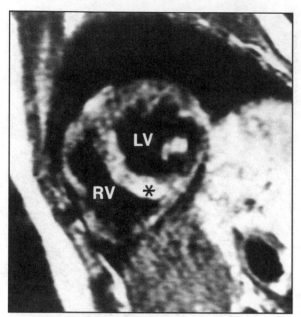

Figure 10. *Magnetic resonance image of a recent inferoseptal myocardial infarction. The heart is seen in short-axis cross-section, depicting the left (LV) and right ventricles (RV). The infarcted area (*) is brighter than the surrounding normal myocardium on this T2-weighted image, suggesting a regional prolongation of T2. (Courtesy of William Stanford, M.D., University of Iowa Department of Radiology.)*

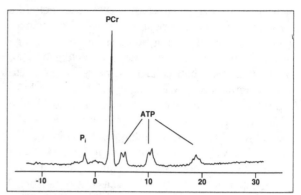

Figure 11. *^{31}Phosphorous MR spectrum obtained with a surface coil from normal skeletal muscle. The peaks representing phosphocreatine (PCr), inorganic phosphate (Pi), and the peaks of the individual phosphorous atoms of adenosine triphosphate (ATP) are clearly seen. (Courtesy of William Thoma, Ph.D., The University of Iowa Department of Radiology.)*

decreasing image brightness (Kaufman et al.). This phenomenon is the cause of the well-recognized "flow void" of patent blood vessels as depicted on MR images. Use of other pulse sequences may make flowing blood look bright on MR images, and turbulent blood may be made to have a dark appearance (Figure 9). These image processing manipulations have produced a variety of promising applications of MR imaging in identification of abnormalities of the peripheral vasculature (Wedeen et al.; Fishman et al.). Atherosclerosis may also be identified using MR techniques (Wesbey et al.; Soila et al.). Although the eventual place of MR in the assessment of peripheral vascular disease is not certain, impressive noninvasive angiograms and an indication of the presence of atherosclerosis may be obtained utilizing advanced MR imaging techniques.

Coronary artery and graft visualization, and myocardial perfusion. Nuclear magnetic resonance methods show the potential of providing information on myocardial perfusion, particularly with the use of paramagnetic contrast agents (Brown and Higgins). The relatively high resolution of newer MR imaging methods may also permit direct evaluation of proximal coronary arterial anatomy and bypass graft patency (Rubinstein et al.).

SPECTROSCOPY

Nuclear magnetic resonance spectroscopy offers abundant information on the concentration and kinetics of several biologically relevant nuclei including the hydrogen nucleus, ^{31}phosphorous, ^{13}carbon, ^{19}fluorine, and ^{23}sodium. Phosphorous spectra (Figure 11) may be used to identify alterations in high energy phosphate pools attendant to acute myocardial ischemia (Massie and Weiner; Robitaille et al.; Kavanaugh et al.). Reaction rates and other kinetic information concerning a variety of chemical reactions may be obtained by spectroscopy of several nuclei (Gadian). Although not widely available at present, MR spectroscopy promises to open a broad diagnostic vista for the clinician caring for the patient with ischemic heart disease (Bottomley).

Acknowledgements

The authors express their gratitude to Steven Fleagle, B.S.E.E., Karim Rezai, M.D., and Byron Vanden-

berg, M.D., for thoughful review of the paper, and Marlene Blakley, Carolyn Frisbie and Ruth Lillie for expert preparation of the manuscript.

Bibliography

Aherne T, Tscholakoff D, Finkbeiner W, et al: Magnetic resonance imaging of cardiac transplants: The evaluation of rejection of cardiac allografts with and without immunosuppression. *Circulation* 74:145, 1986.

Ariet M, Geiser EA, Lupkiewicz SM, Conetta DA, Conti CR: Evaluation of a three-dimensional reconstruction to compute left ventricular volume and mass. *Am J Cardiol* 54:415, 1984.

Armstrong WF: Assessment of myocardial perfusion with constrast enhanced echocardiography. *Echocardiography* 3:355, 1986.

Axelsson B, Msaki P, Israelsson A: Subtraction of scattered photons in single photon computerized tomography. *J Nucl Med* 25:490, 1984.

Bateman TM, Gray RJ, Whiting JS, et al: Prospective evaluation of ultrafast cardiac computed tomography for determination of saphenous vein bypass graft patency. *Circulation* 75:1018, 1987.

Been M, Smith MA, Ridgway JP, et al: Serial changes in the T_1 magnetic relaxation parameter after myocardial infarction in man. *Br Heart J* 59:1, 1988.

Bergmann RS, Lerch RA, Fox KAA, et al: Temporal dependence of beneficial effects of coronary thrombolysis characterized by positron tomography. *Am J Med* 73:753, 1982.

Bergmann SR, Fox KAA, Rand AL, et al: Quantification of regional myocardial blood flow in vivo with $H_2^{15}O$. *Circulation* 70:724, 1984.

Block M, Bove AA, Ritman EL: Coronary angiographic examination with the dynamic spatial reconstructor. *Circulation* 70:209, 1984.

Bottomley PA: Human in vivo NMR spectroscopy in diagnostic medicine: Clinical tool or research probe? *Radiology* 170:1, 1989.

Boyd DP, Gould RG, Quinn JR, et al: A proposed dynamic cardiac 3-D densitometer for early detection and evaluation of heart disease. *IEEE Trans Nucl Sci* NS-26:2724, 1979.

Brown BG, Bolson E, Frimer M, et al. Quantitative coronary arteriography. Estimation of dimensions, hemodynamic resistance, and atheroma mass of coronary artery lesions using the arteriogram and digital computation. *Circulation* 55:329, 1977.

Brown JJ, Higgins CB: Myocardial paramagnetic contrast agents for MR imaging. *Am J Radiol* 151:865, 1988.

Brunken R, Schwaiger M, Grover-McKay M, et al: Positron emission tomography detects tissue metabolic activity in myocardial segments with persistent thallium perfusion defects. *J Am Coll Cardiol* 10:557, 1987.

Brunken R, Tillisch J, Schwaiger M, et al: Regional perfusion, glucose metabolism, and wall motion in patients with chronic electrocardiographic Q wave infarctions: Evidence for persistence of viable tissue in some infarct regions by positron emission tomography. *Circulation* 73:951, 1986.

Caldwell JH, Williams DL, Harp GD, et al: Quantification of size of relative myocardial perfusion defect by single photon emission computed tomography. *Circulation* 70:1048, 1984.

Camici P, Araujo LI, Spinks T, et al: Increased uptake of ^{18}F-fluorodeoxyglucose in postischemic myocardium of patients with exercise-induced angina. *Circulation* 74:81, 1986.

Chandrasekaran K, Aylward PE, Fleagle SR, et al: Feasibility of identifying amyloid and hypertrophic cardiomyopathy with the use of computerized quantitative texture analysis of clinical echocardiographic data. *J Am Coll Cardiol* 13:832, 1989.

Corbett JR, Jansen DE, Lewis SE, et al: Tomographic gated blood pool radionuclide ventriculography: Analysis of wall motion and left ventricular volumes in patients with coronary artery disease. *J Am Coll Cardiol* 6:349, 1985.

Corbett JR, Lewis M, Willerson JT, et al: 99m Tc-pyrophosphate imaging in patients with acute myocardial infarction: Comparison of planar imaging with single photon tomography with and without blood pool overlay. *Circulation* 69:1120, 1984.

Croft BY: *Single Photon Emission Computed Tomography.* Chicago: Year Book Medical Publishers; 1986.

Coulam CM, Erickson JJ, Rollo FD, James AE: *The Physical Basis of Medical Imaging.* New York: Appleton-Century-Crofts; 1981, p. 59.

Cusma JT, Toggart EJ, Folts JD, et al: Digital subtraction angiographic imaging of coronary flow reserve. *Circulation* 75:461, 1987.

DePasquale E, Nody A, DePuey G, et al: Quantitative rotational thallium-201 tomography for identifying and localizing coronary artery disease. *Circulation* 77:316, 1988.

Demer LL, Gould KL, Goldstein RA, et al: Assessment of coronary artery disease severity by positron emission tomography. Comparison with quantitative arteriography in 193 patients. *Circulation* 79:825, 1989.

DeRouen TA, Murray JA, Owen W: Variability in the analysis of coronary arteriograms. *Circulation* 55:324, 1977.

Eisner RL, Noever T, Nowak D, et al: Use of cross-correlation function to detect patient motion during SPECT imaging. *J Nucl Med* 28:97, 1987.

Faber TL, Stokely EM, Templeton GH, et al: Quantification of three-dimensional left ventricular segmental wall motion and volumes from gated tomographic radionuclide ventriculograms. *J Nucl Med* 30:638, 1989.

Farmer D, Lipton MJ, Higgins CB, et al: In vivo assessment of left ventricular wall and chamber dynamics during transient myocardial ischemia using cine-computed tomography. *Am J Cardiol* 55:560, 1985.

Feinstein SB, Lang RM, Dick C, et al: Contrast echocardiographic perfusion studies in humans. *Am J Cardiac Imaging* 1:29, 1986.

Feiring AJ, Rumberger JA, Reiter SJ, et al: Determination of left ventricular mass in dogs with rapid acquisition cardiac CT scanning. *Circulation* 72:1355, 1985.

Feiring AJ, Rumberger JA, Reiter SJ, et al: Sectional and segmental variability of left ventricular function: Experimental and clinical studies using ultrafast computed tomography. *J Am Coll Cardiol* 12:415, 1988.

Fintel DJ, Links JM, Brinker JA, et al: Improved diagnostic performance of exercise thallium-201 photon emission computed tomography over planar imaging in the diagnosis of coronary artery disease: A receiver operating characteristic analysis. *J Am Coll Cardiol* 13:600, 1989.

Fishman MC, Naidich JB, Stein HL: Vascular magnetic resonance imaging. *Radiologic Clinics of North America* 24:485, 1986.

Fitzgerald PJ, McDaniel MD, Rolett EL, et al: Two-dimensional ultrasonic tissue characterization: Backscatter power, endocardial wall motion, and their relationship for normal, ischemic and infarcted myocardium. *Circulation* 76:850, 1987.

Fleagle SR, Johnson MR, Wilbricht CJ, et al: Automated analysis of coronary arterial morphology in cineangiograms: Geometric and physiologic validation in humans. *IEEE Trans on Medical Imaging* 8:387, 1989.

Florentine MS, Grosskreutz CL, Chang W, et al: Measurement of left ventricular mass in vivo using gated nuclear magnetic resonance imaging. *J Am Coll Cardiol* 8:107, 1986.

Freedberg RS, Kronzon I, Rumancik WM, Liebeskind D: The contribution of magnetic resonance imaging to the evaluation of intracardiac tumors diagnosed by echocardiography. *Circulation* 1:96, 1988.

Friedman J, Berman DS, Van Train K, et al: Patient motion in thallium-201 myocardial SPECT imaging: An easily identified frequent source of artifactual defect. *Clin Nucl Med* 13:321, 1988.

Gadian DG: *Nuclear Magnetic Resonance and its Applications to Living Systems*. New York: Oxford University Press; 1982.

Garcia EV: Conventional radionuclide imaging, physics and instrumentation. In: Marcus ML, Skorton DJ, Schelbert HR, Wolf GL, eds. *Cardiac Imaging: Principles and Practice*. Philadelphia: WB Saunders; (in press).

Garcia EV, Van Train K, Maddahi J, et al: Quantification of rotational thallium-201 myocardial tomography. *J Nucl Med* 26:17, 1985.

Garrett JS, Lanzer P, Jaschke W, et al: Measurement of cardiac output by cine-computed tomography. *Am J Cardiol* 56:657, 1985.

Geltman EM, Biello D, Welch MJ, et al: Characterization of nontransmural myocardial infarction by positron tomography. *Circulation* 65:747, 1982.

Geltman EM, Smith JL, Beechler D, et al: Altered regional myocardial metabolism in congestive cardiomyopathy detected by positron tomography. *Am J Med* 74:773, 1983.

Geiser EA, Lupkiewicz SM, Christie LG, et al: A framework for three-dimensional time-varying reconstruction of the human left ventricle: Sources of error and estimation of their magnitude. *Comput Biomed Res* 13:225, 1980.

Gramiak R, Shah PM, Kramer DH: Ultrasound cardiography: Contrast studies in anatomy and function. *Radiology* 92:939, 1969.

Grover-McKay M, Schelbert HR, Schwaiger M, et al: Identification of impaired metabolic reserve in patients with significant coronary artery stenosis by atrial pacing. *Circulation* 74:281, 1986.

Gould KL, Goldstein RA, Mullai NA, et al: Noninvasive assessment of coronary stenoses by myocardial perfusion imaging during pharmacologic coronary vasodilation. VIII. Clinical feasibility of positron cardiac imaging without a cy-

clotron using generator-produced rubidium-82. *J Am Coll Cardiol* 7:775, 1986.

Haendchen RV, Ong K, Fishbein MC, et al: Early differentiation of infarcted and noninfarcted reperfused myocardium in dogs by quantitative analysis of regional myocardial echo amplitudes. *Circ Res* 57:718, 1985.

Heintzen PH: Digital angiocardiography. In: Collins SM, Skorton DJ, eds. *Cardiac Imaging and Image processing*. New York: McGraw-Hill; 1986, p. 239.

Hemmy DC, David DJ, Herman GT: Three-dimensional reconstruction of craniofacial deformity using computed tomography. *Neurosurgery* 13:534, 1983.

Heo J, Hermann GA, Iskandrian A, et al: New myocardial perfusion imaging agents: Description and application. *Am Heart J* 115:1111, 1988.

Higgins CB, Lanzer P, Stark D, et al: Imaging by nuclear magnetic resonance in patients with chronic ischemic heart disease. *Circulation* 69:523, 1984.

Hodgson JM, LeGrand V, Bates ER, et al: Validation in dogs of a rapid digital angiographic technique to measure relative coronary blood flow during routine cardiac catheterization. *Am J Cardiol* 55:188, 1985.

Hoffman EA, Ritman EL: Shape and dimensions of cardiac chamber via computed tomography: Role of imaged slice thickness and orientation. *Radiology* 155:739, 1985.

Holman BL, Goldhaber SZ, Kirsch ZM, et al: Measurement of infarct sizes in single photon emission computed tomography and technetium-99m pyrophosphate: A description of the method and comparison with patient prognosis. *Am J Cardiol* 50:503, 1982.

Huang SC, Phelps ME: Principles of tracer kinetic modeling in positron emission tomography and autoradiography. In: Phelps ME, Mazziotta JC, Schelbert HR, eds. *Positron Emission Tomography and Autoradiography*. New York: Raven Press; 1986, p. 287.

Iwasaki T, Sinak LJ, Hoffman EA, et al: Mass of left ventricular myocardium estimated with dynamic spatial reconstructor. *Am J Physiol* 15:H138, 1984.

Jansen DE, Corbett JR, Buja LM, et al: Quantitation of myocardial injury produced by temporary coronary artery obstruction and reflow with technetium 99m pyrophosphate. *Circulation* 75:611, 1987.

Jaszczak RJ, Floyd CE, Coleman RE: Scatter compensation techniques for SPECT. *IEEE Trans Nucl Sci* NS-32:786, 1985.

Johnson LL, Lerick KS, Coromilas J, et al: Measurement of infarct size and percentage myocardium infarcted in a dog preparation with single photon emission computed tomography, thallium-201, and indium-111-monoclonal antimyosin Fab. *Circulation* 76:181, 1987.

Johnson MR, Collins SM, Marcus ML, Skorton DJ: Quantification of coronary artery stenoses using videodensitometry. *Am J Cardiac Imag* (in press).

Johnston DL, Brady TJ, Ratner AV, et al: Assessment of myocardial ischemia with proton magnetic resonance: Effects of a three hour coronary occlusion with and without reperfusion. *Circulation* 71:595, 1985.

Kaufman L, Crooks L, Sheldon P, et al: The potential impact of nuclear magnetic resonance imaging on cardiovascular diagnosis. *Circulation* 67:251, 1983.

Kavanaugh KM, Aisen AM, Fechner KP, et al: Regional metabolism during coronary occlusion, reperfusion, and reocclusion using ^{31}phosphorous nuclear magnetic resonance spectroscopy in the intact rabbit. *Am Heart J* 117:53, 1989.

Keller AM, Peshock RM, Malloy CR, et al: In vivo measurement of myocardial mass using nuclear magnetic resonance imaging. *J Am Coll Cardiol* 8:113, 1986.

Keller MW, Feinstein SB, Watson DD: Successful left ventricular opacification following peripheral venous injection of sonicated contrast agent: An experimental evaluation. *Am Heart J* 114:570, 1987.

Kersting-Sommerhoff BA, Higgins CB, White RD, et al: Aortic dissection: Sensitivity and specificity of MR imaging. *Radiology* 166:651, 1988.

Khaw BA, Gold HK, Yasuda T, et al: Scintigraphic quantification of myocardial necrosis in patients after intravenous injection of myosin-specific antibody. *Circulation* 74:501, 1986.

Kiat H, Maddahi J, Roy LT, et al: Comparison of technetium 99m methoxyisobutyl isonitryl and thallium-201. Evaluation of coronary artery disease by planar and tomography methods. *Am Heart J* 117:1, 1989.

Knabb RM, Bergmann SR, Fox KAA, Sobel BE: The temporal pattern of recovery of myocardial perfusion and metabolism delineated by positron emission tomography after coronary thrombolysis. *J Nucl Med* 28:1563, 1987.

Lanzer P, Garrett JS, Lipton MJ, et al: Quantitation of regional myocardial function by cine-computed tomography: Pharmacological changes in wall thickening dynamics. *J Am Coll Cardiol* 8:682, 1986.

Lerch RA, Ambos HD, Bergmann SR, et al: Localization of viable, ischemic myocardium by positron-emission tomography with ^{11}C palmitate. *Circulation* 64:689, 1981.

Lewis SE, Devous MD, Corbett JR, et al: Measurement of infarct size in acute canine myocardial infarction by single photon emission computed tomography with technetium 99-m pyrophosphate. *Am J Cardiol* 54:193, 1984.

Liedtke AJ: Alterations of carbohydrate and lipid metabolism in the acutely ischemic heart. *Prog Cardiovasc Dis* 23:321, 1981.

Mahmarian JJ, Pratt CM, Borgen-Neto S, et al: Quantification of infarct size by ^{201}Tl single photon emission computed tomography during acute myocardial infarction in humans. *Circulation* 78:831, 1988.

Mancini GBJ, Vogel RA: Digital subtraction angiography. In: Miller DD, Burns RJ, Gill JB, Ruddy TD, eds. *Clinical Cardiac Imaging*. New York: McGraw-Hill; 1988, p. 203.

Manglos SH, Jaszczak RJ, Floyd CE, et al: Nonisotropic attenuation in SPECT: Quantitative tests of effects and compensation techniques. *J Nucl Med* 28:1884, 1987.

Marcus ML, Skorton DJ, Johnson MR, et al: Visual estimates of percent diameter coronary stenosis: "A battered gold standard". *J Am Coll Cardiol* 11:882, 1988.

Marshall RC, Tillisch JH, Phelps ME, et al: Identification and differentiation of resting myocardial ischemia and infarction in man with positron computed tomography ^{18}F-labeled fluorodeoxyglucose and N-13 ammonia. *Circulation* 64:766, 1981.

Massie B, Weiner MW: Response of myocardial metabolites to graded regional ischemia. ^{31}P NMR spectroscopy of porcine myocardium in vivo. *Circ Res* 64:968, 1989.

McNamara MT, Higgins CB, Schechtmann N, et al: Detection and characterization of acute myocardial infarction in man with use of gated magnetic resonance. *Circulation* 71:717, 1985.

McPherson DD, Aylward PE, Knosp BM, et al: Ultrasound characterization of acute myocardial ischemia by quantitative texture analysis. *Ultrason Imaging* 8:227, 1986.

McPherson DD, Skorton DJ, Kodiyalam S, et al: Finite element analysis of myocardial diastolic function using three-dimensional echocardiographic reconstructions: Application of a new method for study of acute ischemia in dogs. *Circ Res* 60:674, 1987.

Miller DD, Gill JB, Livin E, et al: Fatty acid analog accumulation: A marker of myocyte viability in ischemic-reperfused myocardium. *Circ Res* 63:689, 1988.

Miller JG, Perez JE, Sobel BE: Ultrasonic characterization of myocardium. *Prog Cardiovasc Dis* 28:85, 1985.

Mimbs J, O'Donnell M, Bauwens D, et al: The dependence of ultrasonic attenuation and backscatter on collagen content in dog and rabbit hearts. *Circ Res* 47:49, 1980.

Mimbs JW, Bauwens D, Cohen RD et al: Effects of myocardial ischemia on quantitative ultrasonic back scatter and identification of responsible determinants. *Circ Res* 49:89, 1981.

Moritz WE, Pearlman AS, McCabe DH, et al: An ultrasonic technique for imaging the ventricle in three dimensions and calculating its volume. *IEEE Trans Biomed Eng* 30:482, 1983.

Neely JR, Rovetto MJ, Oram JF: Myocardial utilization of carbohydrate and lipids. *Prog Cardiovasc Dis* 15:289, 1972.

Pflugfelder PW, Wendland MF, Holt WW, et al: Acute myocardial ischemia: MR imaging with Mn-Tp. *Radiology* 167:129, 1988.

Pohost GM, Canby RC: Nuclear magnetic resonance imaging: Current applications and future prospects. *Circulation* 75:88, 1987.

Port SC, Oshima M, Ray G, et al: Assessment of single vessel coronary artery disease: Results of exercise electrocardiography, thallium-201 myocardial perfusion imaging and radionuclide angiography. *J Am Coll Cardiol* 6:75, 1985.

Ranky PG: *Computer Integrated Manufacturing*. Englewood Cliffs, New Jersey: Prentice Hall International; 1986.

Reiter SJ, Rumberger JA, Feiring AJ, et al: Precision of right and left ventricular stroke volume measurements by rapid acquisition cine computed tomography. *Circulation* 74:890, 1986.

Reiter SJ, Rumberger JA, Stanford W, Marcus ML: Quantitative determination of aortic regurgitant volumes by cine computed tomography. *Circulation* 76:728, 1987.

Rellas JS, Corbett JR, Kulkarni P, et al: Iodine-123 phenylpentadecanoic acid: Detection of acute myocardial infarction and injury in dogs using iodinated fatty acid and single-photon emission tomography. *Am J Cardiol* 52:1326, 1983.

Ritman EL, Kinsey JH, Robb RA, et al: 3-dimensional imaging of heart, lungs, and circulation. *Science* 210:273, 1980.

Robb RA, Morin RL: Principles and instrumentation for dynamic x-ray computed tomography. In: Marcus ML, Skorton DJ, Schelbert HR, Wolf GL, eds. *Cardiac Imaging: Principles and Practice*. Philadelphia: WB Saunders; (in press).

Robitaille PM, Merkle H, Sublett E, et al: Spectroscopic imaging and spatial localization using adiabatic pulses and applications to detect transmural metabolite distribution in the canine heart. *Magnetic Resonance Med* 10:14, 1989.

Rubinstein RI, Askenase AD, Thickman D, et al: Magnetic resonance imaging to evaluate patency of aortocoronary bypass grafts. *Circulation* 76:786, 1987.

Rumberger JA, Feiring AJ, Lipton MJ, et al: Use of ultrafast CT to quantitate regional myocardial perfusion: A preliminary report. *J Am Coll Cardiol* 9:59, 1987.

Schelbert HR, Henze E, Keen R, et al: C-11-palmitate for the noninvasive evaluation of regional myocardial fatty acid metabolism with positron computed tomography. IV. In vivo evaluation of acute demand induced ischemia in dogs. *Am Heart J* 106:736, 1983.

Schelbert HR, Phelps ME, Huang SC, et al: N-13-ammonia as an indicator of myocardial blood flow. *Circulation* 63:1259, 1981.

Schon HR, Schelbert HR, Robinson G, et al: C-11-labeled palmitic acid for the noninvasive evaluation of regional myocardial fatty acid metabolism with positron computed tomography. I. Kinetics of C-11-palmitic acid in normal myocardium. *Am Heart J* 103:532, 1982.

Schwaiger M, Brunken R, Grover-McKay M, et al: Regional myocardial metabolism in patients with acute myocardial infarction assessed by positron emission tomography. *J Am Coll Cardiol* 8:800, 1986.

Sechtem U, Pflugfelder P, Higgins CB: Quantification of cardiac function by conventional and cine magnetic resonance imaging. *Cardiovasc Intervent Radiol* 10:365, 1987.

Sechtem U, Pflugfelder PW, Cassidy MM, et al: Mitral or aortic regurgitation: Quantification of regurgitant volumes with cine MR imaging. *Radiology* 167:425, 1988.

Seldin DW, Johnson LL, Blood DK, et al: Myocardial perfusion imaging with technetium 99m SQ30217: Comparison with thallium-201 and coronary anatomy. *J Nucl Med* 30:312, 1989.

Sia STB, Holman BL: Dynamic myocardial imaging in ischemic heart disease: Use of technetium-99m isonitriles. *Am J Cardiac Imag* 1:125, 1987.

Skorton DJ: Ultrasound tissue characterization: Can the state of the myocardium be assessed directly yet noninvasively? *J Am Coll Cardiol* 13:92, 1989.

Skorton DJ, Melton HE Jr, Pandian NG, et al: Detection of acute myocardial infarction in closed-chest dogs by analysis of regional two-dimensional echocardiographic gray-level distributions. *Circ Res* 52:36, 1983.

Sobel BE, Geltman EM, Tiefenbrunn AJ, et al: Improvement of regional myocardial metabolism after coronary thrombolysis induced with tissue type plasminogen activator or streptokinase. *Circulation* 69:983, 1984.

Sobel BE, Weiss ES, Welch MJ, et al: Detection of remote myocardial infarction in patients with positron emission transaxial tomography and intravenous ¹¹C-palmitate. *Circulation* 55:853, 1977.

Soila K, Nummi P, Ekfors T, et al: Proton relaxation times in arterial wall and atheromatous lesions in man. *Invest Radiol* 20:411, 1986.

Sporn V, Balini NP, Holman L, et al: Simultaneous measurement of ventricular function and myocardial perfusion using the technetium 99m isonitriles. *Clin Nucl Med* 13:77, 1988.

Stanford W, Brundage BH, McMillan R, et al: Sensitivity and specificity of assessing coronary bypass graft patency with ultrafast computed tomography: Results of a multicenter study. *J Am Coll Cardiol* 21:1, 1988.

Syrota A: Evaluation of cardiac receptors. In: Marcus ML, Skorton DJ, Schelbert HR, Wolf GL, eds. *Cardiac Imaging: Principles and Practice*. Philadelphia: WB Saunders; (in press).

Tamaki N, Yonekura Y, Mukai T, et al. Segmental analysis of stress thallium myocardial emission tomography for localization of coronary artery disease. *Eur J Nucl Med* 9:99, 1984.

Tillisch J, Brunken R, Marshall R, et al: Reversibility of cardiac wall-motion abnormalities predicted by positron tomography. *N Engl J Med* 314:884, 1986.

Underwood SR, Walton S, Laming PJ, et al: Left ventricular volume and ejection fraction determined by blood pool emission tomography. *Brit Heart J* 53:216, 1985.

Utz JA, Herfkens RJ, Heinsimer JA, et al: Valvular regurgitation: Dynamic MR imaging. *Radiology* 168:91, 1988.

Van Rossum AC, Visser FC, Sprenger M, et al: Evaluation of magnetic resonance imaging for determination of left ventricular ejection fraction and comparison with angiography. *Am J Cardiol* 62:628, 1988.

Vered Z, Barzilai B, Mohr GA, et al: Quantitative ultrasonic tissue characterization with real-time integrated backscatter imaging in normal human subjects and in patients with dilated cardiomyopathy. *Circulation* 5:1067, 1987.

Vered Z, Mohr GA, Barzilai B, et al: Ultrasonic integrated backscatter tissue characterization of remote myocardial infarction in human subjects. *J Am Coll Cardiol* 13:84, 1989.

Vogel R, LeFree M, Bates E, et al: Application of digital techniques to selective coronary arteriography: Use of myocardial contrast appearance time to measure coronary flow reserve. *Am Heart J* 107:153, 1984.

Vyska K, Machulla HJ, Stremmel W, et al: Regional myocardial free fatty acid extraction in normal and ischemic myocardium. *Circulation* 78:1218, 1988.

Wedeen VJ, Meuli RA, Edelman RR, et al: Projective imaging of pulsatile flow with magnetic resonance. *Science* 230:946, 1985.

Wesbey GE, Higgins CB, Hale JD, Valk PE: Magnetic resonance applications in atherosclerotic vascular disease. *Cardiovasc Intervent Radiol* 8:342, 1986.

White CW, Wright CB, Doty DB, et al: Does the visual interpretation of the coronary arteriogram predict the physiological significance of a coronary stenosis? *N Engl J Med* 310:819, 1984.

Wisenberg G, Pflugfelder PW, Kostuk WJ, et al: Diagnostic applicability of magnetic resonance imaging in assessing human cardiac allograft rejection. *Am J Cardiol* 60:130, 1987.

Wisenberg G, Prato FS, Carroll SE, et al: Serial nuclear magnetic resonance imaging of acute myocardial infarction with and without reperfusion. *Am Heart J* 115:510, 1988.

Wolfkiel C, Ferguson JL, Chomka EV, et al: Measurement of myocardial blood flow by ultrafast computed tomography. *Circulation* 76:1262, 1987.

Yonekura Y, Tamaki N, Senda M, et al: Detection of coronary artery disease with N-13 ammonia and high resolution positron emission computed tomography. *Am Heart J* 113:645, 1987.

Zir LM, Miller SW, Dinsmore RE, et al: Interobserver variability in coronary angiography. *Circulation* 53:627, 1976.

12 Clinical Approach to Hyperlipidemia

CHAPTER

Neil J. Stone

LIPID AND LIPOPROTEIN METABOLISM

Knowledge of lipid and lipoprotein metabolism is crucial for understanding atherosclerosis and clinical outcomes such as angina pectoris, myocardial infarction (MI), intermittent claudication, and thrombotic brain infarction. Atherosclerosis is the condition in which the inner layers of the artery walls become thick and irregular due to fatty deposits comprised chiefly of cholesterol (Small). Whereas cells of normal lining or intima of blood vessels contain less than 5% dry weight as lipid, the deposits or plaques of atherosclerosis contain 30-65% dry weight as lipid (mainly in the form of cholesterol and phospholipid).

With the unaided eye, pathologists can classify the signs of atherosclerosis into two major types. The earliest lesions, called *fatty streaks*, contain about 25% lipid. Fatty streaks can be seen in coronary arteries after puberty. During fatty streak development, cells are stimulated to take in more cholesterol than they can excrete. In diet-induced hypercholesterolemia, monocytes percolate through the endothelium and transform into cholesterol-filled macrophages. Plaque formation is aided and abetted by smooth muscle cells, platelets and endothelial cells that release growth factors which hasten development of the fatty arterial plaques. Other factors, such as hypertension, cigarette smoke, and turbulence occurring at vessel branch points, can injure the endothelium and also set in motion this process (Ross). The fatty streaks, however, do not invariably grow into cholesterol-laden plaques. They do progress to intermediate lesions and, finally, to raised plaques in persons who are susceptible either by individual genetic makeup or by diet-induced high blood cholesterol levels. There is strong evidence based on experimental studies in animals that cholesterol plays a key role both in the initiation and maintenance of atherosclerosis.

The second type of hallmark of coronary atherosclerosis is the atheromatous, lipid-rich *fibrous plaque*. These plaques are formed from progressive deposition of cholesterol in an orderly fashion, with the older cholesterol deposits at the base of the plaque and the newer ones at the surface. A simple atheroma may evolve into a complicated plaque with deposits of calcium and thrombus formation by ingrowth of the vessel into the plaque, setting the stage for hemorrhage into the plaque and resulting vessel blockage.

Since lipids are established as playing a causal role in atherosclerosis, all physicians concerned with cardiovascular disease must understand the guidelines set forth by the Adult Treatment Panel of the National Cholesterol Education Program (NCEP) (Adult Treatment Panel 1988). These were designed to promote the detection, evaluation, and treatment of the high-risk patient in the population and should be viewed as complementary to evolving population strategies.

DEFINITIONS

Cholesterol was discovered in bile by Chevreul in 1816. (*Chole* means "bile" and *steros* means "solid.") It has the multi-ring nuclear structure of the steroid family and is a key part of cell membranes, the D vitamins, and adrenal steroids. Most tissues synthesize cholesterol, but in humans this occurs chiefly in the liver and intestine. Plasma cholesterol concentrations are tightly regulated by removal processes keyed to specific liver and extrahepatic cell receptors. Cholesterol is cleared from the body by excretion into bile or conversion to bile acids. Cholesterol is only seen in animal fat; it is not found in plants. Blood cholesterol can be measured in a non-fasting state.

Triglycerides are storage forms of energy consisting of long-chain fatty acids attached to a glycerol backbone. These fatty acids can be saturated or unsaturated, a distinction important in determining whether a dietary fat can raise or lower the blood cholesterol level. Triglyceride levels increase postprandially and are affected by stress, which helps explain their great variability. Blood triglyceride levels must be measured with the patient fasting 12-14 hours, at stable weight for three weeks, and on a stable diet.

Lipids are insoluble in plasma water and must be transported on large macromolecules called *lipoproteins*. Examples of triglyceride-rich lipoproteins are chylomicrons, very low density lipoproteins (VLDL), and intermediate-density lipoproteins (IDL). Examples of cholesterol-rich lipoproteins are chylomicron remnants, low-density lipoproteins (LDL), and high-density lipoproteins (HDL). *Apoproteins* play key roles in the synthesis, processing, and disposal of lipoproteins. These are the protein subunits of the protein-phospholipid complex that packages lipids in the circulation. Knowledge of major apoproteins such as apo AI, AII (major proteins of HDL); apo B100 or LDL B (major protein of LDL); and apo CII and the isoforms of apo E (apoproteins needed for metabolism of VLDL and chylomicron remnants) is already important in understanding genetic susceptibility to coronary atherosclerosis.

Long-chain dietary fat is broken down in the gut and repackaged in intestinal cells as *chylomicrons*. These large, triglyceride-laden particles are responsible for transient, postprandial lipemia. Chylomicrons are processed by aid of an enzyme called *lipoprotein lipase*. This is found in muscle and adipose tissue capillaries. Levels of it are increased by exercise and decreased in insulinopenic diabetes and hypothyroidism.

Endogenously produced triglyceride from liver and intestine circulates on *VLDL*. This family of particles is processed by lipoprotein lipase as well. When levels are sampled 12-14 hours after a meal, the fasting triglyceride level reflects basal levels of VLDL. The half-life of chylomicrons is measured in minutes and that of VLDL in hours; this explains the marked daily variations in triglyceride levels. Carbohydrate, fatty acids (raised due to increased catecholamines or uncontrolled diabetes), elevated basal insulin levels (obesity, estrogens), and augmented hepatic fatty acids (alcohol) stimulate VLDL overproduction from the liver. Non-genetic factors causing impaired clearance include uremia, myxedema, and poorly controlled diabetes.

VLDLs are metabolized to *IDL* or *VLDL remnants*, whose apo E serves as a marker that can bind to the same LDL receptor that also recognizes apo B. Indeed, apo E is needed for the efficient conversion of VLDL remnants to LDL and the efficient disposal of chylomicron remnants by the liver. Moreover, genetic variation in apo E may play a role in susceptibility to coronary artery disease (CAD). The apo E^4 allele is associated with higher levels of LDL cholesterol (LDL-C), as seen in Finns, who have high levels of cholesterol and coronary artery disease (CAD), and is seen less frequently in octogenarians (Davignon et al.). The opposite appears to be true for the apo E^2 allele. Further studies of apo E should better characterize its ability to modulate the susceptibility to atherosclerosis.

Most of *LDL* is produced from the intravascular conversion of VLDL through IDL to LDL, the cholesterol-laden particles whose complex interaction with the arterial wall results in coronary atherosclerosis. The concentration of LDL is regulated by the LDL receptors, which recognize apo B. These LDL receptors are specified by commonly inherited genes. When a person inherits a mutant copy (or copies), deficient or absent LDL receptors are seen. This leads to hypercholesterolemia of a magnitude in proportion to the defect in LDL receptors. When plasma LDL levels rise, scavenger cells are needed to degrade LDL. These macrophages soon become swollen with cholesterol and convert to foam cells, which are prominently seen in arterial plaques.

Factors other than the absolute amount of native, circulating LDL may be important in the genesis of human atherosclerosis. Sniderman and colleagues (1980) emphasize the coronary-prone situation of an elevated apo B in the face of a normal or near-normal LDL-C level. Indeed, when measured, apo B is shown in most studies to be superior to LDL-C in separating patients with angiographic coronary artery disease from those without CAD. Of particular interest to the cardiologist, LDL apo B along with HDL cholesterol (HDL-C) were the most important predictors of subsequent atherosclerosis in saphenous vein bypass grafts (Campeau 1984). In addition, those persons with a preponderance of small, dense LDL particles (usually in association with increased VLDL and IDL and reduced HDL) have a markedly increased risk of MI (Austin et al.). Finally, modified or oxidized LDL is highly cytotoxic and its uptake by macrophages to form fatty streaks could link the key elements of the lipid-infiltration and endothelial-injury hypotheses (Steinberg et al.). The implications of these developments for therapy are exciting to contemplate, but must await further studies.

Finally, *HDLs* are secreted from the liver and intestines and also are formed from surface materials generated by efficient triglyceride-rich lipoprotein metabolism. Apo AI is the major apoprotein and accounts for 30% of the mass of HDL. HDLs play a key role in triglyceride metabolism by serving as a reservoir for apoproteins such as apo CII, which are needed to activate lipoprotein lipase. When triglyceride levels are high due to impaired catabolism, HDL levels are usually low. HDLs play a key role in cholesterol metabolism, as they function in reverse cholesterol transport and may also inhibit uptake of LDL by the cell. Moreover, since the initial observation that men with MI have low levels of HDL-C, numerous epidemiologic and angiographic studies have confirmed that low HDL-C is a powerful, independent predictor of CAD. In the Framingham Study, a significant effect of HDL-C on MI was seen, even among the group with the lowest levels of cholesterol (Abbott et al.). Families with markedly elevated HDL-C have little CAD.

CAD RISK: WHICH LIPIDS AND LIPOPROTEINS TO MEASURE

The recent NCEP guidelines rely for case finding on non-fasting blood cholesterol measurements, which are inexpensive and easy to obtain. Elevated values must be confirmed at least once for greater precision. Risk factor status for CAD is required to place the cholesterol results in perspective (Table 1). A simple classification scheme determines the necessary follow-up action (Table 2). A blood cholesterol level <200 mg/dl is classified as desirable. A level of 200-239 mg/dl is classified as borderline high and a level ≥240 is classified as high. This latter cutpoint defines a value roughly corresponding to the 75th percentile for the adult US population. The basis of these cutoffs is, in large part, derived from the data set of more than 361,662 primary screenees from the Multiple Risk Factor Intervention Trial (Martin et al.). This landmark effort confirmed and extended previous observations. With increasing cholesterol levels, the risk of CAD rose in exponential fashion, with strikingly higher rates at levels above 240 mg/dl. Below 200 mg/dl, the risk seemed lower, but there did not appear to be a so-called threshold above which risk commenced. Although atherosclerosis is seen in persons

Table 1. Factors (Other than Low-density Lipoprotein Cholesterol) Used to Determine High-Risk Status

Definite CAD (definite prior MI or documented myocardial ischemia)
 or
 Two or more of the following risk factors:
    Male sex
    Family history of premature CAD (definite MI or sudden death in a parent or sibling before the age of 55)
    Cigarette smoking
    Hypertension
    Low HDL cholesterol
    Diabetes mellitus
    History of definite cerebrovascular or peripheral vascular disease
    Severe obesity (>30% overweight)

CAD = coronary artery disease; HDL = high-density lipoprotein; MI = myocardial infarction.

with values of 150-200 mg/dl, rates of CAD are low and CAD occurs later in life in this group.

Risk factors are those personal traits or lifestyles that convey an increased risk of developing CAD. Along with cholesterol testing, all adults should be checked for the presence of hypertension, cigarette smoking, diabetes, severe obesity (>30% overweight), family history of CAD in a parent, sibling or child before age 55, and either cerebrovascular or peripheral vascular disease. Other traits considered by many as danger signals for CAD (but not included in the NCEP listing of risk factors) include sedentary lifestyle, aggressive, hostile response to stress, and hormonal factors (early menopause without hormonal replacement or the birth control pill) (Grundy et al. 1987).

Recently, it was suggested that HDL-C be measured in all adults because low HDL-C levels (<35 mg/dl) are a major risk factor for CAD. The NCEP guidelines considered measurement of HDL-C in asymptomatic persons with borderline (and no risk factors) or desirable cholesterol levels optional because of the low rates of CAD in this group. Routine measurement of HDL-C is difficult to justify because (1) in the absence of other risk factors, the risk for CAD is only minimally increased until the cholesterol level exceeds 240 mg/dl; (2) many of the causes of a low HDL-C level (obesity, diabetes, cigarette

Table 2. Screening Guidelines Based on Non-fasting Cholesterol Level*		
Cholesterol (mg/dl)	CAD or Two Risk Factors	Recommendations for Evaluation and/or Diet
<200	Absent	Repeat within 5 years
<200	Present	Same as above†
200-239	Absent	Reevaluate annually Step 1 diet‡
200-239 or	Present	Measure lipoproteins: HDL-C, LDL-C
240 or more	Present/absent	Detailed assessment

*Based on average of two cholesterol values; if they differ by >30 mg/dl, a third value is taken.
†Some physicians may wish to check HDL-C when CAD is strongly suspected.
‡Some physicians may wish to check HDL-C in men.
CAD = coronary artery disease; HDL-C, LDL-C = high- and low-density lipoprotein cholesterol, respectively.
Modified from NCEP guidelines (*Arch Intern Med* 148:36, 1988).

smoking, antihypertensive drugs, and family history of CAD) by themselves put the patients into the high-risk category, mandating measurement of HDL-C anyway; (3) the increased costs with generalized testing are significant because patients must be fasting and tests must be repeated; (4) methods of estimating HDL-C are not well standardized—many laboratories use precipitation of non-HDL lipoproteins with high concentrations of phosphotungstic acid-magnesium, which can systematically underestimate HDL; and (5) data indicating that treatment of HDL per se makes a difference in coronary outcome are lacking; there is no good animal model and no clinical trials have looked at HDL-C alone (Grundy et al. 1989). Nonetheless, determination of a lipoprotein profile may be valuable in defining risk of CAD in a young adult man with a borderline-high cholesterol level, even if he has no other risk factors. The HDL-C level in a healthy woman with a borderline-high cholesterol level is less likely to prove useful due to her lower risk status.

Because the presence of CAD or risk factors for CAD increase the risk of CAD at any given cholesterol value, they can be expected to influence greatly the decisions regarding further evaluation and treatment. For example, in the MRFIT trial, the risk of CAD for hypertensive smokers with the lowest cholesterol values is similar to the risk of CAD for normotensive nonsmokers with the highest cholesterol

values. Dietary studies show that hypertensive smokers respond less well to cholesterol-lowering diets than their nonsmoking, normotensive counterparts (Caggiula et al.).

The NCEP recommended further evaluation when an individual has confirmed blood cholesterol values of ≥240 mg/dl or has confirmed borderline cholesterol values of 200-239 mg/dl *and* either definite CAD or two or more risk factors for CAD (Table 2). If two values for cholesterol differ by more than 30 mg/dl, a third measurement should be performed. The action required once blood cholesterol and risk factor status for CAD are determined is shown in Table 2.

Those at higher risk for coronary events require specific therapy. Lipoprotein analysis is used to guide total risk assessment and therapy. Fortunately, total cholesterol, triglycerides and HDL-C can be measured on a single fasting blood sample. The following formula is used to calculate the LDL-C value:

LDL-C = total cholesterol − (HDL-C) − (triglyceride/5)

(This assumes a specimen obtained after a 12-16-hour fast, a triglyceride level <400 mg/dl and the absence of the rare familial type III disorder.)

Since risk assessment and therapy depend on the LDL-C level, its value should be repeated within one to six weeks. If values vary by >30 mg/dl, a third determination should be made. Table 3 shows how to proceed after LDL-C values are determined. Sec-

Table 3. Use of Low-density Lipoprotein Cholesterol Levels to Guide Decisions for Diet and Drug Therapy

LDL-C* (mg/dl)	CAD or Two Risk Factors	Action Recommended
Desirable		
<130	Absent	Repeat cholesterol measurements in 5 yr. General dietary, risk factor education
<130	Present	Reevaluate yearly Step 1 diet†
Borderline high-risk LDL-C		
<130		Step 1 diet
130-159	Present	Clinical evaluation Step 1 diet Set goal LDL-C of <130 mg/dl
High-Risk LDL-C		
≥160	Absent	Clinical evaluation Step 1 diet Set goal LDL-C of <160 mg/dl
≥160	Present	Clinical evaluation Step 1 diet Set goal LDL-C of <130 mg/dl

Clinical evaluation includes ruling out secondary causes of high cholesterol level and screening family members.
*LDL-C determined by formula; average of two or three measurements is used for greater precision.
†NCEP would simply repeat cholesterol measurement in five years. This reflects the author's practice.
Abbreviations as in Table 2

ondary causes of high blood cholesterol levels are grouped into categories of diet, diseases, and drugs to aid in their systematic appraisal (Table 4). Also, family members should be screened for blood cholesterol and risk factors. Conversely, screening relatives of those who present with CAD is particuarly revealing because previously undetected risk factors are highly prevalent in siblings of such patients (Becker et al.).

SYNDROMES OF FAMILIAL HYPERLIPOPROTEINEMIA

An enriched sample of cases of familial forms of hyperlipidemia is seen in survivors of acute MI. Goldstein, Hazzard and coworkers (1973) showed that one of five survivors under age 60 had a simply inherited form of hyperlipidemia and one third had either a cholesterol or triglyceride level above the upper 5% cutoff for their age. Consideration of hyperlipidemia in patients with MI is important, but cholesterol values may underrepresent the pre-event state if the patient is not sampled within the first 24 hours. After this time, triglyceride values begin to rise and cholesterol values fall over the next four weeks. Reliable lipid values are not obtained again for at least 8-12 weeks, when patients are recovered and on stable diet and exercise regimens.

Several familial syndromes are worthy of review. *Familial hypercholesterolemia* (FH) is a clinical disorder linked since the time of William Osler with premature CAD. It is a striking example of how valuable the sophisticated biochemical skills of the geneticist are to the cardiologist. Familial hypercholes-

Table 4. Secondary Causes of Altered Blood Lipids and Lipoproteins

Diet
  Saturated fat
  Dietary cholesterol
  Excess calories
Medications
  Estrogens
  Steroids
  Thiazides
  Chlorthalidone
  Androgens
Diseases
  Hypothyroidism
  Nephrosis
  Obstructive liver disease
  Diabetes mellitus
  Porphyria (rare)
  Myeloma (rare)

terolemia (Table 5) is inherited as an autosomal dominant trait with a high degree of penetrance. Heterozygotes have a single dose of mutant allele specifying a receptor protein with either absent or defective binding or faulty internalization. An animal model, the Watanabe rabbit, exhibits these same features of receptor deficiency (Goldstein et al. 1983). In the United States, the minimum gene frequency is estimated at 1 in 225. Among survivors of MI under age 60, the frequency of FH (heterozygous form) is 4.1%. Heterozygous FH is diagnosed when LDL-C values exceed the upper 5% cutoffs for age and similar degrees of LDL excess are seen in first-degree relatives. Tendon xanthomas are found in about 80% of cases and are almost pathognomonic. They characteristically involve the Achilles tendons and the tendons overlying the metacarpals (Figures 1 and 2). Many patients recall episodes of acute tendinitis in their teens. Superior and inferior pole corneal arcus in Caucasians under age 35 usually signifies FH, but corneal arcus in older and non-Caucasian populations has no predictive value. Xanthelasma (lipid deposits under the eyes) predict underlying FH in only about 50% of cases (Stone).

The patient with heterozygous FH typically has a cholesterol level of 325-450 mg/dl that characteristically does not respond to cholesterol-lowering diet. Heterozygous FH must be recognized because of the

predilection for premature CAD. At the outset of the Framingham Study, six of 5,127 subjects had cholesterol values >400 mg/dl and detectable xanthomas. All of these subjects died from CAD before age 50. A more systematic observation was carried out on the 116 kindred and over 1,000 relatives studied at the National Institutes of Health (Stone et al.). For those with the FH trait, 29.5% were found to have CAD, compared with only 10.5% of adult relatives without the FH trait. The expectation of CAD by age 40 for affected male relatives was one in six; by age 60, it was more than one in two. When compared with nonaffected men in the same kindred, it was as if CAD had developed 20 years earlier than expected (Figure 3). Although CAD occurred less often and later in women than in men, affected female relatives also had a greater risk of CAD after age 45 (Figure 4).

Homozygous cases, with a gene frequency of one in a million, have a double dose of one of the mutant alleles or, rarely, have two different mutant alleles. These severe defects result in LDL binding and internalization that is markedly impaired, preventing normal feedback of cholesterol synthesis by peripheral cells. The serum cholesterol level is usually 600-1,000 mg/dl. Affected homozygous children have characteristic interdigital web xanthomas and tuberous and tendon xanthomas. If untreated, these lesions are prominent by age 10. Homozygous children have distinctive cardiovascular findings. Basal systolic murmurs are invariably heard; over time, they progress to represent hemodynamically significant aortic stenosis. The aortic stenosis is unique and due to intracellular lipid infiltration of the aortic cusps. In one patient with a peak systolic gradient of 108 mm Hg, atherosclerotic plaquing was found to extend from the higher part of the sinuses of Valsalva to the aortic ring. In these cases, there is almost always greater plaquing in the ascending aorta than in the abdominal aorta—the reverse of the usual situation (Allen et al.). Two-dimensional echocardiography may be used to document stenosis of the supravalvular aortic ring and further suggest cases of ostial coronary stenosis (Beppu et al.). Coronary disease is rapidly progressive in the untreated patient. These patients have limited potential to respond to receptor-enhancing medication. Therapeutic options include plasma exchange and liver transplantation. A dramatic example of modern therapy for FH was seen in the report of a six-year-old girl homozygous for FH and with severe CAD who underwent combined liver and heart transplantation.

Table 5. Familial Forms of Hyperlipidemia Associated with an Increased Risk of Coronary Artery Disease

Genetic Lipid Abnormality	% of Total
I. Studies of survivors of myocardial infarction before age 60*	
Familial combined hyperlipidemia	11.3
Familial hypercholesterolemia	4.1
Familial hypertriglyceridemia	5.2
Polygenic hypercholesterolemia	5.5
II. Studies of patients with angiographic coronary disease before age 60†	
Lp(a) excess (11.5% with other dyslipidemias)	33.3
Hypertriglyceridemia with low HDL-C	14.5
Combined hyperlipidemia with low HDL-C	12.5
Low HDL-C (<10th percentile)	7.0
Combined hyperlipidemia (TG + LDL-C)	5.0
Hypertriglyceridemia (TG >90th percentile)	3.0
High LDL-C with low HDL-C	2.0
Hypercholesterolemia (LDL-C >90th percentile)	1.0

*Goldstein JL: Genetic aspects of hyperlipidemia in coronary heart disease. *Hosp Pract* 2:53, 1973.
†Genest J, Martin-Munley S, McNamara JR, Salem DN, Schaefer EJ: Frequency of genetic dyslipidemias in patients with premature coronary artery disease. *Arteriosclerosis* 9:701a, 1989.
TG = triglycerides; other abbreviations as in Table 2.

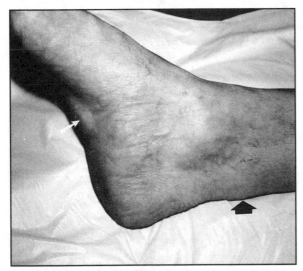

Figure 1. *Achilles and flexor hallicus longus tendon xanthomas (arrows) in a patient with heterozygous familial hypercholesterolemia.*

Her LDL-C level declined by 81%, from 988 to 184 mg/dl, with a marked increase in her fractional catabolic rate. This remarkable case study highlights the importance of hepatic LDL receptors in controlling excess LDL-C levels (Bilheimer et al.).

Familial combined hyperlipidemia (FCHL) is the commonest monogenic lipid disorder among survivors of acute MI. In the Seattle study, 11.3% of survivors under age 60 were affected (Goldstein, Schrott et al. 1973). The disorder appears to be inherited as an autosomal dominant trait. It is first expressed in adulthood, unlike FH, where affected children are easily detected. In kindred with this disorder, there are multiple combinations of elevated lipids, with relatives in successive generations having elevated cholesterol or triglycerides or both. Elevated cholesterol and triglyceride levels combined are very common. Xanthomas are not seen, because the elevations of cholesterol and triglyceride are not severe. Elevated apo LDL-B may target those who present with high triglyceride levels as having FCHL rather than familial hypertriglyceridemia or a secondary cause of high triglycerides. In one study, in which apo LDL-B was

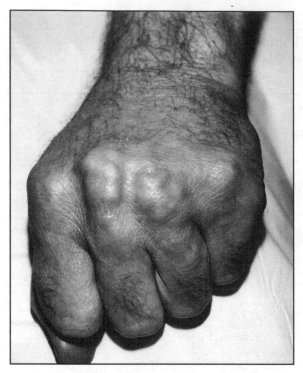

Figure 2. *Extensor tendon xanthomas occurring in tendons overlying the metacarpals in a patient with heterozygous familial hypercholesterolemia.*

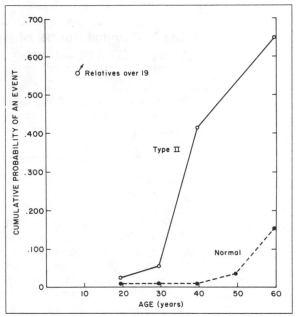

Figure 3. *Cumulative probability by decade of fatal or nonfatal coronary artery disease events in first-degree male relatives with heterozygous familial hypercholesterolemia. (From Stone et al. 1974. See Bibliography. With permission of the American Heart Association.)*

measured in patients with triglyceride elevations, it appeared that those with elevated plasma LDL-B had a significantly higher prevalence of CAD (Sniderman et al. 1982). Use of apo LDL-B as a more sensitive marker for those with familial tendency to CAD was demonstrated in one study of offspring born to parents with premature CAD. Athough 33% of the children were shown to have elevated levels of apo LDL-B, only 10% were shown to have clearly abnormal levels of LDL-C (Sniderman et al. 1985).

Familial dyslipidemic hypertension must also be considered when families are seen with early familial hypertension and multiple forms of lipid/lipoprotein abnormalities (Hunt 1989). Elevated insulin levels may explain the interrelationships between the dyslipidemia (low HDL, high LDL-C and/or triglyceride levels), obesity, and hypertension found in these families.

Familial type III or familial dysbetalipoproteinemia is a rare disorder. It results from an inherited apo E disorder resulting in accumulation of IDL in plasma. Affected relatives are homozygous for apo E^2/E^2 allele. This genotype is seen in 1% of the population. The diagnosis is confirmed by a VLDL cholesterol/triglyceride ratio exceeding 0.3, and the clinical

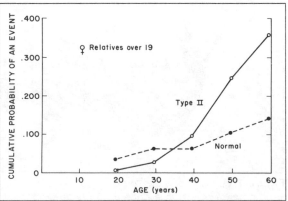

Figure 4. *Cumulative probability by decade of fatal or nonfatal coronary artery disease events in first-degree female relatives with heterozygous familial hypercholesterolemia. (From Stone et al. 1974. With permission of the American Heart Association.)*

setting. The clinical disorder, however, characterized by tuboeruptive xanthomas along with digital and palmar crease xanthomas, striking elevations of both cholesterol and triglyceride levels, and premature coronary and peripheral vascular disease, is rarely seen; thus, the clinical expression must depend on other environmental, genetic or endocrine factors (Breslow).

Familial hypertriglyceridemia (FHTG) was identified in 5.2% of survivors of acute MI under age 60 in the Seattle study. It has an autosomal mode of inheritance and is expressed in adulthood. Genetic and clinical studies of FHTG are impaired, however, by absence of distinguishing clinical features and the common occurrence in the population of elevated triglyceride levels due to diet, obesity, alcohol intake, and medications such as steroids, estrogens, and diuretics. Elevated triglycerides in these families without association with low HDL, elevated apo B, or premature CAD do not appear to be associated with premature CAD.

In *familial low HDL*, the HDL-C level is significantly lower in men than in women after puberty. Familial hypoalphalipoproteinemia is a common, autosomal dominant disorder characterized by HDL-C values below the 10% cutoffs based on age- and sex-specific normal values. This trait is linked to premature CAD, and among consecutive patients undergoing coronary angiography who prove to have CAD, a low HDL-C level is often the most frequent lipid/lipoprotein abnormality found. Additionally, a low HDL-C level may be a marker for an arteriopathy causing childhood stroke (Daniels et al.). Genetic analysis using DNA probes has shown a strong association between the absence of a restriction site near apo AI and both premature CAD and familial hypoalphalipoproteinemia. This polymorphism on chromosome 11 between AI and CIII may be a useful marker for both premature CAD and familial hypoalphalipoproteinemia (Ordovas et al.).

Dramatic premature CAD is seen when apo AI is abnormal. Premature CAD is seen in cases of apo AI and CIII deficiency and in some cases of Tangier's disease. Not all cases of genetic low HDL level are associated with premature CAD, however. Although HDL-C can be as low as 11 mg/dl, premature CAD is not seen in apo AI Milano or in fish-eye disease—HDL deficiency associated with severe corneal opacification (Schaefer). As in epidemiologic studies in which populations with low HDL-C and an otherwise low risk profile for CAD have low rates of CAD,

genetic HDL deficiency appears least likely to be associated with early CAD when there is a paucity of other risk factors.

In *familial Lp(a) excess*, high levels of Lp(a), an LDL that is linked to a protein called apo (a), are associated strongly with premature MI and with CAD at angiography in Caucasian patients (Dahlen et al; Rhoades et al.). Lp(a) has striking sequence similarity to plasminogen, but whether this has functional consequence is not known. Lp(a) is apparently not toxic unless LDL levels are above a certain threshold. The presence of high levels of Lp(a), then, may affect the decision regarding which level of LDL-C to treat aggressively. Thus, although many cholesterol-lowering drugs do not affect the Lp(a) level, the strategy of reducing LDL-C is still a reasonable way to reduce CAD risk, even though the Lp(a) level is not affected.

OTHER LIPID AND LIPOPROTEIN DISORDERS

HYPERTRIGLYCERIDEMIA

Borderline hypertriglyceridemia is defined as a triglyceride value of 250-499 mg/dl. Definite hypertriglyceridemia is defined by values ≥500 mg/dl (NIH Consensus Conference 1984). Although most studies indicate that elevated triglyceride values are not independent risk factors for CAD, some have begun to reexamine the relationship between triglycerides and CAD (Brunzell and Austin). In analyses specific to women, in particular, elevated triglyceride values may be useful markers of risk of CAD. The Framingham Study showed that elevated triglyceride levels were independent predictors in older women. In one study of patients undergoing coronary angiography for suspected CAD, triglycerides and apo B levels were the only factors that correlated with severity of disease (Sedlis et al.). Hypertriglyceridemia, then, is of concern when associated with either a personal or family history of abnormal lipids/lipoproteins (elevated LDL-C and/or low HDL-C levels), a personal or family history of CAD, or when levels are elevated such that pancreatitis (occurring when triglyceride levels exceed 1,500 mg/dl) may occur.

LOW HDL CHOLESTEROL

High-density lipoprotein cholesterol is a major inverse risk factor for CAD. Low values for HDL-C greatly affect treatment decisions regarding LDL-C and are one factor favoring the use of drugs to treat high LDL-C. While low HDL-C is usually due to a genetic cause, secondary causes (Table 6) are common. Reduction of obesity, cessation of cigarette smoking, and regular exercise for the sedentary are general measures that can be recommended to all persons, and physicians should not overlook the opportunity to do so in those with low HDL levels. In hypertensive patients on beta blockers, the use of alpha blockers, angiotensin converting enzyme (ACE) inhibitors, or calcium channel blockers can, in many cases, be substituted for nonspecific beta blocker therapy, with improvement in HDL-C (although a switch to a more selective beta blocker may be preferred for cases of CAD).

When there is a primary elevation of LDL, a goal LDL-C level can be set. For those without CAD or two risk factors, the LDL-C goal is <160 mg/dl. For those with CAD or two risk factors, the LDL-C goal is <130 mg/dl. The recommended goals are set to be minimal goals. In cases of CAD in particular, lower levels can be encouraged and easily achieved, resulting in even further reduction of CAD risk.

DIETARY TREATMENT

EFFECT OF DIET ON CAD

The link between diet and CAD is seen in animal data gathered from regression experiments in rhesus monkeys, epidemiologic studies in man comparing populations, migration studies looking at CAD rates in those who move from an area of low CAD prevalence to high CAD prevalence, studies within high-risk populations, and finally, intervention studies. Strong correlations between dietary saturated fat intake and serum cholesterol levels were noted in the landmark

Seven Countries study (Keys). A striking finding was the corresponding strong correlation between saturated fat intake and CAD. These results are confirmed by the International Atherosclerosis Project, which examined autopsy data from over 23,000 persons from 14 countries (McGill). In this study, severity of atherosclerosis correlated significantly with dietary fat intake and advanced lesions correlated significantly with the mean population serum cholesterol level. The Ni-Hon-San Study examined dietary habits of Japanese living in Japan, Hawaii, and San Francisco and compared these against their differing rates of CAD (Robertson et al.). Migration from Japan eastward was associated with an increase in saturated fat and dietary cholesterol intake as well as increasing death rates from CAD, confirming the key role of diet.

Moreover, two prospective studies, the Chicago Western Electric study (Shekelle et al.) and the Zutphen trial (Kromhout et al.), both with detailed dietary records and lipid assessments at baseline, showed that 20-year rates for CAD were highly correlated with dietary cholesterol intake despite small effects on blood cholesterol values. These studies also showed that regular consumption of fish in the diet was associated with lower rates for CAD. Thus, regular consumption of fish, especially in place of saturated fat, is recommended. Fish oil capsules, whose benefits, negative aspects and long-term safety have still to be determined by further research, are not recommended. The usefulness of fish oil capsules in preventing restenosis after angioplasty is still unconfirmed (Dehmer et al.; Reis et al.).

Finally, two intervention trials give compelling evidence that a diet lower in saturated fat and dietary cholesterol can lower lipid and lipoprotein values and also reduce risk of CAD. The Oslo Study diet-heart trial (Hjermann et al.) examined hard end points for CAD in middle-aged men with severe hypercholesterolemia who were randomized to receive either diet

---

Table 6. Secondary Causes of Low High-density Lipoprotein (HDL) Cholesterol Levels (<35 mg/dl)

Cigarette smoking
Sedentary lifestyle
Obesity (particulary where waist/hip ratio >1.0)
Medications such as thiazide diuretics, nonspecific beta blockers, androgenic steroids, progestins
Excess polyunsaturated fat diets

and smoking advice or no intervention. The intervention group showed a 13% fall in blood cholesterol levels and a decline in smoking frequency, with a 47% lower incidence of sudden death and MI than the control group. The Leiden trial (Arntzenius et al.) looked at the value of vegetarian diet in moderately hypercholesterolemic men with angina who underwent coronary angiography before diet and two years later. Disease progression was significant in patients whose total/HDL cholesterol ratios were greater than 6.9; yet no coronary lesion growth was seen in patients who had values <6.9 or in whom higher values were significantly lowered by diet.

THE STEP 1 AND STEP 2 DIETS

Saturated fat, dietary cholesterol and calorie excess leading to obesity are the nutritional habits leading to elevated blood cholesterol levels in Western countries. The Step 1 diet is recommended by the NCEP panel as the initial dietary intervention to achieve the total cholesterol and LDL-C goals. The key alterations include lowering total fat to 30% of calories, saturated fat to less than 10% of calories, and dietary cholesterol to 300 mg/day. Polyunsaturated fats contain linoleic acid, an essential fatty acid. Nonetheless, they are restricted to no more than 10% of calories as well. No restrictions are placed on monounsaturated fats (olive oil, canola oil) which, unlike polyunsaturated fats, do not appear to reduce the HDL-C level. In the average person ingesting 40% fat, 17% saturated fat, and 500 mg of dietary cholesterol per day, blood cholesterol levels could be reduced by as much as 30 mg/dl. On the other hand, humans are characterized by their great variability in response to cholesterol-lowering diets, so each patient's response must be assessed individually.

In more practical terms, this amounts to about 11 g of saturated fat per 1,000 calories consumed daily. The six categories that account for fat in the diet can be remembered with the mnemonic MEDICS, which stands for *m*eats, *e*gg *y*olks, *d*airy produc*s*, *i*nvisible fats (animal and vegetable fats in baked goods and products such as non-dairy coffee whiteners), *c*ooking and table fats, and *s*nacks (Stone and VanHorn). Table 7 is a list of foods high in saturated fat and cholesterol, and alternate choices in each of these categories.

The patient's cholesterol level should be measured at four to six weeks and at three months after starting the diet. For those with average values for HDL-C,

a cholesterol level of 240 mg/dl corresponds to an LDL-C level of 160 mg/dl; a level of 200 mg/dl corresponds to a an LDL-C of 130 mg/dl. The cholesterol values can be used as surrogates for LDL-C in following progress on diet, with less frequent LDL-C determinations performed if a simple correlation is seen. Those with elevations of LDL-C level >225 mg/dl in whom additional dietary restriction would not be expected to permit LDL-C goals to be met can go more quickly to drug therapy. For others, if repeat tests show that the cholesterol and LDL-C goals are not achieved and adherence seems satisfactory, then the Step 2 diet is recommended. A registered dietitian may facilitate adherence to diet by dealing with issues such as variety, meal preparation including substitutions for ethnic foods, and eating out. The Step 2 dietary pattern restricts saturated fat further to ≤7% of total calories and limits dietary cholesterol to ≤200 mg/day. For those with hypertriglyceridemia, the initial step should always be dietary because reduction of obesity, a regular exercise program and limitation of calories from alcohol can greatly reduce triglyceride values.

Insoluble fiber is useful in relieving constipation, but only soluble fiber, which contains beta glucan, is effective in lowering blood cholesterol (although to a mild degree). Oat bran, rolled oats, broccoli, brussels sprouts, grapefruit, apples and beans such as pinto and navy varieties are good sources of soluble fiber. Psyllium powders used for constipation are also good sources of soluble fiber and lower cholesterol levels to a modest degree. However, while soluble fiber is beneficial, it is not a panacea. Breakfast cereals or commercial muffins combining the cholesterol-raising effects of a saturated oil like coconut or palm oil with the beneficial effects of oat bran make little sense. Patients must be warned about the side effects of abdominal bloating and increased flatus that occur if too large a quantity of fiber is ingested. Alcohol raises the HDL-C as well as triglyceride levels. In addition, the so-called coronary protective effect may merely reflect selection bias of older studies; nondrinkers are often cardiac patients who have been told not to drink. Alcohol can raise blood pressure, contribute to obesity, and cause significant problems if its use is not regulated; therefore, it is not recommended to those with low HDL-C levels. However, if triglyceride levels are not significantly elevated (over 500 mg/dl), there is no reason to proscribe alcohol in non-alcoholics.

Diet adherence and diet success vary greatly from patient to patient. For those with mild hypercholes-

Table 7. Dietary Sources of Saturated Fats and Possible Substitutes

Category	Item	Saturated fat (g)	Cholesterol (mg)
Meats			
	Ground beef patty cooked, regular, 4 oz	9.2	102
	Turkey, light, roasted, skinless, 4 oz	1.2	78
Eggs			
	Egg yolk, one	1.7	275
	Commercial egg substitute	0	0
Dairy			
Cheese	American cheese, 1 oz	6	30
	Substitute cheese	1	
Milk	Milk, whole, 1 cup	5.1	33
	Milk, skim, 1 cup	0.6	5
Cream	Ice cream, 1 cup	9	60
	Nonfat yogurt, 1 cup	0.3	Trace
Invisible fats (as in baked goods, snacks)			
	Donut, 1 piece	5	20
	French fries, 1 order	7	15
	Fruits	0	0
Cooking/table fats:			
	Butter, 1 T	7	30
	Soft diet margarine, 1 T	1	0
	Hard margarine (stick), 1 T	2.1	0
	Coconut oil, 1 T	11.8	0
	Corn oil, 1 T	1.7	0
Snacks			
	Peanuts, dry-roasted, ¼ cup	3.1	0
	Popcorn, salted, buttered, 3 cups	2.7	12
	Popcorn, 3 cups	Trace	0
	Chocolate chip cookies, two	1.3	8

Values are approximate and taken from standard food tables.

terolemia ($\geq$240 mg/dl), physician endorsement, prescription and encouragement of the Step 1 diet may be remarkably successful. In many patients, successful lipid reduction can be expected to occur within three to six months. Physicians should expect gradual change because adherence to a new lifestyle is best ushered in slowly. For nonresponders, a low-cholesterol diet may be insufficient to achieve the minimal goal levels. In these cases, more frequent contact with the registered dietitian can best determine if these persons are truly "biologic" hyporesponders (Katan et al.). Frequent reasons for dietary failure include insufficient motivation or knowledge on how to eat when food is prepared outside of the home, high-fat snacks such as peanuts, ice cream and snack chips, and increased alcohol usage during stressful times. Periodic monitoring with blood or LDL-C values provides the needed feedback for continued progress toward goal values. Patients who may prefer drug therapy without a reasonable dietary trial should be warned that cholesterol-lowering medication is never curative and the convenience of a pill must be balanced against the cost not only in dollars but in potential side effects.

Table 8. Lipid-Lowering Drug Therapy

Name	Mechanism	Effect	Comment
Cholestyramine (Questran)	Binds bile acids in the gut; LDL catabolism is increased	TC ($--$) LDL-C ($--$) HDL-C ($+$) VLDL-C ($+$)	Constipation problem, so start with low doses and move up slowly
Colestipol (Colestid)	--- Same as above ---		
(Remember that both these resins also can bind drugs in the gut, e.g., digoxin, thyroxin, and antibiotics.)			
Niacin (vitamin B$_3$)	Inhibits FFA release; leads to decreased LDL and VLDL synth.	TC ($--$) LDL-C ($--$) HDL-C ($++$) VLDL-C ($--$)	Initial flush seen in all; better in 80%. Low-dose aspirin inhibits flush. Watch LFTs, uric acid & glucose. Avoid in ulcer patient.
(Niacinamide is not a substitute for niacin as lipid-lowering agent!)			
Gemfibrozil (Lopid)	Stimulates LPL Increased C in bile	TC ($-$) LDL-C ($-$) HDL-C ($++$) VLDL-C ($---$)	Lowers CAD risk in men with high TC, TG and low HDL-C. Gallstone risk.
Lovastatin (Mevinolin)	HMG CoA reductase inhibitor	TC ($---$) LDL-C ($---$) HDL-C ($++$) VLDL-C ($--$)	Take with food. Watch liver enzymes; beware of myositis and do not use with gemfibrozil for this reason.
Probucol (Lorelco)	Inhibits synthesis of cholesterol Increased LDL clearance by non-receptor mechanism	TC ($--$) LDL-C ($--$) HDL-C ($--$) VLDL-C ($+/-$)	Assoc. with decrease in xanthomas; Significance of low HDL unclear

Number of plus and minus signs indicates degree. TC = total cholesterol; FFA = free fatty acid; LPL = lipoprotein lipase; LFTs = liver function tests; other abbreviations as in Table 2.

DRUG THERAPY

The cutpoints for initiating drug therapy were set high in guidelines so as to discourage drug usage. Drug therapy should be carefully considered for those without CAD or two risk factors if the LDL-C levels remain above 190 mg/dl despite rigorous diet over at least six months. For those with CAD or two risk factors and an LDL-C level that persists above 160 mg/dl, medication should also be considered. In the former case, the LDL-C goal is ≤160 mg/dl; in the latter, high-risk case, the minimal LDL-C goal for drug therapy is <130 mg/dl. If drug therapy with a single agent does not achieve the LDL-C goal and lower LDL-C by 15% or more, then another agent should be chosen. If LDL-C is lowered by 15% or more, and goal LDL-C levels are not met, it may be reasonable to add a second medication if further doses of the current drug would not be well tolerated.

The ideal cholesterol-lowering drug would effectively lower LDL-C and triglyceride levels and raise HDL-C level. It would be proven by clinical trials to reduce both total mortality and hard end points for CAD. It would not aggravate other factors that contribute to the coronary risk factor profile. It would have no long-term toxicity. It would be an inexpensive, easily taken medication relatively free of side effects. Unfortunately, no such medication exists. The efficacy, safety, and tolerability of the various lipid-lowering medications in use at present are reviewed herein.

RESINS

The bile acid-binding resins or sequestrants are important drugs of first choice. Although not absorbed, they stimulate hepatic production of LDL receptors as well as hepatic cholesterol synthesis. They are known as cholestyramine (Questran) and colestipol (Colestid). The dosage form is a powder which as Questran contains 4 g of active medication, and as Colestid contains 5 g. Similar doses of cholestyramine are also available in a flavored bar form (Cholybar). These resin forms are equivalent in their effects. As mentioned earlier, they lower LDL-C levels moderately, raise HDL-C slightly, and have been associated in several trials in men with and without CAD with lower rates of new cases of CAD. In the Lipid Research Clinics Primary Prevention Trial, after an average follow-up of 7.4 years, the group treated with cholestyramine and diet had reductions in total cholesterol and LDL-C levels that were 8.5% and 12.6% greater than those seen in the placebo group. The treated group had a 19% reduction in risk of the primary end point, which was definite CAD death and/or definite nonfatal MI. Moreover, the incidence rates for new positive exercise tests, angina, and coronary bypass surgery were reduced by 25%, 20% and 21%. For every 1% lowering of cholesterol, there was a 2% reduction of CAD events in the range of cholesterol lowering studied (Lipid Research Clinics Program). The effect of reducing CAD incidence was seen after two years. There was a 7% reduction in all-cause mortality in the cholestyramine group, which was not significant. The excess mortality seen in the treatment group was confined to violent and accidental deaths. Furthermore, a carefully done but small angiographic study compared cholestyramine and diet versus placebo and diet in 116 men and women. Progression of coronary narrowing was significantly decreased in the treated group compared with controls (Brensike et al.).

Although remarkably safe, resins are not popular with patients because of their gritty texture, the inconvenience of carrying and consuming a packet of powder when out of the home, and troublesome gastrointestinal side effects such as bloating, constipation with large bulky stools, and aggravation of hemorrhoids. Considerable efforts at patient education may be required for successful adherence to the moderate to high doses used in patients with FH. For many patients with only moderate hypercholesterolemia, lower doses can be used and are usually well tolerated. Resins should not be drugs of first choice if triglyceride levels are elevated above 250 mg/dl, because they can elevate triglyceride values significantly. Resins can be used once triglyceride values are controlled by diet and exercise or by drugs such as niacin or gemfibrozil.

Resin therapy requires patient education because resins bind other medications, particularly commonly prescribed drugs such as thyroxin, digoxin, and antibiotics. Patients should remember to take these and other drugs at least 1 hour *before* taking the resin or 4 or more hours *after* taking the resin. Although drug adherence can be a problem, the remarkable safety record of the drug makes it an excellent choice in the patient who is young, motivated, and without bowel complaints.

NIACIN

Niacin, also known as nicotinic acid or vitamin B3, decreases synthesis of lipoproteins from the liver and thereby lowers VLDL and LDL. It increases HDL-C values. Niacin comes in tablet form or in a modified, sustained-release form. The usual initial dose is either 100 mg of the USP niacin or 250 mg as the sustained-release form. Some persons with mild-moderate hypercholesterolemia respond well to lower dosages of niacin (500-1,000 mg/day), while those with moderate to severe high cholesterol ($\geq$240 mg/dl) may require $\geq$1-3 g/day. The dosage must be built up slowly, with monitoring of lipid and other blood chemistries as the dosage is increased. Niacinamide (nicotinamide), another form of the vitamin, does not lower lipids as effectively as niacin. Unwittingly, patients may switch to niacinamide, with poor results. In the Coronary Drug Project (Canner et al.), niacin lowered cholesterol levels by about 10% and significantly reduced risk of nonfatal MI by about 27% compared with placebo at the end of the trial period. Although not given further, the group receiving niacin in the study has been shown on long-term follow-up to have a significantly improved survival rate. Furthermore, the Cholesterol Lowering Atherosclerosis

Study (Blankenhorn et al.) showed that niacin and resin together, given to men after coronary bypass surgery who could tolerate medication, significantly reduced the progression of CAD in both native circulation and bypass grafts. In fact, regression was seen in 16% of resin plus niacin users, versus just 2% of placebo-treated controls. In the treatment group, LDL-C levels were lowered to just under 100 mg/dl and the HDL-C levels were raised to over 60 mg/dl.

Long-term safety with niacin seems reasonable; the drug has been used for decades. Side effects are more likely with the higher doses, and at least one study suggests that the modified forms may cause liver side effects more easily than unmodified niacin. Nonetheless, niacin is not more widely used owing to its poor tolerability. Niacin is a potent vasodilator that elicits prostaglandin-mediated flushing and itching. In many, the intensity of the reaction can be reduced by taking aspirin just before niacin (usually required for a month or so) and taking the niacin with food. Tolerance to flushing develops in about 80%. Ulcer disease is aggravated and niacin therapy can raise uric acid, liver enzyme levels and, rarely, muscle enzyme levels. It can worsen glucose tolerance in type II diabetics. Thus, chemistry values must be monitored every six to eight weeks as increasing doses of niacin are used. In doses of ≤ 1 g, niacin is often well tolerated and at this low dose can be effective in some patients (Luria). In persons with combined hyperlipidemia, niacin is the drug of choice. For patients in whom cost is an issue, unmodified niacin is extremely inexpensive and clearly the drug of choice. Also, its record in patients with known CAD who have had either an MI or bypass surgery with proven atherosclerotic plaques by coronary angiography makes it an attractive choice in these patients.

FIBRATES

Fibric acid derivatives have a predominant effect on facilitating triglyceride disposal through lipoprotein lipase as well as moderate decreases in VLDL production by the liver (Vega and Grundy). Clofibrate is a first-generation fibrate which, owing to its lithogenicity and adverse effects, is not recommended. Gemfibrozil is a second-generation fibrate that was recommended initially by the Food and Drug Administration for triglyceride-lowering and, more recently, due to the results of the Helsinki Heart Study, for coronary prevention in those with elevated cholesterol

and triglyceride (type IIb phenotype) and low HDL-C (Frick et al.). Gemfibrozil comes as 300- and 600-mg tablets. It is taken twice daily; the usual dosage is 600 mg twice daily. Gemfibrozil lowers LDL-C levels, but is particularly effective in lowering triglyceride levels and raising HDL-C. This drug should be considered particularly in the patient with an elevated LDL level who has concomitant raised triglyceride and low HDL-C levels. In those with normal LDL-C and elevated triglyceride levels, the LDL-C level may increase as VLDL is converted to LDL.

The Helsinki trial showed gemfibrozil treatment to be associated with a significant lowering of CAD risk (a decrease of 34% in the incidence of CAD) in middle-aged Finnish men with initial cholesterol levels averaging 280 mg/dl. As also seen in the Lipid Research Clinics Trial, the effects in the treatment group became apparent after the second year of therapy. Another similarity was the lack of difference between treated and control groups with respect to mortality risk. Gemfibrozil's beneficial cardiac effects appeared to be due both to the lowered LDL-C as well as the raised HDL-C levels. Gastrointestinal symptoms increased mildly in those taking gemfibrozil. Although the number of operations for gallstones was not significantly increased, more abdominal operations were performed in the treatment group. These drugs are still considered to increase the risk of gallstones, albeit slightly.

Fenofibrate is a third-generation fibrate that has more prominent LDL-C lowering effects than its predecessors and lowers uric acid through a renal action. It has been used extensively in Europe and may soon become available in the U.S. The dose is 100 mg three times daily (Brown et al. 1986).

HMG CoA REDUCTASE INHIBITORS

A new class of drug works directly by increasing LDL receptor activity. Known as hydroxymethylglutaryl Co-enzyme A (HMG CoA) reductase inhibitors, this class promises to be a powerful addition to our cholesterol-lowering armamentarium (Grundy 1988). The only one currently available is lovastatin. Other HMG CoA reductase inhibitors may be introduced on the market in the next five years. Lovastatin comes as 20-mg tablets, which should be taken with food in order to achieve optimal blood levels. For dosage levels >20 mg, twice-daily dosing is more effective than once-daily dosing. The exact dosage is determined by the pre-treatment LDL-C value. These drugs are very effective in lowering LDL-C levels. They lower triglyceride and raise HDL-C levels as well. They are well tolerated in general, with fewer side effects than resins (Lovastatin Study Group III). Lovastatin was only recently introduced into clinical usage, so its long-term safety is not known and no studies of effects on CAD incidence are available. Nonetheless, since the beneficial effect on CAD with lipid-lowering therapy is due to an improved lipid/lipoprotein profile, lovastatin's effects on reducing CAD should be considerable. Chemistry profiles that include liver enzyme tests must be followed regularly because a reversible elevation of liver enzyme levels (usually seen after the third month of therapy) is seen in about 2% of patients receiving lovastatin. Muscle soreness or tenderness should prompt clinical evaluation and CK tests because a small number of cases of myositis and rhabdomyolysis have been reported. Most of these cases were patients who had taken lovastatin in combination with cyclosporine, gemfibrozil or niacin. Although gemfibrozil and lovastatin are a poweful combination for those with familial combined hyperlipidemia, combination therapy with these drugs must be undertaken with great caution due to the increased incidence of myositis and the possibility of rhabdomyolysis and acute kidney failure. Although baseline eye examinations with slit-lamp examination for cataracts is appropriate, the concern about increased cataract incidence has not been confirmed in ongoing studies.

Since gemfibrozil and niacin both may raise blood sugar levels, use of lovastatin may be preferred in type II diabetics who present with combined elevations of cholesterol and triglyceride levels. The ability to lower LDL-C considerably, coupled with its good tolerability, make lovastatin a good choice in the patient with multiple illnesses or medications and the patient with severe hypercholesterolemia.

PROBUCOL

Probucol comes in 250- and 500-mg tablets. It has a unique non-LDL-receptor mechanism of action. The usual maintenance dose is 500 mg twice daily. It lowers LDL-C mildly and does not affect triglyceride levels. It also lowers the level of HDL-C to a variable degree, the significance of which is uncertain. Studies in severe cases of FH have documented xanthoma

regression. It is not clear whether the HDL lowering should be considered an adverse effect. No clinical trial data indicate probucol's efficacy against CAD or its long-term safety. Its ability to retard atherosclerosis in rabbits with genetic high cholesterol (they resemble adults with FH) suggests that further studies will define its role in the treatment of lipids and atherosclerotic disease. It is well tolerated; the tendency toward mild diarrhea counterbalances the tendency toward constipation from resins, with which it is frequently combined (Dujovne et al.). It should not be given to those with a long QT interval and it should be discontinued if QT lengthening occurs.

D-thyroxine and neomycin were not recommended by the NCEP for routine use as lipid-altering drugs.

SPECIAL SITUATIONS

If the LDL-C level is higher than the dietary goals but is not high enough for the drug goals, certain patients judged at increased risk for CAD may utilize small doses of resin therapy to achieve successful lowering of LDL-C with few side effects.

The patient with a normal LDL-C level and an HDL-C level <35 mg/dl presents a difficult therapeutic problem. In the asymptomatic person, it is reasonable to adhere to the Step 1 diet, noting the need to reduce obesity, stop cigarette smoking and develop a regular, aerobic exercise program. Patients must be counseled that the rise in HDL-C will be slow. For the patient with multiple risk factors or with active CAD, a more aggressive approach is recommended by some physicians. Niacin may be a particularly attractive choice here.

In addition, combination therapy is often beneficial in patients with very high levels of LDL-C, those with combined elevations of cholesterol and triglycerides, and those in whom side effects at higher dosages limit usage of maximal doses of just one drug. Combinations that are beneficial for those with very high levels of LDL-C (e.g., patients with genetic familial hypercholesterolemia) include resins plus niacin, resins plus lovastatin, and resins plus gemfibrozil. In patients with FH that is very resistant to monotherapy, double drug therapy can lower the LDL-C level by as much as 35-50% (Kane et al.; Illingworth). For severely resistant disease, triple drug therapy can lower LDL-C into the normal range and has also been shown in some cases to be associated with regression of xanthomas (Malloy et al.; Witzum et al.).

Bibliography

Abbott RD, Wilson PWF, Kannel WB, Castelli WP: High density lipoprotein cholesterol, total cholesterol screening, and myocardial infarction. *Arteriosclerosis* 8:207, 1988.

Adult Treatment Panel: Report of the National Cholesterol Education Program Expert Panel on Detection, Evaluation, and Treatment of High Blood Cholesterol in Adults. *Arch Intern Med* 148:36, 1988.

Allen JM, Thompson GR, Myant NB, et al: Cardiovascular complications of homozygous familial hypercholesterolemia. *Br Heart J* 44:361, 1980.

Arntzenius AC, Kromhout D, Barth JD, et al: Diet, lipoproteins, and the progression of coronary atherosclerosis. The Leiden Intervention Trial. *N Engl J Med* 312:805, 1985.

Austin MA, Breslow JL, Hennekens CH, et al: Low density lipoprotein subclass patterns and risk of MI. *JAMA* 260:1917, 1988.

Becker DM, Becker LC, Pearson TA, et al: Risk factors in siblings of people with premature coronary heart disease. *J Am Coll Cardiol* 12:1, 1988.

Beppu S, Minura Y, Sakakibara H, et al: Supravalvular aortic stenosis and coronary ostial stenosis in familial hypercholesterolemia: Two-dimensional echocardiographic assessment. *Circulation* 67:878, 1983.

Bilheimer DW, Goldstein JL, Grundy SM, Starzl TE, Brown MS: Liver transplantation to provide low-density-lipoprotein receptors and lower plasma cholesterol in a child with homozygous familial hypercholesterolemia. *N Engl J Med* 311:1658, 1984.

Blankenhorn DH, Nessim SA, Johnson RL, et al: Beneficial effects of combined colestipol-niacin therapy on coronary atherosclerosis and coronary venous bypass grafts. *JAMA* 257:3233, 1987.

Brensike JF, Levy RI, Kelsey SF, et al: Effects of therapy with cholestyramine on progression of coronary arteriosclerosis: Results of the NHLBI Type II Coronary Intervention Study. *Circulation* 69:313, 1984.

Breslow JL: Molecular genetics of lipoprotein disorders. *Circulation* 69:1190, 1984.

Brown MS, Kovanen PT, Goldstein JL: Regulation of plasma cholesterol by lipoprotein receptors. *Science* 212:628, 1981.

Brown WV, Dujovne CA, Farquhar JW, et al: Effects of fenofibrate on plasma lipids. Double-blind, multicenter study in patients with type IIA or IIB hyperlipidemia. *Arteriosclerosis* 6:670, 1986.

Brunzell JD, Austin MA: Plasma triglyceride levels and coronary disease. *N Engl J Med* 320:1273, 1989.

Caggiula AW, Christakis G, Farrand M, et al. for MRFIT: The Multiple Risk Factor Intervention Trial (MRFIT). *Prev Med* 10:443, 1981.

Campeau L, Enjalbert M, Lesperance J, et al: The relation of risk factors to the development of atherosclerosis in saphenous-vein bypass grafts and the progression of disease in the native circulation. *New Engl J Med* 311:1329, 1984.

Canner PL, Berge KG, Wenger NK, et al: Fifteen year mortality in Coronary Drug Project patients: Long term benefit with niacin. *J Am Coll Cardiol* 8:1245, 1986.

Dahlen GH, Guyton JR, Attar M, et al: Association of lipoprotein Lp(a), plasma lipids and other lipoproteins with coronary artery disease documented by angiography. *Circulation* 74:758, 1986.

Daniels SR, Bates S, Lukin RR, et al: Cerebrovascular arteriopathy (arteriosclerosis) and ischemic childhood stroke. *Stroke* 13:360, 1982.

Davignon J, Gregg, RE, Sing CF: Apolipoprotein E polymorphism and atherosclerosis. *Arteriosclerosis* 8:1, 1988.

Dehmer GJ, Popma JJ, van den Berg EK, et al: Reduction in the rate of early restenosis after coronary angioplasty by a diet supplemented with N-3 fatty acids. *N Engl J Med* 319:733, 1988.

Dujovne CA, Krehbiel P, Decoursey S, et al: Probucol with colestipol in the treatment of hypercholesterolemia. *Ann Int Med* 1:477, 1984.

Frick MH, Eto O, Haapa K, et al: Helsinki Heart Study: Primary prevention trial with gemfibrozil in middle-aged men with dyslipidemia. *N Engl J Med* 317:1237, 1987.

Garber AM, Sox HC, Littenberg B: Screening asymptomatic adults for cardiac risk factors: The serum cholesterol level. *Ann Intern Med* 110:622, 1989.

Goldstein JL, Hazzard WR, Schrott HG, Bierman EL, Motulsky AG: Hyperlipidemia in coronary heart disease I. Lipid levels in 500 survivors of myocardial infarction. *J Clin Invest* 52:1533, 1973.

Goldstein JL, Kita T, Brown MS: Defective lipoprotein receptors and atherosclerosis: Lessons from an animal counterpart of familial hypercholesterolemia. *N Engl J Med* 309:288, 1983.

Goldstein JL, Schrott HG, Hazzard WR, Bierman EL, Motulsky AG: Hyperlipidemia in coronary heart disease. II. Genetic analysis of lipids in 176 families and delineation of a new inherited disorder, combined hyperlipidemia. *J Clin Invest* 52:1544, 1973.

Gordon DJ, Probstfield JL, Garrison RJ, et al: High density lipoprotein cholesterol and cardiovascular disease. Four prospective American studies. *Circulation* 79:8, 1989.

Grundy SM: Cholesterol and coronary heart disease: A new era. *JAMA* 256:2849, 1986.

Grundy SM: HMG-CoA reductase inhibitors for treatment of hypercholesterolemia. *N Engl J Med* 319:24, 1988.

Grundy SM, Goodman DS, Rifkind BM, Cleeman JI: The place of HDL in cholesterol management. A perspective from the National Cholesterol Education Program. *Arch Intern Med* 149:505, 1989.

Grundy SM, Greenland P, Herd A, et al: Cardiovascular and risk factor evaluation of healthy American adults. *Circulation* 75:1340A, 1987.

Hjermann I, Velve Byre K, Holme I, et al: Effect of diet and smoking intervention on the incidence of coronary heart disease: Report from the Oslo Study Group. *Lancet* 2:1303, 1981.

Hulley SB, Rosenman RH, Bawol RD, Brand RJ: Epidemiology as a guide to clinical decision. The association between triglyceride and coronary heart disease. *N Engl J Med* 302:1383, 1980.

Hunt SC, Wu LL, Hopkins PN, et al: Apolipoprotein, low density lipoprotein subfraction and insulin associations with familial combined dyslipidemia. *Arteriosclerosis* 9:335, 1989.

Huttunen J, Kaitaniemi P, Koskinen P, et al: Lipid alterations and decline in the incidence of coronary heart disease in the Helsinki Study. *JAMA* 260:641, 1988.

Illingworth DR, Rapp JH, Phillipson BE, Connor WE: Colestipol plus nicotinic acid in treatment of heterozygous familial hypercholesterolaemia. *Lancet* 1:296, 1981.

Illingworth DR: Mevinolin plus colestipol in therapy for severe heterozygous familial hypercholesterolemia. *Ann Intern Med* 101:598, 1984.

Kane JP, Malloy MJ, Tun P, et al: Normalization of low density lipoprotein levels in heterozygous familial hypercholesterolemia with combined drug regimen. *N Engl J Med* 304:251, 1981.

Katan MB, Beynen AC, deBries JH, Nobels A: Existence of consistent hypo- and hyperresponders to dietary cholesterol in man. *Am J Epidemiol* 123:221, 1986.

Keys A, ed: Coronary Heart disease in seven countries. *Circulation* 41 (Suppl I):I–1, 1970.

Lasser NJ, Mellies MJ, Palmer RH, et al: Effects of fenofibrate on plasma lipids: Double-blind, multicenter study in patients with type IIA or IIB hyperlipidemia. *Arteriosclerosis* 6:670, 1986.

Kromhout D, Arntzenius AC, Kempen-Voogd N, et al: The inverse relation between fish consumption and twenty year mortality from coronary heart disease. *N Engl J Med* 312:1205, 1985.

Levy RI, Brensike JF, Epstein SE, et al: The influence of changes in lipid values induced by cholestyramine and diet on progression of coronary artery disease: Results of the NHLBI Type II Coronary Intervention Study. *Circulation* 69:325, 1984.

Lipid Research Clinics Program: The Lipid Research Clinics Primary Prevention Trial Results. I. Reduction in incidence of coronary heart disease. *JAMA* 251:351, 1984.

Lovastatin Study Group III: A multicenter comparison of lovastatin and cholestyramine in the therapy of severe primary hypercholesterolemia. *JAMA* 260:359, 1988.

Luria MH: Effect of low-dose niacin on high-density lipoprotein cholesterol and total cholesterol/high-density lipoprotein cholesterol ratio. *Arch Intern Med* 148:2493, 1988.

Malloy MJ, Kane JP, Kunitake ST, Tun P: Complementarity of colestipol, niacin, and lovastatin in treatment of severe familial hypercholesterolemia. *Ann Intern Med* 107:616, 1987.

Martin MJ, Hulley SB, Browner WS, et al: Serum cholesterol, blood pressure, and mortality: Implications from a cohort of 361,662 men. *Lancet* 2:933, 1986.

McGill HC Jr, ed: *The Geographic Pathology of Atherosclerosis.* Baltimore: Williams & Wilkins; 1968.

Ordovas JM, Schaefer EJ, Salem D, et al: Apolipoprotein A-1 gene polymorphism associated with premature coronary artery disease and familial hypoalphalipoproteinemia. *N Engl J Med* 314;671, 1986.

Reis GJ, Boucher TM, Sipperly ME, et al: Randomized trial of fish oil for prevention of restenosis after coronary angioplasty. *Lancet* 2:177, 1989.

Rhoads GG, Dahlen GH, Berg K, Morton NE, Danneberg AL: Lp(a) lipoprotein as a risk factor for myocardial infarction. *JAMA* 256:2540, 1986.

Robertson TL, Kato H, Rhoads GG, et al: Epidemiology studies of coronary heart disease and stroke in Japanese men living in Japan, Hawaii, and California. *Am J Cardiol* 39:239, 1977.

Ross R: The pathogenesis of atherosclerosis—an update. *N Engl J Med* 314:488, 1986.

Schaefer EJ: Clinical, biochemical, and genetic features of familial disorders of high density lipoproteins. *Arteriosclerosis* 4:303, 1984.

Sedlis SP, Schechtman KB, Ludbrook PA, Sobel BE, Schonfeld G: Plasma apoproteins and severity of coronary artery disease. *Circulation* 73:978, 1986.

Shekelle RB, Shyrcock AM, Paul O, et al: Diet, serum cholesterol, and death from coronary heart disease: The Western Electric Study. *N Engl J Med* 304:65, 1981.

Small DM: Progression and regression of atherosclerotic lesions. Insights from lipid physical biochemistry. *Arteriosclerosis* 8:103, 1988.

Sniderman A, Shapiro S, Marpole D, et al: Association of coronary atherosclerosis with hyperapobetalipoproteinemia (increased protein but normal cholesterol levels in human plasma low density (B) lipoproteins). *Proc Natl Acad Sci USA* 77:604, 1980.

Sniderman AD, Teng B, Genest J, et al: Familial aggregation and early expression of hyperapobetalipoproteinemia. *Am J Cardiol* 55:291, 1985.

Sniderman AD, Wolfson C, Teng B, et al: Association of hyperapobetalipoproteinemia with endogenous hypertriglyceridemia and atherosclerosis. *Ann Intern Med* 97:833, 1982.

Steinberg D, Parthasarathy S, Carew T, Khoo JC, Witzum JL: Beyond cholesterol: Modifications of low density lipoprotein that increase its atherogenicity. *N Engl J Med* 320:915, 1989.

Stone NJ, Levy RI, Fredrickson DS, Verter J: Coronary artery disease in 116 kindred with familial type II hyperlipoproteinemia. *Circulation* 49:476, 1974.

Stone NJ, Van Horn LV: Controlling cholesterol levels through diet. *Postgrad Med* 83:229, 1988.

Stone NJ: Type II hyperlipoproteinemia. In: Rifkind B, Levy RI, eds. The hyperlipoproteinemias. Diagnosis and Therapy. New York: Grune & Stratton; 1977, p. 113–136.

Treatment of Hypertriglyceridemia. National Institutes of Health Consensus Development Conference Summary. *JAMA* 251:1196, 1984.

Vega GL, Grundy SM: Gemfibrozil therapy in primary hypertriglyceridemia associated with coronary heart disease. *JAMA* 253:2398, 1985.

Witzum JL, Simmons D, Steinberg D, et al: Intensive combination drug therapy of familial hypercholesterolemia with lovastatin, probucol, and colestipol hydrochloride. *Circulation* 79:16, 1989.

13 Angina Pectoris

Edward J. Brown
Robert A. Kloner

DIAGNOSIS AND EVALUATION OF ANGINA PECTORIS

THE CLINICAL HISTORY

Chest pain is a frequent patient complaint, and its differential diagnosis is extensive (Table 1). A careful and thorough clinical history can provide important clues that may significantly narrow the diagnostic possibilities. The location, quality and duration of the chest pain as well as associated symptoms can all help the clinician determine the cause of chest pain.

Angina pectoris is the subjective symptom patients experience with transient episodes of myocardial ischemia (Table 2). It is typically described as substernal chest discomfort, pressure, heaviness, squeezing, or burning, radiating to the shoulders, arms (left greater than right), neck, jaw, and epigastrium; it is exacerbated by exertion, relieved by rest or within a few minutes of use of sublingual nitroglycerin. The discomfort usually lasts at least 15 seconds and less than 15 minutes. Chest pain lasting only a few seconds is usually not angina pectoris. Angina pectoris is often a visceral sensation and, as such, may be difficult for the patient to describe and locate precisely. In fact, if a physician asks the patient to describe the "pain," the patient may correct the physician and use a description such as discomfort. A positive Levine's sign suggests angina; it is characterized by the patient clenching his fist over his sternum when describing the sensation of discomfort. Occasionally, patients will describe angina as occurring initially in the arms, jaws, or shoulders and then radiating to the chest. Rarely, angina will occur only in those areas and not the chest. When trying to elicit a history of exercise-induced angina, it is often useful to ask the patient whether there are certain activities (such as walking up a hill, climbing stairs, or running) which reliably and predictably bring on the chest discomfort.

Angina pectoris can occur in the absence of exertion. This form of myocardial ischemia may be due to coronary artery spasm (Prinzmetal's angina) that results in an episodic decrease in coronary blood flow. Other factors can precipitate angina pectoris at rest, including severe anemia, which leads to decreased blood oxygen-carrying capacity; fever; arrhythmias, especially tachycardia; hyperthyroidism; and drugs, such as catecholamines, which increase myocardial oxygen consumption at rest. A history of cold- or emotion-induced angina should be sought, as these have been associated with vasospastic elements of coronary artery disease. Angina at rest may also be a presenting feature of unstable angina. In the history, it is important to establish the frequency and severity of angina. The patient should be asked to describe how many times angina occurs per day, week and month; how many nitroglycerin tablets the patient uses during these times; and the severity of the angina on a $1+$ to $10+$ scale ($1+$ being very minimal sensation of chest discomfort, $10+$ the most severe). In taking the history, it is important to ask the patient whether previous diagnostic procedures to evaluate coronary artery disease (exercise stress testing, cardiac catheterization) were performed.

Symptoms accompanying chest pain, and the way chest pain is relieved, can be helpful to know in establishing a diagnosis of angina pectoris. Angina pectoris precipitated by exertion is generally relieved after 1-5 minutes in a standing or sitting position. A supine position may aggravate angina pectoris because it promotes increased venous return, which results in increased myocardial wall stress, a major determinant of myocardial oxygen consumption. Angina pectoris often abates within 1/2-2 minutes after the patient

Table 1. Conditions Causing Chest Pain and Differential Aspects

Noncardiovascular Disorders	Differentiating Features
Neuromuscular	
Costochondritis and other chest wall syndromes	Pain exacerbated with inspiration Chest wall tenderness
Radicular syndromes	Radicular distribution to pain Rash of herpes zoster
Inflammatory syndromes of the shoulder joint	Pain on palpation and exacerbated by arm movement
Gastrointestinal	
Esophageal disease and hiatal hernia	Reflux of food Not exertionally related. Eating may exacerbate pain Relief with antacids Note: Nitroglycerin may relieve esophageal spasm.
Peptic ulcer or gastritis	Epigastric pain worse approximately 3 hrs after eating Relieved by antacids, not exertionally related
Gallbladder disease	Right upper quadrant abdominal pain and tenderness. Not exertionally related
Psychologic	
Psychoneuroses	Panic disorders associated with hyperventilation Not exertionally related
Psychosomatic complaints	
Cardiovascular Disorders	
Coronary Artery Disease	
Fixed atherosclerotic disease	Exercise-induced angina
Prinzmetal's angina	Angina at rest. Transient ST elevation
Mixed angina	Elements of exertional angina plus vasospastic angina (cold induced, emotion induced, variable threshold angina)
Syndrome X	Typical angina without angiographic evidence of epicardial coronary artery disease or spasm. Presumably due to small vessel abnormality.
Aortic Stenosis	Pain is typical of angina. Typical systolic ejection murmur. Delayed carotid upstrokes
Hypertrophic obstructive cardiomyopathy	Pain may be typical of angina. Characteristic murmurs—changes with maneuvers. Brisk carotid upstrokes
Primary myocardial disease	Pain may mimic angina
Pericarditis	Pain is sharper. Pleuritic component to pain. Pain worse with lying down, better with sitting up. Friction rub
Dissecting aortic aneurysm	Pain sharp, tearing, prolonged; often occurs in back or interscapular areas. Check for unequal pulses
Mitral valve prolapse syndrome	Transient pain, not necessarily related to exertion Midsystolic click-murmur on physical exam

(continued)

Table 1. Conditions Causing Chest Pain and Differential Aspects (continued)	
Pulmonary Disorders	
Pulmonary embolus-infarction	Tachypnea, dyspnea, cough, pleuritic pain Signs of RV failure if embolus is massive
Pulmonary hypertension	Pain may be exertional and mimic angina Signs of RV failure
Pneumothorax	Sudden onset of pain and dyspnea. Pain may have pleuritic component. Percussion reveals hyperinflation. Tracheal shift
Pleuritis	Pain is sharp and exacerbated by inspiration
Intrathoracic tumor	Not exertional

takes a nitroglycerin tablet. However, esophageal spasm, a condition that can cause chest pain, may also be relieved by the administration of nitroglycerin. Pain relieved when the patient leans forward or that limits respiratory excursion is generally not due to angina pectoris but is more characteristic of pericarditis.

An assessment of cardiac risk factors can be helpful when evaluating patients with chest pain. Angina pectoris is a very unlikely cause of chest pain in patients in their 20s; it is a more likely explanation for chest pain in patients in their 60s. Similarly, a positive family history of heart disease or a diagnosis of diabetes mellitus, hyperlipidemia, hypertension, or cigarette smoking increases the chances that a patient with chest pain is suffering from angina pectoris. Young women who smoke cigarettes and use oral contraceptives have an increased risk of ischemic heart disease; in this group of patients with chest pain, the diagnosis of angina pectoris or myocardial ischemia should be seriously considered.

THE PHYSICAL EXAMINATION

In the absence of an active episode of chest pain there are physical findings that aid in differentiating ischemic chest pain from chest pain due to other causes. Xanthomas, if present, suggest hyperlipidemia and increase the likelihood that the patient has coronary artery disease (CAD). Carotid or femoral bruits suggest the presence of peripheral vascular disease; if the peripheral arteries have atherosclerotic lesions, it is likely that the coronary arteries are also involved. As noted, hypertension is a risk factor for CAD and in-

creases the likelihood that the patient has ischemia-related chest pain.

There may be transient physical findings during an attack of angina. The skin is typically cold and clammy and the patient is often diaphoretic. S_3 (uncommon) and S_4 (common) diastolic gallops are sometimes heard during an attack of angina pectoris (Cohn et al. 1971). A transient systolic murmur, which may result from ischemic papillary muscle dysfunction, is a helpful finding if present (Martin et al.).

Other physical findings that suggest chest pain secondary to ischemia are pulsus alternans, a precordial bulge (best appreciated if the patient is in the left lateral position), elevated blood pressure and heart rate (Proudfit et al.), and a paradoxically split second heart sound. Although these findings are not always present during angina pectoris, their transient presence during an episode of chest pain is diagnostically very helpful.

Other physical signs suggest that chest pain is not angina pectoris. A tender area over the precordium that reproduces the chest pain when palpated suggests pain of musculoskeletal origin. A murmur of mitral valve insufficiency and/or a systolic click suggests mitral valve prolapse, a condition that can cause angina-like chest pain. A marfanoid body habitus should raise the suspicion that aortic dissection underlies chest pain. A typical systolic murmur and delayed carotid upstroke suggest significant aortic valve stenosis, which can cause angina.

SYNDROME X

"Syndrome X" refers to chest pain that suggests angina but occurs in the presence of angiographically

Table 2. Typical Features of Angina Pectoris

Clinical History
    Description
        Heavy, pressing, squeezing or burning chest discomfort
    Location
        Substernal, anterior chest with or without radiation
    Duration
        >15 seconds, <15 minutes
    Radiation
        Jaw, arms (left>right), back, epigastrium, neck
    Precipitating factors
        Cold, exertion, anxiety, meals
    Associated symptoms
        Breathlessness, fatigue, nausea, palpitations, diaphoresis
    Pain relief
        Resting in a standing or sitting position, nitroglycerin, usually takes 1–5 minutes
    Associated risk factors
        Age, sex, cigarette smoking, hypertension, hypercholesterolemia, positive family history for athero-
        sclerotic heart disease, diabetes mellitus
Physical Examination
    Physical findings present chronically
        Xanthelasma and xanthomas, carotid or femoral bruits, hypertension
    Physical findings present during active ischemia
        Cold and clammy skin, diaphoresis, transient S_4 gallops, transient mitral regurgitation murmur, pulsus
        alternans, transient precordial bulge, tachycardia, transient hypertension, paradoxical splitting of S_2
    Physical findings that suggest chest pain is not due to angina pectoris
        Tender precordium, systolic murmur consistent with mitral valve prolapse, a marfanoid body habitus,
        which increases the likelihood that chest pain is due to aortic dissection

patent coronary vessels and in the absence of spasm of the large epicardial coronaries. Some patients with this syndrome are thought to have an inadequate vasodilator reserve and cannot increase coronary flow or reduce coronary vascular resistance as normally occurs with atrial pacing. The defect is thought to reside in small resistance vessels, which cannot be seen on coronary angiography. Exercise tolerance tests with thallium imaging may be positive for ischemia.

In general, the prognosis of such patients is excellent. Calcium channel blockers and nitrates reduce the frequency and severity of chest pain.

INITIAL MANAGEMENT OF PATIENTS WITH CHEST PAIN

Most patients evaluated for chest pain are seen initially in a physician's office or an emergency room. Following the history and physical examination, a decision as to additional evaluation and therapy must be made (Figure 1). The information gathered from

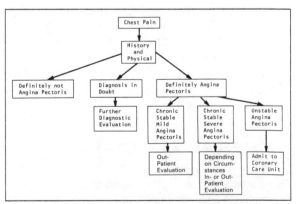

Figure 1. *Initial management strategy for patients with chest pain.*

the history and physical examination may allow the physician to exclude the diagnosis of angina pectoris with no further investigation. For example, the chest pain may clearly be due to a recently acquired chest wall bruise. A second possible decision is that the chest pain may be due to angina pectoris; in this case, further diagnostic evaluation is necessary. A third possibility is that the chest pain is definitely angina pectoris. In this case, the next step is to classify the condition as either chronic stable (mild or severe) angina pectoris or unstable angina pectoris. Chronic stable angina pectoris is present in patients whose chest pain has remained unchanged in terms of severity, frequency, and duration over a period of several weeks to several months. Mild angina pectoris typically occurs only after unusual exertion and does not require the patient to alter lifestyle to prevent the pain. Severe chronic stable angina occurs frequently and causes the patient to modify daily routine in order to exclude strenuous activities.

Patients with mild chronic stable angina, when seen for the first time, usually do not require hospitalization, and evaluation and treatment can be performed on an outpatient basis. Patients with severe chronic stable angina, when seen for the first time, may or may not require hospitalization for evaluation and treatment. The decision to hospitalize depends on the severity of the disease and must be made on an individual basis. Certainly, patients having five to 10 daily episodes of angina pectoris precipitated by very minimal exertion would be most safely evaluated in the hospital.

Patients categorized by the history and physical exam as having unstable angina pectoris should be hospitalized. There is no precise definition of unstable angina that is universally accepted. However, all definitions have a common concern; the state of blood supply to the myocardium is tenuous, and myocardial infarction is likely to follow if no treatment is instituted. Features common to all definitions of unstable angina include new onset of angina; more severe, prolonged or frequent episodes of angina superimposed on chronic stable angina; and angina occurring at rest.

Differentiating chest pain due to myocardial ischemia and myocardial infarction from chest pain due to other causes is one of the most difficult problems in clinical medicine (Table 1). Because the number of patients complaining of chest pain is large, it is impractical to admit all of them to coronary care units for further cardiac evaluation. However, to send home a patient actually suffering from a myocardial infarction or unstable angina with a diagnosis of chest pain of noncardiac origin can be a fatal mistake. Thus, one must have a low threshold for admitting patients when there is any reasonable doubt as to the correct diagnosis. An important point to remember is that patients with an acute myocardial infarction often have a vague feeling of uneasiness that is difficult for them to describe. For most people, an emergency visit is not a regular event, and the fact that they felt worried enough to come to an emergency room is itself an important sign that something is very wrong, whether or not the problem is well stated.

LIMITATIONS OF THE HISTORY AND PHYSICAL EXAMINATION

Many important decisions about the evaluation and treatment of patients with angina pectoris are made on the basis of the initial history and physical exam. For this reason, it is important to be aware of how accurately these tools can reflect the presence and degree of coronary artery disease. Proudfit et al., Cohn (1979), and Banks et al. demonstrated that even the most skillfully and carefully conducted clinical history has limitations. In a series of 188 patients classified clinically as having unstable angina pectoris, Alison et al. found that 10.6% had normal coronary arteries when coronary angiography was performed. Similar proportions of patients with normal coronary arteries have been found in other series of patients with the clinical diagnosis of unstable angina pectoris (Fischl et al.; Conti et al.).

At the other end of the spectrum are patients with silent myocardial ischemia. Some patients with severe CAD and frequent episodes of myocardial ischemia can be asymptomatic and thus beyond diagnosis by the clinical history (see Chapter 14).

Thus, classification of patients with angina pectoris from the history and physical examination may lead to inaccuracies in some cases. However, in spite of their shortcomings, the history and physical examination remain the most frequently used screening tests in cardiac diagnosis and, when properly done, are helpful in diagnosing and staging most patients with angina pectoris.

LABORATORY TESTS

Patients classified as having angina pectoris should undergo further studies to confirm the diagnosis and to stage the extent of their disease. Contemporary cardiology now offers the physician many noninvasive and invasive cardiac diagnostic procedures for this purpose. A proper understanding of the infor-

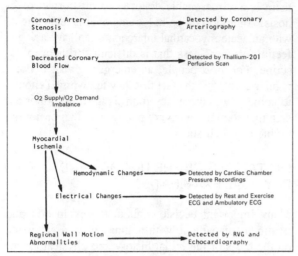

Figure 2. *Schematic showing the pathophysiology of myocardial ischemia and the type of information recorded by the various cardiac diagnostic techniques. RVG = radionuclide ventriculography.*

mation that can be obtained from each of the available procedures, as well as their limitations, is necessary if the physician is to choose the proper test or combination of tests for each patient.

As shown in Figure 2, angina pectoris begins with a decrease in coronary blood supply, usually caused by a stenotic lesion. Coronary arteriography allows visualization of the coronary artery and the extent of stenosis. Thallium-201 imaging is a measure of the amount of blood passing through a stenotic lesion, relative to blood passing through the remainder of the heart. Occasionally, regions of myocardium perfused by severely stenosed coronary arteries can have normal perfusion—perhaps because enough blood is passing through the stenosis to meet the regional myocardial oxygen demands, or perhaps because blood is reaching the area through collateral vessels. Thallium-201 imaging will detect the adequacy of perfusion to a region. Electrocardiography detects the electrical events associated with myocardial ischemia, which appear as ST-segment depression or elevation. Regional wall motion abnormalities that occur when myocardial tissue becomes ischemic can be detected and measured by M-mode and two-dimensional echocardiography, radionuclide ventriculography, and gated magnetic resonance imaging techniques. Thus, the many tests available to the physician provide diagnostic and quantitative information

in different forms. (See individual chapters addressing these tests.)

Because cardiologic diagnostic studies are expensive and in some cases associated with risk to the patient, care and skill must be used when choosing the most appropriate means of evaluating each patient.

Resting Electrocardiogram

The resting electrocardiogram should be a part of the evaluation of any patient with suspected or proven angina pectoris. The presence of Q waves indicates an old myocardial infarction, which is usually, although not always, secondary to CAD. (Emboli or trauma can also cause myocardial infarction.) Other abnormalities, such as intraventricular conduction delays, atrial or ventricular arrhythmias, or ST-T–wave changes are not specific and can be related to conditions other than coronary disease. However, in the presence of chest pain, they increase the suspicion that the pain is related to myocardial ischemia. Occasionally during an attack of angina pectoris, there will be transient ST-segment depression, which is a very specific finding for myocardial ischemia. A normal ECG either during chest pain or between episodes of pain does not exclude myocardial ischemia and is a frequent finding in patients with angina pectoris. Transient ST-segment elevation associated with rest pain is observed in Prinzmetal's variant angina, due to vasospasm.

Exercise Stress Testing

Patients categorized as having suspected or known stable CAD should undergo exercise stress testing as a part of their evaluation. In patients with chest pain of uncertain etiology, the exercise stress test is used as a diagnostic tool.

An exercise stress test positive for myocardial ischemia is good evidence that chest pain is angina pectoris (see also Chapter 6). A negative test does not entirely exclude angina pectoris but makes the diagnosis unlikely. Exercise tests are not simply negative or positive. A stress test that is negative after 10 minutes of vigorous exercise is more likely to exclude significant CAD than a "negative" exercise test that is terminated after only 2 or 3 minutes of exercise. "Positive" also encompasses a wide range of results. Stress tests that are positive with chest pain and 3-4 millimeters of ST depression after only 2-3 minutes of exercise are more likely to represent significant CAD than positive tests with 1 millimeter of upsloping ST depression after 10 minutes of exercise. The latter tests are more likely to represent false-positive results.

An exercise stress test must be interpreted in the context of the information obtained from the history and physical examination, because its predictive value varies with the population being studied (Bayes' theorem). In a population with a statistically low incidence of CAD, such as pre-menopausal non-smoking women with chest pain, the predictive ability is very low (Rifkin and Hood). However, in studies of patients with a high likelihood of CAD, such as men over the age of 60 with multiple risk factors, the predictive value is higher. Thus, in the latter group, a positive stress test is likely to be associated with the presence of CAD, while a negative test is likely to reflect the absence of CAD.

In patients with a diagnosis of angina pectoris, exercise stress testing can provide prognostic information and information about the extent of disease. The degree of positivity is related to the extent of CAD (Goldman et al.; Cheitlin et al.; Lavine et al.). A patient with a very positive test (severe ST depression early during exercise, hypotension) and, therefore, a high probability of left main or severe multi-vessel CAD should be considered for cardiac catheterization and possible revascularization. Alternatively, a patient who develops only 1 millimeter of ST depression after 10 minutes of exercise has a low likelihood of left main or three-vessel coronary disease and may not need to undergo cardiac catheterization.

Angina pectoris is a poor marker of the extent and severity of CAD. Many patients with known CAD and angina pectoris have frequent episodes of "silent ischemia." In this group of patients, exercise stress testing is particularly important for estimating disease severity (see Chapter 14).

Ambulatory (Holter) Electrocardiography

Ambulatory electrocardiography has been available for almost 30 years for the detection of cardiac arrhythmias. Recently, technological improvements have expanded the capabilities of Holter monitoring, and it is now possible to continuously record changes in ST segments (see Chapter 6). ST-segment depression is associated with myocardial ischemia and can be recorded during symptomatic angina pectoris or during episodes of asymptomatic or "silent ischemia." An ambulatory ECG can be useful for diagnostic purposes in patients with chest pain suggestive of Prinzmetal's angina and may establish the diagnosis in such cases. A second indication for this test is for diagnosis of chest pain in patients who are unable to perform a stress test. A third indication is the evaluation of post-infarction patients with angina, in order to look for a correlation between ventricular arrhythmias and ST depression—a combination believed to be associated with increased mortality. A fourth indication is to assess the efficacy of antianginal therapy (ACC/AHA Task Force Report). Indications for ambulatory ECG may expand in the future. Evidence is accumulating that the technique may be useful for predicting future cardiac events, for the evaluation of asymptomatic patients with CAD, and for the diagnosis of patients with chest pain (Kennedy and Wiens).

Thallium-201 Myocardial Perfusion Scintigraphy

Thallium-201 perfusion imaging is usually done in conjunction with exercise stress testing (see also Chapters 5 and 6). While exercise electrocardiography depends on ischemia-related electrical changes, thallium-201 depends on differences in myocardial perfusion. Areas of the myocardium supplied by stenotic vessels do not receive as much blood as surrounding, normally perfused areas and appear as thallium image defects or "cold spots." Infarcted myocardium receives very little blood and also appears as a "cold spot" on a thallium image. Thallium defects due to ischemia or infarct can be differentiated when repeat scans are obtained 3 hours or more after the initial exercise images. Infarcts will still appear as thallium defects while defects due to reversible ischemia will "fill in" due to the redistribution phenomenon.

Thallium-201 stress imaging has a sensitivity of 85–90% and a specificity of 65–70% for the detection of significant coronary artery disease. Exercise testing without thallium-201 is generally reported to have a somewhat lower sensitivity and a lower specificity. The value of combining diagnostic techniques was demonstrated in a multicenter study that evaluated thallium-201 imaging and exercise ECG. Ritchie et al. demonstrated that in a group of 190 patients, 148 of whom had significant CAD, exercise ECG detected 73% of the patients with significant disease and thallium-201 imaging detected 76%. Thus, sensitivities were similar. Specificity was also found to be similar: 86% for exercise ECG and 88% for thallium-201 imaging. However, when the two studies were combined, sensitivity was significantly improved to 91%, better than either test alone. Specificity was not improved.

Due to the extra cost of adding thallium-201 imaging to an exercise stress test, it should not be routinely ordered. If a patient has a strongly positive exercise ECG, thallium-201 imaging adds little diagnostic information. One of the most common indications for thallium-201 perfusion imaging is the evaluation of patients with an abnormal resting ECG. In the presence of abnormal resting ST segments due to left bundle branch block, left ventricular hypertrophy, digoxin, or conduction abnormalities, the diagnostic value of exercise electrocardiography is greatly decreased and thallium-201 imaging should be performed when exercise testing is done. Thallium-201 imaging is also indicated in patients undergoing evaluation for chest pain and who have equivocal ECG changes with exercise.

There are also indications for thallium-201 imaging in patients with known coronary artery disease. In patients with severe CAD, it is generally believed that resting coronary blood flow is normal in the absence of angina pectoris or an acute myocardial infarction. However, Gerwitz et al. and Wackers et al., using thallium-201 imaging, have demonstrated that this may not be true. In patients with severe CAD, some defects that appear on initial images following injections at rest fill in on delayed images, suggesting decreased perfusion at rest. Although it is not clear what the best course is for patients with resting perfusion abnormalities, it is likely that they will benefit most from intensive medical therapy and should be strongly considered for revascularization surgery.

Patients with very severe left ventricular dysfunction and congestive heart failure due to diffuse CAD generally are not recommended for coronary artery bypass surgery because of the high mortality rate. This is particularly true in the absence of angina pectoris. Coronary angiography and left ventriculography usually reveal severe three-vessel coronary artery disease with diffuse hypokinesis or akinesis. However, how much of the left ventricular dysfunction is due to scar and how much to reversible ischemia is difficult to determine. Thallium-201 perfusion imaging that demonstrates perfusion defects that fill in over time suggests reversibly ischemic tissue. If ex-

tensive areas of reversibly ischemic tissue can be demonstrated in this group of very ill patients, coronary artery bypass surgery may result in clinical improvement (Atkins et al.).

Thallium-201 perfusion imaging can be useful in the evaluation of a stenosis of uncertain hemodynamic significance noted on coronary angiography. A lesion of 40-60% may or may not limit flow with exercise. A corresponding thallium-201 perfusion defect with exercise would support the hemodynamic significance of the lesion, while a negative scan would be good evidence that the lesion was not responsible for flow limitations or, by inference, ischemia.

Restenosis of coronary artery lesions following initially successful percutaneous transluminal angioplasty occurs in one of four patients. Early detection of restenosis frequently leads to second and even third or fourth attempts at successful angioplasty. Stress thallium-201 exams can be useful in detecting restenosis by revealing ischemia in the distribution of dilated coronary arteries.

For patients unable to exercise adequately, thallium examinations can be performed with dipyridamole. Both intravenous dipyridamole (currently investigational) and oral dipyridamole block the uptake and degradation of adenosine, thus increasing the levels of adenosine, which is a coronary vasodilator. The vasodilation results in large increases in blood flow to myocardium supplied by normal coronary arteries. Blood flow to myocardium supplied by stenosed coronary arteries is either unchanged or decreases. The imbalance of flow to the heart can be detected by thallium imaging, and redistribution images can be used to differentiate ischemic from infarcted tissue. Image quality and sensitivity and specificity of dipyridamole thallium imaging are comparable to results obtained during exercise thallium-stress testing (Iskandrian et al.).

Exercise Echocardiography

Several medical centers are involved in the development of exercise echocardiography. Like radionuclide ventriculography, echocardiography detects changes in regional wall motion that occur during myocardial ischemia. The stress used to induce myocardial ischemia can be atrial pacing, pharmacologic (dopamine or dipyridamole), cold pressor, or, most commonly, exercise. Using upright bicycle stress, echocardiograms can be obtained during peak exercise; if treadmill stress is used, echocardiograms are obtained in the supine position immediately after exercise. Most exercise imaging is done with a two-dimensional echocardiogram. The normal response to exercise is for all segments of the myocardium to become hyperdynamic. Myocardial segments that become hypokinetic or akinetic during exercise are consistent with ischemia. A major advantage to exercise echocardiography is that wall thickening, the most specific marker of myocardial ischemia, is evaluated. The major problem is the limited success in obtaining adequate images. It is likely that exercise echocardiography will continue to evolve and eventually will be used routinely for the evaluation of cardiac patients.

Ambulatory Ventricular Function Monitoring

It is now possible to continuously monitor left ventricular function in patients using an ambulatory ventricular function monitor ("VEST"). The VEST can be worn by patients and is a nonimaging nuclear detector. Technetium-99^m–labelled red blood cells are utilized and the detector, positioned over the heart, collects beat-to-beat variations in counts. Gated counts are summed over 15-30 seconds and a continuous global left ventricular ejection fraction is reported. Patients can wear the VEST for a period of 4-6 hours. Experience with this new device is limited but several clinical applications are possible. First, the VEST may be useful for the evaluation of patients with chest pain of unknown etiology. It appears that for the detection of myocardial ischemia, the VEST is more sensitive than stress or ambulatory electrocardiography. Second, the functional significance of coronary artery obstructions can be evaluated. Patients with CAD and multiple severe obstructions are more likely to experience large decreases in left ventricular ejection fraction with exercise. Third, data from a 4-6–hour VEST examination may provide important prognostic information that can be helpful to guide the therapy of patients with CAD. Fourth, VEST information can help define the limits of exercise for patients with CAD. Fifth, VEST data can be used to assess the efficacy of antianginal therapy.

Cardiac Catheterization

With the development of percutaneous transluminal coronary angioplasty (PTCA), cardiac catheterization evolved from a purely diagnostic tool to a therapeutic device (see Chapter 9 and 16). Cardiac catheterization is indicated for diagnostic reasons in patients with chest pain and to evaluate patients with known coronary artery disease. As noted earlier, most patients with chest pain can be diagnosed with a thorough history, physical examination, and noninvasive testing. However, in some patients, the results of noninvasive testing are equivocal. For example, some patients are unable to perform a stress test due to physical limitations. In this group, cardiac catheterization may be indicated to provide a diagnosis or at least to exclude CAD as a cause of chest pain.

Patients with severe angina pectoris that cannot be controlled with medications are candidates for revascularization with either surgery or angioplasty. This group needs catheterization to define coronary anatomy. Patients with strongly positive stress tests frequently undergo cardiac catheterization to exclude left main CAD. Although it is difficult to predict cardiac events on the basis of coronary anatomy, knowledge about the coronary anatomy can be helpful in making therapeutic decisions. Patients with a left main stenosis, a proximal left anterior descending coronary stenosis, or multiple lesions in all three major coronary arteries, are often considered for surgery. Lesser disease involving one or two vessels is more often treated medically or with coronary angioplasty.

Cardiac catheterization provides anatomic information and should only be interpreted in the context of other data derived from the history, physical exam, and noninvasive testing.

NATURAL HISTORY AND PATHOPHYSIOLOGY OF ANGINA PECTORIS

NATURAL HISTORY OF PATIENTS WITH ANGINA PECTORIS

The goals of therapy for angina pectoris are to relieve symptoms and to prolong life. To evaluate the effect of therapy on longevity, one must know the natural history of untreated angina pectoris. If coronary arteriography has been performed, natural history studies of patients with angina pectoris that are based on coronary anatomy can be useful when dealing with individual patients. Follow-up studies in the 1960s, before the widespread use of current medical and surgical therapies, showed that patients with one-vessel disease had an annual mortality rate of <4%. In patients with two-vessel disease, this figure increased to 7-10% and in those with three-vessel disease, to

10-12%. Patients with left main coronary artery obstructions had a yearly mortality of 15-25% (Humphries). Left ventricular dysfunction worsens the prognosis.

Often, patients with angina pectoris are managed without knowledge of the coronary anatomy. In such patients, natural history studies based on the clinical history or noninvasive criteria can be helpful. An example is the subset of patients with unstable angina pectoris. Using a definition of unstable angina that includes both accelerating symptoms and ST-segment changes during chest pain, Mulcahy et al. followed 101 patients treated with only bed rest and sublingual nitrates, and found a 9% rate of nonfatal myocardial infarction and a 4% incidence of death within the first 28 days. At the end of one year, the incidence of nonfatal myocardial infarction was 12% and the incidence of cardiovascular death was 10%. Natural history studies such as this are helpful as guidelines when making diagnostic and therapeutic decisions for patients presenting with unstable angina pectoris and unknown coronary anatomy.

PATHOPHYSIOLOGY OF ANGINA PECTORIS

Atherosclerotic coronary artery disease results from a buildup of lipid, foam cells, smooth muscle hyperplasia and dystrophic calcification within the intima of the coronary vasculature, resulting in luminal narrowing. The luminal narrowing compromises blood flow to the heart, leading to myocardial ischemia and the clinical syndromes of angina pectoris, silent ischemia, myocardial infarction, or sudden death. Risk factors for the development of atherosclerotic heart disease include hypercholesterolemia, decreased high-density lipoprotein levels, tobacco smoking, hypertension, diabetes, male sex, older age, family history of CAD, obesity, and a sedentary lifestyle.

While fixed narrowing of the coronary arteries is due to atherosclerotic plaque, variable obstruction of the coronary arteries may occur with increased coronary artery tone and coronary vasospasm. Figure 3 shows the spectrum of coronary artery disease. On the left-hand side of the figure is Patient A, who suffers from fixed atherosclerotic narrowing. This patient is likely to experience typical effort- or exercise-induced angina pectoris associated with ST-segment depression on the ECG. On the right-hand side of the figure is Patient C, who suffers from pure coronary artery vasospasm. This patient typically has focal vasospasm of a segment of a coronary artery and ex-

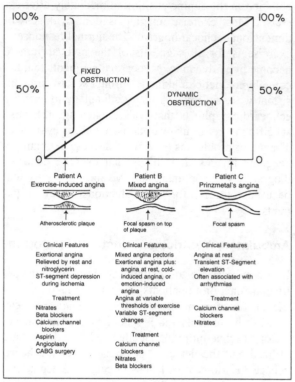

Figure 3. *Causes of myocardial ischemia. (Modified from Muller J.* Cardiology Reference Book, *2nd Edition. New York: CoMedica, Inc; 1984.)*

periences angina at rest with transient ST elevation on the ECG (Prinzmetal's angina). Between these two ends of the spectrum are patients who experience mixed angina pectoris, with elements of both exertion-related angina and rest angina (Patient B). Clinical indications that a patient has a vasospastic component to angina pectoris include emotion-induced or cold-induced angina, and variable-threshold exercise-induced angina. Such a patient has a mixture of fixed atherosclerotic narrowing plus vasospasm on top of the narrowing. Variable-threshold exercise-induced angina results when variable degrees of vasospasm alter the degree of narrowing of a coronary artery with a degree of fixed atherosclerosis. For example, a patient with a fixed atherosclerotic narrowing of 70% of a coronary lumen may be able to exercise on a treadmill for 7 minutes before developing angina on one day; on a second day, when the patient's vasomotor tone is high, and his 70% narrowing is now a 90% narrowing due to vasospasm on top of the atherosclerotic plaque, he may only be able to exercise for 3 minutes before experiencing angina.

What factors determine coronary tone? Recently, it has been appreciated that endothelial derived relaxing factor (EDRF), believed to be nitric oxide, is released from the endothelium into the smooth muscle of the vessel to allow vascular relaxation. EDRF release is stimulated by exposure of normal coronary arteries to acetylcholine (Ach). In patients with atherosclerosis, local administration of Ach does not result in normal EDRF release, due to an abnormality or destruction of the endothelium, and vasoconstriction occurs instead of vasodilation. Thus, patients with atherosclerosis may have an abnormality in EDRF production or release, which could predispose areas of the coronary vasculature to spasm. In addition, an endothelial derived vasoconstricting agent (endothelin) has recently been discovered. Other possible explanations for changes in coronary tone include alterations in the sympathetic nervous system, spasm induced by thromboxane, and serotonin. Also, some patients with vasospasm in other arteries, such as those with Raynaud's phenomenon, have been observed to demonstrate coronary vasospasm. Finally, there may be interactions that occur between platelets and the endothelial wall and contribute to coronary vasospasm.

Coronary angioscopy has provided direct visualization of in vivo coronary arteries in patients and has helped to clarify the pathophysiology of coronary artery disease. Various coronary syndromes have been observed to correlate with specific lesions observed by coronary angioscopy. Forrester et al. demonstrated that the coronary arteries in patients diagnosed as having stable angina had a smooth endothelial surface free of thrombus; those in patients with accelerating angina had ulcerations and a roughened endothelial lining; and those in patients with unstable rest angina often had thrombus.

An understanding of the pathophysiology of myocardial ischemia must take into account that myocardial ischemia represents an imbalance of oxygen supply to the heart and the oxygen demand of the heart. Myocardial ischemia is exacerbated by decreases in oxygen supply and increases in oxygen demand. Conversely, antianginal therapy works primarily by improving oxygen supply or reducing oxygen demand.

Factors That Influence Myocardial Oxygen Supply

Delivery of oxygen to the myocardium depends on both the amount of blood flowing through the coronary arteries and the ability of the myocardial cells to extract oxygen from the blood. Unlike other organs of the body, the heart has the unique property of nearly maximal oxygen extraction at rest; thus, there is little capability for increasing myocardial oxygen supply by increasing myocardial oxygen extraction. Myocardial oxygen supply can be adjusted to meet oxygen demands by changing coronary blood flow, which can and does fluctuate depending on the needs of the myocardium.

The amount of blood flowing through the coronary arteries depends on both the perfusion pressure and the resistance across the coronary vascular bed:

$$\text{CBF} = \frac{\text{Ao pressure} - \text{RA pressure}}{\text{Coronary vascular resistance}}$$

where CBF = coronary blood flow; Ao = aortic; and RA = right atrial. Because of the high intramural pressures during systole, resistance to flow is high and relatively little blood is delivered to the left ventricular myocardium during systole. Most flow occurs during diastole; therefore, aortic diastolic pressure and the duration of diastole are important determinants of myocardial blood flow. Factors that increase the aortic diastolic pressure or prolong the time spent in diastole will increase the blood supply to the myocardium. Conversely, factors that reduce diastolic pressure or, as is true of tachycardia, shorten the time the ventricle spends in diastole, reduce the blood supply to the myocardium.

A second determinant of myocardial oxygen supply is coronary artery resistance. The coronary arteries are not rigid pipes, but flexible tubes that exist in a state of tone. Relaxation of the vessels will decrease resistance to flow and increase coronary blood flow, while contraction (or spasm) of the vessels will increase resistance and decrease coronary blood flow. The factors that control coronary vascular resistance are incompletely understood. External compression of the vessels is important, particularly during systole when the high intramyocardial pressure increases resistance almost to the point of stopping flow. During diastole the end-diastolic ventricular pressure, if elevated, can increase intramyocardial pressure and, therefore, increase resistance and decrease flow through the coronary arteries.

Other influences that control coronary vascular resistance include neural, hormonal, and local metabolic factors. Present and future investigations should increase our knowledge of the mechanism and relative contributions of these factors and lead to thera-

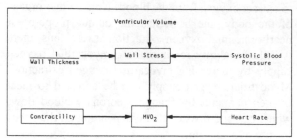

Figure 4. *Major determinants of myocardial oxygen demand (MVO₂).*

peutic interventions aimed at reducing coronary vascular resistance and increasing coronary blood flow.

Factors That Influence Myocardial Oxygen Demand

Unlike the skeletal muscles, the heart depends almost exclusively on aerobic metabolism for its energy. Myocardial oxygen consumption is thus almost identical to the total metabolic requirements of the heart. There are three major determinants of myocardial oxygen consumption (Braunwald et al.) (Figure 4). The first is systolic wall tension development, which, when increased, increases myocardial oxygen demand. Systolic wall tension is directly related to systolic arterial pressure and intraventricular radius and inversely related to wall thickness. The second factor is heart rate, which, when faster, increases myocardial oxygen demand. The third major factor is contractility. Increased contractility leads to increased myocardial oxygen demand. A frequently used noninvasive index of myocardial oxygen demand is the "double product," which is obtained by multiplying the heart rate by the systolic blood pressure. Inaccuracies arise when using this index because it does not consider contractility, intraventricular volume, or wall thickness.

TREATMENT OF ANGINA PECTORIS

When planning a treatment program, it is important to consider the factors that influence myocardial oxygen supply and those that influence myocardial oxygen demand. The ideal therapeutic regimen maximizes myocardial oxygen supply, minimizes myocardial oxygen demand, and is devoid of any adverse side effects.

Table 3. General Treatment Measures for Patients with Angina Pectoris

Alter risk factors
    Lower cholesterol intake
    Control hypertension
    Discontinue smoking
    Weight loss
    Control diabetes mellitus
    Less stressful lifestyle
Avoid activity that precipitates angina pectoris
Exercise
Treat severe anemia
Treat hyperthyroidism

Multiple treatment options exist for patients with angina pectoris. Over the past few years treatment of angina pectoris has reduced patient symptomatology and improved survival. Choosing the best treatment or combination of treatment modalities for a given patient is an increasingly complicated task because of the many available options. Treatment goals should be to eradicate episodes of myocardial ischemia, decrease the progression of disease, and prevent future cardiac events.

GENERAL TREATMENT MEASURES

In all patients presenting with angina pectoris, there are some general measures that should be instituted (Table 3). Although the efficacy of altering risk factors is controversial, such measures should be recommended to all patients. A low-cholesterol, low-saturated fat diet should be started, particularly by patients with elevated serum lipids. There is accumulating evidence that reduction in serum cholesterol can prevent future cardiac events in patients with angina pectoris and perhaps cause atherosclerotic lesions to regress. (See p. 195.)

Hypertension, if present, should be controlled. There are two reasons to correct an abnormal blood pressure: first, to alter a risk factor and possibly slow the progress of coronary artery disease; and second, to decrease myocardial oxygen demand, which depends in part on the systolic blood pressure. Control becomes particularly important in severely hypertensive patients presenting with unstable angina pectoris.

Patients who smoke cigarettes should be encouraged to stop. It is clear that cigarette smoking leads to an increased incidence of atherosclerotic heart disease. Thus, one reason to encourage patients to discontinue smoking is to reverse or at least slow the progress of atherosclerosis. A second reason is to halt the acute adverse effects of cigarette smoking on the heart. Nicotine released in cigarette smoke causes a release of endogenous catecholamines, which in turn step up myocardial oxygen demand by causing increases in heart rate, blood pressure, and myocardial contractility. Catecholamines can also decrease coronary blood supply by stimulation of coronary artery alpha receptors, which results in coronary artery vasoconstriction. An additional adverse effect of nicotine-related catecholamine release is increased platelet aggregation. Carbon monoxide, abundant in cigarette smoke, increases blood levels of carboxyhemoglobin and decreases the capacity of the blood to deliver oxygen to myocardial tissue. Thus, it is not surprising that cigarette smoking leads to decreased exercise tolerance as measured by treadmill testing (Aronow).

The effect of exercise on patients with angina pectoris remains a controversial issue. Certainly, exercise that precipitates angina pectoris should be discouraged. Patients with unstable angina pectoris should not exercise at all but should be restricted to bed rest. Exercise increases myocardial oxygen demand, which may exceed myocardial oxygen supply and, thus, precipitate angina pectoris in patients with CAD. Although it is agreed that a long-term exercise program can improve a patient's sense of well-being, its ability to slow or reverse atherosclerosis or to improve collateral blood supply to the myocardium remains unknown.

A study by Kramsch et al. demonstrated a reduction in coronary atherosclerosis in exercised monkeys fed an atherogenic diet, as compared with sedentary monkeys also fed an atherogenic diet. Redwood et al. showed that patients with chronic stable angina participating in exercise programs can exercise for a longer period of time before developing angina pectoris. In part, this effect is due to the ability of the heart to maintain peripheral muscle oxygenation at a lower myocardial oxygen demand (see Chapter 35). This effect may be due to a decrease in systemic vascular resistance secondary to exercise and the ability of trained muscles to increase their oxygen extraction efficiency. The improved exercise tolerance following exercise training may also be due to an increase in collateral flow and, thus, an increase in oxygen supply (Redwood et al.; Sim and Neill).

At present, exercise can be prescribed to angina patients at minimal risk with the promise that at the very least, it can increase their sense of well-being. Before enrolling in an exercise program, the patient should have an exercise tolerance test to help determine the safety of such a program. Future studies should demonstrate whether or not exercise has an effect on collateral development and atherogenesis in humans.

The risk that exercise will precipitate sudden death or a myocardial infarction is minimal. Ellestad et al., Irving and Bruce, and Doyle and Kinch reported a generally safe experience with exercise treadmill testing. Therefore, particularly in cooperative patients, an exercise program can be an important component of a treatment program for angina pectoris.

Although it is difficult to alter patients' lifestyles, it is helpful to suggest that patients avoid stressful situations, particularly if these situations regularly precipitate angina pectoris.

Systemic conditions such as severe anemia and hyperthyroidism can worsen angina pectoris and should be treated if present.

NITRATES

Nitrates (Table 4) have been and continue to be the mainstay of pharmacologic treatment for angina pectoris. They are relatively inexpensive and are associated with very few side effects. Nitrates are prescribed in patients with angina to relieve symptoms; there is no evidence that nitrates slow disease progression or improve survival. Therefore, there is little reason to prescribe long-acting nitrates in asymptomatic patients unless they are experiencing episodes of silent myocardial ischemia. Nitrates can be used prophylactically before activities that usually precipitate episodes of angina pectoris.

The administration of nitrates produces a transient decrease in myocardial oxygen demand by reducing venous tone and, therefore, preload. With lower filling pressures, the heart size is decreased and myocardial wall stress, a major determinant of myocardial oxygen demand, is reduced. To a lesser extent, nitrates reduce arterial tone and, therefore, afterload, which also reduces wall stress.

In some patients, nitrates can have a detrimental effect. Decreased arterial tone, while beneficial for

Table 4. Dosage and Kinetics of Nitroglycerin and Long-Acting Nitrates

Medication	Usual Recommended Dosage (mg)	Onset of Action (min)	Peak Action (min)	Duration
Sublingual NTG	0.15–0.6	2–5	4–8	10–30 min
Lingual NTG spray	0.4	2–5	4–8	10–30 min
Sublingual ISDN	2.5–10	5–20	15–60	45–120 min*
Buccal NTG	1–3	2–5	4–10	30–300 min†
Oral ISDN	10–80	15–45	45–120	2–6 hr‡
Oral NTG	2.5–26	20–45	45–120	2–6 hr‡
Oral PET	10–40	60	80–120	3–6 hr
NTG ointment (2%)	½–2 in.	15–60	30–120	3–8 hr
NTG patches (transdermal)	10–30	30–60	60–180	Up to 24 hr

NTG = nitroglycerin; ISDN = isosorbide dinitrate; PET = pentaerythritol tetranitrate.
*Up to 3 to 4 hours in some studies.
†Effect persists as long as tablet is intact.
‡Some short-term dosing studies have demonstrated effects to 8 hours.

Modified from Frishman WH: Pharmacology of the nitrates in angina pectoris. *Am J Cardiol* 56(Suppl):81, 1985. With permission.

myocardial oxygen demand, can decrease coronary artery perfusion and, thus, myocardial oxygen supply. Therefore, caution should be observed when administering nitrates to patients with low blood pressure. Similarly, in patients with low filling pressures or preload, nitrates can further lower pressures and cause a dangerous decrease in cardiac output.

The effect of nitrates on the coronary vessels is less well understood than their effects on the peripheral vasculature. Cohn et al. (1977) showed that nitrates can increase flow to myocardium supplied by stenotic coronary arteries if the areas are also supplied by well-developed collateral vessels. The clinical importance of this increased flow, however, is not known. If coronary artery spasm contributes to atherosclerotic-related angina pectoris, nitrates may be helpful in relieving this spasm.

It is important to stress to patients that nitrates are not analgesics. Patients must be reassured that they will not develop a tolerance to the pain-relieving effects of intermittent therapy and they should be encouraged to take nitrates whenever they experience angina pectoris.

Sublingual Nitroglycerin

The least expensive nitrate preparation and the drug of choice for an acute attack of angina pectoris is sublingual nitroglycerin. The usual dose is 0.3–0.4 mg. Patients with angina pectoris should be instructed to carry nitroglycerin with them at all times and to take the medication as soon as pain occurs. The onset of action is usually in 1–3 minutes, with a duration of action of 10–15 minutes. If the angina is not relieved, the dose may be repeated one or two times at 5-minute intervals. For more prolonged or unresponsive pain, patients should be instructed to seek medical attention. Nitroglycerin can also be taken before regular activities known to precipitate angina. Because nitroglycerin decreases blood pressure, patients should be instructed to sit down when taking the medication, in order to avoid syncope. Nitroglycerin is light-sensitive and should be stored in dark containers. Nitroglycerin tablets should be discarded and replaced every six months. There is a sublingual spray formulation of nitroglycerin that delivers a 0.4-mg dose and also is used for acute attacks.

Isosorbide Dinitrate

This long-acting preparation comes in sublingual, oral, and chewable forms. Although there are few studies documenting the efficacy of these agents, in general, the onset of action (15–30 minutes) is longer than that of sublingual nitroglycerin. The duration of action is generally 2–3 hours. The indication for this medication is frequent angina pectoris. It was initially recommended that doses be given every 3–4 hours for an adequate therapeutic response. However, tolerance to frequent dosing may occur, and some physicians recommend that this drug be given on a thrice daily basis. Because the onset of action is delayed, isosorbide dinitrate probably should not be prescribed for acute attacks of angina pectoris.

Nitroglycerin Ointment

Like isosorbide dinitrate, nitroglycerin ointment should be used to prevent angina; its onset of action is too slow to treat an acute attack of angina pectoris. Whether or not the duration of action is longer than that of isosorbide dinitrate has not been well documented. The drug is effective for nocturnal angina. A second advantage is that if the patient becomes hypotensive, the remaining medication can be wiped off. It is messy, however, and not a convenient medication to prescribe to ambulatory patients.

Nitroglycerin Patches (Transdermal Nitroglycerin)

This is the newest form of nitroglycerin delivery. The drug is applied to a patch, which delivers nitroglycerin over a 24-hour period. Like other long-acting nitroglycerin preparations, this form of medication should not be used for acute attacks but to prevent attacks in patients with frequent episodes of angina pectoris. Studies with the patch by Parker and Fung suggested that while patches may be efficacious during the first 4 hours of administration, efficacy as determined by treadmill walking times is gone at 24 hours. In another study, patients receiving one to two weeks of nitroglycerin patch therapy had no difference at all in exercise treadmill times compared with placebo times, suggesting that tolerance to nitroglycerin had developed. However, a recent study by the Transderm-Nitro Study Group showed that intermittent patch-wearing—12 hours on, beginning in the morning, and 12 hours off at night—was effective as

judged by exercise treadmill time during short- and long-term therapy. Larger doses—15-20 mg/24 hr—were necessary to achieve the desired effectiveness. Some physicians advise that patients on chronic nitrate therapy have "nitrate free" intervals during the day to help reduce the phenomenon of tolerance. N-acetylcysteine also has been shown to reduce nitrate tolerance.

Intravenous Nitroglycerin

Intravenous nitroglycerin administration should be considered in patients with unstable angina pectoris that fails to respond to other nitrate preparations and beta blocking drugs. It has the advantage of rapid onset of action and certain absorption; the dose can be tailored to the needs of the particular patient to assure that blood pressure is not too severely lowered and that excessive reflex tachycardia does not occur. For acute ischemia, patients can be started on a continuous infusion of 5–15 μg/min. This continuous infusion can be increased by 5–10 μg/min every 3–5 minutes until the angina resolves, headache occurs, or the mean arterial blood pressure drops by more than 20 mm Hg.

Because nitroglycerin is in part absorbed by polyvinylchloride (PVC) administration sets, non-PVC infusion sets made of less pliable polyethylene are used.

Side Effects

Headache, flushing, and hypotension are the most common side effects and can often be relieved by lowering the dose of nitrate and, in the case of sublingual nitroglycerin, instructing the patient to sit when taking medication. Severe hypotension can be deleterious because of a lowered coronary perfusion pressure and decreased coronary blood supply. For these reasons, nitrates should be used with caution in hypotensive patients. Reflex tachycardia increases oxygen demand, and, therefore, excessive tachycardia should be avoided. Beta-blocking drugs can be helpful in abolishing the reflex tachycardia.

BETA BLOCKADE

The beta-blocking drugs work by competing with endogenous catecholamines for beta-adrenergic receptor sites. The beta receptors are subdivided into two types: $beta_1$ and $beta_2$. $Beta_1$ receptors, when stimulated, cause increased heart rate, increased contractility, and accelerated atrioventricular conduction. Other non-cardiac effects include increased insulin release and increased muscle glycogenolysis. $Beta_2$ receptors, when stimulated, cause bronchodilation, dilation of peripheral blood vessels, and uterine smooth muscle relaxation.

Beta-blocking drugs affect the factors that influence both oxygen supply and oxygen demand, and not all of their effects are beneficial. Beta blockade can actually decrease myocardial oxygen supply by blocking the vasodilating $beta_2$ receptors located in the walls of the coronary arteries, thereby increasing coronary vascular resistance and decreasing coronary blood flow. The hypotensive effect of beta blockers can contribute to a reduction of coronary blood flow by reducing aortic pressure. Another potentially adverse effect is an increase in ventricular volume, which results in increased wall tension and, therefore, increased myocardial oxygen demand.

Beneficial effects of beta blockade include decreases in heart rate and contractility, factors that lead to a decrease in myocardial oxygen demand. Schrumpf et al. demonstrated that beta-blocking drugs shift the oxygen-hemoglobin curve to the right, resulting in an increased delivery of oxygen to the myocardium. Back et al. showed that beta blockers may also have a beneficial effect on coronary blood flow in ischemic areas by redistributing blood flow from subepicardium to subendocardium. Overall, the effect of beta blockade in most patients is favorable. Only in the failing or near-failing heart does beta blockade sometimes have a detrimental effect. In such conditions, increases in left ventricular size and wall tension lead to an increase in myocardial oxygen demand and can also increase the severity of angina pectoris.

In addition to relieving angina pectoris, beta blockers have been shown to reduce the morbidity and mortality in patients with coronary artery disease if administered following an acute myocardial infarction. Timolol, used by the Norwegian Multicenter Study Group, was begun 7–28 days after the onset of myocardial infarction. Follow-up of 945 timolol-treated patients and 939 placebo-treated patients for a mean of 17 months demonstrated a reduction in both mortality and reinfarction in the drug-treated patients. In a similar study (BHAT) by the National Heart, Lung, and Blood Institute, propranolol or placebo was administered to 3,837 patients 5–21 days after acute myocardial infarction. The propranolol-treated group had a reduced mortality compared to the placebo group.

Metoprolol and atenolol have also been shown to reduce postinfarction mortality in large clinical trials. Early intravenous administration of metoprolol following the thrombolytic agent tissue plasminogen activator was shown to reduce the rate of reinfarction and ischemic events.

Whether patients with coronary artery disease and a remote myocardial infarction or no history of myocardial infarction will also benefit in these ways from beta blockade is not known. Because some patients receiving beta blockers will suffer from side effects, it is probably not correct to administer beta blockers to patients with CAD and mild or no angina pectoris who have not had a recent myocardial infarction. Rather, in this group of patients, beta blockade should be reserved to treat symptoms when other methods of treatment are ineffective.

Beta-blocking drugs currently available in the United States are listed in Table 5. Four beta-blocking drugs have been approved for treatment of angina pectoris. Propranolol was the first beta blocker available in the United States. It can be effectively administered twice daily in doses ranging from 40–320 mg/day; a long-acting preparation is available for once-daily dosing. Nadolol has a long half-life and can be administered once daily. Unlike propranolol, which is lipophilic, nadolol is hydrophilic. Hydrophilic substances do not easily penetrate the central nervous system and theoretically are associated with a decreased incidence of CNS side effects. Atenolol is another hydrophilic beta-blocking drug that can also be administered once daily in a dose of either 50 mg or 100 mg; it is selective for $beta_1$ receptors. Metoprolol, like propranolol, is lipophilic and is a twice-daily beta blocker that is effective at doses ranging from 100-400 mg/day. At low doses metoprolol is cardioselective and blocks only $beta_1$ receptors. However, in doses above 100 mg/day, some degree of $beta_2$-receptor blockade is also present.

Seven additional beta-blocking drugs are available but thus far none has been FDA-approved for treatment of angina pectoris. Timolol is a lipophilic beta blocker that is administered twice daily at a dose range of 10–60 mg/day. Pindolol is a beta blocker that has intrinsic sympathomimetic activity and has less of a tendency to lower heart rate than other beta-blocking drugs. Labetalol is a nonselective beta-blocking drug that also has selective $alpha_1$-receptor blocking properties. Because of the latter property, a greater lowering of blood pressure would be expected with this

Table 5. Dosages and Selected Pharmacologic Properties of Currently Available Beta-Blocking Agents

Drug generic name (trade name)	Usual daily oral dose (mg) Range	No. of Daily Doses	Cardio-selective	ISA*	Lipid Solubility	Plasma Half-life (hr)	Primary Route of Elimination
Propranolol**° (Inderal)	160–480	2–4	No	No	High	3.2–6	Hepatic
Nadolol** (Corgard)	40–320	1	No	No	Low	12–24	Renal and biliary (90% unchanged)
Timolol° (Blocadren)	20–40	2	No	Minimal	Low to intermediate	3–5	Hepatic and renal (20% unchanged)
Metoprolol**° (Lopressor)	100–200	2–3	Yes	No	Intermediate	3–4	Hepatic
Atenolol**° (Tenormin)	50–200	1	Yes	No	Low	6–9	Renal (<40% unchanged) and hepatic
Pindolol (Visken)	7.5–22.5	3	No	Yes	Intermediate	3–4	Renal (~40% unchanged) and hepatic
Acebutolol (Sectral)	400–1,200	2–4	Yes	Yes	Low	4–6	Hepatic and renal
Labetalol† (Normodyne or Trandate)	300–1,200	3	No	(Yes)‡	Low to intermediate	3–4	Hepatic
Esmolol (IV)			Yes	No		9 min	Red blood cell

Note: The beta blockers penbutolol (Levatol) and carteolol (Cartrol) were licensed recently by the FDA for the treatment of hypertension.
**Currently indicated for the treatment of angina pectoris.
*ISA = intrinsic sympathomimetic activity
† Labetalol possesses combined beta-blocking and relatively mild alpha-blocking activity (beta-blocking potency at least four times the alpha-blocking potency)
‡Partial agonism of B_2 receptors
° Approved for long-term administration following myocardial infarction to reduce cardiac mortality and/or risk of reinfarction.
(Modified from Shub C et al., 1985. With permission. See Bibliography.)

drug than is seen with other beta-blocking drugs. Acebutolol is a third hydrophilic beta blocker and also has mild sympathomimetic activity. Like metoprolol, at low doses acebutolol is a selective beta$_1$-receptor blocker. Esmolol is an intravenous beta blocker with rapid onset of action and an elimination half-life of 9 minutes. Currently it is indicated only for treatment of supraventricular tachycardias. It has been used to safely treat stress tachycardia in patients with unstable angina as well as myocardial infarction. Its advantage is that if side effects develop, they can be rapidly terminated by discontinuing the infusion of the drug. Carteolol and penbutolol, which became available in

1988, are indicated for hypertension. Both are non-selective beta blockers with sypathomimetic activity.

In patients adequately beta-blocked, heart rate at rest should be in the 50s or 60s and should not go above 90–110 beats/min with moderate exercise. Increased doses of beta blockers after these heart-rate goals are achieved can be beneficial because, while the negative chronotropic or heart-rate slowing effect may not increase, negative inotropy does.

The side effects of beta-blocking drugs are listed in Table 6. The negative inotropic effects that can lead to congestive heart failure in the failing or near-failing ventricle have been covered. In some patients,

Table 6. Adverse Effects of Beta-Blockade Therapy

Cardiac
   Congestive heart failure
   Excessive heart rate slowing
   Propranolol withdrawal syndrome
Noncardiac
   Fatigue
   Mental depression
   Insomnia
   Hallucinations
   Bad dreams
   Gastrointestinal upset
   Raynaud's phenomenon
   Bronchoconstriction
   Worsening of insulin-induced hypoglycemia
   Sexual dysfunction
   Further renal function deterioration in patients with renal disease

mild congestive heart failure precipitated by beta-blocking drugs can be reversed with digitalis; thus, the addition of digitalis may allow continuance of beta blockade, and such patients can benefit with improved exercise tolerance and reduced angina pectoris. Excessive heart-rate slowing can be a serious problem with beta-blocker administration. In some patients, probably those with intrinsic sinus node disease, rates at rest can fall to the 40s, 30s and even lower. In these cases, either the beta-blocking drug must be discontinued or, in some instances, the heart rate can be supported with permanent cardiac pacing.

Abrupt withdrawal of beta blockers can precipitate acute myocardial ischemia. The basis for this phenomenon is unclear, and different theories have been proposed. First, underlying coronary atherosclerosis may have progressed during therapy. Second, the patient may have increased his or her level of activity and not appropriately reduced it when the drug was stopped. Third, there may be a physiologic rebound effect involving increased sympathetic stimulation soon after the drug is stopped. If beta-blocker therapy is to be discontinued, it should be tapered gradually. In hospitalized patients with chronic stable angina pectoris, administering one half the usual dose for 24 hours and discontinuing it on day two is a safe approach. In patients with unstable angina pectoris, beta blockade should not be discontinued without compelling reasons.

Other adverse effects can sometimes be avoided by changing from one beta-blocking drug to another.

CALCIUM CHANNEL BLOCKERS

Four calcium channel-blocking agents are now available in the United States: nifedipine, verapamil, diltiazem and nicardipine (Table 7). Calcium is important in the regulation of both myocardial and vascular smooth muscle contraction and relaxation and in the generation of the membrane action potential, particularly in the cells of the sinoatrial and atrioventricular nodes. The calcium-blocking drugs decrease the availability of intracellular calcium, which can result in decreased vasoconstriction in the coronary, peripheral and pulmonary vasculature; decreased myocardial contractility; decreased rate of depolarization in the SA node; and slowed conduction in the AV node.

Several effects of calcium channel-blocking agents are potentially beneficial for patients with angina pectoris. First, by reducing the rate of SA node depolarization, heart rate is slowed and myocardial oxygen demand is decreased (seen with verapamil and diltiazem but not with nifedipine or nicardipine). Second, myocardial contractility and, subsequently, myocardial oxygen demand are decreased. Third, decreased smooth muscle tone in peripheral arteries results in vasodilation, decreased afterload, and decreased myocardial oxygen consumption. There also may be a small reduction in preload. Fourth, decreased coronary artery tone results in increased coronary blood flow and increased myocardial oxygen supply. The control and movement of calcium in the myocardial cells, the smooth muscle cells in the coronary arteries, and smooth muscle cells in the peripheral arteries are different and are affected differently by various calcium-blocking agents.

These differences translate into varying clinical responses. Unlike the beta blockers, which differ from each other primarily in side-effect profiles, the calcium blockers offer a range of therapeutic options, and selection of the appropriate calcium blocker should depend on the desired clinical response. All of the calcium blockers are effective for the treatment of angina pectoris. They are particularly effective for angina pectoris caused by coronary spasm, but they are also effective for the treatment of angina caused purely by a fixed lesion or for angina due to fixed plus vasospastic narrowing (mixed angina pectoris).

Table 7. Calcium Channel Blockers

	Frequency of Administration	Daily Dosage	Indicated for Treatment of Angina
Nifedipine			
(Procardia, Adalat)	tid, qid	30–160 mg	Yes
	qd (long-acting form)	30–90 mg	Yes
Verapamil			
(Calan, Isoptin)	tid	240–480 mg	Yes
	qd (long-acting)	240 mg	No
Diltiazem			
(Cardizem)	tid, qid	120–360 mg	Yes
	bid (long-acting)	180 mg	No
Nicardipine			
(Cardene)	tid	60–120 mg	Yes

Table 8. Adverse Effects of Calcium Channel Blockers

Cardiac
  Congestive Heart Failure
  Palpitations
  Hypotension
  Bradycardia
  Lightheadedness

Noncardiac
  Flushing
  Headache
  Weakness
  Nausea
  Constipation/Diarrhea
  Nasal Congestion
  Cough
  Wheezing
  Peripheral Edema

Calcium-blocking agents can be used alone or combined with nitrates or beta-blocking drugs. For most patients, calcium blockers and beta blockers are equally effective; frequently, the choice of which agent to use depends on other conditions the patient may have, or on side effects (Table 8). For example, a patient with angina and asthma or peripheral vascular disease who is unable to tolerate beta blockers can be successfully treated with calcium blockers. In a patient with a recent myocardial infarction and angina pectoris, a beta blocker would be a better choice, because beta blockers, unlike the calcium blockers, have a prophylactic effect postinfarction, as discussed above.

Nifedipine is a potent coronary and peripheral artery vasodilator. Although, in vitro, nifedipine will block the SA and AV nodes, the lower in vivo doses usually do not have this effect. In vivo, the sympathetic reflex stimulation that results from vasodilation-induced hypotension may actually increase heart rate and conduction. The increase in heart rate after nifedipine administration tends to be a short-lived phenomenon and, with chronic administration of the drug, heart rate eventually returns to baseline. Similarly, although nifedipine's direct action is to decrease myocardial contractility, afterload reduction plus reflex sympathetic stimulation induced by peripheral vasodilation may increase myocardial contractility. The usual starting dose of nifedipine is 10 mg three times/day. The usual effective dose is 10–20 mg three times/day, which can be increased to 20–30 mg three to four times/day if necessary. More than 180 mg daily is not recommended. A once-daily preparation of nifedipine (Procardia XL) has been shown to result in very steady plasma concentrations, which, by virtue of a unique gastrointestinal absorption system, may alleviate some of the previously observed vasodilator side effects such as headache, flushing, palpitations, and dizziness. Peripheral edema remains a side effect in the once-daily formulation. In one study, tolerance to this form of therapy was not observed.

Verapamil is a potent inhibitor of SA node depolarization and AV node conduction. Myocardial contractility is also decreased in vivo, with relatively less peripheral vasodilation than is seen with nifedipine. The usual starting dose of verapamil is 80 mg three times/day. The usual effective dose is 320–480 mg/day. More than 480 mg/day is not recommended. A once-daily formulation of verapamil is available. Verapamil may exacerbate AV conduction abnormalities, increase heart failure, and cause gastrointestinal side effects including constipation and ileus.

Diltiazem has actions intermediate between those of nifedipine and verapamil. Compared to verapamil, diltiazem causes less reduction in myocardial contractility and less depression of the SA and AV nodes. Compared to nifedipine, diltiazem causes less peripheral vasodilation. Diltiazem appears to dilate both the coronary arteries and the peripheral arteries. The recommended starting dose of diltiazem is 30 mg four times/day. Many patients can tolerate a starting dose of 60 mg three or four times/day. The dose can be gradually increased to 360 mg daily in divided doses three or four times/day. Vasodilator side effects, as described above, may occur, and in some studies diltiazem has exacerbated existing congestive heart failure. A twice-daily slow release form is available.

Nicardipine is a dihydropyridine derivative which has similarities to nifedipine. The drug has a more selective vasodilatory effect in the coronary vasculature than in the systemic vasculature. It is more selective for vascular smooth muscle than cardiac muscle. Nicardipine is equally as effective in reducing angina pectoris as other calcium blockers and beta blockers; it has been shown to reduce the frequency of rest angina. The drug also has been shown to be efficacious in the treatment of hypertension. Nicardipine has minimal negative inotropic and dromotropic effects. The usual starting dose is 20 mg three times/day, which can be increased to 40 mg three times/day. The most common side effects with this drug are pedal edema and dizziness (about 7% of patients), headache, asthenia, flushing, palpitations, nausea and dyspepsia. Some patients (7%) developed increased angina in short-term trials when the drug was started or dosage increased.

ASPIRIN AND ANTICOAGULATION

There is now evidence to support the theory that atherosclerotic plaque rupture, platelet aggregation, and thrombus formation occur in the pathogenesis of unstable angina. Therefore, it is not surprising that antiplatelet and anticoagulant therapies are effective in the treatment of unstable angina. Large randomized trials have documented the benefit of aspirin for the treatment of unstable angina, and it is now evident that aspirin decreases the incidence of myocardial infarction, cardiac death, and refractory angina. The benefits of aspirin treatment continue for months after unstable angina is stabilized. Full-dose heparin in the first few days after the onset of unstable angina is also effective treatment (and probably more effective than aspirin during this time period). Heparin, like aspirin, decreases the incidence of myocardial infarction and refractory angina in unstable angina patients. A combination of aspirin plus heparin offers no advantage to heparin alone and increases the incidence of serious bleeding complications (Theroux et al.). Thus, for unstable angina, heparin therapy for the first few days is appropriate. Before heparin is discontinued, aspirin should be started and continued indefinitely. The optimal dose of aspirin appears to be ≤325 mg/day. (Less information about the treatment of chronic stable angina with aspirin is available. However, it is reasonable to treat all chronic stable angina patients with aspirin 325 mg/day unless they experience aspirin-related side effects.)

The future treatment of unstable angina may include thrombolytic agents, and trials are underway to evaluate the role of thrombolysis in unstable angina treatment.

INTRAAORTIC BALLOON COUNTERPULSATION

For patients with severe unstable angina pectoris not responding to the measures discussed above, intraaortic balloon counterpulsation can often be effective in relieving ischemia (Weintraub et al.). Intraaortic balloon counterpulsation relieves angina pectoris by decreasing systolic blood pressure and, therefore, myocardial oxygen demand; at the same time it increases diastolic blood pressure and accordingly, increases coronary perfusion pressure and myocardial oxygen supply.

The problems with this technique are its frequent complications, most of which are due to vascular damage and thrombosis. More serious complications include perforation of the aortic wall and ischemia distal to the site of insertion in the femoral artery. Severe peripheral vascular disease, aortic aneurysms, aortic insufficiency, and uncontrollable arrhythmias are all relative contraindications to use of intraaortic balloon counterpulsation. This technique should be reserved for patients who continue to have unstable angina pectoris in spite of other measures discussed. Because complications are more likely to occur the longer the balloon is in place, insertion of the balloon should be followed soon by coronary angiography and possibly by coronary artery bypass surgery.

PERCUTANEOUS TRANSLUMINAL CORONARY ANGIOPLASTY (PTCA)

When introduced in 1977, balloon coronary angioplasty was used to treat angina in patients with one-vessel coronary artery disease involving proximal, noncalcified, discrete coronary stenoses (see Chapter 16). Early success rates were 60% and in-hospital complications were almost 10%. Death followed coronary angioplasty in 1.2% of cases and emergency surgical revascularization was performed in 5.8% of patients. It was estimated that only 10–15% of patients with indications for coronary bypass surgery were candidates for coronary angioplasty.

Over the past 10 years the indications and success rates for coronary angioplasty have dramatically changed. Increased experience with the procedure and technical improvements in angioplasty catheters have led to a growth in the number of procedures to a level that now exceeds the number of coronary bypass operations that are performed annually. Coronary angioplasty is now being performed for multi-vessel coronary artery disease, multiple lesions in the same vessel, recurrent angina after coronary bypass surgery, complex, nondiscrete coronary stenoses, and totally occluded coronary arteries. Compared to coronary angioplasty 10 years ago, the patients undergoing this procedure tend to be older and have greater left ventricular dysfunction, and are more likely to have had a prior myocardial infarction. However, although the patients undergoing angioplasty generally have more cardiac disease, the procedure's success rates have improved: successful dilation of a stenosis has increased to 88%, the incidence of nonfatal myocardial infarction has decreased to 4.3%, and the need for emergency coronary bypass surgery has decreased to 3.4%. Mortality following coronary angioplasty remains at 1.0%.

Restenosis of dilated coronary arteries continues to be a problem. Symptomatic restenosis occurs in 20-25% of patients. Angiographic studies suggest the restenosis rate may be 30-35% or even higher in patients with a stenosis at the origin of the left anterior descending coronary artery. Restenosis can be managed with repeat coronary angioplasty. The rate of restenosis after a second angioplasty is similar to that after the first angioplasty. Many cardiologists consider repeat angioplasty for restenosis to be part of the long-term strategy for patients undergoing this form of therapy, and not necessarily a complication of the procedure.

There are several unanswered questions about coronary angioplasty and its role in the management of patients with coronary artery disease. What are the long-term benefits of coronary angioplasty versus those of coronary bypass surgery in patients with multi-vessel coronary disease? Is there a role for coronary angioplasty in the treatment of asymptomatic patients with silent myocardial ischemia? What is the role of coronary angioplasty in the treatment of minimally symptomatic coronary artery disease; does coronary angioplasty protect such patients from future cardiac events? Many of these questions are being addressed by ongoing trials and at least partial answers will be available in the coming months.

CORONARY ARTERY BYPASS SURGERY

As with any treatment strategy for patients with angina pectoris, coronary artery bypass surgery must be evaluated both for its ability to relieve symptoms and for its ability to alter the natural history of coronary artery disease and improve survival.

Compared to medical therapy, coronary bypass surgery can more effectively relieve symptoms, and it results in a greater improvement in quality of life. At the end of five years, 70% of patients undergoing coronary bypass surgery can expect a decrease in symptoms and 50% can expect to be asymptomatic. Patients should be considered for bypass surgery for relief of medically refractory angina pectoris. Individual patient lifestyles should also be considered. Patients who choose to lead inactive lives and who, on medical therapy, have only occasional episodes of angina pectoris should not be sent for bypass surgery for the purpose of symptom relief. However, patients with frequent angina pectoris, particularly those who are unable to perform their usual daily activities and who are not responding to maximal medical therapy and who are not candidates for angioplasty, are appropriate surgical candidates. The evolving role of coronary angioplasty for the relief of angina pectoris and the benefits and efficacy compared to coronary bypass surgery are currently being investigated.

To recommend coronary artery bypass surgery for the purpose of altering the natural history of coronary

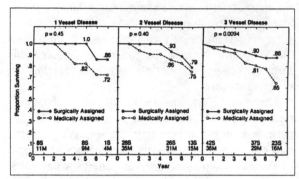

Figure 5. *Seven-year cumulative survival rates for medical (M) and surgical (S) patients with ejection fractions <0.50 (p = 0.012). (From Passamani et al. 1985. With permission. See Bibliography.)*

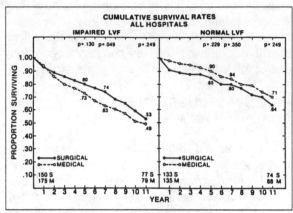

Figure 6. *Eleven-year cumulative survival for patients without left main coronary artery disease, according to whether left ventricular function (LVF) was impaired or normal. Numbers of patients at risk at bottom of figure. Survival among patients with impaired LVF differed significantly at seven years but not at 11 years. M = medical; S = surgical. (From Detre K et al: N Engl J Med 311:1333, 1984. With permission.)*

disease and improving survival is a more complex decision. Three large randomized trials that have provided useful guidelines for making this decision are the Veterans Administration Cooperative Trial, the European Cooperative Surgery Study Group and the Coronary Artery Surgery Study (CASS). Patients who can expect a survival benefit from coronary bypass surgery include those with left main coronary stenosis, three-vessel coronary disease (particularly if they have left ventricular dysfunction), severe symptoms, or a positive exercise test (Figures 5 and 6). There is less evidence that patients with two-vessel coronary disease can expect a survival benefit. However, it appears that patients with mild to moderate angina, two-vessel disease with a proximal left anterior descending coronary artery lesion, or a strongly positive exercise test can expect a survival benefit with surgery.

When approaching the individual patient, a decision regarding coronary bypass surgery is often difficult. Medications and coronary angioplasty are also very effective therapies, and the large randomized trials comparing various treatments often do not include patients identical to the one you are caring for. Patients with left main coronary disease, or patients with three-vessel disease, ischemia, and left ventricular dysfunction, present the clearest indications and should undergo bypass surgery. Whether or not coronary angioplasty confers a survival benefit in patients with three-vessel disease remains to be determined. Patients with one- or two-vessel coronary disease, particularly those with mild or no ischemic symptoms, present a treatment dilemma. If a given patient in this group has proximal left anterior de-

scending coronary disease, substantial ischemia, and left ventricular dysfunction, a strong argument can be made for considering coronary bypass surgery, if angioplasty is not feasible.

For bypass surgery the operative mortality rate is 1.3%, with a range of almost 0% in patients with one-vessel disease and normal ventricular function to 3.5% in patients with three-vessel disease and left ventricular dysfunction (Rahimtoola 1981). Vein grafts have a patency rate of 70–86% six to 12 months after surgery. Graft failure during the first six months is most often due to thrombosis, while graft failure occurring beyond one year is usually due to fibrosis or atherosclerosis developing in the vein graft. At the end of 10 years, more than 50% of vein grafts are occluded. The use of internal mammary artery grafts has increased survival and decreased ischemic symptoms compared with vein grafting. The patency of internal mammary grafts is better than that of vein grafts; 90% are patent 10 years after surgery.

APPROACH TO UNSTABLE ANGINA PECTORIS

Unstable angina refers to a wide range of conditions triggered by severe transient myocardial ischemia. While a precise definition is lacking, Rahimtoola (1985) has proposed three clinical subgroups of patients: patients with anginal pain of recent onset (within six months); patients with anginal pain at rest; and patients with continuing pain after an acute myocardial infarction. Although more than 50% of patients with a clinical diagnosis of unstable angina have left main or three-vessel coronary artery disease, 10% have normal arteries or mildly obstructive coronary artery disease, and 25% have one-vessel disease.

The reasons for the instability associated with unstable angina are not completely understood. Rapid progression of underlying coronary atherosclerosis has been proposed. Intermittent coronary artery occlusion due to spasm, platelet aggregation, and thrombus formation have also been associated with unstable angina. Angioscopy has revealed disrupted, fissured atherosclerotic plaques in some patients with unstable angina.

Even with aggressive therapy, the prognosis of patients with unstable angina is not good. The incidence of nonfatal myocardial infarction within the first few weeks after diagnosis of unstable angina is as high as 15%. The two-week mortality rate is 3% and at one year, 10%.

Goals of therapy are to decrease myocardial ischemia, prevent myocardial infarction, preserve left ventricular function, and prevent death. Patients with unstable angina should be admitted to the hospital and restricted to bed rest. Patients with transient ST-segment changes associated with angina are easily diagnosed. However, patients without ST changes frequently require further diagnostic evaluation. In addition to bed rest, treatment should be directed toward any factor that might aggravate ischemia (anemia, hypoxia). Pharmacologic treatment with nitrates, beta blockers, calcium blockers, or anticoagulants should be instituted and tailored to individual patient requirements. Intravenous nitroglycerin is often the first drug of choice but requires careful monitoring of blood pressure and heart rate. If necessary, intraaortic balloon pumping should be initiated. With few exceptions, patients should proceed to cardiac catheterization and, if appropriate, coronary artery revascularization via bypass surgery or balloon angioplasty.

ATHEROSCLEROTIC REGRESSION AND SLOWING OF PROGRESSION

Perhaps one of the most intriguing new concepts for treatment of coronary artery disease is that of slowing atherosclerotic progression or even causing atherosclerotic regression. The Cholesterol-Lowering Atherosclerosis Study (CLAS) randomized men, aged 40–59, who had previous coronary bypass surgery, to placebo or colestipol-plus-niacin therapy. Coronary angiograms were reviewed over a two-year period. The drug regimen lowered total plasma cholesterol by 26% and LDL cholesterol by 43%. Only 10% of patients receiving colestipol plus niacin developed new native coronary lesions while 22% of patients receiving placebo developed new lesions. Drug therapy also reduced the number of lesions that progressed in patients. Treated patients exhibited less progression of stenosis in bypass grafts as well. There was evidence of actual atherosclerotic regression in coronary arteries in 16% of treated patients versus only 2% of placebo patients.

There is also evidence that certain calcium blockers may slow the progression of atherosclerosis. Loaldi et al. studied the effects of propranolol, nifedipine, and isosorbide dinitrate on atherosclerosis in patients with effort angina and known coronary artery disease. Over a two-year period, they observed that progression of old narrowings and appearance of new narrowings were fewer in the nifedipine patients (31% and 10%, respectively) than in propranolol (53% and 34%) or isosorbide dinitrate (47% and 29%) patients. Nifedipine also was associated with regression of percent stenosis in a larger number of lesions than the other drugs.

The concept of atherosclerotic regression and slowing of progression with cholesterol-lowering agents and calcium blockers will likely continue to be tested in large multicenter trials.

Bibliography

Abrams J: Transdermal nitroglycerin and nitrate tolerance. *Ann Intern Med* 104:424, 1986.

Abrams J: The use of nitroglycerin and long-acting nitrates in angina pectoris. In: Weiner DA, Frishman WH, eds. *Therapy of Angina Pectoris*. New York: Marcel Dekker, Inc; 1986, p. 53–82.

ACC/AHA Task Force Report: Guidelines for ambulatory electrocardiography. *J Am Coll Cardiol* 13:249, 1989.

Alison HW, Russel RO Jr, Mantle FA, et al: Coronary anatomy and arteriography in patients with unstable angina pectoris. *Am J Cardiol* 41:204, 1978.

Aronow WS: Smoking, carbon monoxide, and coronary heart disease. *Circulation* 48:1169, 1973.

Atkins GW, Pohost GM, DeSanctis RW, et al: Selection of angina-free patients with severe left ventricular dysfunction for myocardial revascularization. *Am J Cardiol* 46:697, 1980.

Back JD, Gross GJ, Warltier DC, et al: Comparative effects of cardioselective versus noncardioselective beta blockade on subendocardial blood flow and contractile function in ischemic myocardium. *Am J Cardiol* 44:647, 1979.

Banks DC, Raftery ED, Oran S: Clinical significance of the coronary arteriogram. *Br Heart J* 33:863, 1971.

Blankenhorn DH. Regression of atherosclerosis. In: Braunwald E, ed. *Heart Disease Update 4* ed. Philadelphia: W.B. Saunders; 1988, p. 73.

Blankenhorn DH, Nessin SA, Johnson RL, et al.: Beneficial effects of combined colestipol-niacin therapy on coronary atherosclerosis and coronary venous bypass grafts. *JAMA* 257:3233, 1987.

Braunwald E, Ross J Jr, Sonnenblick EH: Myocardial energetics. In: Braunwald E, Ross J Jr, Sonnenblick EH, eds. *Mechanisms of Contraction of the Normal and Failing Heart.* Boston: Little Brown; 1976, p. 171.

Cannon RO, Bonow RO, Bacharach SL, et al: Left ventricular dysfunction in patients with angina pectoris, normal epicardial coronary arteries, and abnormal vasodilator reserve. *Circulation* 71:218, 1985.

CASS Principal Investigators and their Associates: Coronary artery surgery study (CASS): A randomized trial of coronary artery bypass surgery. Survival data. *Circulation* 68:939, 1983.

Cheitlin MD, Davia JE, deCastro CM, et al: Correlations of "critical" left coronary artery lesions with positive submaximal exercise tests in patients with chest pain. *Am Heart J* 89:305, 1975.

Cheitlin MD: Finding the high-risk patient with coronary artery disease. *JAMA* 259:2271, 1988.

Cohn PF: Severe asymptomatic coronary artery disease. A diagnostic, prognostic and therapeutic puzzle. *Am J Med* 62:565, 1977.

Cohn PF: *Diagnosis and Therapy of Coronary Artery Disease.* Boston: Little Brown; 1979, p. 311.

Cohn PF, Maddox DE, Holman BL, et al: Effect of sublingually administered nitroglycerin on regional myocardial blood flow in patients with coronary artery disease. *Am J Cardiol* 39:672, 1977.

Cohn PF, Vokonas PS, Williams RA, et al: Diastolic heart sounds and filling waves in coronary artery disease. *Circulation* 44:196, 1971.

Conti CR, Brawley RK, Griffith LS, et al: Unstable angina pectoris: Morbidity and mortality in 57 consecutive patients evaluated angiographically. *Am J Cardiol* 32:745, 1973.

Detre K, Holubkov R, Kelsey S, et al: Percutaneous transluminal coronary angioplasty in 1985–1986 and 1977–1981. The National Heart, Lung, and Blood Institute Registry. *N Engl J Med* 318:265, 1988.

Detre KM, Takaro T, Hultgren H, Peduzzi P, and the Study Participants: Long-term mortality and morbidity results of the Veterans Administration Randomized Trial of Coronary Artery Bypass Surgery. *Circulation* 72(suppl V): V–84, 1985.

Doyle JT, Kinch SH: The prognosis of an abnormal electrocardiographic stress test. *Circulation* 41:54, 1970.

Ellestad MH, Allen W, Wan MC, et al: Maximal treadmill stress testing for cardiovascular evaluation. *Circulation* 39:517, 1969.

Epstein SE, Stampfer M, Beiser GD, et al: Effect of a reduction in environment temperature on the circulatory response to exercise in man. Implications concerning angina pectoris. *N Engl J Med* 280:7, 1969.

Erikssen J, Enge I, Forfand K, et al: False positive diagnostic tests and coronary angiographic findings in 105 presumably healthy males. *Circulation* 54:371, 1976.

European Coronary Surgery Study Group: Long-term results of prospective randomized study of coronary artery bypass surgery in stable angina pectoris. *Lancet* 2:1173, 1982.

Forrester JS, Litvack F, Grundfest W, Hickey A: A perspective of coronary disease seen through the arteries of a living man. *Circulation* 75:505, 1987.

Fischl SJ, Herman MV, Gorlin R: The intermediate coronary syndrome: Clinical, angiographic and therapeutic aspects. *N Engl J Med* 228:1193, 1973.

Freedberg AS, Spiegel, ED, Riseman JEF: Effects of external heat and cold on patients with angina pectoris: Evidence for the existence of a reflex factor. *Am Heart J* 27:611, 1941.

Frishman WH, Charlap S, Goldberger J, et al: Comparison of diltiazem and nifedipine for both angina pectoris and systemic hypertension. *Am J Cardiol* 56:41H, 1985.

Gerstenblith G, Ouyang P, Achuff SC, et al: Nifedipine in unstable angina: A double blind, randomized trial. *N Engl J Med* 306:885, 1982.

Gerwitz H, Beller JGA, Strauss WH, et al: Transient defects of resting thallium scans in patients with coronary artery disease. *Circulation* 59:707, 1979.

Goldman S, Tselos S, Cohn K: Marked depth of ST-segment depression during treadmill exercise test: Indicator of severe coronary artery disease. *Chest* 69:729, 1976.

Goldstein RE, Redwood DR, Rosing DR, et al: Alterations in the circulatory response to exercise following a meal and their relationship in postprandial angina pectoris. *Circulation* 44:90, 1971.

Greenberg MA, Grose RM, Neuburger N, Silverman R, Strain JE, Cohen MV: Impaired coronary vasodilator responsiveness as a cause of lactate production during pacing induced ischemia in patients with angina pectoris and normal coronary arteries. *J Am Coll Cardiol* 9:743, 1987.

Gruentzig A: Transluminal dilation of coronary artery stenosis. *Lancet* 1:263, 1978.

Gruentzig AR, King SB, Schlumpf M et al: Long-term follow-up after percutaneous transluminal coronary angioplasty: The early Zurich experience. *N Engl J Med* 316:1127, 1987.

Hamby RI, Katz S: Percutaneous transluminal coronary angioplasty: Its potential impact on surgery for coronary artery disease. *Am J Cardiol* 45:1162, 1980.

Humphries JO: Expected course of patients with coronary artery disease. In: Rahimtoola SH, ed. *Coronary Bypass Surgery.* Philadelphia: FA Davis Company; 1977, p. 48.

Irving JB, Bruce RA: Exertional hypotension and postexertional ventricular fibrillation in stress testing. *Am J Cardiol* 39:849, 1977.

Iskandrian AS, Heo J, Askenase A, et al: Dipyridamole cardiac imaging. *Am Heart J* 115:1132, 1988.

Kennedy HL, Wiens RD: Ambulatory (Holter) electrocardiography and myocardial ischemia. *Am Heart J* 117:164, 1989.

Kent KM, Bonow RO, Rosing DR, et al: Improved myocardial function during exercise after successful transluminal coronary angioplasty. *N Engl J Med* 306:441, 1982.

Kent K, et al: Percutaneous transluminal coronary angioplasty (PTCA): Update from NHLBI Registry. *Circulation* 62(Suppl III):160, 1980.

Killip T, Passamani E, Davis KB, Gillespie MJ, Killip T, and the CASS Principal Investigators and their Associates: A randomized trial of coronary bypass surgery. *Circulation* 72(Suppl V): V-102, 1985.

Kirshenbaum JM, Kloner RA, Antman EM, Braunwald E: Use of ultra-short acting beta-blocker in patients with acute myocardial ischemia. *Circulation* 72:873, 1985.

Kramsch DM, Aspen AJ, Abramowitz BM, et al: Reduction of coronary atherosclerosis by moderate conditioning exercise in monkeys on an atherogenic diet. *N Engl J Med* 305:1483, 1981.

Lavine P, Kimbiris D, Segal BL, et al: Left main coronary artery disease: Clinical, arteriographic, and hemodynamic appraisal. *Am J Cardiol* 30:791, 1972.

Loaldi A, Polese A, Montorsi P, et al: Comparison of nifedipine, propranolol and isosorbide dinitrate on angiographic progression and regression of coronary arterial narrowings in angina pectoris. *Am J Cardiol* 64:433, 1989.

Martin CE, Shaver JA, Leonard JJ: Physical signs, apexcardiography, phonocardiography, and systolic time intervals in angina pectoris. *Circulation* 46:1098, 1972.

Maseri A: Mixed angina pectoris. *Am J Cardiol* 56:30E, 1985.

Mock MB, Fisher LD, Holmes DR, et al: Comparison of effects of medical and surgical therapy on survival in severe angina pectoris and two-vessel coronary artery disease with and without left ventricular dysfunction. A Coronary Artery Surgery Study Registry Study. *Am J Cardiol* 61:1198, 1988.

Mudge GH Jr, Grossman W, Mills RM Jr, et al: Reflex increase in coronary vascular resistance in patients with ischemic heart disease. *N Engl J Med* 295:1333, 1976.

Mulcahy R, Daly L, Graham I, et al: Treatment of chronic stable angina: Natural history and determinants of prognosis. *Am J Cardiol* 48:525, 1981.

Murphy ML, Hultgren HN, Detre K, et al: Treatment of chronic stable angina: A preliminary report of survival data of the randomized Veterans Administration Cooperative Study. *N Engl J Med* 297:621, 1977.

National Heart, Lung, and Blood Institute: Cooperative Trial. Preliminary report. The beta-blocker heart attack trial. *JAMA* 246:2073, 1981.

The Norwegian Multicenter Study Group: Timolol-induced reduction in mortality and reinfarction in patients surviving acute myocardial infarction. *N Engl J Med* 304:801, 1981.

Parker JO, Fung HL: Transdermal nitroglycerin in angina patients. *Am J Cardiol* 54:471, 1984.

Parker JO. Nitrate Tolerance. *Am J Cardiol* 56:281, 1985.

Passamani E, Davis KB, Gillespie MJ, Killip T, and the CASS Principal Investigators and their Associates: A randomized trial of coronary artery bypass surgery: Survival of patients with a low ejection fraction. *N Engl J Med* 312:1665, 1985.

Pepine C: Nicardipine, a new calcium channel blocker: Role for vascular selectivity. *Clin Cardiol* 12:240, 1989.

Pitt B, Strauss HW: Clinical application of myocardial imaging with thallium. In: Strauss HW, Pitt B, ed. *Cardiovascular Nuclear Medicine*, Pt 2. London: C.V. Mosby Company; 1979, p. 243.

Proudfit WL, Hodgman JR: Physical signs during angina pectoris. *Prog Cardiovasc Dis* 10:283, 1968.

Proudfit WL, Shirey EK, Sheldon WC, et al: Certain clinical characteristics correlated with extent of obstructive lesions demonstrated by selective cine coronary arteriography. *Circulation* 38:947, 1968.

Rahimtoola SH: Coronary bypass surgery for chronic angina-1981: A perspective. *Circulation* 65:225, 1982.

Rahimtoola SH: A perspective on the three large multicenter randomized clinical trials of coronary bypass surgery for chronic stable angina. *Circulation* 72(Suppl V): V-123, 1985.

Rahimtoola SH: Unstable angina: Current status. *Mod Concepts Cardiovasc Dis* 54:19, 1985.

Redwood RD, Rosing DR, Epstein SE: Circulatory and symptomatic effects of physical training in patients with coronary artery disease and angina pectoris. *N Engl J Med* 286:959, 1972.

Rifkin RD, Hood WB Jr: Bayesian analysis of electrocardiographic exercise stress testing. *N Engl J Med* 297:681, 1977.

Ritchie JL, Zaret BL, Strauss HW, et al: Myocardial imaging with thallium-201: A multicenter study in patients with angina pectoris or acute myocardial infarction. *Am J Cardiol* 42:345, 1978.

Robertson WS, Feigenbaum H, Armstrong WF, et al: Exercise echocardiography: A clinically practical addition in the evaluation of coronary artery disease. *J Am Coll Cardiol* 2:1085, 1983.

Sampson JJ, Cheitlin MD: Pathophysiology and differential diagnosis of cardiac pain. *Prog Cardiovasc Dis* 13:507, 1971.

Schrumpf JD, Sleps DS, Wolfson S, et al: Altered hemoglobin-oxygen affinity with long-term propranolol therapy in patients with coronary artery disease. *Am J Cardiol* 40:76, 1977.

Shub C, Vlietstra RE, McGoon MD: Selection of optimal drug therapy for the patient with angina pectoris. *Mayo Clin Proc* 60:539 1985.

Sim DN, Neill WA: Investigation of the physiological basis for increased exercise threshold after physical conditioning. *J Clin Inves* 54:763, 1974.

Stadel BV: Oral contraceptives and cardiovascular disease. *N Engl J Med* 305:612, 1981.

Stone PH: Calcium antagonists for Prinzmetal's variant angina, unstable angina and silent myocardial ischemia: Therapeutic tool and probe for identification of pathophysiologic mechanisms. *Am J Cardiol* 59:101B, 1987.

Theroux P, Ouimet H, McCums J, et al: Aspirin, heparin, or both to treat acute unstable angina. *N Engl J Med* 319:1105, 1989.

Transderm-Nitro Trial Study Group: Intermittent transdermal nitroglycerin therapy in the treatment of chronic stable angina. *J Am Coll Cardiol* 13:786, 1989.

Vatner SF: Correlation between acute reduction in myocardial blood flow and function in conscious dogs. *Circ Res* 47:201, 1980.

The Veterans Administration Coronary Artery Bypass Surgery Cooperative Study Group: Eleven-year survival in the Veterans Administration Randomized Trial of Coronary Bypass Surgery for stable angina. *N Engl J Med* 311:1333, 1984.

Vetrovec GW, Parker VE, Cole S, et al.: Nifedipine gastrointestinal therapeutic system in stable angina pectoris. Results of a multicenter open-label crossover comparison with standard nifedipine. *Am J Med* 83(Suppl 6B):24, 1987.

Von Dohlen TW, Rogers WB, Frank MJ: Pathophysiology and management of unstable angina. *Clin Cardiol* 12:363, 1989.

Wackers FJ, Lie KL, Liem KL, et al: Thallium-201 scintigraphy in unstable angina pectoris. *Circulation* 57:738, 1978.

Weintraub RM, Voukydis PC, Aroestry JM, et al: Treatment of preinfarction angina with intraaortic balloon counterpulsation and surgery. *Am J Cardiol* 34:809, 1974.

White HD, Polak JF, Wynne J, Holman BL, Antman EM, and Nesto RW: Addition of nifedipine to maximal nitrate and beta-adrenoreceptor blocker therapy in coronary artery disease. *Am J Cardiol* 55:1303, 1985.

Winniford MD, Kennedy PL, Wells PJ, Hillis LD: Potentiation of nitroglycerin-induced coronary dilation by N-acetylcysteine. *Circulation* 73:138, 1986.

14 Silent Myocardial Ischemia

Thomas L. Shook

Myocardial ischemia occurs when myocardial oxygen demand exceeds myocardial oxygen supply. Angina pectoris is the symptom complex classically associated with transient myocardial ischemia. However, ischemia can occur with or without angina. *Silent* myocardial ischemia is simply myocardial ischemia occurring in the absence of chest pain or anginal equivalents (dyspnea, nausea, or pain in locations other than the chest). Symptoms occur late (or not at all) in a series of events beginning with the initiation of anaerobic metabolism and followed by: (1) impairment of myocardial cellular function and local electrophysiologic disturbances; (2) abnormal left ventricular diastolic performance; (3) abnormal left ventricular systolic performance; and (4) surface electrocardiographic abnormalities.

Clinical understanding of the inconstant relationship between myocardial ischemia and symptoms has been markedly enhanced by recent epidemiologic and methodologic discoveries. First, ischemia severe enough to cause completed myocardial infarction (MI) can be entirely silent. Follow-up data from the Framingham Study suggest that 35% of myocardial infarctions in women and 28% in men are clinically unrecognized. About one half of these are entirely asymptomatic and one half are accompanied by few or atypical symptoms. These data doubtless underestimate the true incidence of silent MI, since non-Q-wave MIs, those manifested by development of new conduction disturbance, and silent MIs followed by sudden cardiac death are not included. Very likely, one third of all myocardial infarctions are truly asymptomatic.

A second major advance in the understanding of myocardial ischemia has been the development of methods to accurately monitor ST-segment changes during ambulatory ECG (AECG, or Holter monitoring). Use of these techniques has revealed that patients with coronary artery disease have frequent episodes of characteristic ischemic ST-segment change during daily activity. Approximately 75% of all episodes of myocardial ischemia detected by AECG are silent. Moreover, these episodes tend to occur at relatively low heart rates and during sedentary activities. Prompted by these findings, additional important observations have followed from the use of conventional exercise ECG testing, radionuclide scintigraphy, exercise echocardiography, and other techniques. These studies are beginning to have important prognostic and therapeutic implications.

PATHOPHYSIOLOGY

General features of the pathophysiology of myocardial ischemia have been discussed (see Chapter 13). Myocardial ischemia occurs when myocardial oxygen demand exceeds myocardial oxygen supply. When one or all of the determinants of myocardial oxygen demand (systolic wall stress, heart rate, and myocardial contractility) increase(s), myocardial blood supply normally increases to meet demand. The presence of flow-limiting atheromatous plaque in epicardial coronary arteries limits increases in flow, resulting in inadequate perfusion and conversion from aerobic to anaerobic metabolism. Subsequently, abnormalities of cellular function are manifested by impaired ion flux and local electrophysiologic disturbances. Next, elevation of left ventricular end-diastolic pressure and a fall in the rate of ventricular relaxation occur, indicative of ventricular diastolic impairment. This is followed by impaired systolic performance as manifested by regional or global contractile failure. Surface ECG abnormalities—ST-segment depression or elevation—occur late in this sequence of events. Generally, angina is an even later manifestation of ischemia. However, all of the above ischemic events may be present without any symptoms whatsoever.

Why are some episodes of myocardial ischemia symptomatic and others not? Silent ischemia may simply represent *brief or less severe* ischemia. Also, the difference in *pain perception* or central transmission of pain may vary from individual to individual or within the same individual during different circumstances. For example, diabetic patients may have a neuropathic basis for painless ischemia. Also, myocardial infarction may destroy or alter cardiac nerve endings. Finally, different relationships between disturbed myocardial blood *supply* and superimposed, changing myocardial *demand* may determine whether or not an episode is symptomatic.

The observation that silent myocardial ischemia occurs during daily activities and at heart rates considerably lower than those provoking ischemia during treadmill exercise has fostered speculation that changing myocardial blood supply may also be important in the pathophysiology of silent myocardial ischemia. Normal coronary arteries are capable of both dilation and constriction in response to multiple neurohumoral stimuli. It is now apparent that diseased epicardial coronary arteries retain the capacity for changing coronary vasomotor tone in spite of their involvement with atherosclerosis. Unfortunately, while atherosclerotic coronary arteries may still respond normally to direct vasodilators, such as nitroglycerin and calcium channel blockers, certain neurohumoral substances depend upon normal endothelium to mediate their vasodilating properties. When endothelium is damaged, these substances may have paradoxical vasoconstrictor properties (Ludmer et al.).

In addition to demonstrating that most episodes of myocardial ischemia during daily activities are asymptomatic and that they tend to occur at relatively low heart rates, ambulatory AECG recordings show a marked circadian variation in frequency and duration of silent ischemia (Rocco et al. 1987). AECG recordings demonstrate a significant peak of events in the morning hours. This circadian peak closely parallels the peak time of onset of myocardial infarction (Figure 1), and circadian peaks of endogenous catecholamines, platelet aggregability (Tofler et al.), and platelet alpha$_2$-adrenoreceptor affinity (Mehta et al.). Coronary arteries already narrowed by atherosclerotic plaque may have heightened vasoconstrictor sensitivity due to the loss of endothelial-mediated vasodilation at certain times of the day. These findings have also supported speculation that many episodes of silent myocardial ischemia are prompted by reduc-

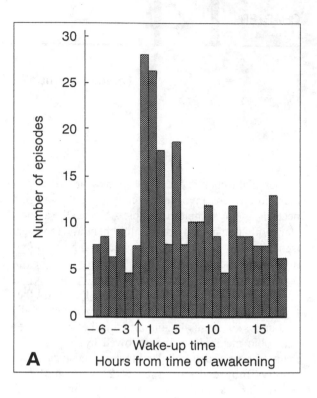

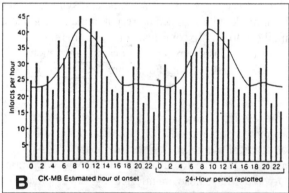

Figure 1. *A: Hourly distribution of number of episodes of myocardial ischemia, corrected for time of awakening. The peak incidence of ischemia occurs within the first 2 hours of awakening. (From Rocco et al. 1987. With permission.) B: Hourly frequency of onset of myocardial infarction in 703 patients. A prominent circadian rhythm is present, with primary peak incidence at 9 a.m. and secondary peak at 8 p.m. (From Muller et al. With permission. See Bibliography.)*

tions in myocardial blood supply as much as by increases in myocardial oxygen demand.

METHODS OF DETECTION OF SILENT MYOCARDIAL ISCHEMIA

Detection of silent myocardial ischemia has relied heavily on ECG (exercise and ambulatory) and radionuclide studies.

AMBULATORY ECG

ST-segment changes suggestive of myocardial ischemia were demonstrated in Norman Holter's original description of ambulatory ECG monitoring in 1961. However, early use of ambulatory monitoring was primarily limited to detection of arrhythmias until the studies of Stern and Tzivoni, and Schang and Pepine in the 1970s. These studies demonstrated frequent asymptomatic ischemic ST-segment changes on AECG monitor recordings in patients with known or suspected coronary artery disease. However, these early studies were criticized because of concerns about technical aspects of the recording and playback systems utilized. Specifically, poor frequency-response characteristics or marked phase-shift of some Holter recording and playback systems may cause artifactual ST-segment deviations (Bragg-Remschel et al.). With the advent of frequency-modulated (FM) systems and improved direct recording (AM) systems, these limitations can be overcome (Shook, Balke, et al.).

When patients with known coronary artery disease are monitored, they are frequently observed to have multiple episodes of characteristic ischemic ST-segment depression, 70–90% of which are asymptomatic (Figure 2). Studies suggest that most patients with coronary artery disease and angina also have episodes of silent myocardial ischemia. There is, however, a very wide range of episode duration, number, and total time of ischemia. It is difficult to predict from clinical features which patients will have silent myocardial ischemia and which will not. Similarly, it is very difficult to predict from exercise testing the frequency or severity of myocardial ischemia as assessed by ambulatory recording (Shook et al. 1989). Radionuclide studies also appear to predict poorly the presence of silent ischemia on AECG recording (Reed et al.).

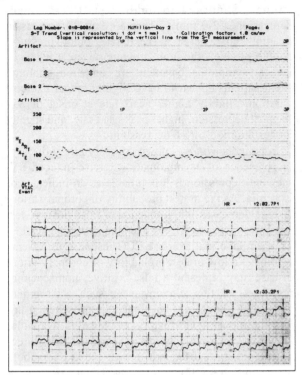

Figure 2. *Episodes of ST-segment depression detected by ambulatory ECG in a patient with known coronary artery disease. These episodes were asymptomatic.*

EXERCISE ECG TESTING

Graded exercise accompanied by transient ST-segment depression on the electrocardiogram is widely accepted as a sign of myocardial ischemia. The presence of angina is useful as confirmatory evidence of myocardial ischemia, but ECG evidence alone is sufficient to diagnose ischemia. Such changes and their "severity" are commonly believed to be important indicators of the severity of obstructive coronary artery disease and its prognosis. Approximately one third to one half of exercise tests in patients with known coronary artery disease are not accompanied by angina. Clinical characteristics (age, sex, previous myocardial infarction, extent of coronary artery disease, presence or absence or type of drug therapy) are similar in patients with silent and symptomatic positive exercise tests (Stern et al.). There appears to be no difference in the number or sequence of ECG leads involved or the degree of maximal ST-segment depression in silent and symptomatic patients with strongly abnormal treadmill tests (ST-segment depression >2.0 mm). There are few differences in treadmill characteristics (heart rate, blood pressure, double product, duration of exercise, etc.) when silent and symptomatic patients are compared, although silent patients appear to have slightly longer exercise duration, slightly higher heart rate at onset of ST-segment depression, higher peak heart rate, and slightly longer duration of ST depression.

In patients *without* known coronary artery disease, the presence of asymptomatic exercise-induced ST-segment depression is less reliable as an indicator of ischemia. As the pretest probability of coronary artery disease decreases, the frequency of false-positive test responses increases (Bayes' theorem—see Chapter 13). Thus an abnormal exercise ECG response in patients who have a low pretest probability of coronary artery disease may represent a false-positive, nonischemic, response. In this circumstance, such ST-segment depression should *not* be termed silent ischemia unless additional confirmatory evidence is available. However, such patients *are* at increased risk (three- to fivefold) for subsequent cardiac events and should have additional follow-up testing (Giagnoni et al.).

RADIONUCLIDE STUDIES

Both thallium stress-redistribution scintigraphy and exercise radionuclide ventriculography improve the sensitivity and specificity of exercise ECG for detection of exercise-induced myocardial ischemia. This is the case whether or not symptoms are present. As discussed in Chapters 5 and 6, the utility of these studies for the *diagnosis* of coronary artery disease is also dependent upon the pretest likelihood. In patients with *known* coronary artery disease, however, additional confirmatory and quantitative evidence of physiologically significant ischemia can be obtained by radionuclide studies. In the absence of angina, additional confirmation of ischemia can be very helpful clinically. The results of exercise testing, even when confirmed by radionuclide studies, do not clearly predict the frequency and extent of silent ischemia detected by ambulatory monitoring (Reed et al.).

Important studies using positron emission tomography (PET) confirmed the presence of transient hypoperfusion during spontaneous episodes of asymptomatic ST-segment depression in patients with typical angina and a positive exercise test (Deanfield et al. 1984) (Figure 3). These findings validated the concept of significant ischemia accompanied by pain-

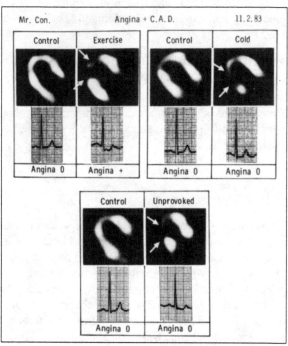

Figure 3. *Tomographic slices through the mid-left ventricle showing the regional myocardial uptake of rubidium-82 (^{82}Rb) in the posterior wall, free wall, anterior wall and interventricular septum. This demonstrates the distribution of regional perfusion during control, cold pressor test, unprovoked ST depression and exercise. Evidence of regional ischemia occurred during all three tests and supported the ST-segment changes as evidence of ischemia whether or not chest pain occurred. CAD = coronary artery disease. (From Deanfield et al. 1984. With permission. See Bibliography.)*

less ST depression. In particular, PET defects indicative of spontaneous asymptomatic reductions in myocardial blood flow were found to be readily provoked by mental stress. These studies support the hypothesis that ambulatory ischemia is often triggered by decrements in blood supply, as well as increases in myocardial demand. Clinical application of PET scanning is promising but largely undeveloped.

FREQUENCY OF SILENT MYOCARDIAL ISCHEMIA

As previously noted, approximately one third of all myocardial infarctions are truly asymptomatic. Findings from ambulatory ECG studies were recently re-

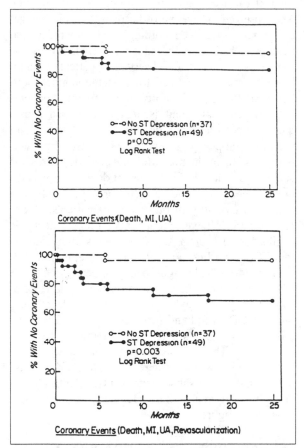

Figure 4. *Kaplan-Meier curves comparing the probability of not experiencing (top) an acute ischemic event (death, myocardial infarction, unstable angina), or (bottom) a progressive ischemic event (death, MI, unstable angina, or revascularization). Follow-up of 37 patients without ST-segment depression (open circles) and 49 patients with ST-segment depression (closed circles) on ambulatory monitoring. (From Rocco et al. 1988. With permission.)*

viewed by Rozanski and Berman. In 10 studies, 75% (range 61–81%) of all episodes of ambulatory ischemia detected by monitoring were silent. The methods used for analysis and definition of ischemic changes have changed somewhat over the course of these studies. Nonetheless, patients with known coronary artery disease appear to have approximately a 3:1 ratio of silent-to-symptomatic episodes of ischemia during daily activity. Episodes characteristically last for approximately 24 minutes and demonstrate a mean of 1.5 mm of ST-segment depression. Depending upon the patient population studied, there is a wide range in the number of episodes and total duration of ischemia per 24 hours of monitoring. Most patients with chronic, stable angina have some evidence of silent ischemia. About one third have frequent episodes (>6/48 hrs).

Hospitalized patients with unstable angina have a high frequency of asymptomatic ST-segment depression during continuous AECG monitoring. Almost 90% of episodes occur silently. In one study, 37 of 70 patients hospitalized for unstable angina had ST-segment depression detected on continuous monitoring (Gottlieb et al. 1986). They had a mean daily duration of 157 minutes of ST-segment change.

Cohn has proposed a classification scheme describing three types of patients with transient myocardial ischemia: *Type I*—totally asymptomatic persons; *Type II*—patients asymptomatic after myocardial infarction; and *Type III*—patients with coexisting angina and silent myocardial ischemia. His estimates suggest that 2–4% of totally asymptomatic middle-aged men have provocable silent myocardial ischemia. Thus, there are probably one million to two million men (and probably a similar number of women) in the United States who have totally asymptomatic, significant myocardial ischemia. Approximately 20–30% of post-MI patients have evidence of provocable asymptomatic myocardial ischemia (Type II). Thus, 50,000–100,000 persons per year are found to have silent ischemia after myocardial infarction. Probably 80–90% of patients with angina (Type III) have coexistent silent myocardial ischemia (approximately 3 million persons in the U.S.).

PROGNOSIS

Assessment of prognosis governs many important management decisions in patients with known or suspected coronary artery disease. Much is known about the determinants of prognosis in such patients. Until recently, little has been known about the prognostic implications of the presence of silent myocardial ischemia. There is growing concern that the presence of ischemia, regardless of accompanying symptoms, may significantly affect prognosis.

The degree of resting left ventricular dysfunction (ejection fraction) is the most powerful determinant of prognosis in patients who have had a myocardial infarction; however, in these patients and, more specifically, in patients without prior myocardial infarction, a number of other features are also important. The extent of coronary artery disease as assessed by coronary angiography can be an important predictor of prognosis. For example, high-grade stenosis of the left main coronary artery was shown early on in the Coronary Artery Surgery Study to be a significant determinant of prognosis (see Chapter 13). Angiography alone, however, is limited because visual interpretation of the coronary angiogram often poorly reflects the pressure gradient across coronary stenosis and, accordingly, coronary blood flow reserve. Thus, it provides limited *physiologic* information. Exercise testing has proved to be an important predictor of subsequent cardiac events, largely because of its ability to quantify the extent of inducible myocardial ischemia. A number of exercise test variables have been shown to predict adverse events. The depth, duration and time of onset of ST-segment depression and total exercise time, have been found to predict an adverse prognosis. Recently, it was observed that the presence of inducible ischemia on exercise testing, regardless of the presence of symptoms, affects prognosis. Follow-up data from the Coronary Artery Surgery Study suggest that the prognosis of patients with the same angiographic extent of coronary artery disease and the same extent of abnormality on exercise testing is independent of the presence of angina (Weiner et al. 1987).

Abnormal exercise findings in patients after myocardial infarction have been shown in multiple studies to define a group at high risk for cardiac death, recurrent myocardial infarction, and unstable angina. This unfavorable prognosis applies equally to patients with silent or symptomatic ischemia on exercise testing.

Studies using thallium scintigraphy also support the concept that patients with exercise-induced ischemia have an adverse prognosis regardless of the presence of chest pain. Asymptomatic patients after myocardial infarction have widely different rates of subsequent cardiac events depending on whether inducible myocardial hypoperfusion is present during exercise (59% event rate in the next 15 months) or absent (6% event rate) (Gibson et al.). In another group of patients with typical angina and ischemia on thallium scintigraphy at low work load, the cardiac event rate was equivalent in patients without symptoms or with typical angina. Thus, both conventional exercise testing and thallium scintigraphy indicate adverse prognosis if exercise-inducible ischemia is present, whether silent or symptomatic.

Does the presence of spontaneous silent ischemia on ambulatory monitoring affect prognosis? Stern and Tzivoni's early studies found an increased rate of sub-sequent cardiac events in follow-up of patients who were observed to have out-of-hospital ischemic changes on ambulatory ECG recording, as compared to patients who had no such changes. A markedly worse prognosis has also been observed in patients with silent ischemia hospitalized for unstable angina (Gottlieb et al. 1986, 1987). Forty-three percent of patients with evidence of silent ischemia developed subsequent myocardial infarction or required surgery or balloon angioplasty, compared with 12% of patients without silent ischemia. Multiple logistic regression analysis revealed that ST-segment depression was the most potent prognostic variable for the prediction of long-term mortality in this group of patients. Rocco et al. (1988) followed 86 patients with chronic stable angina for an average of 12.5 months after ambulatory ECG recording. Patients with ST depression during monitoring had a significantly increased incidence of cardiac death, infarction, or unstable angina compared with patients who exhibited no ST depression. Similarly, DeWood and Rozanski reported three-year follow-up with 59 patients who had ambulatory ECG monitoring. Those patients who demonstrated silent ischemic ST-segment changes had a *fivefold* increase in the incidence of subsequent events. Silent ischemia on ambulatory monitoring appears to adversely affect prognosis (Figure 4).

THERAPY OF SILENT MYOCARDIAL ISCHEMIA

Multiple studies have demonstrated that drug therapy using conventional antianginal agents can markedly reduce or eliminate silent ischemia detected by ambulatory ECG recording. Nitrates (hourly sublingual nitroglycerin, transdermal nitroglycerin), beta blockers (propranolol, atenolol, labetalol and metoprolol), and calcium channel blockers (nifedipine, verapamil, and diltiazem) have all been efficacious in reducing episodes of silent ischemia. In one study, a combination of propranolol and nifedipine was superior to either drug alone in reducing the total number of ischemic episodes. Not unexpectedly, successful balloon coronary angioplasty has also been documented to abolish silent myocardial ischemia as detected by AECG monitoring.

The observation that asymptomatic ST depression detected during ambulatory monitoring occurs at relatively low heart rates has prompted the hypothesis that silent myocardial ischemia is a consequence of reduced myocardial oxygen supply due to enhanced coronary vasomotor tone. Theoretically, treatment strategies with nitrates or calcium channel blockers should prove superior; however, studies have not yet demonstrated clear-cut superiority of any class of antianginal agents. Few direct comparisons of antianginal agents for the treatment of silent ischemia exist.

The marked circadian variation in ischemic activity is another important consideration in the design of potential therapies for silent ischemia. Long-acting beta blockers, for example, have been demonstrated to suppress both morning and evening peaks in myocardial ischemic activity. Ultimately, drugs or drug preparations found to be successful in suppressing the morning surge of ischemia may be preferred.

The precise role for drug, percutaneous interventional, or surgical therapy of silent myocardial ischemia awaits demonstration that the adverse prognosis associated with the presence of silent ischemia can be altered. As yet, such studies have not been performed. As is true for any asymptomatic disorder, general recommendations for therapy (and attendant costs, risks, and morbidity) await a consensus that there are significant prognostic benefits. Substantial evidence that silent ischemia adversely affects prognosis has been reviewed; however, no trials have yet demonstrated that medical treatment of active ischemia improves prognosis. Surgical treatment has been demonstrated to improve survival in certain groups of patients with coronary artery disease. Importantly, patients with three-vessel coronary artery disease and evidence of inducible ischemia do derive benefit from surgery; patients with equivalent coronary artery disease but *no ischemia* do not (Weiner et al. 1987). Since the presence of ischemia on exercise testing alters prognosis, *independently of symptoms*, a logical but unproven conclusion is that medical therapy designed to eliminate or decrease ischemia should favorably affect prognosis.

Indications for use of ambulatory ECG as a guide to therapy remain unclear. Ultimately, AECG may be used as a routine tool to "tailor" therapy to assure adequate control of daily ischemia for an individual's level of activity and lifestyle.

Bibliography

Bala Subramanian V, Lahir A, Green HL, et al: Ambulatory ST-segment monitoring: Problems, pitfalls, solutions, and clinical application. *Br Heart J* 44:419, 1980.

Bala Subramanian V, Bowles MJ, Davies A, Raftery E: Calcium channel blockade as primary therapy for stable angina pectoris. A double-blind, placebo-controlled comparison of verapamil and propranolol. *Am J Cardiol* 50:1158, 1982.

Bala Subramanian V, Bowles MJ, Khurmi NS, et al: Rationale for the choice of calcium antagonists in chronic stable angina: An objective double-blind, placebo-controlled comparison of nifedipine and verapamil. *Am J Cardiol* 50:1173, 1982.

Bragg-Remschel DA, Anderson CM, Winkle RA: Frequency response characteristics of ambulatory ECG monitoring systems and their implications for ST segment analysis. *Am Heart J* 103:20, 1982.

Cohn PF: The concept and pathogenesis of active but asymptomatic coronary artery disease. *Circulation* 75(Suppl II):1, 1987.

Dargie HJ, Lynch PG, Krikler DM, et al: Nifedipine and propranolol: A beneficial drug interaction. *Am J Med* 71:676–682, 1981.

Deanfield JE, Selwyn AP, Chierchia S, et al: Coronary artery spasm as a cause of acute myocardial ischemia in man. *Chest* 5:625, 1975.

Deanfield JE, Shea M, Ribiero P, et al: Transient ST-segment depression as a marker of myocardial ischemia during daily life. *Am J Cardiol* 54:1195, 1984.

DeWood MA, Rozanski A: Long-term prognosis of patients with and without silent ischemia (abstr). *Circulation* 94:II-59, 1986.

Falcone C, DeServi S, Poma E, et al: Clinical significance of exercise-induced silent myocardial ischemia in patients with coronary artery disease. *J Am Coll Cardiol* 9:295, 1987.

Frishman WH, Charlip S, Kimmel B, et al: Diltiazem, nifedipine, and their combination in patients with stable angina pectoris. Effects on angina, exercise tolerance and the ambulatory electrocardiographic ST segment. *Circulation* 77:774, 1988.

Frishman W, Teicher M: Antianginal drug therapy for silent myocardial ischemia. *Am Heart J* 114:140, 1987.

Giagnoni E, Secchi MB, Wu SC, et al: Prognostic value of exercise EKG testing in asymptomatic, normotensive subjects: A prospective matched study. *N Engl J Med* 309:1085, 1983.

Gibson RS, Watson DD, Craddock GB, et al: Prediction of cardiac events after uncomplicated myocardial infarction: A prospective study comparing predischarge exercise thallium-201 scintigraphy and coronary angiography. *Circulation* 68:321, 1983.

Gordon DJ, Ekelund LG, Karon JM, et al: Predictive value of the exercise tolerance test for mortality in North American men. The Lipid Research Clinics Mortality Follow-up Study. *Circulation* 74:252, 1986.

Gottlieb SO, Weisfeldt ML, Ouyang P, Mellits ED, Gerstenblith G: Silent ischemia as a marker for early unfavorable outcomes in patients with unstable angina. *N Engl J Med* 314:1214, 1986.

Gottlieb SO, Weisfeldt ML, Ouyang P, et al: Silent ischemia predicts infarction and death during 2 year follow-up of unstable angina. *J Am Coll Cardiol* 10:756, 1987.

Hlatky MA: Exercise stress testing to screen for coronary artery disease in asymptomatic persons. *J Occupational Med* 28:1020, 1986.

Holter NJ: New method for heart studies: Continuous electro-cardiography of active subjects over long periods is now practical. *Science* 134:1214, 1961.

Imperi GA, Lambert CR, Coy K, et al: Effects of titrated beta blockade (metoprolol) on silent myocardial ischemia in ambulatory patients with coronary artery disease. *Am J Cardiol* 60:519, 1987.

Kannel WB, Abbott RD: Incidence and prognosis of unrecognized myocardial infarction: An update on the Framingham study. *N Engl J Med* 311:1144, 1984.

Khurmi NS, Bowles MJ, O'Hara MJ, Raftery EB: Effect of propranolol on indices of intermittent myocardial ischemia assessed by exercise testing and ambulatory ST-segment monitoring. *Clin Cardiol* 9:391, 1986.

Koonlawee N, Intarachot V, Singh P, Josephson MA, Singh BN: Characteristics and clinical significance of silent myocardial ischemia in unstable angina. *Am J Cardiol* 58:26B, 1986.

Ladenheim ML, Pollock BH, Rozanski A, et al: Extent and severity of myocardial hypoperfusion as predictors of prognosis in patients with suspected coronary artery disease. *J Am Coll Cardiol* 7:464, 1986.

Ludmer PL, Selwyn AP, Shook TL, et al: Paradoxical vasoconstriction induced by acetylcholine in atherosclerotic coronary arteries. *N Engl J Med* 315:1046, 1986.

Mehta J, Malloy M, Lawson D, Lopez L: Circadian variation in platelet alpha$_2$ - adrenoceptor affinity in normal subjects. *Am J Cardiol* 63:1002, 1989.

Muller JE, Stone PH, Turi ZG, et al., and the MILIS Study Group: Circadian variation in the frequency of onset of acute myocardial infarction. *N Engl J Med* 313:1315, 1985.

Multiple Risk Factor Intervention Trial Research Group: Exercise electrocardiogram and coronary heart disease mortality in the Multiple Risk Factor Intervention Trial. *Am J Cardiol* 55:16, 1985.

Nademanee K, Intarachot V, Josephson MA, Singh BA: Circadian variation in occurrence of transient overt and silent myocardial ischemia in chronic stable angina and comparison with Prinzmetal's angina in man. *Am J Cardiol* 60:494, 1987.

Nesto RW, Kowalchuk GJ: The ischemic cascade: Temporal sequence of hemodynamic, electrocardiographic and symptomatic expressions of ischemia. *Am J Cardiol* 57:23C, 1987.

Quyyumi AA, Wright C, Mockus L, Fox KM: Effect of partial agonist activity in beta blockers in severe angina pectoris: A double blind comparison of pindolol and atenolol. *Br Med J* 289:951, 1984.

Quyyumi AA, Wright C, Mockus L, et al: Effects of combined alpha and beta adrenoceptor blockade in patients with angina pectoris. A double blind study comparing labetalol with placebo. *Br Heart J* 53:47, 1985.

Reed DC, Stone PH, Shook TL, et al., and the ASIS Group: Discordance between radionuclide, Doppler echo, angiographic and ambulatory ECG markers of ischemia. *J Am Coll Cardiol* 13:2A, 1989.

Rocco MB, Barry J, Campbell S, et al: Circadian variation of transient ischemia in patients with coronary artery disease. *Circulation* 75:395, 1987.

Rocco MB, Nabel EG, Campbell S, et al: Prognostic importance of myocardial ischemia detected by ambulatory monitoring in patients with stable coronary artery disease. *Circulation* 78:877, 1988.

Rozanski A, Berman DS: Silent myocardial ischemia. I. Pathophysiology, frequency of occurrence, and approaches toward detection. *Am Heart J* 114:615, 1987.

Rozanski A, Bairey CN, Krantz DS, et al: Mental stress and the induction of silent myocardial ischemia in patients with coronary artery disease. *N Engl J Med* 318:1005, 1988.

Schang ST Jr, Pepine CJ: Transient asymptomatic ST-segment depression during daily activity. *Am J Cardiol* 39:396, 1977.

Selwyn AP, Fox F, Eves M, et al: Myocardial ischaemia in patients with frequent angina pectoris. *Br Med J* 2:1594, 1978.

Shell WE, Kirowitz CF, Rubins SB, See J: Mechanisms and therapy of silent ischemia: The effect of transdermal nitroglycerin. *Am Heart J* 112:229, 1986.

Shook TL, Balke CW, Kotilainen PW, et al: Comparison of amplitude-modulated (direct) and frequency-modulated ambulatory techniques for recording ischemic electrocardiographic changes. *Am J Cardiol* 60:895, 1987.

Shook TL, Valvo V, Hubelbank M, Feldman CL, Stone PH: Validation of a new algorithm for detection and quantification of ischemic ST-segment changes during ambulatory electrocardiography. *IEEE: Computers in Cardiology* 276:57, 1987.

Shook TL, Glasser SP, Crawford MH, Bhatia SJS, Stone PH, and the ASIS Group: Discordance between ambulatory electrocardiography and exercise testing for assessment of the severity of ischemia. *Circulation* 76(IV): IV–362, 1989.

Starling MR, Crawford MH, Kennedy GT, O'Rourke RA: Exercise testing early after myocardial infarction: Predictive value for subsequent unstable angina and death. *Am J Cardiol* 46:909, 1980.

Stern S, Weisz G, Gavish A, Keren A, Tzivoni D: Comparison between silent and symptomatic ischemia during exercise testing in patients with coronary artery disease. *J Cardiopulmonary Rehab* 12:507, 1988.

Stern S, Tzivoni D: Early detection of silent ischemic heart disease by 24-hour electrocardiogram monitoring of active subjects. *Br Heart J* 36:481, 1974.

Tofler GH, Brezinski D, Schafer AI, et al: Concurrent morning increase in platelet aggregability and the risk of myocardial infarction and sudden cardiac death. *N Engl J Med* 316:1514, 1987.

Tzivoni D, Gavish A, Zin D, et al: Prognostic significance of ischemic episodes in patients with previous myocardial infarction. *Am J Cardiol* 62:661, 1988.

Weiner DA, McCabe C, Hueter DC, Ryan TJ, Hood WB Jr: Predictive value of chest pain as an indicator of coronary disease during stress testing. *Am Heart J* 96:458, 1978.

Weiner DA, Ryan TJ, McCabe CH, et al: Significance of silent myocardial ischemia in ambulatory patients with coronary artery disease. *Am J Cardiol* 59:725, 1987.

Willich SN, Pohjola-Sintonen S, Bhatia SJS, et al: Suppression of silent ischemia by metroprolol without alteration of morning increase of platelet aggregability in patients with stable coronary artery disease. *Circulation* 79(III):II-557, 1989.

15 Acute Myocardial Infarction

James M. Hagar
Robert A. Kloner

Acute myocardial infarction (MI) is one of the most widespread serious health problems in Western society. In the United States alone, approximately 1,500,000 persons develop myocardial infarction annually. Approximately 500,000 deaths annually are attributable to acute MI, amounting to one fourth of all deaths in the U.S. (AHA 1988).

Sixty percent of acute MI-related deaths occur suddenly in the first hour of infarction, before medical attention is sought. Sudden death often occurs before histologic evidence of necrosis has developed and is usually due to ventricular arrhythmias, chiefly ventricular fibrillation. The advent of prehospital resuscitation, coronary care units, and defibrillators in the early 1960s markedly reduced the in-hospital mortality and lowered the overall case fatality rate for acute MI, mostly by controlling arrhythmias. Trials of beta-blocking drugs since the 1970s demonstrated improved survival following infarction in patients treated with these agents. However, until the advent of thrombolytic therapy, no pharmacologic intervention was shown to be able to limit infarct size.

In recent years, it has become clear that acute thrombotic occlusion is present in most cases of myocardial infarction. Thrombolytic therapy and other methods to reperfuse infarcting myocardium have been demonstrated to decrease infarct size, wall motion abnormalities, complications, and mortality. Reperfusion therapy has become the standard of care for acute MI in appropriate patients, and the ability to salvage infarcting myocardium has become a clinical reality.

DIAGNOSIS OF MYOCARDIAL INFARCTION

HISTORY

The typical history of a patient with acute MI is one of severe substernal chest pressure, described as an intolerable crushing or constricting pain. The sensation of myocardial ischemia, transmitted via visceral sympathetic nerves, is often difficult for the patient to describe precisely, in spite of the severity of the discomfort. Typically the pain is localized beneath the sternum with radiation to the inner aspect of the left arm, but pain in the jaw, neck, epigastrium, arm only, or back is not uncommon. Retrospectively, a history of new or worsening angina preceding the infarction by hours to weeks can be elicited in approximately half of patients. Such symptoms may be mild, however, and medical attention is often not sought. The pain of acute MI is distinguished from angina pectoris by a duration of longer than 20–30 minutes and lack of relief with rest or nitroglycerin (although the pain may be lessened somewhat). There are often associated symptoms of diaphoresis, weakness, or a feeling of impending doom. Vagal symptoms of nausea, vomiting, and abdominal cramps often occur, particularly in the setting of inferior wall infarction. When heart failure supervenes, dyspnea and cough with pink frothy sputum is prominent, and when decreased forward cardiac output occurs, due either to extensive right or left ventricular infarction, weakness and altered mentation may be noted. Some patients experience only nonspecific symptoms and perceive only that they have "indigestion." In 20% of patients, particularly in diabetics, myocardial infarction is completely silent, diagnosed only by routine electrocardiography or when complications (heart failure, arrhythmias) later develop (Kannel and Abbott).

PHYSICAL EXAMINATION

The patient typically appears anxious, restless, and diaphoretic. The skin often is cool and clammy.

Bradycardia may be present, especially in patients with vagal reactions, and the pulse is irregular if atrial or ventricular arrhythmias are present. In patients with severe pump failure, hypotension, tachycardia, oliguria and peripheral cyanosis are noted. Low-grade fever is common in the first few days. Lung examination may reveal basilar rales or wheezes indicating congestive heart failure, although absence of rales does not exclude significant pulmonary venous congestion. Jugular venous distention and hepato-jugular reflux can be seen in patients with biventricular failure, but if found without evidence of left-sided heart failure, suggest right ventricular infarction. The cardiac impulse is often faint and diffuse, or systolic bulging along the sternal border can be felt when a large segment of anterior wall is dyskinetic. A loud fourth heart sound is invariably present and is often palpable; a third heart sound may be audible if congestive failure is present. A blowing, usually holosystolic, murmur of mitral insufficiency is sometimes heard, indicative of papillary muscle ischemia or infarction. Pericardial friction rubs occur frequently in the first days of myocardial infarction, are transient and intermittent, and usually indicate transmural infarction.

DIFFERENTIAL DIAGNOSIS

There are a number of disorders which may be confused with acute myocardial infarction (Table 1). These usually can be suspected from a careful history and physical examination. The clinician must maintain a high level of suspicion for potentially life-threatening disorders for which specific therapy must be given. This includes, in particular, aortic dissection, which is frequently fatal within hours if not recognized, and pulmonary embolism. In cases of pericarditis, peptic ulcer disease, or aortic dissection, a mistaken diagnosis of myocardial infarction could lead to administration of thrombolytic therapy, with disastrous results.

ELECTROCARDIOGRAPHIC FINDINGS

The electrocardiogram is of central importance in the diagnosis of acute MI (Table 2). Evolutionary changes diagnostic of myocardial infarction will be seen on serial tracings in approximately two thirds of patients with acute MI, with the remainder having only ST- and T-wave depression. The initial ECG, however, will show only mild or nonspecific abnormalities as often as half the time, and is normal in about 20% of cases.

In the classic pattern, initial hyperacute T-wave peaking followed by ST-segment elevation develops promptly after onset of ischemia in the leads facing the area of injury. As cell death occurs, R-wave height is lost and pathologic Q waves (defined as >0.04 seconds in duration and 25% of total QRS height) develop over hours to days. ST-segment elevation decreases toward baseline and finally returns to normal simultaneously with the development of symmetrical T-wave inversion over subsequent days. Posterior infarction produces an "inverted" pattern, with ST-depression instead of elevation, T-wave peaking, and development of R waves in V_1 and V_2. Right ventricular infarction is manifested electrocardiographically as ST-elevation in right-sided precordial leads, especially V_3r-V_4r, and sometimes in V_1. These changes should be sought in all cases of inferior infarction, with which they are frequently associated.

T-wave inversions may persist for weeks or months. When ST-segment elevation persists, a large area of dyskinesis is suggested (Arvan and Varat), and if it is present late after recovery from infarction, ventricular aneurysm should be suspected. Months to years after infarction, Q waves often diminish in size or sometimes disappear, particularly with inferior infarction. These changes are shown in Figure 1. ST depression may be seen in leads remote from the area of infarction, particularly anterior ST depression with inferior infarctions. This finding often indicates posterolateral extension of infarction (Goldberg et al. 1981), but could also indicate "ischemia at a distance" (Schuster and Bulkley 1981) due to obstruction of the left anterior descending coronary or simply reciprocal ST changes without remote ischemia. Following early reperfusion, such as that associated with thrombolytic therapy, ST elevation resolves rapidly, development of Q waves is accelerated, and arrhythmias such as accelerated idioventricular rhythm may occur.

In many cases, ST-segment depression or elevation and T-wave inversion are present on the initial ECG, and persist for 48 hours or more. ST segments gradually normalize and enzyme release occurs, but pathologic Q waves never develop. This may indicate nontransmural necrosis. The finding of non-Q-wave infarction, previously called nontransmural or subendocardial infarction, has important diagnostic and therapeutic implications, as discussed later in this chapter.

Table 1. Disease Entities That May be Confused with Myocardial Infarction	
Angina pectoris	Pain less severe and of shorter duration, usually <20 minutes; relieved with rest and nitroglycerin
Aortic dissection	Pain is sharp, tearing and extremely severe; typically radiates to back. Neurologic signs, loss of pulses, or aortic insufficiency often develop. Mediastinum widened on chest x-ray. Myocardial infarction may occur if dissection extends into coronary artery; diagnosis confirmed by CT scan or aortography
Pulmonary embolism	Dyspnea, tachycardia and hypoxemia are prominent; pain is usually pleuritic, especially when pulmonary infarction develops, but may resemble angina in bland infarction; ECG is nonspecific, LDH may be elevated but not CK; diagnosis confirmed by lung scan or pulmonary angiogram
Pericarditis	May be preceded by viral illness; pain is sharp, positional, pleuritic and relieved by leaning forward. Pericardial rub often present; diffuse ST elevation occurs without evolution of Q waves; CK usually normal but rises in some cases; responds to anti-inflammatory agents
Myocarditis	May be preceded by viral illness; pain is generally vague and mild if present. Total CK and MB often elevated. Conduction abnormalities and sometimes Q waves occur
Muscoloskeletal disorders	Includes costochondritis, cervical osteoarthritis, radiculitis. Pain is atypical, stabbing, localized, may be pleuritic; reproduced by motion or palpation; ECG changes absent
Gastrointestinal disorders	Esophageal reflux is often made worse with recumbency or after meals, may be associated with regurgitation and relieved by antacids. Episodes of spasm may be brought on by cold liquids, relieved by nitroglycerin, and may closely resemble angina or infarction. Diagnosis may be confirmed by upper GI series, endoscopy or esophageal manometry. Peptic ulcer disease, pancreatitis and cholecystitis may occasionally mimic infarction; abdominal tenderness is present, with radiation to back and elevated amylase in pancreatitis; sonography can confirm cholecystitis
Pneumothorax	Onset abrupt with sharp pleuritic chest pain and dyspnea; breath sounds absent, chest x-ray confirms
Pleuritis	Pain is sharp and increases on inspiration; friction rub or dullness may be present; other respiratory symptoms and underlying pulmonary infection usually present

The suggested nomenclature for locating infarct site by ECG is shown in Figure 1, Table 2 and Chapter 3. Useful inferences concerning the involved coronary artery can often be made (Figure 1; Blanke et al.; Fuchs et al.), but anatomic variation and collateral flow in the presence of multivessel disease frequently make such estimations inexact.

The electrocardiographic diagnosis of acute myocardial infarction may be mimicked by a variety of conditions. ST-segment elevation occurs without infarction in coronary spasm, where it is rapidly reversible, and in pericarditis, which produces diffuse ST elevation. In distinction from myocardial infarction, the ST elevation in pericarditis returns to base-

Table 2. Localizing Myocardial Infarction

LOCATION	ECG LEADS INVOLVED	PROBABLE ARTERY INVOLVED
Anteroseptal	V_1-V_2	Proximal left anterior descending (LAD), septal perforators
Anteroapical	V_2-V_4	LAD or its branches
Anterolateral	V_4-V_6, I, aVL	Mid-LAD or circumflex
Extensive anterior	V_1-V_6	Proximal LAD
High lateral	I, aVL	Circumflex
Inferior	II, III, aVF	Right coronary; less often circumflex or distal LAD
Posterior	Mirror image in V_1 and V_2 (ST depression, peaked T, tall R, loss of S waves)	Posterior descending
Right ventricular	V_1 and reversed chest leads rV_3-rV_4	Right coronary

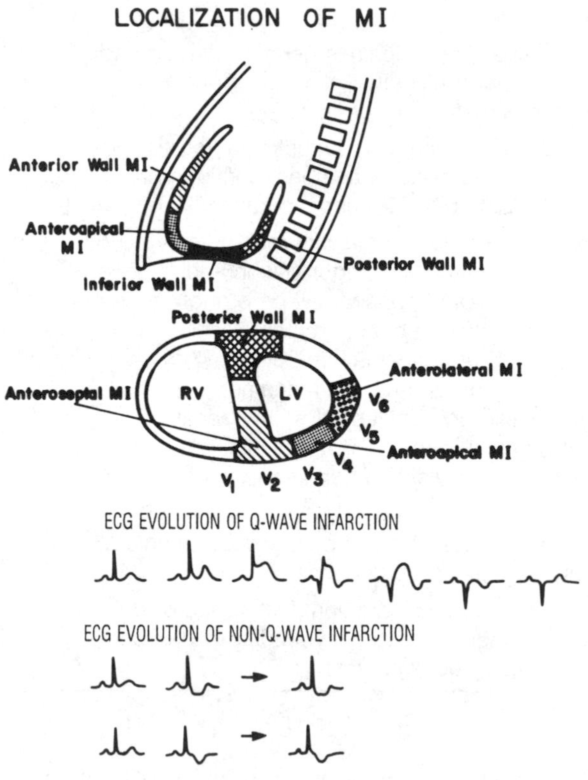

LOCALIZATION OF MI

ECG EVOLUTION OF Q-WAVE INFARCTION

ECG EVOLUTION OF NON-Q-WAVE INFARCTION

Figure 1. *Nomenclature for the localization of myocardial infarction. ECG evolution of Q-wave infarction showing development of Q waves. ECG evolution of non-Q-wave infarction showing persistent ST-T–wave abnormalities.*

line before T-wave inversion occurs, and PR-segment depression is often seen. J-point elevation seen in early repolarization, a normal variant, is sometimes confused with acute infarction, but evolutionary changes and cardiac enzyme elevations do not occur. ST-segment depression and T-wave changes from left ventricular hypertrophy, digitalis, hypokalemia, hyperventilation and many other conditions may suggest ischemia (Marriott). Q waves are found without infarction in patients with bypass tracts, hypertrophic cardiomyopathy, and dilated cardiomyopathy, as well as chronic lung disease and neuromuscular disorders (Goldberger). Likewise, the typical changes of infarction may be masked by other ECG abnormalities, particularly left (but not right) bundle branch block.

It has been traditional to equate ST elevation with transmural myocardial injury, ST depression with subendocardial ischemia, and development of Q waves with transmural necrosis of myocardium. While these concepts are clinically useful, the actual situation is more complex. For example, development of transient Q waves has been documented after reversible ischemia and following thrombolytic therapy (Bateman et al.). In particular, it has been appreciated that anatomically transmural infarction may not lead to Q waves on ECG, and that many nontransmural infarctions *do* manifest Q waves on the surface ECG, usually when they encompass >50% of the thickness of the ventricular wall (Raunio et al.). Thus, the terms Q wave and non-Q-wave infarction should be used clinically, and transmural or nontransmural applied pathologically.

LABORATORY DIAGNOSIS

Determination of serum levels of enzymes released from damaged myocytes is crucial to the diagnosis of myocardial infarction. Each enzyme has its own time course, use and limitations. Enzyme tests are the subject of excellent reviews (Lee and Goldman; Puleo and Roberts).

1) *Creatine kinase (CK)* is present in high concentration in muscle cells. Serum levels rise within 6–8 hours after onset of infarction, peak within 24 hours, and return to normal within 48–96 hours. Peak level is higher and occurs earlier (8–12 hours) when coronary reperfusion is achieved. Peak and duration of elevation are increased in larger infarcts but peak level does not correlate with infarct size following reperfusion, due to enzyme "washout." Total CK rises after any type of muscle trauma, such as intramuscular injections or rhabdomyolysis, as well as in hypothyroidism, renal failure or stroke. CK is optimally sampled on admission, then 12 hours and 24 hours later.

2) The *MB isoenzyme of CK* is currently the enzymatic mainstay in the diagnosis of myocardial infarction. It is found only in minute amounts in noncardiac tissues, and does not increase following skeletal muscle trauma. Its levels rise and peak slightly earlier than the total CK, and normalize in 36–72 hours. The usual electrophoretic assay reliably detects levels >5 IU/ml, but optimum specificity is achieved when a cutoff of 5% of total CK or 13 IU/ml is used. The subset of patients (15–20%) with elevated CK-MB but normal total CK should be considered to have myocardial infarction if a typical rise and fall in total CK levels is seen and clinical presentation is compatible, as mortality risk is increased in such patients (Hong et al.; White et al. 1985). Cardiac release of CK-MB may occur with peri-myocarditis, defibrillation, cardiac surgery, cardiac contusion, or prolonged severe ischemia without infarction. Elevations of CK-MB have also been noted in myopathies, hypothyroidism, and following strenuous exercise. False-positive tests sometimes occur in the setting of chronic renal failure, rhabdomyolysis, isoenzyme variants, or with some immunoassay methods which detect BB isoenzyme from CNS and kidney.

3) *Lactate dehydrogenase (LDH)* and its five isoenzymes rise within 24–48 hours of infarction, peak in 3–5 days and persist for 7–10 days. LDH is present ubiquitously and rises in muscle, liver, and hematologic disorders. A ratio of LDH_1/LDH_2 of >1.0 (or 0.76 if lower specificity is acceptable) is relatively specific for myocardial necrosis, although hemolysis also raises LDH_1. LDH isoenzymes are useful when CK-MB is negative and infarction is believed to have occurred at least 2–4 days earlier.

4) *Serum glutamic oxaloacetic transferase (SGOT)* is another nonspecific marker for myocyte necrosis, peaking 48–72 hours after infarction. It is of little or no clinical utility.

5) Assays for the three *isoforms of CK-MM* are becoming available. The MM_3 isoform appears and disappears earlier than the other isoforms, and earlier than MB; it could ultimately prove to be of value in assessing reperfusion, infarct extension, and postoperative infarction.

6) *Myoglobin* appears and disappears in serum and urine very early in infarction, and peaks in 3–20 hours. Its place in clinical practice is unclear, but it might have a potential role in very early diagnosis of infarction.

7) Other laboratory abnormalities are associated with acute MI. Marked hyperglycemia or ketoacidosis are common in diabetics, are sometimes the only symptoms of myocardial infarction, and can occur even in non-insulin-requiring or borderline diabetics. Leukocytosis, sometimes with increased band forms, may persist for up to a week. Serum lipids are altered variably and do not accurately reflect the true profile for weeks after myocardial infarction.

CHEST X-RAY

The chest roentgenogram is of value in the initial assessment of the myocardial infarction patient, but has limitations (see also Chapter 4). Cardiomegaly, when present, could indicate pre-existing heart disease which has led to ventricular dilatation. When pulmonary artery wedge pressure is acutely ≥16 mm Hg, pulmonary vascular redistribution is noted, and interstitial and alveolar edema become manifest above wedge pressures of 22–25 mm Hg. Although important findings, the presence of pulmonary congestion or pulmonary edema does not always correlate with the patient's current hemodynamic status. Radiographic findings lag behind the clinical picture by up to 12 hours when the onset of heart failure has been abrupt, and persist for up to several days after failure has been treated.

RADIONUCLIDE STUDIES

In cases where the triad of history, ECG and enzymes is insufficient to confirm the diagnosis of acute MI or when infarct location is uncertain, as in association with left bundle branch block, radionuclide studies are of value. These are described in detail in Chapter 5. ^{99m}Technetium-pyrophosphate scanning is useful in this setting. The tracer binds to accumulated calcium within irreversibly damaged myocardium. Sensitivity is highest when scanning is performed between 24–72 hours after infarction, and in transmural infarcts, and is significantly lower in nontransmural infarction. Newer infarct-avid agents, particularly imaging with ^{111}indium-labeled antimyosin Fab fragments, have improved sensitivity for detecting Q-wave infarcts (Volpini), but false-positive tests have been noted in cases of dilated cardiomyopathy (Obrador et al.).

Myocardial perfusion imaging agents, ^{201}thallium and newer ^{99m}technetium isonitrile derivatives, accumulate within myocardium in proportion to regional blood flow and demonstrate and localize defects in ischemic or infarcted areas. New infarct, old infarct and persistent ischemia can not be distinguished with a single study. Thallium's most important use is in conjunction with exercise in the postinfarct assessment of inducible ischemia. Radionuclide angiography with ^{99m}Tc-labeled red blood cells can localize and quantify areas of left or right ventricular wall motion abnormality and global ventricular function, which is related to prognosis.

Positron emission tomography (PET), since it reflects regional myocardial metabolism and uptake of glucose and fatty acids, as well as regional blood flow, has provided exciting insights into the pathophysiology of myocardial infarction and reperfusion not available by other modalities. It holds great promise in the differentiation of stunned or hibernating myocardium from infarcted myocardium, infarct sizing, and diagnosis of residual ischemia following infarction. Development of longer-lived radionuclides and nuclides not requiring a cyclotron for production may allow dissemination of this technique beyond a few research centers.

ECHOCARDIOGRAPHY

Two-dimensional and Doppler echocardiography is of considerable value in the diagnosis of essentially all the complications of acute MI (Kloner and Parisi; Feigenbaum), and can provide prognostic information as well (see Chapters 7 and 8). A regional wall motion abnormality can be demonstrated in nearly all patients with acute MI, and the location and extent of infarction and degree of left and right ventricular dysfunction can be reliably assessed. Echocardiography is an essential aid in the diagnosis of the mechanical complications of myocardial infarction, including papillary muscle rupture, ventricular septal rupture, ventricular aneurysm and pseudoaneurysm, ventricular mural thrombus, pericardial effusion, and infarct expansion. Newer uses include tissue characterization, visualization of coronary artery lumina, and detection of return of wall motion following reperfusion.

OTHER STUDIES

Magnetic resonance imaging (MRI) of the cardiovascular system is being recognized as valuable in a variety of disease states. With gated cine images, ventricular volumes, global and regional wall motion, and ventricular mass can be assessed accurately. Infarcted and viable myocardium can be distinguished and infarct size estimated (Johnson et al.). Flow imaging allowing visualization of flow velocities, and perfusion imaging using tracers hold promise as well. The need to transport patients limits MRI's use in the critically ill, however. The full potential of this modality and its role in routine clinical practice remain to be fully explored (see also Chapter 11).

PATHOLOGY AND PATHOGENESIS OF MYOCARDIAL INFARCTION

Most myocardial infarctions occur in the territory of an atherosclerotic coronary artery, when plaque disruption leads to platelet aggregation, thrombus formation and spasm, causing acute reduction of blood flow and myocardial ischemia. When ischemia is sufficiently severe and prolonged, infarction results. Because therapeutic interventions in modern cardiology are increasingly directed toward modifying the cellular and molecular events of ischemia and infarction, a sound understanding of these events is important.

Within seconds of coronary artery occlusion, cellular metabolism shifts to anaerobic glycolysis. Contraction ceases and high energy stores of creatine phosphate, then ATP, become depleted (Jennings and Reimer). Eventually, injury becomes irreversible, proceeding as a wavefront of cell death from subendocardium toward subepicardium (Reimer and Jennings), and culminating in a transmural infarct. The duration of ischemia necessary for completion of cell death averages from 2 to 6 hours in experimental studies; it may be longer in vivo if infarction progresses in a "stuttering" fashion. The rate of necrosis and infarct size is determined by 1) the size of the coronary bed, 2) the amount of collateral flow and residual antegrade flow to the ischemic region, and 3) how soon reperfusion occurs, if at all. An intervention that lessens cardiac work and heart rate during ischemia (for example, a beta blocker or negative inotropic drug) might delay the rate of progression of necrosis but does not limit ultimate infarct size if there is no reperfusion.

In the absence of reperfusion, light microscopic evidence of cellular injury is first seen within 6–8 hours. Mild white cell infiltration begins at the edge of the infarct within 12 hours, and by 24 hours, clear myocyte disruption and coagulative necrosis are evident. Mononuclear cell infiltration and myocyte removal begin by the fourth day, making the infarct susceptible to expansion or rupture. Collagen deposition begins at the periphery after 10–12 days, and healing with dense scar formation is essentially complete in four to six weeks in all but very large infarcts (Waller).

When reperfusion occurs early in the course of infarction, a different sequence of events ensues. Restoration of flow of oxygenated blood leads to large increases in tissue water, sodium, and calcium, and explosive disruption of irreversibly injured myocytes, which are unable to regulate their cell volume. Salvage of ischemic but viable myocardial cells occurs in the mid-myocardial and subepicardial layers of the ventricular wall, often resulting in a subendocardial infarction. Ventricular arrhythmias often increase, white cell infiltration is accelerated, and intramural hemorrhage occurs within the infarct zone. Pharmaco-

logic interventions aimed at blunting such effects could potentially enhance the myocardial salvage that occurs with reperfusion (Braunwald and Kloner).

The onset of severe ischemia leads initially to increased diastolic stiffness and elevation of end-diastolic pressure. The involved wall becomes akinetic or dyskinetic and compromises systolic function, although compensatory hyperkinesis of the remaining myocardium preserves global function acutely in smaller infarcts. Greater losses of functioning myocardium lead to progressively more severe ventricular dysfunction, with subsequent dilatation and remodeling due to abnormal wall stress within the infarcted segment. In general, infarction of >10% of ventricular mass leads to reduction in ejection fraction; to dilatation and congestive failure when ≥25% is lost; and to cardiogenic shock or death with loss of ≥40%, whether the loss occurs from a single or multiple insults.

PATHOPHYSIOLOGY OF CORONARY THROMBOSIS

Coronary angiography early in acute myocardial infarction (deFeyter et al.), and angioscopy (Forrester et al. 1987), have provided a great deal of insight into the complex events that occur within an infarct-related coronary artery. Acute thrombotic occlusion is found in 80–90% of cases of Q-wave infarction studied within 4–6 hours of onset, and in fewer non-Q-wave infarcts (DeWood et al. 1980, 1986). Coronary occlusion is usually the result of instability of an underlying atherosclerotic plaque and its dynamic interaction with mediators of vascular tone, platelets, and the clotting cascade, as shown in simplified form in Figure 2. Fissuring, rupture or hemorrhage into an atheromatous plaque (Davies and Thomas) appears to often be the initiating event, exposing collagen, atheroma, and tissue thromboplastins to circulating platelets and clotting factors. Platelet aggregation further promotes thrombosis and leads to vasoconstriction via release of thromboxane A_2, thus overwhelming endogenous vasodilators such as prostacyclin and endothelial derived relaxation factor. Luminal obstruction results from the combination of atheromatous plaque, intraluminal thrombus, platelets, and variable degrees of spasm.

A totally occluding thrombus is the usual proximate cause of myocardial infarction; when subtotal, unstable angina is more often the result. Spontaneous thrombolysis occurs in one third to one half of infarct-

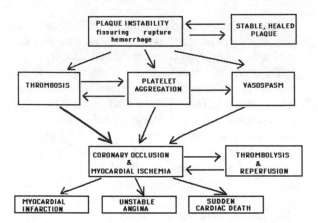

Figure 2. Pathogenic mechanisms in unstable coronary syndromes.

related arteries over hours to days following infarction. Non-Q-wave infarction is often the result of such spontaneous lysis, although such an infarct may also result from an initially subtotal occlusion or a transmural infarct that fails to produce a Q wave. Clot lysis leaves behind a fixed stenosis of varying severity and unstable morphology which is prone to reocclusion or may heal with incorporation of thrombus and progression of stenosis.

NON-ATHEROSCLEROTIC ETIOLOGIES

A wide variety of disorders other than atherosclerosis can occasionally lead to myocardial infarction; these account for a few percent of cases, and are shown in Table 3 (Cheitlin et al.). Vasculitides have been reported to produce coronary occlusion, including lupus erythematosus, polyarteritis nodosa, and Kawasaki disease (which leads to the late sequela of coronary artery aneurysm). Coronary anomalies, emboli, hypercoagulable states and aortic diseases involving the coronary arteries also cause myocardial infarction on occasion. Myocardial infarction sometimes occurs in persons with normal coronaries without evidence of any of these disorders, usually heavy smokers or cocaine users.

Myocardial infarction and sudden death associated with cocaine use have been increasingly recognized. The mechanisms are not fully defined, but coronary spasm, often with resultant thrombus formation, is most likely (Frishman et al; Isner et al. 1986). It was recently reported that intranasal cocaine caused vasoconstriction of coronary arteries and reduced coronary blood flow, actions which appeared to be

Table 3. Causes of Myocardial Infarction Without Coronary Atherosclerosis

Vasculitis
   Systemic lupus erythematosus
   Polyarteritis nodosa
   Takayasu's arteritis
   Mucocutaneous lymph node syndrome
   Luetic aortitis
Anomalous Origin of Coronary Artery
Acquired Coronary Artery Abnormalities
   Trauma
   Aortic dissection
   Coronary artery dissection
   Iatrogenic
Coronary Spasm
   Variant angina
   Cocaine abuse
   Nitroglycerin withdrawal
Coronary Artery Embolus
   Infective endocarditis
   Mitral valve prolapse
   Atrial myxoma
   Atrial or ventricular thrombus
Hypercoagulable States
   Polycythemia vera
   Thrombocytosis

mediated by alpha-adrenergic stimulation (Lange et al.). A direct effect on myocardium has also been implicated (Karch and Billingham), and arterial intimal hyperplasia has been reported in a few cases. Coronary arteriography and ergonovine testing is usually normal, and recurrent infarction can occur with continued drug use.

REPERFUSION THERAPY FOR MYOCARDIAL INFARCTION

Since the 1960s, management of the patient with known or suspected myocardial infarction has focused on early prehospital supportive care and CCU monitoring. This has reduced the mortality associated with acute MI by one half or more, almost entirely due to treatment of primary ventricular arrhythmias (Killip and Kimball; Goldman). However, most sudden deaths still occur before medical attention is sought. Mortality due to pump failure and cardiogenic shock, which are related to infarct size, has not been appreciably altered by such conventional therapy, and pharmacologic limitation of infarct size has proved disappointing (Rude et al.). However, with the recognition of the importance of thrombosis in the pathogenesis of myocardial infarction, and the wide availability of thrombolytic drugs, there has been a paradigm shift in the treatment of myocardial infarction toward a primary goal of minimizing infarct size.

THE FIBRINOLYTIC SYSTEM

Under normal circumstances, the endogenous fibrinolytic system is responsible for the dynamic equilibrium between thrombosis and thrombolysis. When fibrin is formed and polymerized into thrombus, circulating plasminogen is bound to it. Locally produced tissue plasminogen activator (TPA) eventually induces clot-specific lysis by cleaving this bound plasminogen to its active form, plasmin, which specifically degrades fibrin to degradation products. This process remains localized because of the selectivity of TPA for fibrin-bound rather than unbound circulating plasminogen (fibrin specificity), the relative specificity of plasmin for fibrin rather than fibrinogen, and plasminogen activator inhibitor. However, if plasmin is activated in the systemic circulation, circulating fibrinogen is degraded as well, leading to a hemorrhagic state brought on by fibrinogen depletion and fibrin/fibrinogen degradation products with anticoagulant and platelet inhibiting properties. A systemic lytic state may lead to bleeding at any site, but dissolution of hemostatic plugs in wounds and puncture sites and arterial thrombi in coronary and cerebral vessels occurs whether the agent employed is fibrin-specific or not. Thus, the incidence of serious bleeding at catheterization sites (which accounts for most bleeding episodes in thrombolytic patients) and intracranial hemorrhage does not differ among the agents available for intravenous use.

Commercially available fibrinolytic drugs act at different points in this schema. Recombinant single-chain tissue plasminogen activator (rt-PA) maintains the same relative fibrin specificity of the native protein, although at the massive intravenous doses used clinically, a mild lytic state can be observed. Streptokinase (SK), a bacterial protease, combines with both fibrin-bound and circulating plasminogen to form an active complex which activates other plasminogen and leads to degradation of both fibrin and fibrinogen. Anisoylated plasminogen-streptokinase activator complex (APSAC, also known as anistreplase) is ini-

tially inactive, binds to fibrin, and is then deacylated to the active complex. This confers some fibrin specificity at low doses, but fibrinogenolysis equal to streptokinase occurs at the doses used for coronary thrombolysis. Urokinase (UK) activates plasminogen directly. It is not antigenic and produces a slightly less severe lytic state than does streptokinase. Its inactive precursor, called pro-urokinase (pro-UK) or single-chain urokinase plasminogen activator (scu-PA), is converted to urokinase by plasmin. Both agents have some degree of fibrin specificity. Newer agents under development will ideally maintain high degrees of fibrin specificity and fibrinolytic efficacy.

THROMBOLYTIC THERAPY

The clinical and pharmacologic features of thrombolytic regimens that have undergone clinical trials are compared in Table 4. Streptokinase and APSAC, being antigenic, induce hypotension with rapid infusion, occasional allergic phenomena, and antibody-mediated resistance if the agent is administered a second time within three to six months. Systemic fibrinogenolysis, as expected, is severe with SK, APSAC and UK, lasting from 12–36 hours; it is mild and usually clinically insignificant with rt-PA. Agents differ in circulating half-life, being very brief with rt-PA and scu-PA (though activity at the site of thrombus may be longer), and more prolonged with other agents. Accordingly, it is currently recommended that a 100-mg dose of rt-PA be given as an initial bolus of 10 mg and then an infusion to provide a total of 60 mg in the first hour for a rapid lytic effect; and 20 mg/hr for 2 successive hours, with full anticoagulation initiated prior to the end of the infusion. Urokinase and APSAC can be given as an intravenous bolus, and SK is given over 1 hour to avoid hypotension; anticoagulation is delayed 4–8 hours to prevent excess bleeding. Shorter half-life and absence of a prolonged lytic state may explain the higher rate of reocclusion noted especially with shorter infusions of rt-PA; prolonged maintenance infusion reduces this problem.

Intracoronary thrombolysis achieves vessel patency in 70–75% of patients; since the total thrombolytic dose is lower, there is a less severe lytic state produced, and patency is achieved typically within 30 minutes. Intravenous fibrinolytic agents have somewhat lower efficacy; for SK, patency rate (assessed at end of infusion) is 50–60%; for UK and APSAC, it is in the 60–70% range. Efficacy of SK and APSAC

Table 4. Comparison of Thrombolytic Agents						
Thrombolytic Agent	IC SK	IV SK	APSAC	UK	SCU-PA	rt-PA
Half Life (min)	—	23	90	16	7	5
Systemic lytic state	1+	4+	4+	3+	2+	1+
Dose: Bolus	none	none	30 mg	2,000,000 U	?	10 mg
Infusion	1 hr	1 hr	—	—		3 hr*
Total dose	160,000 U	1,500,000 U	30 mg	2,000,000 U		100 mg
Reperfusion rate (%)	70-75	50-60	60-70	60	60-70	65-75
Reocclusion rate (%)	20	15	10	10	NA	20
Antigenicity	yes	yes	yes	no	no	no
Simultaneous heparin	no	no	no	no	yes	yes
Cost per dose	—	$93	$1700	$2200	NA	$2330

IC SK = intracoronary streptokinase; IV SK = intravenous steptokinase; APSAC = anisoylated plasminogen streptokinase activator complex; U = urokinase; SCU-PA = single chain urokinase plasminogen activator (prourokinase); rt-PA = recombinant tissue-type plasminogen activator (single and double chain). Reperfusion rate assessed at 90 minutes following infusion, if agent given within 4 hours. Lytic state is arbitrary scale, 1+ to 4+. Cost is September 1989 AMFAC average wholesale price. NA = data not available. *See text.

Adapted from Marder and Sherry. See Bibliography.

depends upon how long after MI onset they are given. In the TIMI-I trial, patency with SK was achieved in 50% of arteries when given within 3 hours after symptom onset, but in substantially fewer when given later. Vessel patency is highest with rt-PA, equal to that of intracoronary therapy, and does not diminish when given later. With all intravenous agents, successful reperfusion typically requires 45 minutes of treatment.

Restoration of coronary flow is often associated with a decrease in ST-segment elevation (sometimes to normal), marked improvement or resolution of chest pain, and increased incidence of arrhythmias. These arrhythmias include increased numbers of ventricular premature beats, ventricular tachycardia or fibrillation, paroxysmal sinus bradycardia, AV block, or accelerated idioventricular rhythm (Goldberg et al. 1983). Accelerated idioventricular rhythm, in particular, has been considered characteristic of reperfusion. However, these "indicators" of reperfusion are not able to discriminate between patients who have and have not reperfused with enough accuracy to be clinically useful (Califf, Topol et al. 1988), except in the small minority of patients with complete resolution of ST-segment elevation within 90 minutes of treatment.

Selection of patients for thrombolytic therapy involves weighing the anticipated benefits against the risk of serious adverse effects of treatment for a given patient. Thus, patient selection is somewhat individualized and indications continue to evolve. However, general guidelines can be offered.

Patients to be considered for thrombolytic therapy have chest pain lasting longer than 30 minutes, not relieved by nitroglycerin, and associated with ST-segment elevation (in order to distinguish the pain from unstable angina and variant angina). More than 80% of patients meeting these criteria will have a completely occluded infarct-related artery at initial presentation. Thrombolytic therapy in patients with ST-depression infarcts and in unstable angina is currently investigational, and may be less effective (Ambrose and Alexopoulos), since coronary occlusion is more often subtotal in these cases.

Patients with anterior infarctions have shown the greatest survival benefit from thrombolysis, while inferior infarcts have failed to show benefit in many of the clinical trials (since smaller infarct size and low mortality makes it difficult to demonstrate improved survival). However, preservation of ventricular function occurs regardless of infarct site, and mortality reduction does occur in larger inferior infarcts, such as when posterior or lateral extension or reciprocal precordial ST depression is present. Thus, all patients with acute ST-elevation infarcts are potential candidates.

Table 5. Contraindications to Thrombolytic Therapy

Absolute

  Major trauma or surgery within two months
  History of cerebrovascular accident or tumor
  Active internal bleeding
  Severe uncontrolled hypertension
  Active peptic ulcer disease
  Puncture of a non-compressible vessel

Relative

  Age over 75
  History of any cerebral pathology
  Prolonged cardiopulmonary resuscitation
  Impaired hemostasis
  History of peptic ulcer disease
  Hemorrhagic diabetic retinopathy

The time from onset of infarction to initiation of treatment is critical in determining whether any benefit will be derived from thrombolytic treatment. Consistent with experimental models, clinical trials demonstrate the greatest benefit in patients treated within the first 2 hours after infarction. Those treated within 4 hours uniformly demonstrate benefit in most studies, and when treatment is given from 4–6 hours after MI onset, treatment benefit is reduced, although present. Late treatment, from 6–12 and even up to 24 hours after onset, has not translated into clinical benefit in most studies except the ISIS-2 trial. However, in cases where an infarct is "stuttering," late treatment may be justified, and it has theoretical benefits that may not be detectable until further trials are conducted.

Contraindications to thrombolytic therapy, listed in Table 5, include any condition predisposing to major bleeding complications. Hypertension can usually be rapidly controlled, but otherwise would contraindicate thrombolytic therapy. A history of cerebral ischemia particularly predisposes to bleeding and is a strong contraindication. Cardiopulmonary resuscitation would not lead to increased bleeding risk if it was brief (< 1 minute) and without significant trauma.

Major bleeding, especially cerebral bleeding, is the most serious complication of thrombolytic therapy. While fibrin-specific agents produce little systemic lytic effect, major bleeding complications due to disruption of hemostatic plugs at the sites of invasive procedures, in the CNS, and elsewhere, are no less

likely. In studies where invasive procedures are employed in the study protocol, bleeding episodes occur in most patients, and bleeding requiring transfusion occurs in 11–30% (TAMI, TIMI-I). Administration of heparin simultaneously with infusion of the thrombolytic agent also predisposes to excessive bleeding without improving efficacy. When invasive procedures are minimized, bleeding episodes are uncommon; the incidence of any bleeding episodes can be expected to be 3.5–5% (GISSI, ISIS-2) with bleeding requiring transfusion in 0.3–0.5%. Intracerebral bleeding has varied in incidence, from 0.1% and 0.2% in the ISIS-2 and GISSI trials, respectively, to 0.5% in the TIMI-II trial among patients receiving 100 mg rt-PA and 1.9% in the subset of patients treated with 150 mg rt-PA. Hypertension, advanced age and previous cerebrovascular disease are potent risk factors for intracerebral hemorrhage, which is usually catastrophic when it occurs. In ISIS-2 and other trials, the incidence of stroke in control and treated patients was equal, because while intracranial hemorrhage increased with treatment, thrombotic and embolic stroke was reduced.

Reocclusion, reinfarction, and recurrent ischemia after thrombolytic therapy are significant complications of treatment. Studies using repeat angiography have demonstrated reocclusion of initially reperfused arteries in about 20% of patients with intracoronary SK and 10–15% with intravenous SK, though this varies markedly between studies. The reocclusion rate may be slightly higher, about 20%, with rt-PA. Longer maintenance infusion of the drug (Johns et al.) or combinations of thrombolytic agents may be effective in reducing residual intraluminal thrombus, reocclusion, and recurrent ischemia. The incidence of recurrent infarction in the TIMI-II trial was 6%; 4% in the GISSI trial (which was twice that found in untreated controls); and even lower in the ISAM trial, where routine anticoagulation was used. Recurrent angina occurs in 15–25% of patients following thrombolytic therapy, and was not more frequent in treated than control patients in several studies including GISSI. The incidences of reinfarction and recurrent angina are higher in the subgroup of patients who have been successfully reperfused. It is clear, however, that many reocclusions are either silent or associated with angina rather than reinfarction.

There is no doubt that thrombolytic therapy reduces mortality from myocardial infarction. Hospital mortality is reduced by 35–50%, and further still in patients treated within 2 hours, those with anterior infarctions, younger patients, and when antiplatelet therapy is also given. The survival benefit is maintained after discharge and correlates with infarct artery patency. Conversely, unsuccessful thrombolysis or failure to maintain arterial patency is associated with increased mortality.

Thrombolytic therapy has beneficial effects on global and regional left ventricular function, which is a crucial issue since ventricular function after infarction is a powerful determinant of long-term survival and is the presumed mechanism of mortality benefit from thrombolysis. Such improvements, however, have been difficult to demonstrate, since considerable variability in ventricular function is common in the first days of infarction. Spontaneous reperfusion, collateral blood flow, and subtotal occlusion may lead to preservation of ventricular function, while functional deterioration is associated with persistent total occlusion (Blanke et al.; deFeyter et al.) or with waning of initial compensatory hyperkinesis. After reperfusion, regional wall motion may not improve if there is an underlying severe stenosis or prolonged postischemic dysfunction ("stunning"); the latter can persist for 3–10 days. With these limitations, it is understandable that ventricular function may fail to improve when measured early after thrombolytic therapy. To date, three trials of rt-PA, one with APSAC and one with SK demonstrated improved ejection fraction at discharge after thrombolysis; patients with inferior as well as anterior infarcts showed benefit, and the incidence of congestive heart failure was reduced (Guerci et al.). Likewise, patients having coronary balloon angioplasty after thrombolysis in the TAMI-1 trial showed improved ventricular function with both anterior and inferior infarcts (Bates et al.).

It was initially believed that thrombolysis was acting to "convert" Q-wave into non-Q-wave infarcts, with lower short-term mortality but a high incidence of recurrent ischemia and late reinfarction, which would mandate aggressive intervention in all cases. This has not, however, turned out to be true in all cases. Plaque instability and residual thrombus will lead to reocclusion in some patients, but plaque healing occurs in many, leaving behind a stable lesion and a fixed stenosis varying from insignificant to severe in obstruction. Likelihood of reocclusion and recurrent angina depends to a large extent on how severe this underlying stenosis is, and patients having angina before infarction are more likely to have a severe underlying stenosis (Matsuda et al.). Such considerations have led to the investigation of expectant or "noninvasive" strategies after thrombolysis.

CLINICAL TRIALS OF THROMBOLYTIC THERAPY

There have been dozens of randomized and nonrandomized clinical trials of thrombolytic therapy published, and many more are in progress. Understanding the lessons of each major trial is important to grasping the basis for current recommendations and their limitations. There are many excellent in-depth reviews of such trials (O'Neill et al. 1988; Marder and Sherry; Wasserman and Ross) to which the reader is encouraged to refer.

Early trials of intracoronary SK with small numbers of patients established that patency rates of 70–75% could be achieved, and that efficacy was strongly time-dependent. No survival benefit could be demonstrated, however, unless results of multiple trials were pooled (Yusuf et al. 1985). The exception was the Western Washington trial (Kennedy et al. 1983) which showed improved survival in treated patients at one month and persisting at one year in the subgroup with patent infarct arteries (Kennedy et al. 1985). Intravenous thrombolysis, first with SK then with other agents, was then studied. With larger numbers of patients enrolled and treatment given earlier, significantly improved survival has been demonstrated repeatedly, averaging 35–50% mortality reduction.

The Italian Group for the Study of Streptokinase in Myocardial Infarction trial (GISSI 1986, 1987) enrolled nearly 12,000 patients within 12 hours of onset of symptoms. Mortality was reduced from 12% to 9% in patients treated within 3 hours. A striking 47% decrease in mortality occurred in patients receiving treatment within 1 hour. Benefit was also seen with treatment up to 6 hours, and a trend toward benefit from 6 to 9 hours; benefit persisted at one year follow-up. Subgroup analysis in this study could not show statistically significant survival benefit in patients over age 65 or those with inferior infarction, however.

The TIMI trials compared various strategies for administration of thrombolytic therapy. The phase I trial (Chesebro et al.) compared intravenous SK with rt-PA, after angiography to document an occluded infarct artery, in patients with symptoms of less than 7 hours duration. Reperfusion occurred in 62% of those treated with rt-PA and in 31% of SK treated patients. The much reduced efficacy of streptokinase after 3 hours of symptoms was demonstrated; even when SK was given in less than 3 hours, the reperfusion rate was only 47%. Bleeding complications were comparable between the groups and were frequent at catheterization sites. At 12-month follow-up, mortality was comparable between the groups; mortality was lower in patients with successful reperfusion and sustained arterial patency (Dalen et al.).

The role of immediate angioplasty was then studied in the TIMI phase IIA trial. Patients received thrombolysis within 4 hours of infarction with rt-PA followed either by immediate (2 hours) or delayed (18–48 hours) catheterization and angioplasty (TIMI 1988). Patients having delayed angioplasty had lower bleeding rates, transfusion requirements, need for emergent bypass surgery, and overall adverse clinical event rate. Mortality, arterial patency at discharge, and ventricular function were equal in both groups. It was concluded that immediate angioplasty after thrombolysis as a routine strategy is not necessary and increases complication rates. The European Cooperative Study Group (Simoons et al.), using a similar study design, reached the same conclusion and noted increased mortality as well in the immediate angioplasty group. The TAMI-1 trial (Topol et al. 1987), which randomized patients after successful thrombolysis, was also unable to show a benefit with immediate compared to delayed (7-10 days) angioplasty. In addition, 14% of patients in the delayed group no longer had a significant stenosis by seven days, thus obviating the need for angioplasty.

This strategy was then compared to a "noninvasive" strategy in the TIMI-IIB study (TIMI 1989), involving 3,262 patients. Following thrombolysis, patients received either catheterization at 18–48 hours with angioplasty of suitable lesions, as before (invasive group), or catheterization and angioplasty only if spontaneous or exercise-induced ischemia recurred (noninvasive group). Thirty-three percent of the noninvasively treated patients required cardiac catheterization, and 13% had angioplasty. The noninvasive patients had fewer transfusions, less emergency bypass surgery following angioplasty, and fewer adverse end points than the invasively treated patients, but also had more positive treadmill exercise tests at discharge. Reinfarction, death and ventricular function were comparable between groups. It was concluded that the strategy of deferring angiography and revascularization for spontaneous or inducible is-

chemia does not subject the patient to increased risk of death or reinfarction, and involves fewer complications and reduced cost.

The Second International Study of Infarct Survival (ISIS-2, 1988) was a massive study involving 17,187 patients randomized to treatment with SK, aspirin, both, or neither commencing up to 24 hours after symptom onset; some of the patients undoubtedly had non-Q infarctions or unstable angina. Mortality was reduced 25% by aspirin or SK alone, and 42% by the combination. Remarkably, survival benefit was evident even when treatment began 13–24 hours after admission. Aspirin given alone prevented reinfarction and eliminated the increased reinfarction rate noted in SK-treated patients, without increasing the incidence of serious bleeding. The implications of the ISIS-2 study are profound. The important adjuvant role of aspirin has been convincingly demonstrated, and the trial lends the first firm support to the concept that even delayed reperfusion may be beneficial.

The ASSET (Anglo-Scandinavian Study of Early Thrombolysis, Wilcox 1988) gave rt-PA or placebo plus heparin to 5,011 patients with suspected infarction, and observed a 26% mortality reduction; even those with a normal ECG had a trend toward reduced mortality. Convincing mortality reductions have been demonstrated in most but not all of the large studies. The earlier Intravenous Streptokinase in Acute Myocardial Infarction (ISAM 1986; Schroder et al.) trial failed to show either early or late improvement in survival with SK, and reinfarction rates were increased. Differences may have been obscured, however, because mortality was low in both groups.

Trials with APSAC have shown thrombolytic efficacy with this agent approaching that of intracoronary streptokinase (Anderson et al.). Reocclusion and complication rates are comparable to those of streptokinase, although hypotension occurs less often and is less severe. Improved mortality and preservation of ventricular function have been confirmed (AIMS; Bassand et al.).

When initiation of thrombolytic therapy is delayed more than 6 hours after symptom onset, infarct size limitation, mortality reduction, and preservation of ventricular function have not generally been demonstrated in randomized trials. This is consistent with animal data showing little salvage of myocardium when reperfusion is delayed more than 3 hours. Late treatment may be considered on a case-by-case basis for patients with intermittent or recurrent symptoms, on the supposition that the presence of ongoing pain indicates the presence of ischemic but viable myocardium. The ISIS-2 trial was the first to show mortality reduction in the subgroup of patients treated late. Along with the Western Washington trial, showing marked mortality benefit in spite of no improvement in ventricular function, the possibility is raised that there are other mechanisms by which delayed reperfusion may be beneficial. Myocardium supplied by collateral vessels or at infarct borders may be salvaged by late reperfusion and can lead to some preservation of ventricular function (Rentrop et al.). It is possible that having a persistently patent artery or a rim of viable subepicardial myocardium, though not preserving ejection fraction, may reduce late mortality by preventing infarct expansion (Hochman and Choo), left ventricular remodeling (Hale and Kloner), and aneurysm formation, analogous to the beneficial effects of spontaneous thrombolysis and collateral blood flow (Braunwald 1989). Furthermore, a patent artery increases potential collateral blood flow to other diseased vessels. Incidence of late arrhythmias may be reduced in some patients as well (Sager et al.). Multicenter trials to address some of these issues are now in progress.

The choice of thrombolytic agent in a given circumstance is an unresolved issue. Clinical trials, including side-by-side comparisons of rt-PA and SK have shown higher initial patency rates with rt-PA, although patency rates at discharge are equal. Pooled results of smaller trials suggest that this might translate into greater mortality reduction and preservation of ventricular function with rt-PA (Tiefenbrunn and Sobel); the ongoing GISSI-II and ISIS-3 trials address this question. Because of the extreme cost difference among the available agents, however, cost-effectiveness considerations may also enter into treatment strategies. APSAC, because of its ease of administration, offers the potential advantage of earlier thrombolysis or even prehospital thrombolysis, and may be preferred in some settings for this reason.

ANGIOPLASTY IN MYOCARDIAL INFARCTION

The use of percutaneous transluminal coronary angioplasty (PTCA) in myocardial infarction actually constitutes five different treatment strategies, each with differing indications and safety profiles, and each the subject of randomized trials. These strategies are: 1) primary revascularization by angioplasty; 2) emergent catheterization and angioplasty after thrombolytic therapy; 3) delayed, "routine" angioplasty after thrombolytic therapy; 4) deferred angioplasty, for indications of spontaneous or inducible ischemia after thrombolysis; and 5) "salvage" angioplasty after failed thrombolysis.

Primary revascularization by means of PTCA in acute MI is an attractive alternative to thrombolytic therapy when facilities can be made available in a timely manner. Direct comparison of intracoronary SK with primary angioplasty (O'Neill et al. 1986) demonstrated equal rates of reperfusion, greater improvement of ventricular function, a reocclusion rate of 12%, and less residual stenosis with PTCA. Overall, patency is achieved in 80–90% of cases. In uncontrolled series, early and late mortality is comparable to that seen in patients given thrombolytic therapy (Rothbaum et al.) but markedly increases in patients with advanced age or severe ventricular dysfunction, and increases threefold among those failing PTCA. Compared to elective angioplasty, the rate of reocclusion is higher with emergent angioplasty, but the rate of restenosis may be lower than with elective angioplasty (Simonton et al.), and bleeding risk is minimal compared to thrombolysis. Primary angioplasty, however, is limited to those facilities, estimated to be approximately 8% of hospitals, where catheterization and bypass surgery are immediately available; its best use is for infarction patients with contraindications to thrombolytic therapy.

In contrast, the TIMI-IIA, TAMI-1, and European Cooperative Study Group trials established convincingly that immediate angioplasty as a routine strategy after thrombolysis is of little benefit to stable patients compared with delayed PTCA, as discussed above. When ischemia recurs early after thrombolytic therapy, however, emergency angioplasty can be very effective.

Considerable experience with salvage angioplasty after failed thrombolysis has accumulated from the TAMI trials. This subset of patients in the TAMI-1 trial (Califf, Topol et al.) had a 14% mortality rate and 29% reocclusion rate, with no improvement in ejection fraction. The TAMI-2 trial of rt-PA with urokinase failed to confirm this poor outcome, however; the TAMI-5 trial further investigates the issue. The higher rate of reocclusion when angioplasty follows thrombolysis, compared to primary angioplasty, may be due to bleeding within the plaque (Waller et al.).

This problem would tend to limit the broad use of salvage angioplasty to patients in the highest-risk subsets.

Whether angioplasty is desirable for all patients with a residual stenosis after thrombolysis is less clear. The findings of the TIMI-IIB trial suggest that expectant management and conventional risk stratification are able to detect most patients at high risk after thrombolysis. The corollary of this is that not all residual lesions after thrombolysis seem to require angioplasty. This does not mean, however, that diagnostic angiography in stable patients after thrombolysis does not have value; the anatomic and prognostic information obtained is very useful even if PTCA is not performed, and it remains a reasonable practice.

CORONARY BYPASS SURGERY IN MYOCARDIAL INFARCTION

Coronary artery bypass grafting (CABG) is sometimes required in the setting of acute or recent MI. Patients with early recurrence of rest ischemia in spite of medical therapy are candidates for early surgical intervention if they have three-vessel or left main disease, or other anatomy not suitable for PTCA. Those with failed angioplasty and large areas of jeopardized myocardium or hemodynamic instability are also candidates. Those stabilized medically or having inducible but not rest ischemia may undergo bypass surgery electively. Six percent of patients in the TAMI trials underwent CABG; in the TIMI trials, 10–13% of patients, with or without delayed angioplasty, required CABG after thrombolysis, more often if immediate PTCA was performed. Although the operative mortality is increased in patients undergoing emergency surgery in the acute phase, the increased mortality appears to be limited mainly to those with poor ventricular function, congestive failure, shock, and advanced age; patients without these risk factors have reasonable operative risk (Naunheim et al.).

Primary revascularization by CABG in the first hours of infarction has also been performed with acceptable mortality rates and with long-term results better than those seen with no reperfusion (DeWood et al. 1989). While it is intriguing to consider that such therapy both limits infarct size and offers definitive revascularization, it is clearly impractical for widespread use, and its safety and effectiveness are unlikely to be equal to those of thrombolysis with PTCA in unselected patients.

ADJUNCTIVE THERAPY

Adjunctive pharmacologic therapy during and after thrombolytic therapy is an area of intense interest. Such therapy might delay the progression of myocardial necrosis in order to prolong the time window for effective thrombolysis and enhance salvage of myocardium; maneuvers to decrease afterload and heart rate, and to increase collateral blood flow, such as beta blockers and nitrates, may be useful when given before reperfusion. Adjunctive therapy might limit myocyte injury at the time of reperfusion (discussed in pathobiology section); many agents are under investigation for this purpose, including calcium channel blockers, oxygen radical scavengers, white cell inhibitors, and thromboxane antagonists, but none has shown sufficient promise to warrant clinical use. Further, pharmacologic intervention might enhance the return of function of stunned myocardium and has been shown to prevent coronary reocclusion after thrombolysis or angioplasty; antiplatelet therapy with aspirin and anticoagulation with heparin are in routine clinical use for this purpose and are discussed below.

RECOMMENDATIONS

It must be kept in mind that because of delay in seeking medical attention, contraindications to thrombolysis, or a nondiagnostic initial ECG, only a minority of patients with acute MI are candidates for thrombolytic therapy or acute revascularization—an estimated 15% (Murray et al.) to 37% (GISSI). Therapy is rapidly evolving, and changes in this situation are certain. In particular, new agents and dosing schedules, interventional strategies, and adjunctive therapies are being developed. Indications for administration of thrombolytic therapy to patients over age 70, with unstable angina and ST-depression infarcts, >6 hours after infarction, or with cardiogenic shock, remain to be defined fully.

At present it is recommended that intravenous thrombolysis be administered immediately to all patients age 70 and younger with acute MI accompanied by ST elevation who present within 6 hours of onset of symptoms, if no contraindications exist. Thrombolytic treatment for ST depression or non-Q-wave infarcts is of uncertain efficacy; treatment after 6 hours may be given on an individualized basis if symptoms have been intermittent. Treatment of older patients can be individualized also. If contraindications to IV thrombolysis exist and facilities are available, then emergent catheterization with PTCA or intracoronary thrombolysis is an effective alternative, especially with large infarcts. In the 20–30% of cases where thrombolysis is unsuccessful, emergent "salvage" PTCA might benefit selected patients, but high bleeding and reocclusion rates preclude this as a routine strategy. Delaying angioplasty of significant residual lesions for several days in stable patients reduces complications and does not increase morbidity due to recurrent ischemia. In the 15–25% of patients having spontaneous recurrent ischemia after thrombolysis, and in those having inducible ischemia before discharge, catheterization and potential revascularization are indicated. In those who remain stable and without inducible ischemia, there is evidence that conservative treatment does not subject the patient to increased short-term risk; however, routine diagnostic catheterization for all patients after thrombolysis remains a reasonable strategy.

PHARMACOLOGIC THERAPY

Every patient with acute MI, whether receiving reperfusion therapy or not, is a candidate for "conventional" therapies. These include bed rest in the first days of infarction, supplemental oxygen if hypoxemia is known or suspected, narcotics or anxiolytics if needed for uncontrolled pain or anxiety, and low-dose subcutaneous heparin for prevention of thromboembolism. Though many additional pharmacologic agents are available which could in theory be beneficial during MI, none of them can be considered standard treatment for all patients. Treatment must be individualized, based on known pathogenic mechanisms, the risks and benefits of treatment, and the results of large clinical trials.

BETA BLOCKERS

There are many published trials of beta blockade both early and late after MI. Short-term trials using IV then oral dosing beginning in the first hours of infarction have shown reductions in seven-day mortality and reinfarction rates averaging 15% (Yusuf, Collins et al. 1985; Furberg and Byington) in relatively uncomplicated patients, most of whom did not receive thrombolysis. The benefit-versus-risk of using this

therapy for all patients is controversial. Immediate and delayed initiation of beta blockade were directly compared among patients receiving thrombolytic therapy in the TIMI-IIB trial, where immediate beta blockade reduced the incidence of reinfarction and recurrent ischemia within the first six days, especially in patients receiving thrombolysis within 4 hours and those in the low-risk subset. Early and late mortality were not reduced by immediate beta blockade.

Multiple long-term trials with beta blockers (ISIS-1; BHAT) and analysis of these trials (Furberg and Byington) show unequivocal reduction in long-term mortality averaging 25%, which persists during at least three years of treatment. Both sudden and non-sudden cardiac mortality is decreased, which suggests that beta blockers exert their beneficial effect both by relief of ischemia and by preventing arrhythmias. Agents without intrinsic sympathomimetic activity are probably more effective for this purpose. Currently recommended regimens include timolol 20 mg, propranolol 180–240 mg, and metoprolol 200 mg daily in divided doses, and atenolol 100 mg daily. Contraindications include heart failure, heart block, bradycardia or obstructive lung disease.

High-risk patients, those with large infarcts or transient heart failure are the ones most likely to benefit, but are also the ones most likely to suffer side effects of treatment, particularly heart failure, which increases from 5–15% if there is a history of previous heart failure (Chadda et al.). Experience has shown, however, that most patients with compensated ventricular dysfunction tolerate beta blockade well if monitored carefully. On the other hand, the cost effectiveness of administering beta blockers to all low-risk patients has been questioned, as the incremental benefit is small. Nevertheless, beta blockade remains an effective prophylactic treatment after myocardial infarction, and is a reasonable option for most patients. If desired it can be given safely early after infarction in selected patients, and when given should be continued for at least two to three years, probably indefinitely.

NITRATES

Oral and intravenous nitrates are essential initial therapy in patients with acute myocardial ischemia, including suspected myocardial infarction, recurrent ischemia after infarction, and pulmonary congestion complicating infarction. There is no definite evidence in humans that nitrates alone can limit infarct size in the face of a persistently occluded infarct artery, but they exert potentially beneficial effects by relieving coronary spasm, increasing collateral flow, and reducing subendocardial ischemia by lowering end-diastolic pressure. Pooling of multiple small trials of IV nitrates in myocardial infarction (Yusuf, Collins et al. 1988) has shown reduced mortality in treated patients, suggesting that their broad use is justified. Intravenous nitroglycerin should be given with intensive care unit monitoring, as hypotension may occur, especially when hypovolemia or right ventricular infarction is present; therapy is then continued with oral nitrates to avoid development of tolerance.

CALCIUM CHANNEL BLOCKERS

Experimental evidence indicates potential benefits of calcium channel blockers administered early during infarction or at reperfusion (Kloner and Braunwald). Compared to the clear-cut benefit of beta blockers, however, routine treatment with calcium channel blockers does not decrease mortality after myocardial infarction (Skolnick and Frishman), even when begun very early and in conjunction with thrombolytic therapy (Erbel et al.). One short-term trial of diltiazem after non-Q-wave infarction suggested it confers a lower reinfarction rate, though mortality was not decreased (Gibson et al. 1986). A long-term diltiazem trial (Multicenter Diltiazem Postinfarction Trial) suggested that treatment was harmful in the subset of patients having pulmonary congestion or ventricular dysfunction, and beneficial in the remainder of patients, which could account for the lack of overall benefit. At present, it is not recommended that calcium antagonists be administered routinely, but only if a valid indication for their use exists, such as recurrent ischemia, hypertension, or rate control of atrial fibrillation.

ANTIPLATELET DRUGS

The value of aspirin alone and in conjunction with thrombolysis was most convincingly demonstrated in the ISIS-2 trial. An independent decrease in mortality and reinfarction was found, which was synergistic with thrombolysis, even when treatment was initiated 12–24 hours after onset of chest pain. Bleeding rate does not appear to increase with the combined therapy. Aspirin treatment is clearly beneficial in unstable angina (Lewis et al.), is probably beneficial in secondary prevention after infarction (Harker; Klimt et al.), and may reduce infarction rate in healthy men over age 50 (Physicians' Health Study). It is probable, however, that aspirin does not influence restenosis after PTCA. Thus, low-dose aspirin treatment should be initiated to infarction patients immediately on admission and be continued indefinitely thereafter, unless surgery is planned or a contraindication for its use exists. A dose of 160 mg/day is as effective as higher doses and is better tolerated; even lower doses may be equally or more effective. There is no other antiplatelet agent that can be recommended for use at this time, either alone or in combination with aspirin, but newer, more potent agents are undergoing clinical trials.

ANTICOAGULANTS

Possible uses for anticoagulants in myocardial infarction include: 1) low-dose heparin for prophylaxis of deep venous thrombosis (DVT); 2) full anticoagulation with heparin and warfarin as routine treatment of infarction; 3) use of heparin after thrombolysis or angioplasty; 4) use of heparin in patients with unstable coronary syndromes and recurrent ischemia after infarction; and 5) treatment of patients with known mural thrombosis or embolic stroke after infarction.

It is generally accepted that low-dose subcutaneous heparin is effective in preventing DVT in bed-bound infarction patients; along with early mobilization, this treatment has dramatically reduced the incidence of thromboembolic events in the modern era. Debate over routine anticoagulation for myocardial infarction, a common therapy in the past, has continued for decades. Trials of anticoagulation with heparin and Coumadin in the 1960s and 1970s did not show clear-cut survival benefits, and though a more recent retrospective analysis of these studies suggested a trend toward lower mortality in treated patients (Chalmers et al.), such information is of little relevance today. On the other hand, anticoagulation is important adjunctive treatment in patients with spontaneous ischemia following infarction, unstable coronary syndromes, and immediately following angioplasty—situations where intraluminal thrombus and unstable plaque are likely to be present. A recent study of heparin and aspirin alone or combined for treatment of unstable angina (Theroux et al.) suggests that heparin provides no additional benefit over aspirin alone but increases bleeding complications. Whether this is true in infarction patients requires further study.

Following successful thrombolytic therapy, IV heparin is administered routinely in most centers in order to reduce the rate of reocclusion. With shorter-acting agents such as rt-PA, anticoagulation is initiated prior to the conclusion of the thrombolytic infusion, and several hours following the end of infusion with streptokinase and APSAC; earlier treatment increases bleeding complications without further benefit (Topol et al. 1989). Whether heparin is necessary after streptokinase treatment, and the nature of the interaction between heparin and aspirin, has not been studied in a randomized trial. In the GISSI trial, though, which did not require heparin therapy, the incidence of reinfarction was similar to that reported in other trials. Likewise, the optimum duration of such treatment in patients undergoing deferred or no catheterization is not defined, and there are currently no data to suggest that Coumadin therapy after discharge benefits these patients either. After angioplasty, aspirin therapy plus heparin for 6–24 hours remains fairly routine treatment.

INOTROPIC DRUGS

The use of digitalis in heart failure is discussed in Chapter 23. Its use in acute MI has been debated for many years. In experimental models of infarction, digitalis worsens ischemia when heart failure is not present by increasing oxygen demand, although when heart failure is present, this is offset by a beneficial reduction in wall stress. Detrimental effects are harder to prove in humans. Retrospective studies show increased mortality in infarction patients treated with the drug (Moss et al. 1981), but when adjusted for the increased numbers of poor prognostic variables present in treated patients, higher mortality is not clearly demonstrated (Muller et al. 1986; Bigger et al. 1985). Digitalis is a mainstay of therapy for patients developing atrial fibrillation or flutter. In patients with heart failure due to systolic dysfunction, digitalis is a reasonable option; for very ill patients requiring immediate treatment for pulmonary edema or cardiogenic shock, however, its delayed onset of action and relatively mild inotropic effect make it an agent of second choice. Adverse effects include exacerbation of arrhythmias if hypokalemia or hypomagnesemia are present, and vasoconstriction with excessively rapid IV administration.

Intravenous catecholamines are indicated for treatment of low cardiac output states complicating myocardial infarction when the patient is symptomatic (oliguria, altered mentation, heart failure with hypotension, shock) and intravascular volume is adequate. Contractility of both nonischemic and reversibly injured "stunned" myocardium can be enhanced with these agents. Combination therapy with a vasodilator is often useful if systemic vascular resistance is increased and blood pressure is adequate. The possibility of worsening ischemia and arrhythmias must be weighed against the anticipated benefit, but they are infrequent if high doses and excessive tachycardia are avoided. Dopamine, with potent beta-agonist effects, increases cardiac output and blood pressure as well as renal blood flow; alpha-adrenergic vasoconstriction at high doses can be harmful, however. Dobutamine lacks both the renal and alpha-adrenergic effects of dopamine; it increases heart rate and blood pressure less and lowers pulmonary artery wedge pressure more than dopamine. Dopexamine is a relatively pure beta agonist like dobutamine but retains the beneficial renal effects of dopamine. All these agents should be administered with invasive hemodynamic monitoring.

The phosphodiesterase inhibitors are a new class of non-catecholamine inotropic drugs which have both inotropic and arterial vasodilating properties and produce little or no increase in myocardial oxygen demand or arrhythmias. Amrinone, given by intravenous infusion, may be particulary useful in patients requiring both an inotrope and a vasodilator. Tolerance to its effects occurs with prolonged infusion and thrombocytopenia is a frequent side effect.

ARTERIAL VASODILATORS

Arterial vasodilators are valuable adjunctive therapy for congestive heart failure complicating myocardial infarction, and also for treatment of severe hypertension in this setting. Intravenous agents—nitroglycerin or nitroprusside—are preferred for initial treatment because of their speed of action and ease of titration. Intravenous nitroprusside, with its balanced arterial and venodilating properties, is particularly useful. Excessive reductions in blood pressure, however, may lead to "coronary steal" and worsening of ischemia by diverting blood flow away from ischemic areas. Thiocyanate toxicity is a problem with prolonged use. Intravenous nitroglycerin is very effective for relieving pulmonary congestion and has milder arteriolar effects. Serious hypotension can occur with either agent, but is more likely with nitroprusside. Continuing treatment with an oral vasodilator is reasonable when heart failure is due to significant systolic, rather than diastolic, dysfunction; angiotensin converting enzyme (ACE) inhibitors may be the agents of choice for this purpose. Use of these agents to treat asymptomatic ventricular dysfunction following infarction has been shown to prevent progressive ventricular enlargement, and preserve ventricular function (Sharpe et al.), especially in high-risk patients with persistently occluded arteries (Pfeffer et al.). It is likely, but still unproven, that treatment with these agents will also decrease the incidence of death and late heart failure in such patients. There is evidence that reducing systolic wall stress reduces infarct expansion and thinning, and prevents progressive ventricular remodeling and dilatation.

HEMODYNAMIC COMPLICATIONS OF MYOCARDIAL INFARCTION

CONGESTIVE HEART FAILURE

The onset of myocardial infarction brings with it a prompt decrease both in systolic contractile force in the ischemic zone and diminished compliance, which may lead to clinically evident congestive heart failure. More than half of infarction patients have an elevated pulmonary capillary wedge pressure on admission, often not recognized clinically. This is frequently due only to diastolic dysfunction, requiring elevated pulmonary wedge pressure (15-18 mm Hg or more) to maintain cardiac output. When it is more severe, pulmonary rales, dyspnea, and radiographic vascular congestion occur, but these lag behind the hemodynamic changes. A smaller number of patients, about 15%, present with frank pulmonary edema. Hypotension, when it occurs, may be a manifestation of hypovolemia, increased vagal tone, right ventricular infarction, or cardiogenic shock.

It was observed very early that patients with heart failure and shock had a worse outcome, and the classification system of Killip made use of this fact. Those with rales encompassing 50% of the lung fields or a third heart-sound (class II) had 17% mortality; pulmonary edema (class III) a 38% mortality; and those with cardiogenic shock nearly a 100% mortality, compared with those having none of these findings (class I), who had a 6% mortality. Recognizing that

there is considerable heterogeneity among patients within each Killip class and that clinical indicators sometimes fail to detect significant hypoperfusion or heart failure, classification based on hemodynamics (Table 6) has proven more useful in clinical practice (Forrester et al. 1976). Patients with pulmonary congestion are treated with diuretics and oral or intravenous nitrates to reduce preload, if they are not hypotensive. Arterial vasodilators and possibly digitalis are added if congestion fails to respond. Those with hypoperfusion and low or "normal" filling pressures may improve with careful volume expansion, while those with severely depressed cardiac output and pulmonary congestion, who have the highest mortality rate, may require inotropic support or intraaortic balloon counterpulsation. Invasive hemodynamic monitoring with a pulmonary artery catheter is very valuable in the diagnosis and management of many subsets of infarction patients, and suggested indications for its use are shown in Table 7. It is, however, neither indicated nor desirable in the treatment of uncomplicated patients or those with mild pulmonary congestion resolving rapidly with diuretics.

POSTINFARCTION ANGINA AND INFARCT EXTENSION

Recurrence of angina during recovery from myocardial infarction is associated with higher rates of death and reinfarction, both in the short term and long term (Schuster et al. 1981), and should be considered a strong indication for urgent catheterization and potential revascularization. Early recurrence of angina may indicate instability within a reperfused infarct-related artery, instability in a vessel remote from the infarct, or jeopardized collateral flow; it often portends infarct extension.

Infarct extension occurs in approximately 10% of patients managed conventionally. It is diagnosed by the finding of reappearance of CK-MB after infarction. Prolonged chest pain and new ECG changes are characteristic, but found in only half of patients (Weisman and Healy). Infarct extension may lead to cardiogenic shock, and is associated with a four-fold increased hospital mortality. It is more likely to occur in patients with non-Q-wave infarction, diabetes, early recurrence of chest pain, and prior infarction (Muller et al. 1988), and in women. Analogous to reocclusion and reinfarction following thrombolysis, infarct ex-

Table 6. Clinical and Hemodynamic Subsets in Acute Myocardial Infarction

		HEMODYNAMIC FINDING		HOSPITAL MORTALITY (%)	
	Class and Clinical Finding	CI (L/min/ m²)	PCW (mm Hg)	CLINICAL	HEMODYNAMIC
I	No pulmonary congestion or hypoperfusion	>2.2	<18	1	3
II	Pulmonary congestion only	>2.2	>18	11	9
III	Peripheral hypoperfusion only	<2.2	<18	18	23
IV	Pulmonary congestion and peripheral hypoperfusion	<2.2	>18	60	51

CI = cardiac index; PCW = pulmonary capillary wedge pressure.
Adapted from Forrester et al. 1976. See Bibliography.

Table 7. Indications for Hemodynamic Monitoring in Acute Myocardial Infarction

Diagnosis

   Diagnosis of suspected left ventricular
      failure
   Hypotension
   Right ventricular infarction
   Persistent oliguria or azotemia
   Acute mitral regurgitation
   Suspected ventricular septal rupture
   Uncertain volume status

Treatment

   Congestive heart failure or pulmonary
      edema
   Cardiogenic shock
   Vasodilator therapy
   Intravenous inotropic support

tension usually results from reocclusion of a spontaneously reperfused or subtotally occluded infarct artery.

CARDIOGENIC SHOCK

Cardiogenic shock results from loss of a critical amount of contractile function, leading to hypotension and inadequate tissue perfusion. The resulting decrease in coronary blood flow and increase in vascular resistance further increase ischemia, leading to ongoing necrosis and further worsening of ventricular function in a vicious cycle that is usually fatal. Patients dying from cardiogenic shock uniformly have infarction of 40% or more of the left ventricle (Page et al. 1971), and most have severe three-vessel coronary disease. Cardiogenic shock usually results from extension of the initial infarction at its borders, and expansion of the infarct, with resulting deterioration of ventricular function. It complicates 7-15% of infarctions in the first days after admission and is often heralded by persistent CK-MB release and recurrent chest pain suggesting infarct extension. It is diagnosed when arterial hypotension (<90 mm Hg systolic) and depressed cardiac index (<1.8 L/min/m²) occur with elevated pulmonary artery wedge pressure and signs of hypoperfusion. Other causes of shock, such as papillary muscle rupture, free wall rupture, and ventricular septal defect, must be excluded. Cardiogenic shock occurs more frequently among those with large infarcts, previous infarction, admission ejection fraction <35%, diabetes, and advanced age (Hands et al.).

Treatment of cardiogenic shock is aimed at maintaining cardiac output and perfusion pressure and minimizing ischemia. The inotropic drugs dopamine and dobutamine, as well as amrinone, alone or in combination, will improve contractility. Vasodilators often further improve cardiac output but may worsen coronary perfusion pressure. Intraaortic balloon counterpulsation, discussed below, improves the hemodynamic profile by reducing afterload and increasing cardiac output while simultaneously increasing diastolic blood pressure. None of these treatments, however, diminishes the ultimate mortality rate from cardiogenic shock, which is 65-90%.

The abysmal prognosis of cardiogenic shock has not improved appreciably in the last two decades. It is hoped that early reperfusion will prevent cardiogenic shock or decrease mortality when it occurs. The incidence of cardiogenic shock was reduced in the European Cooperative trial (Van de Werf et al.), the first trial to show this. Other trials including GISSI demonstrated neither a decreased incidence of cardiogenic shock nor decreased mortality when it occurs. Uncontrolled trials of primary angioplasty, on the other hand, suggest that mortality might be reduced by this intervention in selected patients (Ellis et al.). Surgical revascularization also carries a 50-60% mortality rate in this setting, less if the patient has been stabilized medically for a period of time. Although this mortality is high (and the patients somewhat selected), it is probably lower than the mortality expected with medical therapy alone. It is reasonable to think that those cardiogenic shock patients having evidence of reversible ischemia are likely to benefit from revascularization, while those with shock due to necrosis of a critical mass of myocardium without ongoing ischemia will not.

RIGHT VENTRICULAR INFARCTION

Involvement of the right ventricle occurs in roughly one third of inferior wall infarctions when studied pathologically (Isner and Roberts) or noninvasively, but is infrequent in anterior infarction. Hemodynamically significant right ventricular infarction is only seen in about 10% of inferior infarcts, and is characterized by elevated right atrial pressure and depressed cardiac index with normal or low pulmonary wedge pressure. Kussmaul's sign, "square root" right ventricular pressure tracing, and diastolic equalization of pressures are frequent findings, resembling pericardial disease. In fact, it is the action of the pericardium and shifting of the septum that probably contribute most to impairment of left ventricular filling when the right ventricle dilates acutely. ST elevation in the right precordial leads is highly specific, but is transient and may be missed (Bellamy et al.). Hemodynamic monitoring is useful both in diagnosis and treatment.

The manifestations of right ventricular infarction range from mild jugular venous distention to frank shock. Profound hypotension after administration of nitrates is not uncommon. Initial treatment of the hypotensive patient with right ventricular infarction consists of volume expansion, which may be sufficient in mild cases. When equalization of left- and right-sided pressures occurs, no further effect of volume expansion is likely and treatment with dobutamine, which is more effective, becomes necessary if hypoperfusion persists (Dell'Italia et al.). Bradyarrhythmias are best treated by dual chamber pacing; ventricular pacing alone is ineffective. Although shock may be severe, and inotropic support required for several days, both short- and long-term prognosis are good with appropriate therapy—in marked contrast to shock due to left ventricular failure.

NON-Q-WAVE INFARCTION

The subset of patients presenting with myocardial infarction without development of Q waves represents a distinct group of particular concern to the clinician (Klein and Helfant). Non-Q-wave infarction, which pathologically is often subendocardial, tends to be smaller in size than Q-wave infarction. Hospital mortality is half as great, and incidence of heart failure is less. However, infarct extension, recurrent angina, and late death occur more frequently, and reinfarction develops in 21% by nine months and 54% by 57 months (Hutter et al.). As a result, ultimate mortality is equal to or higher than in transmural infarcts. The incidence of multi-vessel disease is high in these patients, the infarct-related artery is typically patent, usually with a high-grade stenosis, and treadmill testing is often positive. These factors argue for early angiography in most or all patients with non-Q-wave infarcts. Those with anterior ECG changes, spontaneous or inducible ischemia, or a history of prior infarction merit intervention; stable patients under age 70 without prior infarction may have a better prognosis (Nicod et al.).

MECHANICAL COMPLICATIONS

The so-called "mechanical" complications of infarction have a common pathogenesis involving disruption of necrotic cardiac tissues, usually with dramatic consequences. The most common form is infarct expansion, which occurs in approximately 30% of infarcts, particularly anterior infarcts. It is characterized by regional dilatation and thinning of the infarcted wall segment. It develops most commonly from three to seven days following infarction, when the infarct tissues are weakest and scar formation has not begun, and is found near the edge of the infarct where shearing forces are greater. Infarct expansion impairs ventricular systolic function, and progression of the expansion process leads to cardiac rupture in some patients (Schuster and Bulkley 1979). Cardiac rupture is most common following first, large, transmural infarctions, usually anterior, that lack collateral flow. It is somewhat more common in women and in patients with a history of hypertension, and is usually located in the free wall of the ventricle. There is experimental evidence that timely reperfusion may prevent infarct expansion and rupture; clinical data, as yet, are lacking. Beta blockade appears to decrease the incidence of cardiac rupture, and it is possible that early vasodilator therapy may do so also.

The patient with cardiac rupture suddenly develops shock and circulatory collapse with electromechanical dissociation and signs of tamponade. Death is often immediate, but if the diagnosis can be made and the patient stabilized (with pericardiocentesis, inotropes, and an intraaortic balloon pump), operative repair, usually with coronary artery bypass, is lifesaving. Occasionally, incomplete rupture occurs, in which pericardium and thrombus seal a site of rupture and form a pseudoaneurysm that communicates with the ventricular cavity through a narrow neck. Pseudoaneurysms can be visualized by echocardiography or left ventriculography. Death is not immediate in such cases; treatment is the same as in rupture.

The pathogenesis of ventricular septal rupture is identical to that of rupture of the free wall. The septal defect is located near the apex in patients with anterior infarction, and in the basal septum following inferior infarction. Clinically, there is abrupt onset of heart failure, ranging from mild to profound, in a previously stable patient, associated with a new holosystolic murmur at the left sternal border, sometimes with a thrill. The diagnosis is confirmed by Doppler echocardiography. Right-heart catheterization rapidly diagnoses septal rupture by demonstrating a step-up in oxygen saturation from right atrium to pulmonary artery, which distinguishes the rupture from papillary muscle rupture and allows shunt calculations. Treatment with inotropes and vasodilators is useful, and intraaortic balloon counterpulsation can decrease the degree of shunting. Immediate surgical repair is recommended if the shunt flow is large ($>2:1$ flow) or if circulatory support is required. In patients who are clinically stable with small shunts, delaying surgery by four to six weeks to allow infarct healing is appropriate.

Papillary muscle rupture results in acute mitral regurgitation and variable hemodynamic compromise depending on whether rupture is partial or complete, and may occur with relatively small infarctions. Rupture of the posteromedial papillary muscle, in the setting of inferoposterior infarction, is more common than anterolateral rupture, which results from anterolateral infarction. Complete rupture of a muscle is rapidly fatal; when partial, stabilization is possible. The patient develops abrupt onset of pulmonary edema, hypotension, and tachycardia. If hypotension is severe, the murmur of mitral insufficiency may be soft and short; in less severe cases a typical loud holosystolic apical murmur is heard. Pulmonary artery catheterization demonstrates markedly increased pulmonary wedge pressure with very large v-waves. Echocardiography can distinguish papillary muscle rupture from dysfunction. Treatment with vasodilators and intraaortic balloon counterpulsation is particularly useful in treating this condition. Urgent mitral valve repair or replacement, often with bypass grafting, is then indicated.

When mitral regurgitation is due to ischemia or infarction of a papillary muscle without rupture, the clinical presentation is variable. The patient may present days to weeks after infarction with symptoms of congestive heart failure and a murmur of mitral regurgitation. If dysfunction is related to intermittent ischemia, repeated bouts of pulmonary edema may occur, with relatively few symptoms between episodes. Many of these patients can be managed medically or undergo revascularization without valve replacement. In other cases, severe chronic mitral regurgitation leads to ventricular dilatation and chronic heart failure. In such patients, coronary bypass alone will not improve the regurgitation, and valve repair or replacement is necessary.

INTRAAORTIC BALLOON COUNTERPULSATION

Intraaortic balloon counterpulsation (IABP) is indicated for the following conditions: 1) stabilization of the hemodynamically unstable patient prior to angiography and bypass surgery; 2) cardiogenic shock unresponsive to medical therapy; 3) acute severe mitral regurgitation or ventricular septal rupture; and 4) persistent angina refractory to maximal medical therapy,

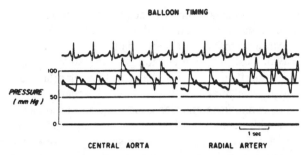

Figure 3. *The effect of initiation of intraaortic balloon pumping (IABP) on central aortic pressure (left panel) and radial artery pressure (right panel). The electrocardiogram shows balloon timing markers in the PR and ST segments. In the left panel the up-stroke of the balloon pulse is timed to coincide with the central aortic dicrotic notch; however, this timing requires slightly earlier balloon inflation, as judged from the radial artery pressure measurement. The minimal diastolic radial arterial pressure during IABP is approximately 5–10 mm Hg below the diastolic radial pressure prior to IABP. (From Leinbach RC, Gold HK: Intraaortic balloon pumping: Use in treatment of cardiogenic shock and acute myocardial ischemia. In: Karliner JS, Gregoratos G, eds. Coronary Care. London: Churchill Livingstone; 1981.)*

pending definitive therapy. Inserted either percutaneously or surgically through the femoral artery, preferably under fluoroscopic guidance, the balloon is positioned in the descending aorta beyond the left subclavian artery and above the renal arteries. The balloon is adjusted to inflate at aortic valve closure (dicrotic notch) and deflate prior to aortic valve opening. Systolic pressure (afterload) and pulmonary wedge pressure (preload) are reduced, while diastolic pressure (coronary perfusion) is raised (Figure 3). Stroke volume rises, myocardial oxygen demand falls and ischemia is reduced. Pulmonary shunting from septal rupture and mitral regurgitation, if present, are reduced. Complications include aortic dissection, embolization, and femoral artery occlusion.

PERICARDITIS

Pericarditis, developing in 10% or less of infarctions, occurs most commonly in the first two to four days after infarction and is due to inflammation associated with transmural necrosis. It occurs more frequently in those with Q-wave infarctions, as well as those with larger and more complicated infarctions (Tofler et al. 1989), and is uncommon after successful thrombolytic therapy. The patient has pain of a positional and pleuritic nature, often with a transient pericardial rub and sometimes with fever or leukocytosis. Electrocardiographic changes are difficult to distinguish from those of the underlying infarction. The syndrome is brief and self-limited, responds to anti-inflammatory agents, and is important to distinguish from recurrent ischemia. The authors prefer aspirin therapy, which has not been shown to inhibit infarct healing; in contrast, steroids and other nonsteroidal anti-inflammatory agents have been shown to cause scar thinning in experimental models. The presence of a small pericardial effusion by echocardiography is seen in 25% of infarction patients and does not indicate pericarditis. The finding of a large effusion or tamponade is more likely to indicate subacute ventricular rupture than pericarditis.

Pericarditis occurring later, from two weeks to three months after infarction, is known as Dressler's syndrome, which is now rarely seen. Pericardial rub, fever, pleural effusions and sometimes pneumonitis can be found. Small pericardial effusions are often noted by echocardiography; large effusions or tamponade are infrequent. The syndrome is probably an autoimmune disorder. Treatment with anti-inflammatory agents is usually necessary. Recurrence is not uncommon and corticosteroids are sometimes required, though the ability of these agents to impair infarct healing should be kept in mind.

VENTRICULAR ANEURYSM

Ventricular aneurysm formation is a late sequela of myocardial infarction. Aneurysms develop most often in the first three months following anterior infarction (Visser et al. 1986) with poor collateral flow, probably as a result of infarct expansion. An aneurysm consists of a thin fibrotic wall which bulges in both diastole and systole; this can sometimes be detected as a precordial bulge on palpation or abnormal cardiac silhouette on chest radiograph. Persistent ST-segment elevation on the ECG indicates dyskinetic wall motion, but a true aneurysm may not be present in all such cases. The diagnosis is best made by echocardiography or ventriculography. The presence of an aneurysm, especially early after infarction, is associated with a markedly increased risk of death, heart failure, angina, ventricular arrhythmias, and embolization. Surgical resection is indicated for patients having intractable heart failure, angina, or arrhythmias, but only if function of the remaining myocardium is good.

Mural thrombus adherent to the infarcted wall is found in a large proportion of necropsy cases of infarction; in clinical series, a third of anterior infarctions have demonstrable mural thrombi, but they are rare in inferior infarction. The thrombi are usually found in areas of severe wall motion abnormality or in ventricular aneurysms, and can be reliably diagnosed by echocardiography, although false-positive studies can occur. The embolic potential of such thrombi is controversial, with a reported incidence of embolic events ranging from 4–52%. Emboli are more likely to occur with protruding and mobile thrombi (Visser et al. 1985), and during the first six weeks following infarction. Anticoagulation is essential for those with such morphology or those with a history of an embolic event (Meltzer et al.). Most authorities recommend anticoagulation for a period of three to six months for all patients with mural thrombus after anterior infarction. Persistence of a thrombus by echocardiogram is common after treatment and does not necessarily indicate continued embolic potential.

ARRHYTHMIC COMPLICATIONS

SUPRAVENTRICULAR ARRHYTHMIAS

Sinus bradycardia occurs in about 20% of cases of acute MI. It is most common in inferior infarction related to sinoatrial node ischemia, and it is not associated with a poorer prognosis. It is often asymptomatic but when severe and accompanied by hypoperfusion or increased ventricular ectopy, chronotropic agents or temporary pacing can be used. Sinus bradycardia is sometimes seen in patients after successful thrombolytic therapy or abrupt reperfusion of the right coronary artery; this is known as the Bezold-Jarisch reflex.

Sinus tachycardia is also common and may be caused by pain, anxiety, left ventricular dysfunction (which may be otherwise unsuspected), congestive heart failure, hypovolemia, pericarditis, exogenous catecholamines, or atrial infarction. Its recognition is important so that the underlying process can be addressed, since tachycardia can increase myocardial oxygen demand, increase infarct size, and raise mortality. Treatment with beta blockers is advisable if tachycardia is attributable to hyperdynamic circulation and not to ven-

tricular dysfunction; invasive hemodynamic monitoring is often necessary to make this distinction.

Atrial premature beats are relatively common, and may indicate atrial dilatation or congestive failure. Atrial fibrillation occurs in about 15% of infarction patients and may be related to atrial ischemia. It is more common in anterior infarction, and in association with ventricular dysfunction; patients manifesting this arrhythmia have a worse prognosis. Atrial fibrillation tends to occur most frequently on the first day of infarction. It is transient but often recurrent, and can lead to profound hemodynamic compromise. Supraventricular tachycardia and atrial flutter are also seen occasionally during infarction. Treatment of these arrhythmias is the same as when they occur in other settings, but it must be prompt to avoid the detrimental effects of the tachycardia.

VENTRICULAR ARRHYTHMIAS

Ventricular arrhythmias are major causes of death during and after myocardial infarction. Sudden arrhythmic death occurs in approximately 15% of patients with acute MI in the first hour, accounting for about 60% of all infarction-related mortality. The cause is usually ventricular fibrillation (VF) or ventricular tachycardia (VT). Most of these events occur before hospital admission but develop in 3–9% of patients after admission, usually within 12 hours of infarction. Ventricular fibrillation occurring within the first 24–48 hours of infarction is usually not associated with severe pump failure or shock and is termed primary. Ventricular fibrillation occurring later during the hospital phase of infarction usually occurs in the setting of infarct extension, severe pump failure or shock, and is termed secondary.

Premature ventricular beats occur in more than 90% of patients with acute MI and do not predict subsequent ventricular fibrillation, even when frequent, early, or paired. In fact, 50–60% of cases of VF occur without preceding high-grade arrhythmias. Primary VF occurs more frequently in younger patients, patients with a first infarction, and almost always within the first 12–24 hours of infarction. It has been associated with higher in-hospital mortality in some studies (Volpi et al.) but not in others (Tofler et al. 1987). It does not, however, signify a poor long-term prognosis for those who survive it. Secondary VF, on the other hand, is associated with extremely high in-hospital and late mortality.

The issue of prophylactic antiarrhythmic therapy in myocardial infarction is unresolved. Since the presence or absence of ventricular premature beats is of no use in determining whether to give lidocaine or not, many recommend that prophylactic therapy should be given to all patients with diagnosed or suspected infarction. Lidocaine is very effective in preventing primary VF (Lie et al.). However, mortality has not been shown to improve with such therapy, probably because immediate defibrillation is routinely available when VF or sustained VT does occur. To the contrary, a trend toward increased mortality is noted when trials of such therapy are pooled (Yusuf, Wittes et al.). The potential for toxicity with lidocaine should not be overlooked. Toxicity is most frequent in the elderly and those with liver disease, heart failure, and hemodynamic compromise. It is most reasonable to recommend prophylactic treatment with lidocaine if begun within 6 hours of infarction in patients younger than 70, in settings where close monitoring and immediate defibrillation are not available, and in other situations, according to an individualized risk-benefit assessment (Goldman and Batsford).

Abrupt coronary reperfusion can lead to increased ventricular arrhythmias, including VT, VF, or accelerated idioventricular rhythm. Once believed useful to noninvasively predict reperfusion after thrombolysis, such arrhythmias are now known to occur almost as frequently when there is no reperfusion (Miller et al.); thus, they can not be used for this purpose. Likewise, the routine administration of lidocaine to patients receiving thrombolytic therapy, though a common practice, is unproven, since the incidence of life-threatening arrhythmias directly attributable to reperfusion is not known (Solimene et al.), and the effectiveness of lidocaine against such arrhythmias is uncertain.

In the late hospital phase of myocardial infarction and following discharge, the presence of premature beats, especially when frequent or in couplets and nonsustained runs, has been shown to be associated with an increased incidence of late sudden death (Bigger et al. 1984; Moss et al. 1979) and are more frequent with increasing degrees of ventricular dysfunction. However, commonly available modalities are poor predictors of future arrhythmic death after infarction. Only about one fourth of the 5–15% of patients ultimately developing sudden death after discharge have such arrhythmias detected on ambulatory monitoring. Programmed ventricular stimulation can identify patients at increased risk of arrhythmic death after infarction (Denniss et al.), and antiarrhythmic therapy guided by electrophysiologic testing can prevent arrhythmic events in high-risk patients (Buxton et al.). However, inducible ventricular tachycardia can be found in as many as 40% of unselected infarction patients, most of whom are at low risk for sudden death (Brugada et al.), and thus can not be recommended for routine use. The signal-averaged ECG can identify a group of patients without late potentials who have a very low risk of arrhythmic complications and require no further investigation, and a moderate risk group with late potentials who might then undergo further evaluation (Turitto et al.). This might prove to be a useful clinical strategy, but for those having only simple ectopic beats, drug treatment is not effective and may actually be harmful (CAST Investigators). The recent finding that thrombolytic therapy reduces the incidence of late potentials (Gang et al.) holds the promise that thrombolysis will lead to a reduction in late arrhythmic deaths.

Unlike patients with simple or nonsustained ventricular arrhythmias, those having sustained, symptomatic ventricular tachycardia or sudden death during the late hospital phase or after discharge have a high incidence of recurrence and death. They warrant aggressive intervention in all cases. Programmed ventricular stimulation with guided antiarrhythmic therapy to suppress inducible ventricular tachycardia (see Chapter 10) appears to be superior to empiric or noninvasively guided antiarrhythmic therapy for this purpose (Mitchell et al. 1987).

CONDUCTION ABNORMALITIES

New abnormalities of atrioventricular conduction develop in 16–25% of patients with myocardial infarction. Patients with a new conduction abnormality during myocardial infarction often progress to complete AV block and have twice the hospital mortality rates than do those without (Roos and Dunning; Hindman et al.; DeGuzman and Rahimtoola). The increased mortality is related to more extensive infarction as well as bradyarrhythmias. AV block in anterior infarction is usually due to extensive necrosis of the conducting system below the bundle of His and associated with bundle branch blocks; in inferior infarction, AV block is usually due to ischemia of the AV node and is often not associated with other conduction abnormalities.

Temporary ventricular pacing (Table 8) is required when a bradyarrhythmia or conduction abnormality results in hypoperfusion. Sinus bradycardia and

Table 8. Indications for Temporary Transvenous Pacing in Acute Myocardial Infarction

Definite

    Complete heart block
    Second-degree AV block, type II
    Second-degree AV block, type I, with hypoperfusion
    Sinus bradycardia despite atropine, with hypoperfusion
    Junctional or idioventricular rhythm with slow ventricular rate and hypoperfusion
    "High-risk" bundle branch block:
        bifascicular block with first-degree AV block
        new bifascicular block

Possible

    Second-degree AV block, type I, with wide QRS
    Overdrive pacing of ventricular tachycardia
    AV synchronous pacing for right ventricular infarction, with hypoperfusion

symptomatic type I second-degree AV block usually respond to atropine but occasionally require pacing. Third-degree block, and type II second-degree block in anterior infarction (and in inferior infarction with wide QRS), require pacing in all cases. Prophylactic temporary pacing is also indicated in patients judged to be at high risk for development of complete AV block. About 30% of patients with new bundle branch blocks will progress to high-grade heart block. Complete heart block often develops suddenly, especially in patients with anterior infarctions. The risk of complete AV block is high in those having prolonged PR interval with new bundle branch block (20–30%) and bilateral (bifascicular or alternating) bundle branch blocks (40%) or new bilateral bundle branch block alone (30%). Risk is moderate in other groups, including those with bifascicular block not known to be new. With none of these factors, or with bundle branch block alone, risk is about 10%. The availability of reliable external pacing may obviate the need for temporary transvenous pacing in moderate risk patients.

Resolution of high-grade AV block occurs in more than 90% of the patients that develop it. Nevertheless, permanent ventricular pacing is required if symptomatic bradyarrhythmias, third-degree block, or type II second-degree blocks persist during recovery from infarction. Those with transient complete heart block in whom a bundle branch block persists had a lower incidence of late sudden death when permanently paced in one study. Permanent pacing should at least be considered in this setting or electrophysiologic studies performed.

POST-MYOCARDIAL INFARCTION CARE

PROGNOSIS AFTER INFARCTION

Discharge of the patient surviving uncomplicated MI typically takes place after 7–10 hospital days, and the safety of this approach has been demonstrated repeatedly. Earlier discharge after thrombolysis may be possible in highly selected patients (Topol et al. 1988). However, death occurs in 5–15% of patients in the first year after infarction, and reinfarction in about the same number. About 50% of patients have three-vessel or left main disease and thus have a significant amount of myocardium at risk. Those patients at high risk for death and recurrent infarction must be identified for early intervention. Many factors have been associated with a poor prognosis (Table 9). Left ventricular dysfunction, severity of coronary disease, a large amount of jeopardized myocardium, and early recurrence of ischemia are the most powerful predictors of subsequent cardiac events. The prognostic importance of arrhythmias has been previously discussed. Combinations of clinical factors can be used to stratify patients into subgroups with two-year mortality ranging from 3–60% (Multicenter Postinfarction Research Group).

The most common strategy for stratifying patients following infarction is use of clinical criteria coupled with low-level treadmill exercise data before discharge, and symptom-limited maximal exercise in four to six weeks (DeBusk et al.). Return to work is then recommended at this point for patients without marked

---

Table 9. Risk Factors After Acute Myocardial Infarction

Congestive heart failure (clinical, hemodynamic, or radiographic)
Left ventricular ejection fraction less than 0.40
Large infarct size (estimated by enzymes, ^{99m}technetium radionuclide scan, electrocardiographic QRS mapping, echocardiographic techniques)
New bundle branch block (any type, including fascicular blocks)
Mobitz II second-degree or third-degree heart block
Anterior infarction
Reinfarction or infarct extension
Ventricular fibrillation or ventricular tachycardia
Ventricular premature beats (especially if frequent or complex)
Supraventricular arrhythmias (other than sinus bradycardia)
Abnormal signal-averaged electrocardiogram
Inducible sustained monomorphic ventricular tachycardia during electrophysiologic study
Postinfarction angina
Inability to perform exercise testing
Angina pectoris, ST-segment elevation or depression, abnormal blood pressure response, or ventricular ectopy induced by exercise testing
Diabetes mellitus
Hypertension or loss of preexisting hypertension
Age >70 years
Female gender

From Hessen SE, Brest AN: Risk profiling the patient after acute myocardial infarction. *Cardiovasc Clinics* 20:284, 1989.

---

ischemia or functional impairment. Those patients having complicated infarcts, early recurrence of spontaneous ischemia, previous infarction or abnormal low-level exercise tests, are considered high risk and referred for angiography. Inability to complete a low-level exercise test or abnormal hemodynamic response are predictors of death and reinfarction, more so than ST-segment response (Krone et al.). The predictive value of low-level exercise testing is enhanced by thallium perfusion scanning, which together have a predictive value equal to or better than angiography (Gibson et al. 1983). Subsequent maximal exercise testing identifies further patients at increased risk. With no abnormalities and normal functional capacity, one-year mortality is 1%, compared to 13% with an abnormal test; this prognostic information has additive value beyond clinical assessment alone (Stone et al.). Such an approach leads to coronary angiography in about half of infarction patients and identifies a group of patients with moderately high risk and a group at extremely low risk.

RISK FACTOR MODIFICATION AND REHABILITATION

In addition to secondary prevention with antiplatelet drugs and beta blockers, intensive effort should be made to modify coronary risk factors in the postinfarction patient. Progression of disease and death after infarction is more common among those with elevated cholesterol, smokers, and women, and is reduced by smoking cessation. Lipid-lowering drugs have been shown to reduce mortality in patients after infarction (Carlson and Rosenhamer; Coronary Drug Project). Decreased rate of progression, and in some cases, regression of coronary atherosclerosis has also been observed following bypass surgery (Blankenhorn et al.). Diabetes and hypertension contribute to increased late mortality as well, and should be controlled optimally. There is every reason to believe that intensive multiple risk factor intervention will improve long-term prognosis and that primary prevention is an attainable goal.

Exercise training of the stable postinfarction patient is intended mainly to avoid the complications of prolonged bed rest and return the patient to a maximum level of functional capacity following discharge (see Chapter 36). It hastens the spontaneous improvement in functional capacity that occurs during convalescence and produces further improvement, which is especially beneficial in patients with marked impairment of exercise capacity on predischarge exercise testing (Greenland and Chu; O'Connor et al.). Exercise training programs are clearly safe for the majority of patients, but concern still exists about deleterious effects of early exercise on infarct healing and ventricular remodeling (Jugdutt et al.) in patients with large infarctions.

Education of the postinfarction patient in the outpatient setting is of great importance. Lifestyle and dietary changes must be reinforced and guidelines concerning return to work given. The postdischarge treadmill test is useful for disability assessment in this setting. Patients may exhibit either excessive anxiety or excessive denial that can hinder their recovery. The physician should be alert for symptoms of depression and social and sexual dysfunction, which are common even after uncomplicated infarction.

WHEN MYOCARDIAL INFARCTION IS RULED OUT

Many patients admitted to coronary care units for acute myocardial ischemia do not develop myocardial infarction. It must be kept in mind that many of these "ruled-out" patients have extensive heart disease and a prognosis as bad as or worse than those with infarction (Schroeder et al. 1980). Risk is particularly high among patients presenting with ischemia-related pulmonary edema, who have 60% mortality in two years (Clark et al.).

Bibliography

AIMS Study Group: Effect of intravenous APSAC on mortality after acute myocardial infarction: Preliminary report of a placebo-controlled clinical trial. *Lancet* 1:545, 1988.

American Heart Association: 1989 Heart Facts. Dallas: American Heart Association National Center; 1988.

Ambrose JA, Alexopoulos D: Thrombolysis in unstable angina: Will the beneficial effects of thrombolytic therapy in myocardial infarction apply to patients with unstable angina? *J Am Coll Cardiol* 13:1666, 1989.

Anderson JA, Rothbard RL, Hackworthy RA, et al: Multicenter reperfusion trial of intravenous anisoylated plasminogen streptokinase activator complex (APSAC) in acute myocardial infarction: Controlled comparison with intracoronary streptokinase. *J Am Coll Cardiol* 11:1153, 1988.

Arvan S, Varat MA: Persistent ST-segment elevation and left ventricular wall abnormalities: A two-dimensional echocardiographic study. *Am J Cardiol* 53:1542, 1984.

Bassand JP, Machecourt J, Cassagnes J, et al (for the APSIM Study Investigators): Multicenter trial of intravenous anisoylated plasminogen streptokinase activator complex (APSAC) in acute myocardial infarction: Effects on infarct size and left ventricular function. *J Am Coll Cardiol* 13:988, 1988.

Bateman TM, Czer LSC, Gray RJ, et al: Transient pathologic Q waves during acute ischemic events: An electrocardiographic correlate of stunned but viable myocardium. *Am Heart J* 106:1421, 1983.

Bates ER, Califf RM, Stack RS, et al, and the TAMI Study Group: Thrombolysis and Angioplasty in Myocardial Infarction (TAMI-I) Trial: Influence of infarct location on arterial patency, left ventricular function and mortality. *J Am Coll Cardiol* 13:12, 1989.

Bellamy GR, Rasmussen HH, Nasser FN, Wiseman JC, Cooper RA: Value of two-dimensional echocardiography, electrocardiography, and clinical signs in detecting right ventricular infarction. *Am Heart J* 112:304, 1986.

Beta-blocker Heart Attack Trial (BHAT) Research Group: Randomized trial of propranolol in patients with acute myocardial infarction. *JAMA* 247:1707, 1982.

Bigger JT Jr, Fleiss JL, Kleiger R, et al: The relationships among ventricular arrhythmias, left ventricular dysfunction, and mortality in the two years after myocardial infarction. *Circulation* 69:250, 1984.

Bigger JT, Fleiss JL, Rolnitzky LM, Merab JP, Ferrick KJ: Effect of digitalis treatment on survival after acute myocardial infarction. *Am J Cardiol* 55:623, 1985.

Blanke H, Cohen M, Schlueter GV: Electrocardiographic and coronary arteriographic correlations during acute myocardial infarction. *Am J Cardiol* 54:249, 1984.

Blankenhorn DH, Nessim SA, et al: Beneficial effects of combined colestipol-niacin therapy on coronary atherosclerosis and coronary venous bypass grafts. *JAMA* 257:3233, 1987.

Braunwald E: Myocardial reperfusion, limitation of infarct size, reduction of left ventricular dysfunction, and improved survival: Should the paradigm be expanded? *Circulation* 79:441, 1989.

Braunwald E, Kloner RA: Myocardial reperfusion: A double edged sword? *J Clin Invest* 76:1713, 1985.

Brugada P, Waldecker B, Kersschot Y, Zehender M, Wellens HJ: Ventricular arrhythmias initiated by programmed stimulation in four groups of patients with healed myocardial infarction. *J Am Coll Cardiol* 8:1035, 1986.

Buxton AE, Marchlinski FE, Flores BT, et al: Nonsustained ventricular tachycardia in patients with coronary artery disease: Role of electrophysiologic study. *Circulation* 75:1178, 1987.

Califf RM, Topol EJ, George BS, et al, and the TAMI Study Group: Characteristics and outcome of patients in whom reperfusion with intravenous tissue-type plasminogen activator fails: Results of the Thrombolysis and Angioplasty in Myocardial Infarction (TAMI) I trial. *Circulation* 77:1090, 1988.

Califf RM, O'Neill W, Stack RS, et al, and the TAMI Study Group: Failure of simple clinical measurements to predict perfusion status after intravenous thrombolysis. *Ann Int Med* 108:658, 1988.

Cardiac Arrhythmia Supression Trial (CAST) Investigators: Preliminary report: Effect of encainide and flecainide on mortality in a randomized trial of arrhythmia suppression after myocardial infarction. *N Engl J Med* 321:406, 1989.

Carlson LA, Rosenhamer G: Reduction of mortality in the Stockholm Ischaemic Heart Disease Secondary Prevention Study by combined treatment with clofibrate and nicotinic acid. *Acta Med Scand* 223:405, 1988.

Chadda K, Goldstein S, Byington R, Curb JD: Effect of propranolol after acute myocardial infarction in patients with congestive heart failure. *Circulation* 73:503, 1986.

Chalmers TC, Matta RJ, Smith H Jr, et al: Evidence favoring the use of anticoagulants in the hospital phase of acute myocardial infarction. *N Engl J Med* 297:1091, 1977.

Cheitlin MD, McAllister HA, de Castro CM: Myocardial infarction without atherosclerosis. *JAMA* 231:951, 1975.

Chesebro JH, Knattrud G, Roberts R, et al: Thrombolysis in Acute Myocardial Infarction (TIMI) Trial, Phase I: A comparison between intravenous tissue plasminogen activator and intravenous streptokinase: Clinical findings through hospital discharge. *Circulation* 76:142, 1987.

Clark LT, Garfein OB, Dwyer EM: Acute pulmonary edema due to ischemic heart disease without accompanying myocardial infarction: Natural history and clinical profile. *Am J Med* 75:332, 1983.

Coronary Drug Project Research Group: Natural history of myocardial infarction in the coronary drug project: Long-term prognostic importance of serum lipid levels. *Am J Cardiol* 42:489, 1978.

Dalen JE, Gore JM, Braunwald E, et al: Six and twelve month follow-up of the Phase I Thrombolysis in Myocardial Infarction (TIMI) Trial. *Am J Cardiol* 62:179, 1988.

Davies MJ, Thomas AC: Plaque fissuring—the cause of acute myocardial infarction, sudden ischemic death, and crescendo angina. *Br Heart J* 53:363, 1985.

DeBusk RF: Specialized testing after recent myocardial infarction. *Ann Int Med* 110:470, 1989.

DeBusk RF, Blomqvist CG, Kouchoukos NT, et al: Identification and treatment of low-risk patients after acute myocardial infarction and coronary-artery bypass graft surgery. *N Engl J Med* 314:161, 1986.

deFeyter PJ, Serruys PW, Wijns W: Early angiography after myocardial infarction: What have we learned. *Am Heart J* 109:194, 1985.

DeGuzman M, Rahimtoola SH: What is the role of pacemakers in patients with coronary artery disease and conduction abnormalities? *Cardiovasc Clin* 13:191, 1983.

Dell'Italia LJ, Starling MR, Blumhardt R, et al: Comparative effects of volume loading, dobutamine and nitroprusside in patients with predominant right ventricular infarction. *Circulation* 72:1327, 1985.

DeWood MA, Spores J, Notske R, et al: Prevalence of total coronary occlusion during the early hours of transmural myocardial infarction. *N Engl J Med* 303:897, 1980.

DeWood MA, Stifter WF, Simpson CS, et al: Coronary arteriographic findings soon after non-Q wave myocardial infarction. *N Engl J Med* 315:417, 1986.

DeWood MA, Notske RN, Berg R Jr, et al: Medical and surgical management of early Q wave myocardial infarction. I. Effects of surgical revascularization on survival, recurrent myocardial infarction, sudden death and functional class at 10 or more years of follow-up. II. Effects on mortality and global and regional left ventricular function at 10 or more years of follow-up. *J Am Coll Cardiol* 14:65, 1989.

De Zwaan C, Willems GM, et al: Enzyme tests in the evaluation of thrombolysis in acute myocardial infarction. *Br Heart J* 59:175, 1988.

Denniss AR, Richards DA, Cody DV, et al: Prognostic significance of ventricular tachycardia and fibrillation induced at programmed stimulation and delayed potentials detected on the signal-averaged electrocardiograms of survivors of acute myocardial infarction. *Circulation* 74:731, 1986.

Dressler W: The post-myocardial infarction syndrome: A report of forty-four cases. *Arch Intern Med* 103:28, 1959.

Ellis SG, O'Neill WW, Bates ER, et al: Implications for patient triage from survival and left ventricular functional analyses in 500 patients treated with coronary angioplasty for acute myocardial infarction. *J Am Coll Cardiol* 13:1251, 1989.

Erbel R, Pop T, Meinertz T, et al: Combination of calcium channel blocker and thrombolytic therapy in acute myocardial infarction. *Am Heart J* 115:529, 1988.

Feigenbaum H: Coronary artery disease. In: *Echocardiography*. Philadelphia: Lea and Febiger; 1986, p. 462.

Force T, Kemper A, Leavitt M, Parisi AF: Acute reduction in functional infarct expansion with late coronary reperfusion: Assessment with quantitative two-dimensional echocardiography. *J Am Coll Cardiol* 11:192, 1988.

Forrester JS, Diamond G, Chatterjee K, et al: Medical therapy of acute myocardial infarction by application of hemodynamic subsets (two parts). *N Engl J Med* 295:1356,1404, 1976.

Forrester JS, Litvack F, Grundfest W, Hickey A: A perspective of coronary disease seen through the arteries of a living man. *Circulation* 75:505, 1987.

Frishman WH, Karpenos A, Molloy TJ: Cocaine-induced coronary artery disease: Recognition and treatment. *Med Clin North Am* 73:475, 1989.

Fuchs RM, Achuff SC, Grunwals L, et al: Electrocardiographic localization of coronary artery narrowings: Studies during myocardial ischemia and infarction in patients with one-vessel disease. *Circulation* 66:1168, 1982.

Furberg CD, Byington RP: Beta-adrenergic blockers in patients with acute myocardial infarction. *Cardiovasc Clin* 20:235, 1989.

Gang ES, Lew AS, Hong M, et al: Decreased incidence of ventricular late potentials after successful thrombolytic therapy for acute myocardial infarction. *N Engl J Med* 321:712, 1989.

Gibson RS, Boden WE, Theroux P, et al: Diltiazem and reinfarction in patients with non-Q wave myocardial infarction: Results of a double-blind, randomized, multicenter trial. *N Engl J Med* 315:423, 1986.

Gibson RS, Watson DD, Craddock GB, et al: Prediction of cardiac events after uncomplicated myocardial infarction: A prospective study comparing predischarge exercise thallium-201 scintigraphy and coronary angiography. *Circulation* 68:321, 1983.

Gillum RF: Acute myocardial infarction in the United States, 1970–1983. *Am Heart J* 113:804, 1987.

Goldberg HL, Borer JS, Jacobstein JG, et al: Anterior ST segment depression in acute myocardial infarction: Indicator of posterolateral infarction. *Am J Cardiol* 48:1009, 1981.

Goldberg S, Greenspoon AJ, Urban PL, et al: Reperfusion arrhythmia: A marker of restoration of antegrade flow during intracoronary thrombolysis for acute myocardial infarction. *Am Heart J* 105:26, 1983.

Goldberger AL: ECG simulators of myocardial infarction. Pathophysiology and differential diagnosis of pseudo-infarct Q wave patterns (Part I) and pseudo-infarct ST-T patterns (Part II). *PACE* 5:106,414, 1982.

Goldman L, Batsford WP: Risk-benefit stratification as a guide to lidocaine prophylaxis of primary ventricular fibrillation in acute myocardial infarction: An analytic review. *Yale J Bio Med* 52:455, 1979.

Goldman L: Coronary care units: A perspective on their epidemiologic impact. *Int J Cardiol* 2:284, 1982.

Greenland P, Chu JS: Efficacy of cardiac rehabilitation services, with emphasis on patients after myocardial infarction. *Ann Int Med* 109:650, 1988.

Gruppo Italiano per lo Studio della Streptochinasi nell' Infarto Miocardico (GISSI): Effectiveness of intravenous thrombolytic treatment in acute myocardial infaction. *Lancet* 1:397, 1986.

Guerci AD, Gerstenblith G, Brinker JA, et al: A randomized trial of intravenous tissue plasminogen activator for acute myocardial infarction with subsequent randomization to elective coronary angioplasty. *N Engl J Med* 317:1613, 1987.

Hale SL, Kloner RA: Left ventricular topographic alterations in the completely healed rat infarct caused by early and late coronary reperfusion. *Am Heart J* 116:1508, 1988.

Hands ME, Rutherford JD, Muller JE, et al, and the MILIS Study Group: The in-hospital development of cardiogenic shock after myocardial infarction: Incidence, predictors of occurrence, outcome and prognostic factors. *J Am Coll Cardiol* 14:40, 1989.

Harker LA: Clinical trials evaluating platelet-modifying drugs in patients with atherosclerotic cardiovascular disease and thrombosis. *Circulation* 73:206, 1986.

Hindman MC, Wagner GS, JaRo M, et al: The clinical significance of bundle branch block complicating acute myocardial infarction. 1. Clinical characteristics, hospital mortality, and one year follow-up; 2. Indications for temporary and permanent pacemaker insertion. *Circulation* 58:679, 1978.

Hochman JS, Choo H: Limitation of myocardial infarct expansion by reperfusion independent of myocardial salvage. *Circulation* 75:299, 1987.

Hong RA, Licht JD, Wei JY, et al: Elevated CK-MB with normal creatine kinase in suspected myocardial infarction: Associated clinical findings and early prognosis. *Am Heart J* 111:1041, 1986.

Hutter AM, DeSanctis RW, Flynn T, Yeatman LA: Nontransmural myocardial infarction: A comparison of hospital and late clinical course of patients with that of matched patients with transmural anterior and transmural inferior infarction. *Am J Cardiol* 48:595, 1986.

ISAM Study Group: A prospective trial of intravenous streptokinase in acute myocardial infarction (ISAM): Mortality, morbidity, and infarct size at 21 days. *N Engl J Med* 314:1465, 1986.

ISIS-1 Collaborative Group: A randomized trial of intravenous atenolol among 16,027 cases of suspected acute myocardial infarction. *Lancet* 2:57, 1986.

ISIS-2 (Second International Study of Infarct Survival) Collaborative Group: Randomised trial of intravenous streptokinase, oral aspirin, both, or neither among 17,187 cases of suspected acute myocardial infarction: ISIS-2. *Lancet* 2:349, 1988.

Isner JM, Roberts WC: Right ventricular infarction complicating left ventricular infarction secondary to coronary heart disease: Frequency, location, associated findings and significance from analysis of 236 necropsy patients with acute or healed myocardial infarction. *Am J Cardiol* 42:885, 1978.

Isner JM, Estes NA, Thompson PD, et al: Acute cardiac events temporally related to cocaine abuse. *N Engl J Med* 315:1438, 1986.

Jennings RB, Reimer KA: Pathobiology of acute myocardial ischemia. *Hosp Pract* 24:89, 1989.

Johns JA, Gold HK, Leinbach RC, et al: Prevention of coronary artery reocclusion and reduction in late coronary artery stenosis after thrombolytic therapy in patients with acute myocardial infarction. *Circulation* 78:546, 1988.

Johnson DL, Thompson RC, Liu P, et al: Magnetic resonance imaging during acute myocardial infarction. *Am J Cardiol* 57:1059, 1986.

Jugdutt BI, Michorowski BL, Kappagoda CT: Exercise training after anterior Q wave myocardial infarction: Importance of regional left ventricular function and topography. *J Am Coll Cardiol* 12:362, 1988.

Kannel WB, Abbott RD: Incidence and prognosis of unrecognized myocardial infarction. *N Engl J Med* 311:1144, 1984.

Karch SB, Billingham ME: The pathology and etiology of cocaine-induced heart disease. *Arch Pathol Lab Med* 112:225, 1988.

Kennedy JW, Ritchie JL, Davis KB, Fritz JK: Western Washington randomized trial of intracoronary streptokinase in acute myocardial infarction. *N Engl J Med* 309:1477, 1983.

Kennedy JW, Ritchie JL, Davis KB, et al: The Western Washington randomized trial of intracoronary streptokinase in acute myocardial infarction. *N Engl J Med* 312:1073, 1985.

Killip T, Kimball JT: Treatment of myocardial infarction in a coronary care unit: A two-year experience with 250 patients. *Am J Cardiol* 20:457, 1967.

Klein LW, Helfant RH: The Q-wave and non-Q wave myocardial infarction: Differences and similarities. *Prog Cardiovasc Dis* 29:205, 1986.

Klimt CR, Knatterud GL, Stamler J, Meier P: Persantine-Aspirin Reinfarction Study part II. Secondary coronary prevention with persantine and aspirin. *J Am Coll Cardiol* 7:251, 1986.

Kloner RA, Braunwald E: Effects of calcium antagonists on infarcting myocardium. *Am J Cardiol* 59:84B, 1987.

Kloner RA, Parisi AF: Acute myocardial infarction: Diagnostic and prognosi applications of two-dimensional echocardiography. *Circulation* 75:521, 1987.

Kloner RA, Przyklenk K, Whittaker P: Deleterious effects of oxygen radicals in ischemia/reperfusion—Resolved and unresolved issues. *Circulation* 80:1115, 1989.

Krone RJ, Gillespie JA, Weld FM, Miller JP, Moss AJ, and the Multicenter Postinfarction Study Group: Low-level exercise testing after myocardial infarction: Usefulness in enhancing clinical risk stratification. *Circulation* 71:80, 1985.

Lange RA, Cigarroa RG, Yancy CW, et al: Cocaine-induced coronary-artery vasoconstriction. *N Engl J Med* 321:1577, 1989.

Lee T, Goldman L: Serum enzyme assays in the diagnosis of acute myocardial infarction. Recommendations based on a quantitative analysis. *Ann Intern Med* 102:221, 1986.

Lewis HD, David JW, Archibald DG, et al: Protective effects of aspirin against acute myocardial infarction and death in men with unstable angina. *N Engl J Med* 309:396, 1983.

Lie KI, Wellens HJ, Van Capelle FJ, et al: Lidocaine in the prevention of primary ventricular fibrillation: A double-blind randomized study of 212 consecutive patients. *N Engl J Med* 291:1324, 1974.

Marder VJ, Sherry S: Thrombolytic therapy: Current status. *N Engl J Med* 318:1512, 1585, 1988.

Marriott HJ: Coronary mimicry: Normal variants, and physiologic, pharmacologic and pathologic influences that simulate coronary patterns in the electrocardiogram. *Ann Int Med* 52:411, 1960.

Matsuda Y, Fujii B, Takashiba K, et al: Presence of angina pectoris before acute myocardial infarction and degree of residual stenosis after coronary thrombolysis. *Am Heart J* 117:1014, 1989.

Meltzer RS, Visser CA, Fuster V: Intracardiac thrombi and systemic embolization. *Ann Int Med* 104:689, 1986.

Miller FC, Krucoff MW, Satler LF et al: Ventricular arrhythmias during reperfusion. *Am Heart J* 112:928, 1986.

Mitchell LB, Duff JH, Manyari DE: et al: A randomized trial of the noninvasive and invasive approaches to drug therapy of ventricular tachycardia. *N Engl J Med* 317:1681, 1987.

Moss AJ, Davis HT, Conrad DL, Decamilla JJ, Odoroff CL: Digitalis-associated cardiac mortality after myocardial infarction. *Circulation* 64:1150, 1981.

Moss AJ, Davis HT, Decamilla J, et al: Ventricular ectopic beats and their relation to sudden and nonsudden cardiac death after myocardial infarction. *Circulation* 60:998, 1979.

Muller JE, Rude RE, Braunwald E, et al, and the MILIS Study Group: Myocardial infarct extension: Occurrence, outcome, and risk factors in the Multicenter Investigation of Limitation of Infarct Size. *Ann Int Med* 108:1, 1988.

Muller JE, Turi ZG, Stone PH, et al, and the MILIS Study Group: Digoxin therapy and mortality after myocardial infarction. Experience in the MILIS study. *N Engl J Med* 314:265, 1986.

Multicenter Postinfarction Research Group: Risk stratification and survival after myocardial infarction. *N Engl J Med* 309:331, 1983.

Multicenter Diltiazem Postinfarction Trial Research Group: The effect of diltiazem on mortality and reinfarction after myocardial infarction. *N Engl J Med* 319:385, 1988.

Murray N, Lyons J, Layton C, Balcon R: What proportion of patients with myocardial infarction are suitable for thrombolysis? *Br Heart J* 57:144, 1987.

Naunheim KS, Kesler KA, Kanter KR, et al: Coronary artery bypass for recent infarction: Predictors of mortality. *Circulation* 78:I-122, 1988.

Nicod P, Gilpin E, Dittrich H, et al: Short and long-term clinical outcome after Q wave and non-Q wave myocardial infarction in a large patient population. *Circulation* 79:528, 1989.

Obrador D, Ballester M, Carrio I, Berna L, Pons-Llado G: High prevalence of myocardial monoclonal antimyosin antibody uptake in patients with chronic idiopathic dilated cardiomyopathy. *J Am Coll Cardiol* 13:1289, 1989.

O'Connor GT, Buring JE, Yusuf S, et al: An overview of randomized trials of rehabilitation with exercise after myocardial infarction. *Circulation* 80:234, 1989.

O'Neill W, Timmis GC, Bourdillon PD, et al: A prospective randomized clinical trial of intracoronary streptokinase versus coronary angioplasty for acute myocardial infarction. *N Engl J Med* 314:812, 1986.

O'Neill WW, Topol EJ, Pitt B: Reperfusion therapy of acute myocardial infarction. *Prog Cardiovasc Dis* 30:235, 1988.

Page DL, Caulfield JB, Kastor JA, DeSanctis RW, Sanders CA: Myocardial changes associated with cardiogenic shock. *N Engl J Med* 285:133, 1971.

Pasternak RC, Braunwald E, Sobel BE: Acute myocardial infarction. In: Braunwald E, ed. *Heart Disease: A Textbook of Cardiovascular Medicine.* Philadelphia: Saunders; 1988, p. 1222.

Pfeffer MA, Lamas GA, Vaaughan DE, Parisi AF, Braunwald E: Effect of captopril on progressive ventricular dilatation after anterior myocardial infarction. *N Eng J Med* 319:80, 1988.

Physicians' Health Study Research Group Steering Committee: Final report on the aspirin component of the ongoing Physicians' Health Study. *N Engl J Med* 321:129, 1989.

Puleo PR, Roberts R: An update on cardiac enzymes. *Cardiol Clin* 6:97, 1988.

Rackley CE, Russell RO Jr, Mantle JA, et al: Modern approach to the patient with acute myocardial infarction. *Curr Probl Cardiol* 1:1, 1977.

Raunio H, Rissanen V, Romppanen T, et al: Changes in the QRS complex and ST segment in transmural and subendocardial myocardial infarctions. A clinicopathologic study. *Am Heart J* 98:176, 1979.

Reimer KA, Jennings RB: The wavefront phenomenon of myocardial ischemic cell death. II. Transmural progression of necrosis within the framework of ischemic bed size (myocardium at risk) and collateral flow. *Lab Invest* 40:633, 1979.

Reimer KA, Jennings RB, Tatum AH: Pathobiology of acute myocardial ischemia: Metabolic, functional and ultrastructural studies. *Am J Cardiol* 52:72, 1983.

Rentrop KP, Feit F, Sherman W, et al: Late thrombolytic therapy preserves left ventricular function in patients with collateralized total coronary occlusions: Primary end point findings of the second Mount Sinai-New York University Reperfusion Trial. *J Am Coll Cardiol* 14:58, 1989.

Roos JC, Dunning AJ: Bundle branch block in acute myocardial infarction. *Eur J Cardiol* 6:403, 1978.

Rothbaum DA, Linnemeier TJ, Landin RJ, et al: Emergency percutaneous transluminal coronary angioplasty in acute myocardial infarction: A 3 year experience. *J Am Coll Cardiol* 10:264, 1987.

Rude RE, Muller JE, Braunwald E: Efforts to limit the size of myocardial infarcts. *Ann Int Med* 95:736, 1981.

Sager PT, Perlmutter RA, Rosenfeld LE, et al: Electrophysiologic effects of thrombolytic therapy in patients with a transmural anterior infarction complicated by left ventricular aneurysm formation. *J Am Coll Cardiol* 12:19, 1988.

Schaper J, Schaper W: Reperfusion of ischemic myocardium: Ultrastructural and histochemical aspects. *J Am Coll Cardiol* 1:1037, 1983.

Schroeder JS, Lamb IH, Hu M: Do patients in whom myocardial infarction has been ruled out have a better prognosis after hospitalization than those surviving infarction? *N Engl J Med* 303:1, 1980.

Schroder R, Neuhaus KL, Leizorovicz A, Linderer T, Tebbe U (for the ISAM Study Group): A prospective placebo-controlled double-blind multicenter trial of intravenous streptokinase in acute myocardial infarction (ISAM): Long-term mortality and morbidity. *J Am Coll Cardiol* 9:197, 1987.

Schuster EH, Bulkley BH: Early post-infarction angina: Ischemia at a distance and ischemia in the infarct zone. *N Engl J Med* 305:1101, 1981.

Schuster EH, Bulkley BH: Expansion of transmural myocardial infarction: A pathophysiologic factor in cardiac rupture. *Circulation* 60:1532, 1979.

Schwaiger M, Brunken RC, Krivokapich J, et al: Beneficial effect of residual anterograde flow on tissue viability as assessed by positron emission tomography in patients with myocardial infarction. *Eur Heart J* 8:981, 1987.

Sharpe N, Smith H, Murphy J, Hannan S: Treatment of patients with symptomless left ventricular dysfunction after myocardial infarction. *Lancet* 1:255, 1988.

Sheehan FH, Doerr R, Schmidt WG, et al: Early recovery of left ventricular function after thrombolytic therapy for acute myocardial infarction: An important determinant of survival. *J Am Coll Cardiol* 12:289, 1988.

Simonton CA, Mark DB, Hinohara T, et al: Late restenosis after emergent coronary angioplasty for acute myocardial infarction: Comparison with elective coronary angioplasty. *J Am Coll Cardiol* 11:698, 1988.

Simoons ML, Betriu A, Col J, et al, for the European Cooperative Study Group for Recombinant Tissue-Type Plasminogen Activator: Thrombolysis with tissue plasminogen activator in acute myocardial infarction: No additional benefit from immediate percutaneous coronary angioplasty. *Lancet* 1:197, 1988.

Skolnick AE, Frishman WH: Calcium channel blockers in myocardial infarction. *Arch Int Med* 149:1669, 1989.

Solimene MC, Ramires JA, Bellotti G, Tranchesi B Jr, Pileggi F: Reperfusion arrhythmias in acute myocardial infarction—fact or coincidence? *Int J Cardiol* 20:341, 1988.

Spirito P, Bellotti P, Chiarella F, Domenicucci S, Semanta A, Vecchio C: Prognostic significance and natural history of left ventricular thrombi in patients with acute anterior myocardial infarction: A two-dimensional echocardiographic study. *Circulation* 72:774, 1985.

Stone PH, Turi ZG, Muller JE, et al: Prognostic significance of the treadmill exercise test performed 6 months after myocardial infarction. *J Am Coll Cardiol* 8:1007, 1986.

Theroux P, Ouimet H, McCans J, et al: Aspirin, heparin, or both to treat acute unstable angina. *N Engl J Med* 319:1105, 1988.

Tiefenbrunn AJ, Sobel BE: The impact of coronary thrombolysis on myocardial infarction. *Fibrinolysis* 3:1, 1989.

TIMI Study Group: Comparison of invasive and conservative strategies after treatment with intravenous tissue plasminogen in acute myocardial infarction. *N Engl J Med* 320:618, 1989.

TIMI Research Group: Immediate versus delayed catheterization and angioplasty following thrombolytic therapy for acute myocardial infarction. TIMI II A results. *JAMA* 260:2849, 1988.

Tofler GH, Muller JE, Stone PH, et al: Pericarditis in acute myocardial infarction: Characterization and clinical significance. *Am Heart J* 117:86, 1989.

Tofler GH, Stone PH, Muller JE, et al: Prognosis after cardiac arrest due to ventricular tachycardia or ventricular fibrillation associated with acute myocardial infarction (the MILIS study). *Am J Cardiol* 60:755, 1987.

Topol EJ: Coronary angioplasty for acute myocardial infarction. *Ann Int Med* 109:970, 1988.

Topol EJ, George BS, Kereiakes DJ, et al, and the TAMI Study Group: A randomized controlled trial of intravenous tissue plasminogen activator and early intravenous heparin in acute myocardial infarction. *Circulation* 79:281, 1989.

Topol EJ, Burek K, O'Neill WW, et al: A randomized controlled trial of hospital discharge three days after myocardial infarction in the era of reperfusion. *N Engl J Med* 318:1083, 1988.

Topol EJ, Califf RM, George BS, et al: A randomized trial of immediate versus delayed elective angioplasty after intravenous tissue plasminogen activator in acute myocardial infarction. *N Engl J Med* 317:581, 1987.

Tsukamoto H, Hashimoto H, Matsui Y, et al: Detection of myocardial reperfusion by analysis of serum creatine kinase isoforms. *Clin Cardiol* 11:287, 1988.

Turitto G, Fontaine JM, Ursell SN, et al: Value of the signal-averaged electrocardiogram as a predictor of the results of programmed stimulation in nonsustained ventricular tachycardia. *Am J Cardiol* 61:1272, 1988.

Van de Werf F, Arnold AE: Intravenous tissue plasminogen activator and size of infarct, left ventricular function, and survival in acute myocardial infarction. *Br Med J* 297:1374, 1988.

Visser CA, Kan G, Meltzer RS, Koolen JJ, Dunning AJ: Incidence, timing and prognostic value of left ventricular aneurysm formation after myocardial infarction: A prospective, serial echocardiographic study of 158 patients. *Am J Cardiol* 57:729, 1986.

Visser CA, Kan G, Meltzer RS, Dunning AJ, Roelandt J: Embolic potential of left ventricular thrombus after myocardial infarction: A two-dimensional echocardiographic study of 119 patients. *J Am Coll Cardiol* 5:1276, 1985.

Volpi A, Maggioni A, Franzosi MG, et al: In-hospital prognosis of patients with acute myocardial infarction complicated by primary ventricular fibrillation. *N Engl J Med* 317:257, 1987.

Volpini M, Giubbini R, Gei P, et al: Diagnosis of acute myocardial infarction by indium-111 antimyosin antibodies and correlation with the traditional techniques for the evaluation of extent and localization. *Am J Cardiol* 63:7, 1989.

Wackers FJ, Terrin ML, Kayden DS, et al, and TIMI Investigators: Quantitative radionuclide assessment of regional ventricular function after thrombolytic therapy for acute myocardial infarction: Results of Phase I Thrombolysis in Myocardial Infarction (TIMI) Trial. *J Am Coll Cardiol* 13:998, 1989.

Waller BF, Rothbaum DA, Pinkerton CA, et al: Status of the myocardium and infarct-related coronary artery in 19 necropsy patients with acute recanalization using pharmacologic (streptokinase, r-tissue plasminogen activator), mechanical (percutaneous transluminal coronary angioplasty) or combined types of reperfusion therapy. *J Am Coll Cardiol* 9:785, 1987.

Waller BF: The pathology of acute myocardial infarction: Definition, location, pathogenesis, effects of reperfusion, complications, and sequelae. *Cardiol Clin* 6:1, 1988.

Wasserman AG, Ross AM: Coronary thrombolysis. *Curr Probl Cardiol* 14:9, 1989.

Weisman HF, Healy B. Myocardial infarct expansion, infarct extension, and reinfarction: Pathophysiologic concepts. *Prog Cardiovasc Dis* 30:73, 1987.

Weld FM, Chu KL, Bigger JT, et al: Risk stratification with low-level exercise testing two weeks after acute myocardial infarction. *Circulation* 64:306, 1981.

White HD, Rivers JT, Maslowski AH et al: Effect of intravenous streptokinase as compared with that of tissue plasminogen activator on left ventricular function after first myocardial infarction. *N Engl J Med* 320:817, 1989.

White RD, Grands P, Califf L, Palmeri ST, Califf RM, Wagner GS: Diagnostic and prognostic significance of minimally elevated creatine kinase-MB in suspected acute myocardial infarction. *Am J Cardiol* 55:1478, 1985.

Wilcox RG, Olsson CG, von der Lippe G, et al, for the ASSET Study Group: Trial of tissue plasminogen activator for mortality reduction in acute myocardial infarction. *Lancet* 2:525, 1988.

Yusuf S, Collins R, Peto R, et al: Intravenous and intracoronary fibrinolytic therapy in acute myocardial infarction: Overview of results on mortality, reinfarction and side effects from 33 randomized trials. *Eur Heart J* 6:556, 1985.

Yusuf S, Collins R, MacMahon S, et al: Effect of IV nitrates on mortality in acute myocardial infarction: An overview of the randomized trials. *Lancet* 1:1088, 1988.

Yusuf S, Peto R, Lewis J, et al: Beta blockade during and after myocardial infarction: An overview of the randomized trials. *Prog Cardiovasc Dis* 27:335, 1985.

Yusuf S, Wittes J, Friedman L: Overview of results of randomized clinical trials in heart disease. I. Treatments following myocardial infarction. *JAMA* 260:2088, 1988.

16 Interventional Cardiology

Stephen Oesterle
Andrew C. Eisenhauer

PERCUTANEOUS TRANSLUMINAL CORONARY ANGIOPLASTY

The first decade of percutaneous transluminal coronary angioplasty (PTCA) was characterized by dramatic technological advances and unparalleled growth in application. Following Dr. Andreas Gruentzig's first description of the technique in the late 1970s (Gruentzig et al. 1979), approximately 200 procedures were performed by 1980. By the end of the last decade, more than 200,000 procedures were performed annually. This exponential growth in application, associated with broadening indications and vastly improved success rates, is largely attributable to technological improvements in the instruments available for performing angioplasty.

Early dilatation devices developed by Gruentzig in conjunction with Schneider-Medintag (Zurich) were neither steerable nor low-profile. Guiding catheters were stiff and had very poor torque. Because of these technical limitations, PTCA was initially targeted at proximal, discrete lesions. Poor steerability precluded routine dilatation of distal stenoses, branch stenoses, and most lesions in the left circumflex coronary artery. Because these early procedures were also tedious and frequently prolonged, angioplasty of multivessel coronary artery disease was rarely attempted.

By the conclusion of the registry of the National Heart, Lung, and Blood Institute in 1982 (Kent et al.), the overall success rate was just over 60%, with single-vessel coronary artery disease representing the vast majority of cases. Around this same time, Simpson introduced a second-generation dilatation device (Advanced Cardiovascular Systems, Santa Clara, California) which was distinguished by an independently moveable guide wire (Simpson et al. 1982).

Dilatation devices could then be tracked over a wire, which could be independently positioned across target stenoses. Although the first intracoronary guide wires were neither steerable nor particularly flexible, multiple advances in engineering and manufacturing produced a family of intracoronary guide wires with various degrees of flexibility and steerability. With the current generation of intracoronary guide wires, it is possible to position a wire in virtually every patent branch of the coronary tree.

Concurrent advances in balloon technology have led to further miniaturization of dilatation devices. New plastic materials have been incorporated into the balloon and shaft allowing for lower crossing profiles and the ability to cross critical stenoses without the need for significant "backup" support from the guiding catheters. Some dilatation balloons are attached directly to the guide wire, adding no more than 0.001–0.002 inches to the crossing profile of the bare wire. These low-profile devices have facilitated the crossing of high-grade stenoses in the most distal aspects of the coronary anatomy.

In comparison to the NHLBI Registry data of 1982, overall success rates for coronary angioplasty are now routinely better than 90%. Improved steerability and lower profiles have expanded the potential for this procedure to include lesions which may be distal, heavily calcified, eccentric, or involving branch vessels. Multi-lesion and multivessel dilatations now represent a substantial proportion of the successful cases.

Long-term benefits have been clearly documented with follow-up now extending beyond 10 years in selected groups of patients (Gruentzig et al. 1987). For most patients with symptomatic single-vessel coronary artery disease, angioplasty offers a very acceptable alternative to coronary artery bypass surgery and, for at least 70% of patients, results in significant improvement in symptoms and reduction in ischemia by objective criteria (Talley et al.). Whether patients with multivessel coronary disease are best treated by angioplasty or surgery remains controversial and is the focus of at least two randomized trials in progress in the United States.

INDICATIONS

Given the refinements in angioplasty equipment, the question is rarely, "Can it be done by balloon angioplasty," but, more frequently, "Should it be done?" The best candidates for PTCA generally have single-vessel disease with stenoses that are proximal, noncalcified, and concentric, and do not involve major side branches. Patients hospitalized with unstable or new-onset angina constitute a large proportion of patients with single-vessel disease. Patients considered for elective PTCA should be moderately to significantly symptomatic with objective evidence of ischemia by treadmill testing, thallium scintigraphy, exercise echocardiography or exercise radionuclide ventriculography.

Many cardiologists offer angioplasty as an alternative to medical therapy in patients who are well controlled with medication but would like to reduce or eliminate the need for taking medications.

Some patients undergoing PTCA are asymptomatic and have had their underlying coronary disease unmasked by surveillance treadmill testing or by the development of serious ventricular arrhythmias. Angioplasty has been offered to these patients with "silent ischemia" when they present with disease anatomically favorable for dilatation.

The application of PTCA in the setting of an acute myocardial infarction remains controversial. Angioplasty can be used either as direct therapy for recanalization or as an adjunct to thrombolytic therapy. These issues will be discussed more extensively in a later section.

Some patients with symptomatic multivessel CAD have several major stenoses, each of which has suitable location and morphology for PTCA; others may have one or two vessels which are ideal for PTCA while the remaining diseased vessels are poor targets because of lesion morphology. Incomplete revascularization, with dilatation of only the putative "culprit" lesion, is frequently advocated as an alternative to bypass surgery. Although many of these patients

Table 1. Relative Contraindications to PTCA
Chronic total occlusion (>3 months)
Long lesions (>2 cm)
Old vein grafts with diffuse disease
Ostial stenoses of the right coronary artery or vein grafts
Stenoses involving major side branches that cannot be protected
Stenoses with associated organized thrombus
Stenoses within *severely* angulated segments
Extensive calcification of the involved arterial segment
Coronary spasm as a predominant component of stenosis (lesion <70%)
Very recent reperfusion with tissue plasminogen activator
Presence of noncritical left main coronary artery disease when firm engagement of a left main guiding catheter is anticipated
Noncritical stenoses (<60%)

can either be relieved or significantly improved, some physicians are critical of this incomplete approach.

Coronary bypass grafts, including reverse saphenous vein grafts and internal mammary artery grafts, can usually be easily dilated; however, restenosis and embolization of vein graft debris are common problems following dilatation (Cote et al.).

RELATIVE CONTRAINDICATIONS

Guidelines for PTCA have been delineated by a joint task force from the American College of Cardiology and the American Heart Association. Tables 1 and 2 present a synthesis of these conservative guidelines and our experience. Although experienced operators can expect initial success rates in excess of 90% for ideal lesions, PTCA for lesions listed in Table 1 will be less successful. Table 1 lists "relative" contraindications. The contraindications do not mean that these lesions should not be done, but that the lesions are less likely to be successfully dilated without complications. (Success is defined as >20% reduction in

Table 2. Absolute Contraindications to PTCA

Unprotected left main coronary artery disease

Extensive myocardial jeopardy, i.e., where vessel occlusion following PTCA would result in loss of >60% of viable myocardium

Coronary stenoses in vessels uninvolved with acute myocardial infarction

Absence of timely surgical standby

luminal diameter with a residual stenosis <50%, and no major complication such as death or the need for coronary bypass surgery during the hospitalization.)

Chronic total occlusions are not likely to be recanalized by conventional balloon angioplasty. Although the risks are low, failure is frequently encountered with the attendant financial loss from used equipment and personnel time. Lesions >2 cm in length are associated with a higher rate of dissection, abrupt closure, and restenosis (Ellis et al. 1988 and 1988a). Ostial stenoses of the right coronary artery or of a bypass graft are associated with poor results because of inability to seat the guiding catheter; balloon dilatations are generally suboptimal and restenosis is encountered more frequently, most likely because of the recoil of the elastic fibers in the aorta.

Most side branches can be protected during angioplasty of an adjacent vessel; however, anatomic variability may preclude protecting major side branches (Oesterle). These unprotected side vessels will either be occluded during angioplasty of the adjacent vessel (20% incidence) or will be left as a potential source of coronary insufficiency. Frequently, they are best treated surgically.

Organized thrombus at the site of dilatation dramatically increases the complications during PTCA (Cameron et al.). Organized thrombus should be addressed adjunctively with intracoronary thrombolytic agents.

Lesions causing <60% stenosis should not be routinely dilated, as they are not likely to cause coronary insufficiency. Dilatation of these lesions is associated with the same risks of vessel occlusion and restenosis (Ischinger et al.). A noncritical stenosis can become a high-grade critical stenosis following restenosis.

ABSOLUTE CONTRAINDICATIONS

Table 2 outlines circumstances whereby PTCA is believed to be contraindicated. Although dilatation of high-grade left main coronary artery stenosis is technically straightforward, complications such as abrupt closure can threaten life. Restenosis in this subset of patients has also been associated with out-of-hospital sudden death. For the very rare patient who requires revascularization and for whom surgery cannot be performed, PTCA can be accomplished by the use of special dilatation catheters which perfuse the distal coronary bed while the balloon is inflated (Stack, Quigley et al.; Turi et al. 1988) or with the circulatory support of a percutaneous cardiopulmonary pump system.

Left main disease can be appropriately treated by PTCA when "protection" exists in the form of a patent bypass graft to the left anterior descending or the left circumflex coronary arteries. In these circumstances the left main disease has been reduced to "single vessel" disease.

The jeopardy of a single dilatation should be assessed before subjecting a patient to PTCA. Frequently, a target vessel for angioplasty is the source of collaterals to another major coronary artery. Abrupt closure immediately after angioplasty can result in massive infarction from compromise of both the target artery and the collateralized artery. Attempts should be made to open the collateralized artery before dilating the target artery. If the collateralized artery cannot be opened with PTCA and the total amount of jeopardized myocardium represents more than 60% of the remaining viable myocardium, surgery should be considered. Elective bypass surgery will generally mean lower risk for the patient in such a situation.

Angioplasty for acute myocardial infarction is extensively discussed in a later section. In the setting of a myocardial infarction, angioplasty of coronary vessels uninvolved with the acute event can lead to catastrophe and should be deferred until the reperfused, "stunned" myocardium in the area of the infarct recovers.

Until a reliable percutaneous solution to abrupt vessel closure is developed, emergency bypass surgery will continue to be necessary for 2-3% of patients at the time of angioplasty. Therefore, *angioplasty is contraindicated in settings where cardiac surgery is not readily available.*

PATIENT MANAGEMENT

The management of patients before, during and after coronary angioplasty is directed predominantly toward the anticipation of potential complications. Planning of the procedure, preparation of the patient, performance of the angioplasty and subsequent patient care all interact to determine the ultimate success of the procedure. Most elective coronary angioplasty is uncomplicated and elaborate precautions may therefore seem "unnecessary." However, many potentially unsuccessful procedures have been successful because of careful planning and anticipatory management.

Surgical Support

Coronary angioplasty and surgical myocardial revascularization are complementary and not competitive. The standby surgical team must be truly supportive and willing to perform cardiac surgery on patients with angioplasty complications under emergency conditions. Early in the development of coronary angioplasty, an operating room was held open for each patient. As angioplasty has improved, a designated, waiting operating room for all patients has become unnecessary. Accordingly, many centers have adopted a tiered approach to surgical standby. There are some patients for whom the potential need for emergency cardiac surgery during angioplasty approaches that associated with routine catheterization. Patients with chronic, well-collateralized occlusions of the right coronary artery, for example, are at low risk. Thus, dilatation of a chronically occluded vessel that supplies a moderate or small amount of myocardium and is well collateralized is very unlikely to require emergency surgical revascularization even if the procedure is unsuccessful. There are complications that may arise, such as guide wire perforation or proximal coronary dissection from the guiding catheter, that require urgent surgical intervention. For these "level 0" angioplasties, an operating room need not be ready and there need be no greater surgical involvement than that for routine cardiac catheterization and angiography.

In the majority of other single-vessel coronary angioplasties, the surgical team simply needs to be aware that angioplasty is taking place and that a complication could arise requiring urgent surgery. In large centers with active cardiac surgical programs, no single operating room need be kept available; an available surgical team on site is sufficient. Single-vessel an-

gioplasty involving the right or circumflex system, where the amount of jeopardized myocardium is relatively small, can fit into this group. With the advent of coronary reperfusion catheters and stents for the control of acute reocclusions that do not respond to redilatation, many more patients may fall into this category requiring "level 1" backup.

If there is concern that significant hemodynamic compromise will result from uncontrollable coronary occlusion, and that immediate surgical revascularization may be necessary, a designated operating room and surgical team should be kept on standby until there is no longer a significant risk of occlusion. Angioplasties of arteries that supply a large myocardial segment—a proximal lesion in a very large circumflex system, left anterior descending lesions proximal to the first significant diagonal branch, or large arteries in patients with severely compromised left ventricular function—are best dealt with using this "level 2" backup. For some patients it is prudent to have an intraaortic balloon pump console available with the electrocardiographic monitoring leads preconnected to the patient and both groins prepped for any easy second arterial access. An occasional patient is best supported on an intraaortic balloon pump during PTCA.

As increasingly complex and complicated angioplasties are performed, several additional support options have been developed. Angioplasty of the left main coronary artery or its hemodynamic equivalent has been carried out in a combined angiographic suite/operating room setting (McAuley et al.). Other institutions keep equipment for open-chest cardiopulmonary bypass and surgery available in the catheterization laboratory. Finally, percutaneous total cardiopulmonary bypass systems have been developed to support hemodynamically unstable patients during potentially dangerous angioplasty procedures (Vogel et al.).

All patients should be fully and openly informed about their PTCA procedure and its potential risks. Written or videotaped educational materials are helpful adjuncts, as is the use of nurse-clinicians to provide further teaching and support. The concept of surgical standby should be discussed with the patient to ensure complete understanding. The patient's oral intake should be managed in preparation for possible intubation and general anesthesia.

Consideration should be given to the presence of dentures or other oral appliances. Relative contraindications to intubation and surgery (such as critical obstructive lung disease) should be kept in mind. Although it is seldom needed, all information relative to the patient's tolerance of emergency intubation, anesthesia, and cardiac surgery should be sought in the preoperative period, as there will be little time to do so should emergency surgery be necessary.

Hospital admission for elective coronary angioplasty need not occur until the day of the procedure in many cases. A stable and free-running intravenous line should be started in the forearm and the patient kept well hydrated (be mindful of the potential for fluid overload in patients with impaired renal or cardiac function). Many pre-procedure regimens for sedation exist and most are satisfactory. Patients should be started on low-dose aspirin before their procedure. Blood products are not routinely reserved for patients undergoing angioplasty.

Management of Patients during PTCA

Control of periodic and unintended occlusion. Successful coronary angioplasty creates controlled, periodic coronary occlusion. The most common problems that an operator must deal with during angioplasty are those arising when control of occlusion is lost. It is difficult to predict the response of an individual patient and individual artery to the resulting ischemia, but prediction can be attempted by evaluating the amount of myocardium that will be ischemic during balloon inflation and estimating its contribution to cardiac performance and hemodynamic stability. Dilatation of a small distal right coronary artery is unlikely to render a large amount of myocardium ischemic during balloon inflation. Nevertheless, elective right coronary dilatation can result in hypotension that is vagally mediated or caused by the Bezold-Jarisch reflex. In a similar fashion, balloon *deflation* can result in paradoxical hypotension or bradycardia (Gacioch et al.). The judicious use of atropine and fluid therapy to correct reflex vasodilation can help to mitigate this problem. On the other hand, the dilatation of certain vessels, such as the proximal left anterior descending coronary, may be associated with hemodynamic compromise simply because they supply a large amount of contracting muscle. The proper choice of inflation times or the use of distal perfusion (Erbel et al.; Turi et al. 1987, 1988) may help in situations where acute depression of left ventricular function occurs. In some patients, the prophylactic use of intraaortic balloon counterpulsation or other cardiopulmonary support may be warranted.

The occurrence of unintended coronary occlusion during PTCA is infrequent, and the ability to gain control over these occlusions has increased. Early in the history of coronary angioplasty, it was feared that coronary embolization from plaque debris might be a significant problem. Plaque embolization is now known to be uncommon in native vessels but can occur in deteriorating, aging saphenous vein bypass grafts. The distal embolization of thrombus occurs more frequently and is reason for caution in the dilatation of arteries containing large amounts of thrombus (Cameron et al.). Some operators advocate prolonged pretreatment with intravenous heparin, some use no adjuvant therapy, and others use local thrombolytic agents (Cohen et al.). Particular caution should be exercised in vessels totally occluded with plaque and subacute thrombus—the notion that a patient with an occluded vessel cannot be "made worse" by an unsuccessful PTCA of a totally occluded artery is untrue. Embolization can compromise collateral flow to the distal vessel and create or worsen ischemia. Unintended but controllable coronary ischemia can also occur from inappropriate or inept manipulation of equipment. The inadvertent injection of air or thrombus from improperly or inadequately flushed catheters can create profound ischemia and hemodynamic collapse or simulate other forms of uncontrollable coronary occlusion. This is entirely preventable by careful attention to equipment setup and manipulation.

Ostial coronary occlusion can result from obstruction by the guiding catheter. This may occur when a minimal ostial narrowing is present or when a guide catheter is deeply seated to provide support for advance of the balloon catheter. The resulting persistent ischemia after balloon deflation is often misinterpreted by inexperienced dilators as a more distal coronary occlusion due to spasm, dissection or embolus. Unseating the catheter, using a guiding catheter with a different configuration, or using a catheter with side holes for coronary perfusion will usually alleviate this problem.

All types of coronary instrumentation, including angioplasty, can produce coronary spasm. Spasm may occur at the site of coronary dilatation and can be associated with continuing ischemia following balloon deflation. Although there are some common angiographic features of spasm, there is no absolutely characteristic appearance—it is often indistinguishable from other forms of occlusion or near-occlusion at the angioplasty site. In such situations, the administration of intracoronary nitroglycerin can sometimes ameliorate ischemia and thus is diagnostic. If spasm at the site of dilatation is resistant to nitroglycerin, redilatation (often at higher pressures, with a larger balloon or for a longer duration) may resolve it.

Vasospasm can occur in the nondilated portions of the instrumented artery or even in the contralateral coronary vessel. Guide catheter tips can produce ostial spasm and profound ischemia. A guide wire tip can cause mechanical irritation and spasm and impede distal flow in a fashion similar to an embolus. These kinds of spasm often respond to repositioning of the offending device and to use of intracoronary nitroglycerin. Occasionally, intraaortic balloon counterpulsation has been associated with the reversal of profound coronary spasm and amelioration of hemodynamic compromise.

Managing coronary dissection. Coronary dissection is probably the most feared management difficulty during coronary angioplasty. It is also the most common. At times, the deep seating of a guiding catheter may cause ostial coronary dissection. Left main dissection with occlusion is rare but often fatal. Prompt balloon dilatation, or the placement of a coronary perfusion ("bailout") catheter and emergency coronary surgery, may salvage the situation (Ferguson et al.). Right coronary ostial dissection with occlusion, because of possible compromise of both the sinoatrial and atrioventricular nodal arteries, is also a dire complication. Ostial dissections are not always associated with complete occlusion and can simply create further reduction in the lumen, with dye staining or irregularities characterizing their angiographic appearance. Their prompt recognition and (usually) surgical management can prevent death. Figure 1 illustrates a proximal dissection precipitated by deep-seating a guiding catheter. More distal coronary dissection may also be instigated by passage of a guide wire tip through an area of disrupted or friable plaque. The guide wire tip or other coronary instrumentation can raise a "flap" and cause luminal compromise or occlusion at any point along the vessel. This accounts for the difficulty in separating guide wire-mediated distal coronary dissection from spasm. Most commonly, however, coronary dissection occurs at the site of dilatation.

It might be argued that most successful angioplasties are associated with dissection simply because the predominant mechanism of angioplasty is to produce a controlled dissection over a limited area (Block et al.; Soward et al.; Mizuno et al.). "Pathologic" dissection results when there is sufficient disruption of plague to collapse the vessel lumen and compromise

distal flow (Waller et al.; Waller). Multiple techniques have been proposed to reduce the incidence of pathologic dissections, including the undersizing or oversizing of balloons, the use of low pressure-long duration inflations, intraprocedural monitoring of balloon/vessel compliance, sequential dilatation with successively larger balloons, or limiting the rate of balloon inflations (Jain et al.; Levin et al.; Simpendorfer et al.). There is no proven "best" strategy—most dilators opt to increase the rate of pressure slowly during inflation and to avoid overdilatation. Interestingly, the presence of an angiographically visible dissection without luminal compromise has been correlated with improved long-term patency (Matthews et al.; Leimgruber et al. 1985, 1986). Characteristics that suggest an increased risk of dissection may include calcification of the vessel, lesion location, and the angiographic appearance of the stenosis (Bredlau et al.; Cowley et al.).

The management of dissection consists primarily of its avoidance; and as PTCA equipment and operators have improved, the rate of uncontrollable dissections has decreased. Yet, there seem to be some arteries where dissection will occur no matter what technique is employed—an operator-independent variable. Under these circumstances, redilatation is the first-line therapy, in most cases using the same balloon inflated for a longer time, at a higher pressure, or both. Occasionally, the substitution of a larger balloon will be required to "tack down" a recalcitrant flap. Figure 2 shows a severe localized dissection at the site of balloon dilatation in a coronary vein graft. Empiric intracoronary nitroglycerin, if permitted by the patient's blood pressure, may help to rule out or treat concomitant coronary spasm. The duration, number, and extent of redilatations that should be used in the management of dissection are functions of operator experience, the degree of ischemia, and the patient's hemodynamic status.

At times, redilatation will not control the dissection. This is one of the most common indications for urgent cardiac surgery after angioplasty. The use of coronary reperfusion catheters may relieve ischemia while preparations for surgery are being made. Coronary stents or laser-balloon "welding" techniques may help to provide further control of coronary dissection in the future. When severe hypotension or hemodynamic compromise occurs, the prompt insertion of an intraaortic balloon or other circulatory assist device may help to achieve hemodynamic stability in preparation for emergency surgery.

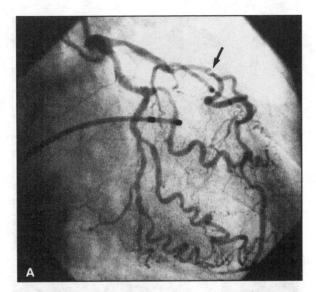

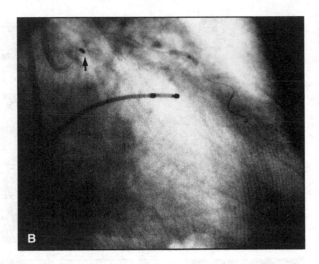

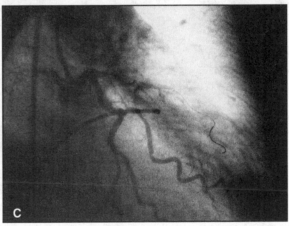

Figure 1. *Proximal dissection in the left anterior descending coronary artery caused by deep seating of the guiding catheter. A. The pre-angioplasty angiogram indicates both proximal LAD plaquing and a distal shelf-like stenosis (arrow) in a tortuous vessel that required forceful seating (B, arrow) of the guide catheter to cross and dilate. C. Disruption of the proximal LAD resulted in acute dissection unresponsive to repeat balloon dilatation and necessitating emergency surgery.*

Post-procedure Management

The most important management problem after coronary angioplasty is long-term restenosis, discussed in detail in the next section of this chapter. The management of acute closure is of paramount concern in the immediate post-angioplasty period.

Routinely following a successful angioplasty (if the procedure has been performed from the femoral approach), vascular access sheaths are left indwelling and the patient is continued on intravenous heparin. Should acute occlusion occur, vascular access is readily available for redilatation. The appropriate duration of systemic heparinization is not known. As a practical matter, most operators leave the vascular sheaths in place from 12-24 hours. Interruption of heparinization and the removal of the sheaths on the day after PTCA is therefore the rule. In the past, most angio-

plasty patients were monitored in intensive care units, as these were the only places in the hospital where arterial catheters could be maintained. Many institutions now have special areas where stable post-angioplasty patients can be followed overnight. This has reduced costs and increased patient comfort.

Under all circumstances, careful monitoring for the development of peri-access bleeding is appropriate. Femoral hematomas can be difficult to detect unless the clinician is alert for their presence. The development of hypotension or a vasovagal reaction several hours after coronary angioplasty should always prompt suspicion of hemorrhage. In most instances bleeding is minimal, but it is uncomfortable and cosmetically unappealing. In some cases, blood loss is significant, and heparinization should be interrupted and the vascular access removed. The development of pseudoaneurysm or arteriovenous fistula is possi-

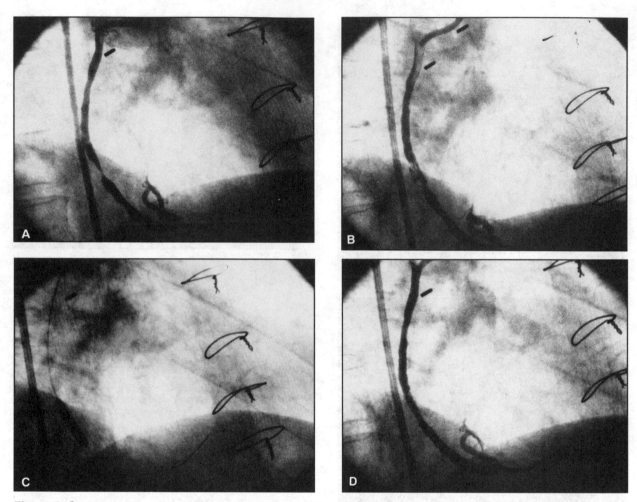

Figure 2. *Severe, localized dissection in an old vein graft. A. The pre-angioplasty angiogram. B. After initial dilatation with a 3.5-mm balloon, there is plaque disruption and luminal compromise. C. Following redilatation with a 4.0-mm balloon for an extended duration, a good result is established (D).*

ble and should be considered. In addition, patients have often undergone diagnostic catheterization before angioplasty and then are kept without their usual oral intake. The subsequent angioplasty procedure entails the use of radiographic contrast material and an ensuing osmotic diuresis. Following angioplasty, therefore, patients tend to be intravascularly volume-depleted and may require vigorous fluid replacement. Thus, the major differential diagnosis in postprocedural hypotension is blood loss versus simple dehydration volume-depletion. Occasionally vasovagal reactions or medication-related bradycardias also account for hypotension.

In the past, there was great concern over the late development of coronary spasm after angioplasty. Pa-

tients were thus routinely kept on nitrates and/or calcium channel blockers in the immediate postprocedure period. The development of significant delayed coronary vasospasm is uncommon. Although some luminal narrowing may often occur (Fishell et al.), its clinical significance is doubtful. Since most patients are managed on calcium channel blockers before their procedure, many are continued on them afterwards. We generally discharge patients on a calcium channel blocker and continue it for at least six weeks. In this way, should the patient develop early restenosis, some protection against angina will be on board. We do not routinely perform predischarge exercise testing in patients with adequate angiographic results. Occasionally, following a very difficult procedure or those with uncertain angiographic results, the performance of a "second look" coronary angiogram is appropriate before sheath removal and hospital discharge. This is also appropriate in patients with recurrent symptoms after dilatation. It should be emphasized to nurses and other monitoring personnel that the development of recurrent ischemic symptoms after dilatation is a medical emergency that is often best dealt with by repeat angiography and angioplasty. It is not a situation in which the administration of nitrates alone is sufficient.

In most instances, the discharge of patients from the hospital can be accomplished 24-36 hours after completion of PTCA. This is predicated on the patient being ambulatory and without complications after removal of the vascular access. Repeat exercise testing or other objective confirmation of the abolition of ischemia can be accomplished on an outpatient basis.

RESTENOSIS

Restenosis after successful balloon dilatation occurs in 20-35% of patients and requires repeat angioplasty (Holmes et al.; Meier et al.; Leimgruber et al. 1986). The majority of cases of restenosis occur in the first two to three months following PTCA and are generally heralded by either recurrent angina or a clearly positive exercise treadmill test (Serruys et al. 1988; Nobuyoshi et al.). Although both thallium scinitigraphy and exercise echocardiography are more sensitive indicators of coronary insufficiency than is treadmill testing alone, their cost makes them less attractive for routine surveillance. Patients who have not developed restenosis at six months will generally have continued patency of the dilated coronary segment for years. Repeat angioplasty for restenosis is associated with favorable results and lower complication rates, but recurrent restenosis can occur (Quigley et al.; Glazier et al.; Bonan). Third dilatations are performed (Teirstein et al.), but a patient is generally declared an angioplasty failure after three dilatations and should be considered for either surgery or experimental intervention (see sections following on new intravascular devices).

Restenosis is rarely a reaccumulation of plaque. It is a sequela of "healing" at the site of dilatation (Faxon et al.). Platelets adhere to the sites of endothelial trauma and may stimulate a complex cascade that leads to restenosis over the course of weeks to months (Harker; Ross; Fuster et al.). The primary "culprit" appears to be *smooth muscle cell proliferation* which is stimulated by various growth mediators released from platelet aggregates, endothelial cells, and local macrophages in response to the local injury from balloon angioplasty. Several mechanical solutions for limiting endovascular injury have been devised, including cutting devices, intravascular stents, and lasers (see below). None of these devices has yet been proven to reduce the incidence of restenosis.

"Biologic" solutions appear to be more promising but as yet are undeveloped. Blocking substances to the various mediators of smooth muscle cell proliferation are being sought. Antiplatelet antibodies are in development which offer the potential of blocking platelet adherence (Coller et al.; Gold et al.). No conventional therapy has significantly altered the incidence of restenosis (Harker and Fuster; Kyrle et al.; Blackshear et al.). Fish oil has recently been proposed as an effective prevention in restenosis; however, the data remain controversial (Dehmer et al.; Grigg et al.).

NEWER INTRAVASCULAR DEVICES

Atherectomy

The Simpson directional atherectomy device (Athero Cath) was developed as an alternative to balloon angioplasty (Simpson et al. 1988; Pinkerton et al.). This percutaneous device has a rigid metal housing which cuts and extracts intracoronary plaque, leaving a relatively smooth surface. Simpson coined the word "atherectomy" and postulated that the type of "controlled" intravascular injury it caused might lead to a reduction in the incidence of restenosis. Figure 3 is a schematic representation of the atherectomy device. The device was recently approved for use in the peripheral vessels but remains an investigational device for coronary artery disease. Although initial data suggest that it reduces the incidence of restenosis, this complication is still a significant problem. Atherectomy may nonetheless emerge as the preferred treatment for friable bypass graft stenoses and complex coronary stenoses involving ulcerations and thrombus. Increased flexibility and further miniaturization will be necessary before it can be used routinely in the coronary circulation.

The transluminal extraction catheter (TEC) is similar to the Simpson directional atherectomy device in that it is an "over the wire" system which cuts and

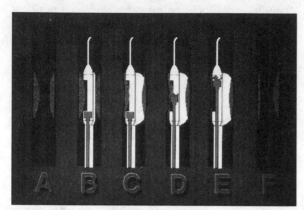

Figure 3. *Schematic representation of atherectomy using the Simpson AtheroCath. In plate B, the device is positioned across the stenosis with the aid of a guide wire. A stabilizing balloon is inflated at low pressures and the rotational cutting device is advanced at 2,000 rpm, "shaving" plaque into the metal housing (C-E). The device can be rotated to shave additional plaque, or withdrawn. (Courtesy of John Simpson, M.D.)*

removes plaque (Stack). It is a cutting device with two blades that revolve in a conical fashion as the device advances. Continuous suction during cutting will theoretically remove the shaved debris (Figure 4). Data have yet to validate its potential to reduce restenosis. Like the Simpson atherectomy device, it appears to have particular promise when applied to vein grafts and thrombus.

The Auth-Rotablator device (Figure 5) is considered an alternative atherectomy device, although pulverization, not atherectomy, is accomplished (Ritchie et al.; Hansen et al.; O'Neill et al.). An abrasive burr

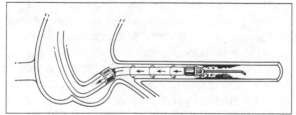

Figure 4. *Schematic representation of the transluminal extraction catheter (TEC). The device consists of a motorized cutting head with triangular blades controlled by a steerable guidewire. The cutting head rotates at 750 rpm, and a suction apparatus removes excised plaque. (From Stack. With permission.)*

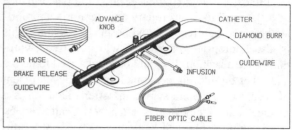

Figure 5. *The Auth-Rotablator device. The diamond burr is rotated at high speed by an air-driven turbine. Rotational speed is monitored with the fiber optic cable. The burr is advanced over an independently moveable guide and "pulverizes" plaque. (Courtesy of David Auth, M.D.)*

is advanced over a wire down the coronary artery at rotation speeds in excess of 150,000 rpm. Atherosclerotic plaque is pulverized into debris less than 10 microns in size. This particulate debris embolizes distally, without apparent micro-infarction. The Rotablator can easily track over a wire and offers flexibility for delivery into branched and distal vessels. Like the TEC device, fixed profiles of the rigid burr necessitate large-lumen guiding catheters for delivery of the device. No data have yet indicated that restenosis will be substantially reduced with the Rotablator.

Stents

Several investigational intracoronary stents are being evaluated in the United States. Sigwart, working in Lausanne, Switzerland, is credited with developing the first intracoronary stent (Sigwart et al. 1987). Although these devices have obvious application in the setting of acute dissection and abrupt vessel closure (Sigwart et al. 1988), enthusiasm has spread for their potential to reduce rates of restenosis (King; Schatz). Elastic recoil of the dilated coronary segment has been implicated as one of the important factors in early restenosis. Rigid stenting of the dilated segment would potentially mitigate this phenomenon. "Tacking" of a major dissection might limit the exposure of damaged intima and media to circulating platelets, and secondarily reduce the stimulation for smooth muscle cell proliferation and attendant restenosis.

Among the metal stents that have now been developed, the Wallstent is the self-expanding stent developed by Sigwart and his colleagues. The Palmaz-Schatz stent is a balloon-expanded stent that has been used both in the periphery and the coronary circulation (Palmaz et al.; Schatz et al.). In clinical trials, both of these stents have been associated with restenosis and late occlusion, although the majority of implanted stents appear to have long-term patency. Experience is too limited to make any conclusions about their ability to meaningfully reduce the incidence of restenosis.

The Gianturco-Roubin stent (Roubin et al.) has been primarily investigated at Emory University. Initial studies evaluated it as a "bail-out" device for acute closure after dissection from balloon angioplasty. The stent has been used as a "bridge" to coronary bypass surgery, maintaining patency of the dissected vessel as the patient is taken for surgery. It is envisioned that this device, like the Wallstent and the Palmaz-Schatz stent, will be used as an alternative to emergency surgery, obviating the need for surgical bypassing of badly dissected coronary segments. It is anticipated that this family of stents will also reduce the incidence of embolization during balloon dilatation of friable vein graft segments (Urban et al.; Serruys et al. 1989).

Flexibility has not been an outstanding feature of the current generation of stents; delivery of these metal devices to branch and distal vessels is not easy. Furthermore, they remain as a foreign body in the coronary circulation and serve as stimulants for platelet adhesion and subsequent development of thrombosis and restenosis.

Laser Angioplasty

Lasers have been used as both an adjunct to balloon angioplasty and as a primary recanalization device in coronary artery disease. The so-called "hot tip" laser device (Laser Probe, Spectraprobe) was the first percutaneous laser system approved for vascular use. The "hot tip" laser is a thermal device with a metal tip (probe) heated by a laser fiber; the thermal energy is used to recanalize diseased vessels (Cumberland et al.; Sanborn et al.). The device can be used as an over-the-wire system or as a blunt probe. Although this type of device is effective in recanalization, the thermal injury from it can be extensive, and it has not been proven to reduce restenosis. It has been primarily used as an adjunct to conventional balloon angioplasty. The Laser Probe opens a channel allowing passage of a wire and low-profile dilatation catheter; the technique is referred to as laser-assisted angioplasty.

Spears (1987) developed an alternative technique using laser assistance as an adjunct to angioplasty. He incorporated a fiberoptic fiber wrapped cylindrically along the central shaft of a dilatation catheter. The balloon is inflated at the target site and continuous-wave laser radiation is concomitantly delivered thought the fiber. The balloon materials are transparent to the laser radiation, and thermal energy is transmitted through the plaque and surrounding tissues to a depth of approximately 3 mm. Desiccation of thrombus and fusion of separated layers of arterial wall can be achieved reliably. This process has been referred to as laser balloon angioplasty (LBA) and has a potential for creating a wide, smooth, thrombus-free lumen. Clinical trials are underway and restenosis rates are yet unknown.

Multiple devices have been developed to "ablate" rather than thermally injure plaque (Litvack et al. 1988). Continuous and pulsed lazing can result in ablation or evaporation of the plaque. The excimer laser offers the potential of ablating variable composition atheromas without thermal damage to the adjacent normal tissue (Grundfest et al.; Forrester et al.; Litvack et al. 1989). The direction and depth of injury are still poorly controlled with all of these systems, however. Coupled with the limitation of small areas of focused ablation, such obstacles have largely precluded the routine use of laser devices. Lasers will clearly be useful as *recanalization* devices. But it is still uncertain whether they will be effective in substantially debulking intracoronary plaque or reducing restenosis.

ANGIOPLASTY IN ACUTE MYOCARDIAL INFARCTION

In the early history of coronary angioplasty, the presence of intracoronary thrombus was considered a near absolute contraindication to the procedure. As operators became more comfortable with the technique, its indications expanded and cardiologists began to use angioplasty to restore patency of coronary arteries that remained severely obstructed after administration of intracoronary thrombolytic therapy (Meyer et al.). It was quickly realized that angioplasty without thrombolytic agents could also be used as primary therapy to restore coronary patency (Hartzler et al.). Using currently available equipment, skilled operators can now successfully and stably recanalize more than 80% of infarct-related vessels in the setting of an acute myocardial infarction (Figure 6). At this time,

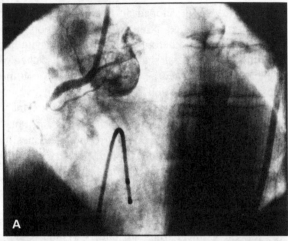

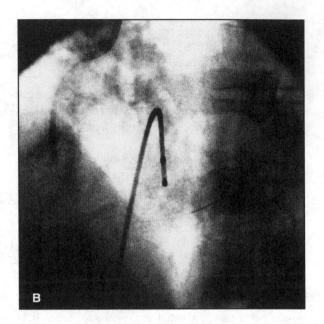

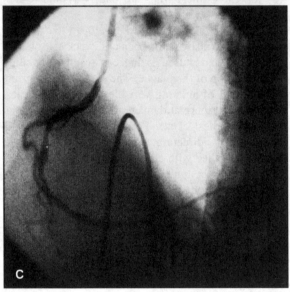

Figure 6. *Direct coronary angioplasty in acute myocardial infarction. A proximally occluded right coronary artery (A) is subjected to balloon dilatation (B), with the initial results shown in (C).*

effective, easily administered, intravenous thrombolytic agents have been developed that also effect successful and stable coronary reperfusion (see Chapter 15). Tissue plasminogen activator (TPA), despite its high cost, has become the mainstay of coronary thrombolytic therapy and its relationship to and interaction with angioplasty have been studied extensively (Topol et al.; Guerci et al.; TIMI).

Coronary angiography performed during myocardial infarction has shown clearly that when thrombolytic therapy is applied to an infarct-related vessel, there is often an underlying residual stenosis after dissolution of the intracoronary thrombus (Meyer et al.). The assumption has been that presence of this residual stenosis might be flow limiting or that it could somehow become biologically active, engendering

rethrombosis. Therefore, concern was raised that simple dissolution of thrombus would not be sufficient to prevent rethrombosis once the thrombolytic agent was cleared. A logical strategy evolved recommending intravenous thrombolytic therapy followed by emergency or urgent coronary angioplasty.

While thrombolytic therapy can be given easily in nearly every emergency room and hospital setting, the performance of emergency coronary angioplasty requires appreciably greater organization, facilities, and personnel. Thus, coronary angioplasty is not always available for all patients. The cost of making it available may be substantial and the benefits uncertain. Fortunately, this dilemma prompted organized and large-scale scientific investigation. Recently concluded randomized trials of TPA with and without routine coronary angioplasty confirm that if thrombolytic therapy is the first line of intervention, routine angioplasty offers no benefit in short-term survival or in improved ventricular function (Topol et al; Guerci et al.; TIMI). In fact, the vascular access required for the performance of PTCA may engender more short-term complications (see also Chapter 15).

Significant clinical issues in the relationship of PTCA to thrombolytic therapy were not addressed in these trials. For example, angioplasty without prior thrombolytic therapy has not yet been compared to thrombolytic therapy in a large-scale prospective trial. In addition, TPA is the only agent extensively evaluated with and without angioplasty. Other thrombolytic agents may not have a similar relationship. In centers where primary angioplasty is used for acute MI patients, mortality has been as low as that reported in large-scale thrombolysis trials (Sinclair et al.; Rutherford et al.; Giorgi et al.). In cardiogenic shock patients, direct coronary angioplasty has been shown to be the intervention of choice; it has achieved significant reductions in mortality compared with historic controls (Lee et al.; O'Neill).

Accumulating data are also indicating that in the setting of acute myocardial infarction, a patent infarct-related artery at the time of hospital discharge may confer an improved prognosis (Stack, Califf et al.). The improvement may be unrelated to the degree of myocardial salvage or ventricular function (Hochman and Choo; Sager et al.). ISIS-2, a large-scale thrombolysis trial, indicated that reperfusion delayed for up to 24 hours after the onset of symptoms may confer a survival advantage (ISIS-2). Delayed direct angioplasty may also be effective (Eisenhauer and Moore; Ellis et al. 1989).

At present, the patient successfully reperfused with TPA should not *routinely* be treated with balloon angioplasty. However, there is danger in assuming that the biologic activities of all other lytic agents will make this conservative approach appropriate with them as well. What should be the intervention strategy for those patients who clinically fail chemical reperfusion, develop recurrent ischemia after reperfusion, have a contraindication to thrombolytic therapy, or who simply cannot receive lytic therapy within 4-6 hours after the onset of infarction? In many institutions, patients in these groups are catheterized emergently and undergo PTCA. It is clear that a significant percentage of patients who receive initial TPA therapy will require such emergent angiography and intervention. Some will need "elective" procedures for

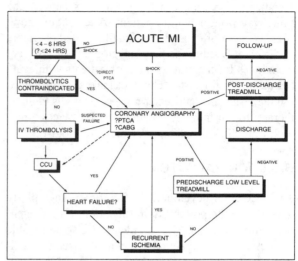

Figure 7. *Flow diagram for the clinical management of acute myocardial infarction. The central concept is that reperfusion should be achieved as quickly as possible. Definition of coronary anatomy is essential in complicated situations (shock, thrombolytic failure, or recurrent ischemia) where mechanical therapy may be helpful. Arrows toward center represent potential transfer from primary to tertiary center. In high-risk patients or those with a complicated clinical course or ongoing ischemia, definition of coronary anatomy and possible mechanical reperfusion are valuable adjuncts.*

symptoms that develop after hospital discharge, and a significant number will require emergency angiography and angioplasty to control recurrent or ongoing ischemia. A flow chart used at The Heart Institute of The Hospital of the Good Samaritan for the management of patients with acute MI is shown in Figure 7. Although it is not necessary to transport every infarct patient to a catheterization laboratory for intervention, every infarct patient *may need* subsequent intervention. And while it is not cost effective to ensure instant local availability of PTCA for all patients, it is desirable to develop systems that give community hospitals direct access to the full range of emergency interventional cardiology services on a regionalized and cost effective basis.

The challenge for the future is not only to develop the best thrombolytic agent, but also to determine how best to combine interventional techniques with thrombolytic reperfusion, and to determine if and when direct intervention without thrombolysis is preferable. In comparing techniques with drugs, one must remember that a drug can be given in essentially the same way from patient to patient. A technique, however, is operator dependent. Equally skilled operators at different institutions may develop subtly different techniques for the management of patients with acute MI during angioplasty. This fact makes it difficult to use the results of multicenter prospective trials to guide therapy for an individual patient; and it places a premium on clinical judgment of the cardiologist.

BALLOON VALVOTOMY

The successful development of coronary angioplasty gave rise to the possibility of dilatation of other stenotic cardiac lesions. Such an idea was also a probable outgrowth of interventional techniques such as balloon atrial septostomy (Rashkind et al.) or blade septostomy (Park et al.) that have been applied in pediatric cardiology.

Consideration was first given to the dilatation of congenital pulmonic stenosis in children through use of a moving, inflated balloon like that used for septostomy (Semb et al.). "Angioplasty-like" static balloon dilatation was first proposed by Kan (Kan et al.). The pathology of congenital valvular pulmonic stenosis involved fusion of valve leaflets or the development of a supravalvular membrane; balloon dilatation of these noncalcified valves might result in commissural splitting and a low incidence of distal embolization. In addition, it was believed that brief occlusions of the pulmonary artery might be well tolerated and that small distal embolizations would be less of a problem in the pulmonary circuit than in the left heart. These assumptions proved true. The first catheters used for pulmonic dilatation were modifications of those developed for peripheral angioplasty. The procedure has been successful and has become the treatment of choice for congenital valvular pulmonic stenosis (Kvelselis et al.; Ali Khan et al.; Radtke et al.).

Interest soon developed in the balloon dilatation, or valvotomy, of adult acquired stenotic valvular heart disease (Lock et al.). Rheumatic mitral and tricuspid stenoses were first attempted (McKay, Lock, et al.; Palacios et al. 1986) with large balloons that permitted transvalvular passage, inflation, and dilatation, resulting in disruption of rheumatic commissural fusion.

High-quality echocardiography and color flow Doppler mapping have facilitated the pre-procedure risk stratification of patients with mitral stenosis and helped in evaluating the results of the balloon valvotomy procedure. As is the case for surgical commissurotomy, ideal valvotomy patients are those whose valvular stenosis is a result primarily of commissural fusion and not of chordal foreshortening and subchordal scarring, and whose valve leaflets are not calcified. Echocardiographic identification of left atrial thrombus, which increases the chance of systemic or cerebral embolization, can also be made before the procedure. A quantitative scoring system has been developed to evaluate patients and to predict results of balloon valvotomy (Wilkins et al.).

Mitral valvotomy is performed typically via the transseptal approach. Arterial and venous access is obtained (usually from the right groin); retrograde, transseptal catheterization of the left heart is performed and a transmitral gradient measured. Following confirmation of mitral stenosis, a balloon flotation catheter is passed from the left atrium to the left ventricle through the mitral valve. A stiff guide wire or guide wires are then passed transseptally to the left ventricle or, in some cases, out into the aorta. The skin tract through the groin and into the femoral vein is enlarged and dilatation of the intraatrial septum is performed with an 8-10 mm balloon. This accommodates the larger balloon catheters needed for effective dilatation. Both single- and double-balloon techniques are employed; several types of balloons have been developed that permit more stable seating within the mitral apparatus (Inoue et al.; Meier et al. 1986). After dilatation and confirmation of a reduction in transvalvular gradient, the mitral valve area is measured using standard catheterization techniques.

Figure 8 illustrates balloon dilatation of the interventricular septum and mitral valve. Contrast ventriculography or echocardiography is employed to assess the change in degree of mitral regurgitation, if any, and oximetry is used to assess the magnitude of the atrial-septal defect produced by dilatation of the interventricular septum.

The short- and long-term results of mitral valvotomy are encouraging. Reported restenosis rates at nine months have been under 5% (Vahanian et al.). Although the technique has been in use for far less time than surgical commissurotomy, the mechanism of balloon valvotomy is similar and the long-term results are expected to be similar (McKay et al. 1987; John et al.). An additional benefit of balloon valvotomy is that it does not involve a sternotomy or a thoracotomy, and it is easily reapplied to appropriate patients. Today, balloon mitral valvotomy is consid-

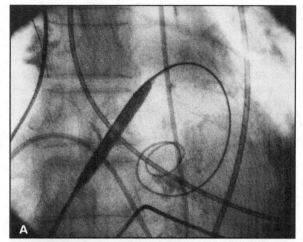

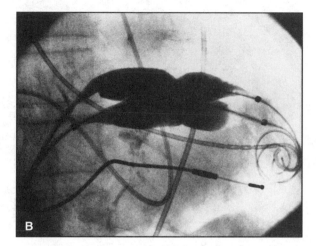

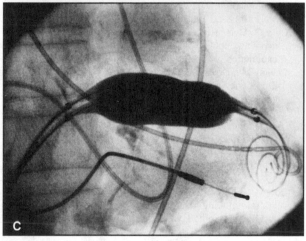

Figure 8. *Transseptal mitral balloon valvotomy. Balloon dilatation of the interatrial septum (A) allows passage of two large valvotomy balloons. Initial inflation (B) reveals a "waist" that largely disappears with full balloon expansion (C). (Courtesy of Carlos Ruiz, M.D.)*

ered by many cardiologists to be the most widely applicable first-line therapy in patients with rheumatic mitral stenosis (Roberts).

Although noncalcific congenital aortic stenosis is effectively treated with balloon valvotomy (Perry et al.), balloon dilatation of acquired aortic stenosis has not fared as well. This experience parallels that of surgical valvotomy of rheumatic aortic valves. It results in part from the way aortic valvotomy has been applied in the United States—to degenerative calcific aortic stenosis, the most common type of adult aortic stenosis. Although it was feared initially that obstruction of the aortic valve orifice would be very dangerous and potentially fatal, this obstruction was quickly shown to be well tolerated if associated with subsequent reduction in aortic stenosis.

Retrograde aortic valvotomy requires crossing of the aortic valve with guide wires and the retrograde passage of a dilating balloon or balloons through the orifice (Figure 9). A high degree of technical success has been achieved with the procedure. In degenerative calcific aortic stenosis, however, the mechanism of reduction in stenosis is the cracking and deformation of areas of calcification in the valve leaflets; the disruption of commissural fusion is less apparent in these valves than in mitral valves (McKay et al. 1986). For this reason, just as in surgical valvotomy, the long-term results of balloon valvotomy in calcific aortic stenosis have been relatively poor. Up to 50% of patients develop restenosis within six months (Block and Palacios). Outside of the U.S., where aortic stenosis is more likely to be rheumatic in origin, better long-term success has been reported with balloon valvotomy (Letac et al.).

In the U.S., valvotomy of the aortic valve should be reserved for patients who are too ill to undergo aortic valve replacement or in patients whose expected survival because of other intercurrent disease

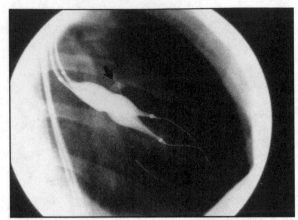

Figure 9. *Cineangiogram of transaortic dilatation of a stenotic aortic valve using the retrograde double-balloon technique. A large amount of asymmetric calcification is noted (arrow).*

(malignancy, for example) is brief. In addition, balloon aortic valvotomy may be used as protective therapy should other major noncardiac surgery be required (Roth et al.). Another potential use is diagnostic: there exists a group of patients with extremely poor ventricular function and aortic stenosis in whom the clinician may question whether relief of aortic obstruction will improve ventricular function or symptoms. A trial balloon valvotomy may be appropriate to determine whether the patient will be a candidate for subsequent valve replacement. Perhaps future advances in valvotomy catheters and better patient selection will give aortic valvotomy an improved long-term success rate and expanded clinical applications.

Bibliography

Ali Khan MA, Yousef SA, Mullins CE: Percutaneous transluminal balloon pulmonary valvuloplasty for the relief of pulmonary valve stenosis with special reference to double-balloon technique. *Am Heart J* 112:158, 1986.

American College of Cardiology/American Heart Association Task Force Report: Guidelines for percutaneous transluminal coronary angioplasty. *J Am Coll Cardiol* 12:529:, 1988.

Blackshear JL, O'Callaghan WG, Califf RM: Medical approaches to prevention of restenosis after coronary angioplasty. *J Am Coll Cardiol* 9:834, 1987.

Block PC, Myler RK, Stertzer S, Fallon JT: Morphology after transluminal angioplasty in human beings. *N Engl J Med* 305:382, 1985.

Block PC, Palacios IF: Clinical and hemodynamic follow-up after percutaneous aortic valvuloplasty in the elderly. *Am J Cardiol* 62:760, 1988.

Bonan R: Angioplasty and restenosis revisited: Diagnosis and management of restenosis. *J Interv Cardiol* 1:69, 1989.

Bredlau CE, Roubin GS, Leimgruber PP, et al. In-hospital morbidity and mortality in patients undergoing elective coronary angioplasty. *Circulation* 72:1044, 1985.

Califf RM, Topol EJ, George BS, et al: Coronary arterial thrombolysis with combined infusion of recombinant tissue-type plasminogen activator and urokinase in patients with acute myocardial infarction. *Circulation* 77:1100, 1988.

Cameron J, Buchbinder M, Wexler L, Oesterle SN: Thromboembolic complications of percutaneous transluminal coronary angioplasty for myocardial infarction. *Cathet Cardiovasc Diagn* 13:100, 1987.

Cohen BM, Buchbinder M, Kozina J, et al: Rethrombosis during angioplasty in myocardial infarction and unstable syndromes: Efficacy of intracoronary urokinase and redilating (abstr). *Circulation* 78(Suppl):II-8, 1988.

Coller BS, Scudder LE, Berger HJ: Inhibition of human platelet function in vivo with a monoclonal antibody. *Ann Intern Med* 109:635, 1988.

Cote G, Myler RK, Stertzer SH, et al: Percutaneous transluminal angioplasty of stenotic coronary artery grafts: 5 years experience. *J Am Coll Cardiol* 9:8, 1987.

Cowley MJ, Dovros G, Kelsey SF, Van Raden M, Detre KM: Emergency coronary bypass surgery after coronary angioplasty: The National Heart, Lung, and Blood Institute's Percutaneous Transluminal Coronary Angioplasty Registry experience. *Am J Cardiol* 53:22C, 1984.

Cumberland DC, Sanborn TA, Tayler DI, et al: Percutaneous laser thermal angioplasty: Initial clinical results with a laser probe in total peripheral artery occlusions. *Lancet* i:1457, 1986.

Dehmer GJ, Popman JJ, Vandenberg EG, et al: Reduction in the rate of early restenosis after coronary angioplasty by a diet supplemented with n-3 fatty acids. *N Engl J Med* 319:733, 1988.

Eisenhauer AC, Moore L: Direct angioplasty in acute myocardial infarction. Benefit of late reperfusion in patients with collateral flow (abstr). *J Am Coll Cardiol* 9:191A, 1987.

Erbel R, Clas W, Busch U, et al: New balloon catheter for prolonged percutaneous transluminal coronary angioplasty and bypass flow in occluded vessels. *Cathet Cardiovasc Diagn* 12:116, 1986.

Ellis SG, Roubin GS, King SB, et al: Angiographic and clinical predictors of acute closure after native vessel coronary angioplasty. *Circulation* 77:372, 1988.

Ellis SG, Roubin GS, King SB, et al: In-hospital cardiac mortality after acute closure after coronary angioplasty: Analysis of risk factors from 8,207 procedures. *J Am Coll Cardiol* 11:211, 1988. (a)

Ellis SG, O'Neill WW, Bates ER, et al: Coronary angioplasty as primary therapy for acute myocardial infarction 6-48 hours after symptom onset: Report of an initial experience. *J Am Coll Cardiol* 13:1122, 1989.

Faxon DP, Sanborn TA, Haudenschild CC: Mechanism of angioplasty and its relation to restenosis. *Am J Cardiol* 60:5B, 1987.

Ferguson TB Jr, Hinohara T, Simpson J, Stack RS, Wechsler AS: Catheter reperfusion to allow optimal coronary bypass grafting following failed transluminal coronary angioplasty. *Ann Thorac Surg* 42:399, 1986.

Fischell TA, Derby G, Tse TM, Stadius M: Coronary artery vasoconstriction routinely occurs after percutaneous transluminal coronary angioplasty—a quantitative arteriographic analysis. *Circulation* 78:1323, 1988.

Forrester JS, Litvack F, Grundfest W, et al: The excimer laser: Current knowledge and future prospects. *J Interv Cardiol* 1:75, 1988.

Fuster V, Badimon L, Cohen M, et al: Insights into the pathogenesis of acute ischemic syndromes. *Circulation* 77:1213, 1988.

Gacioch GM, Topol EJ: Sudden paradoxic clinical deterioration during angioplasty of the occluded right coronary artery in acute myocardial infarction. *J Am Coll Cardiol* 14:1202, 1989.

Giorgi LV, et al: Direct PTCA for acute MI in patients commonly excluded from thrombolytic trials (abstr). *Circulation* 78:11, 1988.

Glazier JJ, Varricchione TR, Ryan TJ, et al: Factors predicting recurrent restenosis after percutaneous transluminal coronary balloon angioplasty. *Am Heart J* 63:902, 1989.

Gold HK, Coller BS, Yasuda T, et al: Rapid and sustained coronary artery recanalization with combined bolus injection of recombinant tissue-type plasminogen activator and monoclonal antiplatelet GIIb/IIIa antibody in a canine preparation. *Circulation* 77:670, 1988.

Grigg LE, Kay TWH, Valentine PA, et al: Determinants of restenosis and lack of effect of dietary supplementation with eicosapentaenoic acid on the incidence of coronary artery restenosis after angioplasty. *J Am Coll Cardiol* 13:665, 1989.

Gruentzig AR, Senning A, Siegenthaler WE: Nonoperative dilatation of coronary-artery stenosis: Percutaneous transluminal coronary angioplasty. *N Engl J Med* 301:61, 1979.

Gruentzig AR, King SB, Schlumpf M, Siegenthaler W: Long-term follow-up after percutaneous transluminal coronary angioplasty. The early Zurich experience. *N Engl J Med* 316:1127, 1987.

Grundfest WS, Litvak F, Forrester JS, et al: Laser ablation of human atherosclerotic plaque without adjacent tissue injury. *J Am Coll Cardiol* 5:929, 1985.

Guerci AD, Gerstenblith G, Brinker JA, et al: A randomized trial of intravenous tissue plasminogen activator for acute myocardial infarction with subsequent randomization to elective coronary angioplasty. *N Engl J Med* 317:1613, 1987.

Hansen DD, Auth DC, Hall M, Ritchie JL: Rotational endarterectomy in normal canine coronary arteries: Preliminary report. *J Am Coll Cardiol* 11:1073, 1988.

Harker LA: Role of platelets and thrombosis in mechanisms of acute occlusion and restenosis after angioplasty. *Am J Cardiol* 60:20B, 1987.

Harker LA, Fuster V: Pharmacology of platelet inhibitors. *J Am Coll Cardiol* 8(Suppl):21B, 1986.

Hartzler GO, Rutherford BD, McConahay DR, et al: Percutaneous transluminal coronary angioplasty with and without thrombolytic therapy for treatment of acute myocardial infarction. *Am Heart J* 106:965, 1983.

Hochman JS, Choo H: Limitation of myocardial infarct expansion by reperfusion independent of myocardial salvage. *Circulation* 75:299, 1987.

Holmes DR, Vlietstra RE, Smith HC, et al: Restenosis after percutaneous transluminal coronary angioplasty (PTCA): A report from the PTCA Registry of the National Heart, Lung, and Blood Institute. *Am J Cardiol* 53:77C, 1984.

Ischinger T, Gruentzig AR, Hollman J, et al: Should coronary arteries with less than 60% diameter stenosis be treated by angioplasty? *Circulation* 68:148, 1983.

ISIS-2 (Second International Study of Infarct Survival): Randomized trial of intravenous streptokinase, oral aspirin, both or neither among 17,187 cases of suspected acute myocardial infarction. *Lancet* 2:349, 1988.

Jain A, Demer LL, Raizner AE, et al: In vivo assessment of vascular dilatation during percutaneous transluminal coronary angioplasty. *Am J Cardiol* 60:988, 1987.

John S, Bashi VV, Jairaj PS, et al: Closed mitral valvotomy: Early results and long-term follow-up of 3,274 consecutive patients. *Circulation* 68:892, 1983.

Kan JS, White RI Jr, Mitchell SE, Gardner TJ: Percutaneous balloon valvuloplasty: A new method for treating congenital pulmonary valve stenosis. *N Engl J Med* 307:540, 1982.

Kent KM, Bentivoglio LG, Block PC, et al: Percutaneous transluminal coronary angioplasty: Report from the registry of the National Heart, Lung, and Blood Institute. *Am J Cardiol* 49:2011, 1982.

King SB III: Vascular stents and atherosclerosis. *Circulation* 79:460, 1989.

Kvelselis DA, Rocchini AP, Snider AR et al: Results of balloon valvuloplasty in the treatment of congenital valvar pulmonary stenosis in children. *Am J Cardiol* 56:527, 1985.

Kyrle PA, Eichler HG. Jager U, et al: Inhibition of prostacyclin and thromboxane A_2 generation by low-dose aspirin at the site of plug formation in man in vivo. *Circulation* 75:1025, 1987.

Lee L, Bates ER, Pitt B, et al: Percutaneous transluminal coronary angioplasty improves survival in acute myocardial infarction complicated by cardiogenic shock. *Circulation* 78:1345, 1988.

Leimgruber PP, Roubin GS, Anderson V, et al: Influence of intimal dissection on restenosis after successful coronary angioplasty. *Circulation* 72:530, 1985.

Leimgruber PP, Roubin GS, Hollman J, et al: Restenosis after successful coronary angioplasty in patients with single-vessel disease. *Circulation* 73:10, 1986.

Letac B, Cribier A, Koning R, Bellefleur JP: Results of percutaneous transluminal valvuloplasty in 218 adults with valvular aortic stenosis. *Am J Cardiol* 62:598, 1988.

Levin DC, Boxt LM, Abben R, et al: Sequential balloon technique in angioplasty of severe coronary arterial obstructions. *Am J Cardiol* 56:789, 1985.

Litvack F, Grundfest WS, Papaioannou T, et al: Role of laser and thermal ablation devices in the treatment of vascular diseases. *Am J Cardiol* 61:81G, 1988.

Litvack F, Grundfest W, Hickey A, et al: Percutaneous coronary excimer laser angioplasty in animals and humans. *J Am Coll Cardiol* 13:61A, 1989.

Lock JE, Khalilullah M, Shrivastava S, Bahl V, Keane JF: Percutaneous catheter commissurotomy in rheumatic mitral stenosis. *N Engl J Med* 313:1515, 1985.

Matthews BJ, Ewels CJ, Kent KM: Coronary dissection: A predictor of restenosis? *Am Heart J* 115:547, 1988.

McAuley BJ, Selmon M, Sheehan D, Simpson J: Coronary angioplasty in a combined catheterization laboratory-operating room setting (abstr). *Circulation* III-217, 1985.

McKay RG, Lock JE, Keane JF, et al: Percutaneous mitral valvuloplasty in an adult patient with calcific rheumatic mitral stenosis. *J Am Coll Cardiol* 7:1410, 1986.

McKay RG, Safian RD, Lock JE, et al: Balloon dilatation of calcific aortic stenosis in elderly patients: Postmortem, intraoperative, and percutaneous valvuloplasty studies. *Circulation* 74:119, 1986.

McKay RG, Lock JE, Safian RD, et al: Balloon dilatation of mitral stenosis in adult patients: Post mortem and percutaneous mitral valvuloplasty studies. *J Am Coll Cardiol* 9:723, 1987.

Meier B, King SB, Gruentzig AR, et al: Repeat coronary angioplasty. *J Am Coll Cardiol* 4:463, 1984.

Meier B, Friedli B, Oberhaenlsi I, Belenger J, Finci L: Trefoil balloon for percutaneous valvuloplasty. *Cathet Cardiovasc Diagn* 12:277, 1986.

Meyer J, Merx W, Schmitz H, et al: Percutaneous transluminal coronary angioplasty immediately after intracoronary streptolysis of transmural myocardial infarction. *Circulation* 66:905, 1982.

Mizuno K, Jurita A, Imazeki N: Pathologic findings after percutaneous transluminal coronary angioplasty. *Br Heart J* 52:588, 1984.

Nobuyoshi M, Kimura T, Nosaka H, et al: Restenosis after successful percutaneous transluminal coronary angioplasty: Serial angiographic follow-up of 229 patients. *J Am Coll Cardiol* 12:616, 1988.

Oesterle SN: Angioplasty techniques for stenoses involving coronary artery bifurcation. *Am J Cardiol* 61:29G, 1988.

O'Neill WW: Primary percutaneous coronary angioplasty: A protagonist's view. *Am J Cardiol* 62:15K, 1988.

O'Neill WW, Bates ER, Kirsh M, et al: Mechanical transluminal coronary endarterectomy: Initial clinical experience with the Auth mechanical rotary catheter. *J Am Coll Cardiol* 13:227A, 1989.

Palacios IF, Lock JE, Keane JF, Block PC: Percutaneous transvenous balloon valvotomy in a patient with severe calcific mitral stenosis. *J Am Coll Cardiol* 7:1416, 1986.

Palacios IF, Block PC, Brandi S, et al: Percutaneous balloon valvotomy for patients with severe mitral stenosis. *Circulation* 75:778, 1987.

Palmaz JC, Sibbitt RR, Tio FO, et al: Expandable intraluminal vascular graft: A feasibility study. *Surgery* 99:199, 1986.

Park SC, Zuberbuhler JR, Neches WH, Lenoa CC, Zoltun RA: A new atrial septostomy technique. *Cathet Cardiovasc Diagn* 1:195, 1975.

Perry SB, Keane JF, Lock JE: Interventional catheterization in pediatric congenital and acquired heart disease. *Am J Cardiol* 61:109G, 1988.

Pinkerton C, Simpson J, Selmon M, et al: Percutaneous coronary atherectomy: Early experiences of a multicenter trial. *J Am Coll Cardiol* 13:108A, 1989.

Quigley PJ, Hlatky MA, Hinohara T, et al: Repeat transluminal coronary angioplasty and predictors of recurrent restenosis. *Am J Cardiol* 63:409, 1989.

Radtke W, Keane JF, Fellows KE, Lang P, Lock JE: Percutaneous balloon valvotomy of congenital pulmonary stenosis using oversized balloons. *J Am Coll Cardiol* 8:909, 1986.

Rashkind WJ, Miller WW: Creation of an atrial septal defect without thoracotomy: Palliative approach to complete transposition of the great arteries. *JAMA* 196:991, 1966.

Ritchie JL, Hansen DD, Vracko R, Auth DC: Mechanical thrombolysis: A new rotational catheter approach for acute thrombi. *Circulation* 73:1006, 1986.

Roberts WC: Good-bye to thoracotomy for cardiac valvotomy. *Am J Cardiol* 59:198, 1987.

Ross R: The pathogenesis of atherosclerosis—an update. *N Engl J Med* 314:488, 1986.

Roth RB, Palacios IF, Block PL: Percutaneous aortic balloon valvuloplasty: Its role in the management of patients with aortic stenosis requiring major noncardiac surgery. *J Am Coll Cardiol* 13:1039, 1989.

Rothbaum DA, Linnmeier TJ, Landin RJ, et al: Emergency percutaneous transluminal coronary angioplasty in acute myocardial infarction: A 3-year experience. *J Am Coll Cardiol* 9:264, 1987.

Roubin GS, Robinson KA, King SB, Gianturco C, et al: Early and late results of intracoronary arterial stenting after coronary angioplasty in dogs. *Circulation* 76:891, 1987.

Rutherford BD, et al: Direct balloon angioplasty in myocardial infarction: Long-term results (abstr). *Circulation* 78:II-502, 1988.

Sager PT, Perlmutter RA, Rosenfeld LE, et al: Electrophysiologic effects of thrombolytic therapy in patients with a transmural anterior infarction complicated by left ventricular aneurysm formation. *J Am Coll Cardiol* 12:19, 1988.

Sanborn TA, Faxon DP, Kellett MA: Percutaneous coronary laser thermal angioplasty. *J Am Coll Cardiol* 8:1437, 1986.

Schatz RA: A view of vascular stents. *Circulation* 79:445, 1989.

Schatz RA, Palmaz JC, Tio FO, et al: Balloon-expandable intracoronary stents in the adult dog. *Circulation* 76:450, 1987.

Semb BKH, Tjonneland S, Stake G, Aabyholm G: Balloon valvulotomy of congenital pulmonary valve stenosis with tricuspid valve insufficiency. *Cardiovasc Radiol* 2:239, 1979.

Serruys PW, Luitjen HE, Beatt KJ, et al: Incidence of restenosis after successful coronary angioplasty: A time-related phenomenon. *Circulation* 77:361, 1988.

Serruys PW, Beatt J, DeFeyter PJ: Stent implantation for the treatment of coronary artery bypass graft stenosis. *J Am Coll Cardiol* 13:107A, 1989.

Sigwart U, Puel J, Mirkovitch V, et al: Intravascular stents to prevent occlusion and restenosis after transluminal angioplasty. *N Engl J Med* 316:701, 1987.

Sigwart U, Urban P, Golf S, et al: Emergency stenting for acute occlusion after coronary balloon angioplasty. *Circulation* 78:1121, 1988.

Simpfendorfer C, Belardi J, Bellamy G, et al: Frequency, management and follow-up of patients with acute coronary occlusions after percutaneous coronary angioplasty. *Am J Cardiol* 59:267, 1987.

Simpson JB, Baim DS, Robert EW, Harrison DC: A new catheter system for coronary angioplasty. *Am J Cardiol* 49:1216, 1982.

Simpson JB, Selmon MR, Robertson GC, et al: Transluminal atherectomy for occlusive peripheral vascular disease. *Am J Cardiol* 61:96G, 1988.

Sinclair IN, McCabe CH, Sipperly ME, Baim DS: Predictors, therapeutic options and long-term outcome of abrupt reclosure. *Am J Cardiol* 61:61G, 1988.

Soward AL, Essed CE, Serruys PW: Coronary arterial findings after accidental death immediately after successful percutaneous transluminal coronary angioplasty. *Am J Cardiol* 56:794, 1985.

Spears JR: Percutaneous transluminal coronary angioplasty restenosis: Potential prevention with laser balloon angioplasty. *Am J Cardiol* 60:61B, 1987.

Stack R: New interventional technology. *Am J Cardiol* 62:12F, 1988.

Stack RS, Califf RM, Hinohara T, et al: Survival and cardiac event rates in the first year after emergency coronary angioplasty for acute myocardial infarction. *J Am Coll Cardiol* 11:1141, 1988.

Stack RS, Quigley PJ, Collins G, et al: Perfusion balloon catheter. *Am J Cardiol* 61:77G, 1988.

Talley JD, Hurst JW, King SB, et al: Clinical outcome 5 years after attempted percutaneous coronary angioplasty in 427 patients. *Circulation* 77:820, 1988.

Teirstein PS, Hoover CA, Ligon RW, et al: Repeat coronary angioplasty: Efficacy of a third angioplasty for a second restenosis. *J Am Coll Cardiol* 13:291, 1989.

TIMI Study Group: Comparison of invasive and conservative strategies after treatment with intravenous tissue plasminogen activator in acute myocardial infarction. Results of the Thrombolysis in Myocardial Infarction (TIMI) Phase II trial. *N Engl J Med* 320:618, 1989.

Topol EJ, Califf RM, George BS, et al: A randomized trial of immediate versus delayed elective angioplasty after intravenous tissue plasminogen activator in acute myocardial infarction. *N Engl J Med* 317:581, 1987.

Turi ZG, Rezkalla S, Campbell CA, Kloner RA: Amelioration of ischemia during angioplasty of the left anterior descending coronary artery with an autoperfusion catheter. *Am J Cardiol* 62:513, 1988.

Turi ZG, Campbell CA, Gottimukkala MV, Kloner RA: Preservation of distal coronary perfusion during prolonged balloon inflation with an autoperfusion angioplasty catheter. *Circulation* 75:1273, 1987.

Urban P, Sigwart U, Golf S, et al: Intravascular stenting for stenosis of aortocoronary venous bypass grafts. *J Am Coll Cardiol* 13:1085, 1989.

Vahanian A. Michel PL, Comier B, et al: Results of percutaneous mitral commissurotomy in 200 patients. *Am J Cardiol* 63:847, 1989.

Vogel RA, Shawl F, Tommaso C: Report of the National Registry of Elective Cardiopulmonary Bypass Supported Coronary Angioplasty. *J Am Coll Cardiol* 1990 (in press).

Waller BF, Gorfinkel HJ, Rogers FJ, Kent KM, Roberts WC: Early and later morphologic changes in major epicardial coronary arteries after percutaneous transluminal coronary angioplasty. *Am J Cardiol* 53:42C, 1984.

Waller BF: "Crackers, breakers, stretchers, drillers, scrapers, shavers, burners, welders and melters." Future treatment of atherosclerotic coronary disease? A clinical-morphologic assessment. *J Am Coll Cardiol* 13:969, 1989.

Wilkins GT, Weyman AE, Abascal VM, Block PC, Palacios IF: Percutaneous mitral valvotomy: An analysis of echocardiographic variables related to outcome and the mechanism of dilatation. *Br Heart J* 60:299, 1988.

17 Valvular Heart Disease

Sylvia A. Mamby
Robert A. Kloner

Although there has been a definite shift in the major causes of cardiac valvular lesions, valvular disease continues to play a substantial role in the spectrum of cardiovascular diseases. While rheumatic fever is no longer the chief etiologic consideration, recent evidence suggests that a resurgence in this disease may be imminent.

Methods used to identify and assess the severity of valvular heart pathology have also changed dramatically. A simpler approach, dominated by noninvasive ultrasound techniques, has made the assessment of valvular function safer and less costly. In addition, follow-up examinations to assess the progression of disease are readily performed. The management of valve conditions has also undergone substantial change. Importantly, there is better understanding of the optimal timing of intervention.

This chapter briefly reviews the presentation, assessment, and management of valvular heart diseases, taking into consideration the significant changes that have occurred in this branch of cardiology.

RHEUMATIC FEVER AND RHEUMATIC CARDITIS

The incidence of heumatic fever has dropped considerably over the past several decades. In the 1940s, there were an estimated 200,000 to 250,000 new cases of rheumatic fever developing in the United States per year, with an average of more than 7,000 new cases in the military alone. In the past 20 years, a decline already observed in North America and Western Europe has accelerated, making rheumatic fever indeed rare in these regions today. Reasons for the decline are debatable; however, improved health care, including the emergence of antimicrobial agents (although the decline predated this era), diminished household overcrowding, and socioeconomic factors, is believed to have contributed.

In recent years, however, several outbreaks of acute rheumatic fever have been reported, in Salt Lake City, Utah; Northeastern Ohio; Western Pennsylvania; and at a naval training center in San Diego, California. Theories to explain this possible resurgence relate to new strains of group A streptococcus with enhanced rheumatogenic potential. Additionally, various genetic markers have been identified which may predispose individuals to rheumatic fever.

Acute rheumatic fever is characterized by exudative and proliferative inflammatory lesions of the connective tissues, particularly the heart, joints, and subcutaneous tissues. Later in the course of the disease, circumvascular inflammatory lesions called Aschoff's nodules develop in the heart and are considered pathognomonic. These nodules consist of central areas of fibrosis within a zone of lymphocytes, plasma cells, and large basophilic cells.

Clinically, rheumatic fever presents as a generalized inflammatory disease complicating upper respiratory infection with Group A beta hemolytic streptococci; it occurs approximately 10–21 days after this infection. It tends to affect young people 5–15 years of age, and is generally uncommon in adults. Although the precise mechanism by which the bacterium triggers the inflammatory response is unknown, current belief favors the theory of autoimmunity, whereby tissue damage is created by the body's own immunologic response to the antecedent streptococcal infection. This idea is supported by the relatively long latency between pharyngitis and acute rheumatic fever.

The Jones criteria (Denny), established to direct the diagnosis of acute rheumatic fever, were revised in 1965. The presence of two major criteria indicates a high probability of the presence of acute rheumatic fever, provided supporting evidence of a preceding Group A streptococcal infection is also present (Table 1). Symptoms include fever, chills, migratory polyarthritis, fatigue, weakness, irritability, and epistaxis. Although clearly nonspecific, a tachycardia out of proportion to fever and persistent during sleep is often present. During the initial attack of rheumatic fever, the incidence of carditis varies from 40–60%. The diagnosis of carditis, however, requires at least one of four manifestations: ① organic heart murmur; ② cardiomegaly; ③ pericarditis; and ④ congestive heart failure. Rheumatic carditis is virtually always associated with a murmur. The physician may auscultate an apical holosystolic murmur of mitral regurgitation, an apical mid-diastolic (Carey-Coombs) murmur, or the diastolic murmur of aortic regurgitation. Since pancarditis is also a feature, a friction rub may be heard on auscultation.

On chest x-ray, an enlarged cardiac silhouette may be due to cardiac chamber enlargement or pericardial effusion. Signs of congestive heart failure may also be evident, namely, pulmonary vascular redistribution, pulmonary interstitial edema, Kerley B lines, and pleural effusion.

Electrocardiographic findings, primarily PR-interval prolongation, are frequently observed. Others include tachycardia, second- and third-degree heart block, diminished voltage of QRS complexes, and prolongation of the QT interval. With pericarditis, the ST segments are elevated; however, with myocarditis,

ST-segment changes are often nonspecific. Supraventricular and ventricular tachyarrhythmias also occur.

Therapy for acute rheumatic fever includes rest and sodium restriction. Although antibiotic therapy neither alters the course of rheumatic fever nor influences the development of carditis, antibiotics are indicated to eradicate the streptococcal infection. The following regimens are suggested: benzathine penicillin G 600,000 units IM for children <27 kg; benzathine penicillin G 1.2 million units for children >27 kg and adults; penicillin V 125–250 mg po qid for 10 days, or erythromycin 250 mg po qid for 10 days. Buffered aspirin 5–8 g/day in divided doses is given. Occasionally, prednisone 40–60 mg/day is given to patients with marked cardiac dysfunction. Both agents reduce the symptoms of rheumatic fever but do not shorten its course, or prevent cardiac sequelae. Long-term rheumatic fever prophylaxis helps prevent recurrent attacks of rheumatic fever and subsequent cardiac damage. The most effective regimen appears to be 1.2 million units benzathine penicillin G monthly. The duration of the prophylaxis is debatable. Some clinicians suggest a lifelong regimen; others favor an individualized approach, since increasing age and disease-free interval from the previous attack are associated with a diminished likelihood of recurrence.

As suggested by the United Kingdom-United States Cooperative Study, lack of severe carditis during the initial attack of rheumatic fever favors the absence of late rheumatic heart disease. Seventy percent of the study patients with mild carditis (mitral regurgitation)

Table 1. Jones Criteria (revised)

Major Manifestations	Minor Manifestations
Carditis	Fever
Polyarthritis	Arthralgia
Chorea	Previous rheumatic fever or rheumatic heart disease
Erythema marginatum	Elevated ESR or positive CRP; leukocytosis
Subcutaneous nodules	Prolonged PR interval
Plus supporting evidence of preceding streptococcal infection; history of recent scarlet fever; positive throat culture for group A streptococcus; increased ASO titer or other streptococcal antibodies.	
ESR = erythrocyte sedimentation rate; CRP = C-reactive protein; ASO = antistreptolysin-O. From: Jones Criteria (revised) for guidance in the diagnosis of rheumatic fever. *Circulation* 32:664, 1965. With permission of the American Heart Association, Inc.	

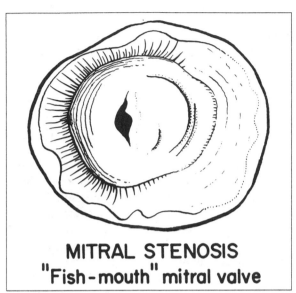

MITRAL STENOSIS
"Fish-mouth" mitral valve

Figure 1. *Looking down into the left atrium at a stenotic mitral valve. The mitral leaflets have thickened, the commissures are fused, and the mitral orifice has a narrowed "fish-mouth" appearance.*

had normal health at 10 years. It should be noted that the development of valvular lesions is gradual, requiring 10–30 years to become manifest. In rheumatic heart disease, the mitral valve is involved in approximately 85% of cases, the aortic valve in 44%, and the tricuspid valve in 10–16%; the pulmonic valve is rarely involved.

LEFT-SIDED VALVULAR HEART DISEASE

MITRAL STENOSIS

By far the most common etiology of mitral stenosis is rheumatic heart disease. Congenital forms of mitral stenosis also occur, but rarely. Typically, rheumatic mitral stenosis is manifested by fusion of the valve leaflet cusps, and thickening and shortening of the chordae (Figure 1). Subsequent calcium deposition within the valve leaflets compounds the problem. The normal mitral valve area is 4–6 cm². The severity of symptoms depends primarily on the degree of stenosis. As the valve area decreases, a greater pressure gradient is required to generate flow from the left atrium to the left ventricle, resulting in substantial left atrial pressures. Elevated left atrial pressure results in increased pulmonary venous and capillary pressures. Once pulmonary capillary pressure exceeds plasma oncotic pressure, transudation of fluid occurs (one of the mechanisms of hemoptysis in this disease). Subsequently, pulmonary arteriolar resistance increases and impedes right ventricular performance. The right ventricle hypertrophies, dilates, and ultimately fails. The left atrium, which also becomes severely dilated in time, may develop atrial fibrillation, losing its effective contraction. Of note, rapid heart rates are poorly tolerated in mitral stenosis, because they allow less time for the already impaired ventricular filling to occur, necessitating even higher left atrial pressures.

The progression of mitral stenosis is chronic and variable. In underdeveloped countries, it may progress quickly in patients presenting in their teens. More commonly, however, symptoms begin in the patient's fourth decade. Mitral stenosis is far more common in women and may become evident with the onset of atrial fibrillation and pregnancy.

Diagnosis

Patients primarily complain of dyspnea, with progressive limitations on physical exertion as mitral stenosis worsens. Patients will also manifest orthopnea, paroxysmal nocturnal dyspnea, fatigue, weakness, and hemoptysis. When pulmonary vascular resistance increases, there may be a transient period during which left-sided symptoms diminish and right-sided symptoms increase. With advanced mitral stenosis, symptoms of right heart failure develop, including nausea, anorexia and right upper quadrant pain (secondary to hepatic congestion), ascites, hoarseness, and peripheral edema. Hoarseness, the primary manifestation of Ortner's syndrome, is created by compression of the left recurrent laryngeal nerve between the enlarged pulmonary artery, the aorta, and the ligamentum arteriosum, and not by the enlarged left atrium, as has often been assumed. Chest pain can occur and has been thought to be related to developing pulmonary hypertension. However, angina due to concomitant coronary artery disease may also be present. In one necropsy study (Reis and Roberts) of patients with mitral stenosis who were >30 years old, 50% had significant narrowing of at least one major epicardial coronary artery.

NB

Physical examination reveals characteristic ruddy cheeks (so-called mitral facies), and usually a normal arterial pulse unless atrial fibrillation is present. Rales may be present depending on the degree of interstitial and alveolar edema. With increased right-sided pressures, jugular venous distention is present, with a prominent a-wave in patients in sinus rhythm. Palpation reveals a normal or reduced left ventricular impulse and, often, a right ventricular heave. Auscultation typically reveals a prominent S_1, a loud P_2 if pulmonary hypertension is present, and an opening snap occurring after the S_2. The murmur is a low-pitched diastolic rumble that begins with the opening snap and becomes loudest just before S_1 (presystolic accentuation) if the patient is in sinus rhythm. The opening snap is a high-pitched sound believed to be created by sudden tensing of, particularly, the anterior mitral valve leaflet by the chordae tendineae after cuspal opening. Its presence implies valve mobility. The interval between A_2 and the opening snap has been used to estimate the severity of mitral stenosis. A shorter interval (<0.06–0.07 sec) suggests higher left atrial pressure, which supports more severe mitral stenosis. The reverse is not always true, however, since in elderly patients or those with systemic hypertension the decline in left ventricular systolic pressure may be prolonged. The diastolic rumble (Table 2) is best heard with the bell of the stethoscope at the apex, with the patient in the left lateral decubitus position. Its prolonged duration, more than its intensity, is a predictor of severe mitral stenosis. Associated murmurs include tricuspid regurgitation with severe right heart failure, and pulmonary regurgitation (Graham Steell murmur) with pulmonary hypertension. These systolic murmurs may be differentiated from mitral regurgitation (not uncommonly associated with mitral stenosis) by their enhancement during inspiration. Other signs of right ventricular failure also may be present, including a tender pulsatile liver, ascites, and peripheral edema.

Electrocardiographic findings, although not specific, may suggest mitral stenosis and include left atrial enlargement (p mitrale), right-axis deviation and right ventricular hypertrophy. Atrial fibrillation may be present, and represents a poor prognostic sign. The chest x-ray demonstrates signs of left atrial enlargement: an elevated left mainstem bronchus, double cardiac density, and prominent left heart border. A severely dilated left atrium suggests concomitant mitral regurgitation. Pulmonary vascular redistribution, interstitial edema, Kerley B lines, and prominence of the right ventricle and pulmonary artery also may be observed. (See also Chapters 3 and 4.)

Echocardiography is the diagnostic tool of choice in mitral stenosis (see also Chapters 7 and 8). The primary M-mode signs are reduction of the E to F slope (reduced left ventricular filling rate), thickening of the mitral valve leaflets, and concordant (rather than the normal discordant) motion of the posterior mitral valve leaflet with the anterior leaflet. Far more useful is two-dimensional echocardiography, which may reveal typical diastolic doming of the mitral valve and restricted leaflet separation, as well as a thickened mitral valve. Echocardiography also reveals an enlarged left atrium and may demonstrate rheumatic involvement of other valves. Doppler echocardiography reveals an increased velocity of transmitral flow. This technique allows an estimation of the severity of mitral stenosis by calculation of the mitral valve half-time, the time necessary for peak transmitral flow velocity to fall to half its value (Figure 2). Echocardiography is also helpful in ruling out other diagnoses in the differential of mitral stenosis, specifically, left atrial myxoma, atrial septal defect, cor triatriatum, ball-valve thrombus in the left atrium, and large mitral valve vegetations. Transesophageal echocardiography may be useful for identifying thrombi in the left atrial appendage (see Chapter 7).

Cardiac catheterization, although not required for the diagnosis of mitral stenosis, is often performed before surgical intervention to evaluate concomitant coronary artery disease in older patients. A study by Sutton et al. evaluating the surgical outcome of groups of patients undergoing either mitral or aortic (or both) valve replacement, with or without preoperative cardiac catheterization, revealed similar operative mortalities and two-year survival rates. However, if cardiac catheterization is performed in the setting of mitral stenosis, typical features are elevated left atrial pressures and a significant left atrial-to-left ventricular diastolic gradient (Figure 3). Elevated right heart pressures may also be observed, with associated tricuspid regurgitation manifested as tall, regurgitant systolic v-waves on the atrial pressure tracing. Although hardly diagnostic, a calcified mitral valve may be revealed on fluoroscopy. (See Chapter 9.)

Therapy

The management of mitral stenosis has changed considerably over the years. Medical management fol-

Table 2. Differential Diagnosis of Mitral Valve Stenosis	
Disease Entity	Differentiating Features
Left atrial myxoma (symptoms and signs, especially diastolic murmur, mimic mitral stenosis)	Auscultatory findings change with body position; signs of systemic illness (weight loss, anemia, fever, emboli); usually no opening snap; tumor plop; characteristic echocardiographic findings
Atrial septal defect (increased flow across tricuspid valve causes diastolic flow murmur)	Fixed splitting of the S_2; absence of left atrial enlargement; absence of Kerley B lines; echocardiography reveals normal mitral valve and large right ventricle; left-to-right shunt by catheterization study
High flow states, such as hyperthyroidism (diastolic flow rumbles across AV valves due to increased amount of blood transversing these valves)	Hyperactive cardiac state; signs of hyperthyroidism; echocardiogram shows normal mitral valve, hyperkinetic left ventricular motion
Mitral regurgitation (with large amounts of blood flowing across the mitral valve during diastole, a diastolic rumble may be present)	Holosystolic murmur of mitral regurgitation (although mitral regurgitation and mitral stenosis may coexist); concomitant S_3, signs of left ventricular enlargement
Cor triatriatum (uncommon congenital malformation consisting of a fibromuscular membrane that divides the left atrium and impedes flow from pulmonary veins to left ventricle)	Murmurs (both systolic and diastolic) are not typical of mitral stenosis; normal mitral valve by echo with characteristic echo in left atrium; left atrial angiography may visualize membrane
Congenital stenosis of pulmonary veins (unusual congenital entity resulting in signs of pulmonary hypertension, pulmonary venous congestion, and right ventricular failure)	No distinctive murmurs; mitral valve normal by echo
Primary pulmonary hypertension (signs of right ventricular failure; more common in women)	No opening snap or diastolic rumble; no left atrial enlargement or elevated pulmonary artery wedge pressure
Large mitral vegetations from endocarditis	Vegetations may be visualized by echocardiography
Ball-valve thrombus formation in the left atrium	Auscultatory findings change with body position; two-dimensional echocardiography may be helpful

lows five general considerations: (1) prophylaxis against infective endocarditis; (2) efforts to limit elevations of left atrial pressure; (3) management of right heart failure; (4) management of atrial fibrillation; and (5) prophylaxis against systemic embolizations.

Antibiotic prophylaxis for dental and surgical procedures is essential. Long-term antibiotic therapy as prophylaxis against recurrent episodes of rheumatic fever is advised primarily in young patients who have had episodes of acute rheumatic fever.

Rapid atrial fibrillation is poorly tolerated and digitalis is useful in slowing the rapid ventricular rate. Beta blockers may be added to digitalis in patients with atrial fibrillation whose ventricular rate is not well controlled on digitalis alone. Alternatively, dil-

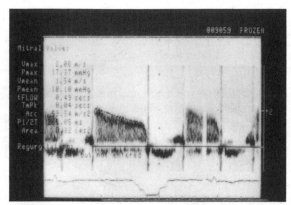

Figure 2. *An on-screen Doppler echocardiographic calculation of the mitral valve half-time.*

tiazem in combination with digoxin exerts good control of ventricular response rates at rest and during exercise. Class IA antiarrhythmics (generally either quinidine or procainamide) may help maintain sinus rhythm in patients previously experiencing atrial fibrillation. Diuretic therapy helps to reduce symptoms of pulmonary congestion and right heart failure, although it must be used with caution, as sharp reduction in venous return may further reduce cardiac output. Oral anticoagulation is indicated in patients with atrial fibrillation or heart failure, or in those who have already experienced either atrial or venous embolic phenomena.

Surgical therapy currently consists of either open commissurotomy or mitral valve replacement. Closed mitral commissurotomy is more frequently performed in developing nations. Indications for surgical inter-

vention include symptomatic patients (New York Heart Association class II or higher) with moderate to severe mitral stenosis (mitral valve area < 1.0 cm^2). An alternative to surgery, however, is percutaneous balloon mitral valvuloplasty, in which a balloon flotation catheter, after insertion across the interatrial septum, is advanced through the stenotic mitral valve and inflated. This technique has been shown to significantly increase mitral valve area and reduce the transvalvular gradient (see also Chapter 16). In patients with favorable mitral valve morphology (determined by echocardiography and consisting of pliable leaflets, minimal calcification, mild thickening only, and mild subvalvular fibrosis [Block 1989]), post-valvuloplasty mitral valve area is ≥ 1.5 cm^2 in about 90% of cases. Mitral regurgitation is unchanged in half of patients and increased by one angiographic grade (e.g., from 1 + to 2 +) in the other half of patients. Follow-up studies show continued clinical improvement in those patients with successful mitral valvuloplasty. Although the technique is still in its early stages, it appears to offer an alternative to patients who are at high operative risk or who refuse surgery, or in women of childbearing age in whom the risk of anticoagulation for valve prosthesis should be avoided. A study by McKay, Lock et al. confirmed that the mechanism of successful balloon mitral valvuloplasty is commissural separation and fracture of nodular calcium. Another study (McKay et al. 1988) demonstrated marked improvement in functional class as confirmed by exercise testing.

MITRAL REGURGITATION

It is important to recognize that the mitral valve apparatus consists of five supportive components: valve leaflets, chordae tendineae, papillary muscles, the left ventricle, and the mitral annulus. The various causes of mitral regurgitation (Table 3) may result from failure of any of these components.

Mitral regurgitation is manifested by significant systolic backflow of blood from the left ventricle into the left atrium across an incompetent mitral valve. This regurgitant load is returned to the left ventricle, resulting ultimately in dilation of both the left ventricle and left atrium. The presentation of acute mitral regurgitation is quite different from chronic mitral regurgitation; left atrial size is the mediator of these differences. In acute mitral regurgitation, initial left atrial size is small; sudden increased pressure in this noncompliant chamber results in pulmonary conges-

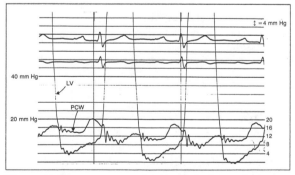

Figure 3. *Pressure wave forms. Note the pulmonary capillary wedge (PCW) tracing against left ventricular (LV) pressure (off-scale) and the significant diastolic gradient between them.*

Table 3. Etiologies of Mitral Valve Regurgitation	
Acute	Chronic
Ruptured chordae tendineae	Rheumatic heart disease
Papillary muscle rupture	Papillary muscle dysfunction
Endocarditis	Mitral valve prolapse (click-murmur syndrome,
Trauma	Barlow's syndrome, floppy mitral valve)
	Endocarditis
	Calcification of the mitral valve annulus
	Accompanying hypertrophic obstructive cardiomyopathy
	Congenital endocardial cushion defect,
	corrected transposition
	Endocardial fibroelastosis
	Severe left ventricular dilatation

tion. In chronic mitral regurgitation, the left atrium has had time to dilate, and it accommodates the regurgitant load. The result is lower left-atrial pressure and far less pulmonary congestion. Limited effective forward output, resulting from the failing dilated ventricle, appears to be the primary mechanism of symptoms in the chronic state.

Diagnosis

In chronic mitral regurgitation, patients may be asymptomatic for 20–30 years, and then present with dyspnea on exertion, orthopnea, weakness and fatigue. A dilated left atrium may result in atrial fibrillation with systemic embolization, although not as often as in mitral stenosis. After long-standing severe mitral regurgitation, left ventricular failure inevitably results in right ventricular failure.

Because left ventricular ejection is actually hyperdynamic in the initial phases of regurgitation, the carotid impulse is brisk, as is the left ventricular impulse. The S_1 is generally soft and the S_2 widely split. An S_3 also may be present. The murmur of mitral regurgitation characteristically is high-pitched and holosystolic, and is most prominent at the apex with radiation to the axilla. Mild mitral regurgitation typically reveals a normal S_1 and a late systolic murmur. Table 4 lists features that help differentiate this murmur from others.

The chest x-ray generally reveals enlargement of both the left atrium and ventricle, and, occasionally, signs of pulmonary congestion. Calcification of the mitral valve annulus may be observed, and is a frequent cause of mitral regurgitation in the elderly. The most common electrocardiographic finding is left atrial enlargement. Atrial fibrillation and evidence of left ventricular hypertrophy may develop over time. In acute mitral regurgitation, as occurs with sudden papillary muscle rupture, signs of ischemia may be the only electrocardiographic finding.

On 2D echocardiography, an enlarged left atrium and a dilated hyperdynamic left ventricle are generally observed. Two-dimensional echo is particularly useful in attempts to establish the cause of mitral regurgitation. It may identify mitral valve prolapse, evidence of rheumatic mitral valvular disease, mitral annular calcification, flail leaflets, vegetations, wall motion abnormalities, or scarred papillary muscles. Doppler echocardiography is the most specific noninvasive tool to identify the presence of mitral regurgitation. With emergence of color flow Doppler, the identification of any valvular regurgitation is further enhanced (see Chapter 8). Color flow Doppler allows mapping of the regurgitant jet into the left atrium as well as an estimation of the severity of regurgitation. Helmcke et al. evaluated 147 patients with color flow Doppler and angiography. Sixty-five patients had no mitral regurgitation by either technique, while 82 patients had mitral regurgitation by both techniques, suggesting a sensitivity and specificity of 100% using angiography as the standard. This study also demonstrated the ability of color flow to accurately estimate severity of mitral regurgitation (see p. *xix*).

Cardiac catheterization in acute mitral regurgitation demonstrates marked elevation of the pulmonary capillary wedge pressure and prominent systolic regurgitant v-waves. Angiographically, regurgitant flow is observed in the left atrium during left ventriculogra-

Table 4. Differential Diagnosis of Mitral Valve Regurgitation	
Disease Entities	Differentiating Features
Ventricular septal defect (murmur may be confused with mitral regurgitation)	Murmur localized over lower left sternal border. Radionuclide studies or Doppler confirm left-to-right shunt. Cardiac catheterization reveals O_2 step up from right atrium to ventricle.
Hypertrophic obstructive cardiomyopathy (or idiopathic hypertrophic subaortic stenosis— IHSS)	Associated mitral regurgitation murmur may be present. However, outflow murmur typical of hypertrophic obstructive cardiomyopathy (HOCM) is present as well, which increases with Valsalva maneuver and amyl nitrite and decreases with squatting, hand grip. Typical echocardiographic features of HOCM.
Aortic stenosis (murmur may be confused with mitral regurgitation)	The murmur is systolic ejection in quality. Confusion occurs when mitral regurgitation is due to prolapse of posterior papillary muscle or rupture of posterior chordae tendineae with radiation of the murmur to the aortic area. In some patients the murmur of aortic stenosis is loudest at the apex. With aortic stenosis, carotid upstroke is delayed, S_2 is soft, single or absent, echocardiographic features of aortic stenosis and calcification of the aortic valve are present.

phy; if mitral regurgitation is severe, the flow may be trackable back into the pulmonary veins. Over time, as the left ventricle fails, end-diastolic pressure will rise and ejection fraction fall. It should be noted, however, that left ventricular ejection fraction is dependent on the cause and duration of mitral regurgitation and may actually be increased in the early phases. Left ventricular regurgitant fraction can be calculated from the formula:

$$\frac{\text{Angiographic cardiac output} - \text{FICK cardiac output}}{\text{Angiographic cardiac output}}$$

If the regurgitant fraction is >60%, severe mitral regurgitation is likely.

Therapy

The primary goal of medical management of mitral regurgitation is afterload reduction. Reduced impedance to left ventricular outflow serves to reduce regurgitation across the mitral valve. In acute mitral regurgitation, this is readily accomplished by use of intravenous nitroprusside and/or intraaortic balloon counterpulsation. Chronic afterload reduction can be achieved with hydralazine or angiotensin converting enzyme (ACE) inhibitors. A low sodium diet and aggressive diuretic therapy are also good supportive measures.

Traditionally, parameters of left ventricular function have been used to guide the timing of intervention for mitral regurgitation. However, measurements of ejection fraction can be misleading, given that end-systolic volumes are smaller due to reduced impedance to left ventricular outflow. Appropriate timing of intervention is critical: premature intervention is associated with operative morbidity and mortality, while delayed intervention can lead to irreversible left ventricular dysfunction. Once mitral regurgitation is corrected, the left ventricle faces increased impedance, having lost the left atrial reservoir as an unloading chamber. Acute severe mitral regurgitation generally requires aggressive surgical intervention. Chronic mitral regurgitation with significant limiting symptoms also calls for intervention provided that left ventricular function is not severely depressed. Table 5 lists guidelines, described by Ross, for patient selection.

Surgical intervention takes two forms: valve reconstruction (annuloplasty) or valve replacement. In

---

Table 5. Guidelines for Selecting Patients With Mitral Regurgitation for Operation

1. The downhill clinical course is relatively gradual in chronic mitral regurgitation once symptoms begin, and left ventricular dysfunction may develop insidiously.
2. With significant *limiting symptoms* and severe mitral regurgitation, operation is usually indicated provided left ventricular function is good or not severely depressed (ejection fraction <40%). Even when left ventricular function is sustained preoperatively, the ejection fraction will deteriorate to some degree after operation.
3. In patients with severe regurgitation who have *few or no symptoms*, operation should be considered to preserve left ventricular function provided serial noninvasive studies of the left ventricle show ejection fraction <55%, fractional shortening <30%, plus either A or B:
   A) End-diastolic diameter approaching 75 mm and end-systolic diameter approaching 50 mm or 26 mm/m² body surface area (end-systolic volume approaching 60 ml/m²).
   B) Both an end-systolic diameter approaching 26 mm/m² and a radius/wall thickness ratio at end-systole × systolic pressure approaching 195 mm Hg.

From Ross. With permission of the American College of Cardiology. See Bibliography.

---

the U.S., valve replacement has been the procedure of choice. However, in recent years, largely because of the technique of Carpentier, there has been a trend toward valve repair where feasible. Clearly, if reconstruction is conceivable and available, the chronic anticoagulation and embolic risks associated with prosthetic valves can be avoided. The only contraindication to reconstruction appears to be severe disease of the anterior mitral valve leaflet or irreparable leaflet or chordal fusion. Transesophageal echocardiography has been useful recently in intraoperative evaluation of mitral valve repair.

Endocarditis prophylaxis is recommended in patients with mitral regurgitation associated with organic disease of the mitral leaflets.

MITRAL VALVE PROLAPSE SYNDROME

Mitral valve prolapse (MVP) has traditionally been thought to be a common entity with an incidence of approximately 5% in normal individuals, although it has been observed in as many as 21% in one series of healthy young women. There has been recent speculation that MVP is actually overdiagnosed. This is not to say that true mitral valve prolapse is rare, but rather that many patients so diagnosed may have a variant of normal, particularly when echocardiographic definitions alone are applied.

Mitral valve prolapse is due to myxomatous degeneration of the mitral valve leaflets, resulting in a marked systolic bowing of the mitral valve leaflets and loss of leaflet coaptation, with subsequent mitral regurgitation. There appears to be some familial tendency for prolapse, as well as associations with disorders including various connective tissue diseases (e.g., systemic lupus erythematosus, polyarteritis nodosa), Wolff-Parkinson-White syndrome, neurocirculatory asthenia, anxiety neurosis, and straightback syndrome, to name just a few. In order to allow some stratification and validation of MVP, Perloff et al. established a set of major and minor criteria for the syndrome (Table 6).

The vast majority of patients with mitral valve prolapse are asymptomatic. However, patients may complain of palpitations, atypical chest pain, fatigue, dyspnea, lightheadedness, and syncope. Physical examination will generally reveal a midsystolic click (and sometimes multiple clicks). The click is often followed by the mid-to-late systolic murmur of mitral regurgitation. The murmur becomes more holosystolic with increasing severity of regurgitation. The electrocardiogram is usually normal, but may reveal nonspecific inferior repolarization changes. Supraventricular tachycardia is the most frequent tachyarrhythmia observed. There has also been an association of mitral valve prolapse with sudden death, although this is rare.

Two-dimensional echocardiography demonstrates the prolapsing motion of either or both mitral valve leaflets into the left atrium during systole. Two-dimensional echo may also reveal prolapse of the tricuspid and/or aortic valves. Doppler echocardiography

Table 6. Minor and Major Criteria for Establishing the Diagnosis of Mitral Valve Prolapse

Minor Criteria	Major Criteria
History	Auscultation
Focal neurologic attacks or amaurosis fugax in the young patient	Mid- to late systolic clicks and a late systolic murmur at the cardiac apex
First-degree relatives with major criteria	Mobile mid- to late systolic clicks at the cardiac apex.
Recurrent supraventricular tachycardia (documented)	Late systolic murmur at the cardiac apex in the young patient
Auscultation	Auscultation plus echocardiograhy
Soft, inconstant, or equivocal mid- to late systolic sounds at the cardiac apex	Apical holosystolic murmur of mitral regurgitation plus echocardiographic criteria (below)
Other physical signs	Two-dimensional/Doppler echocardiography
Low body weight, asthenic habitus	Marked systolic displacement of mitral leaflets with coaptation point at or on the left atrial side of the annulus
Low blood pressure	Moderate systolic displacement of the leaflets with at least moderate mitral regurgitation, chordal rupture, and annular dilatation
Thoracic bony abnormalities	Two-dimensionally targeted M-mode echocardiography
Two-dimensional/Doppler/color flow echocardiography	Marked ($\geq$3 mm) late systolic buckling posterior to the line between points C and D
Moderate superior systolic displacement of mitral leaflets with Doppler mitral regurgitation	
Two-dimensionally targeted M-mode echocardiography	
Moderate (2 mm) late systolic buckling posterior to the line between points C and D	
Holosystolic displacement (3 mm) posterior to the line between points C and D	

(From Perloff JK, Child JS: Clinical and epidemiologic issues in mitral valve prolapse: Overview and perspective. *Am Heart J* 113:1324, 1987. With permission.)

may confirm the presence of associated mitral regurgitation.

Most patients with mitral valve prolapse have a completely benign course. A small number of patients experience cerebral or cerebellar infarction, transient ischemic attacks, seizures, and amaurosis fugax, suggesting an increased risk of systemic embolization in this syndrome. It is important, from a prophylactic standpoint, to try to categorize patients into high- and low-risk categories. In the past, controlled studies demonstrated that male gender, age over 45 years, and the presence of a systolic murmur (before the onset of endocarditis) are three risk factors for the complications of mitral valve prolapse, namely, severe mitral regurgitation and infective endocarditis. More recently, features of the mitral valve itself have

been used to estimate risk. Nishimura et al. found thickening of the mitral valve leaflets to predict the occurrence of infective endocarditis and sudden death.

Mitral valve prolapse-associated cerebral embolic events occur with an estimated incidence of 1/6,000 patients per year. Those patients with severely myxomatous and large mitral valve leaflets are assumed to be at greatest risk (Hart and Easton).

Antibiotic prophylaxis against bacterial endocarditis is strongly advised when mitral regurgitation is present. Beta blockers may be useful for the atypical chest pain associated with mitral valve prolapse as well as the ventricular arrhythmias. Fifteen percent of patients with mitral valve prolapse develop progressive mitral regurgitation with heart failure. These patients should be managed like other patients with mitral regurgitation and may require valve replacement.

MITRAL ANNULAR CALCIFICATION

Calcification of the mitral annulus is frequently idiopathic and is a cause of mitral regurgitation in the elderly. Although considered a degenerative change, it appears to be hastened by certain conditions, including hypertension, aortic stenosis, diabetes, Marfan's syndrome and Hurler's syndrome, and has been associated with hypertrophic obstructive cardiomyopathy. There may be associated calcification of the aortic valve cusps as well. Typical chest x-ray film shows "C"-shaped calcification of the mitral valve annulus. The annular calcification can be diagnosed by echocardiography. If the calcium extends into the conduction system, atrioventricular or intraventricular conduction defects may develop. Nair et al. reported a high prevalence of mitral annular calcification (87%) in patients with symptomatic bradyarrhythmias, including complete AV block, atrial fibrillation with a slow ventricular response, and intermittent sinus arrest. Pacemaker therapy was required in these patients. Functional mitral stenosis has been reported in patients with massive annular calcification.

AORTIC STENOSIS

There are three major varieties of adult valvular aortic stenosis: rheumatic; senile-calcific or degenerative; and congenital bicuspid aortic valve with secondary calcification (Figure 4). In rheumatic aortic stenosis, the major pathologic feature is fusion of the commissures with thickening and fibrosis of the valve leaflets. Patients in their 20s and 30s may have a murmur but symptoms might not occur until ages 50–60. With senile-calcific or degenerative aortic stenosis, calcium accumulates in the pockets of the aortic cusps with eventual fibrosis. Symptoms typically occur at ages 60–70. With congenital bicuspid valve, calcific changes occur earlier in life, presumably secondary to increased turbulence. There is progressive narrowing of the valve orifice over time and symptoms are present at ages 40–50. Congenital aortic stenosis, in which the aortic valve is dome-shaped, causes symptoms early in life. Isolated aortic stenosis in the adult is unlikely to be secondary to rheumatic disease and more likely to be secondary to the congenital bicuspid or senile-calcific variety.

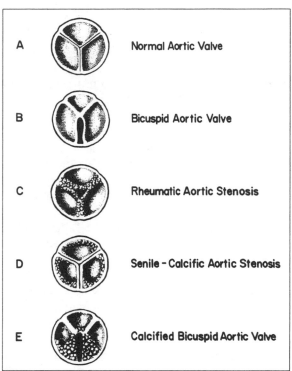

Figure 4. *Pathology of aortic stenosis. (a) Normal tricuspid aortic valve. (b) Bicuspid aortic valve. (c) Rheumatic aortic stenosis. The commissures are fused and the valve leaflets are thickened. (d) Senile-calcific aortic stenosis. Calcium deposits are present within the cusps of the aortic valve without primarily affecting the commissures. (e) Calcified bicuspid aortic valve. (Adapted from Brandenburg RO, Fuster V, Giuliani E: Valvular heart disease. When should the patient be referred? Pract Cardiol 5:50, 1979; and Fuster V, Brandenburg RO, Giuliani E, et al: Clinical approach and management of acquired valvular heart disease. In: Office Cardiology. Cardiovasc Clinics 10:126, 1980. With permission.)*

Obstruction to flow between the left ventricle and aorta also may be due to hypertrophic obstructive cardiomyopathy; sub- or supravalvular stenosis due to an abnormal membrane below or above the valve; or supravalvular stenosis due to a congenital narrowing of the proximal ascending aorta. Supravalvular stenosis has been associated with hypercalcemia and mental retardation. There is an association between aortic stenosis and gastrointestinal bleeding. In one survey of 600 patients, aortic stenosis was significantly more prevalent among patients with idiopathic

GI tract bleeding than among patients with bleeding from a known source (Shoenfeld et al.).

Diagnosis

Aortic stenosis results in increased resistance to flow from the left ventricle. The left ventricle compensates by developing hypertrophy in order to maintain cardiac output. The hypertrophied muscle has diminished compliance, which results in a rise in left ventricular end-diastolic pressure. Left atrial contraction thus becomes more important for filling the left ventricle. Hence, patients with significant aortic stenosis often become more symptomatic when they develop atrial fibrillation and lose the "atrial kick." Myocardial oxygen consumption is increased, largely due to increased left ventricular wall tension (due to increased intracavitary left ventricular pressure), while subendocardial coronary blood flow is compromised because of high subendocardial intramural pressure. Hence, patients may exhibit symptoms and signs of ischemia without having coronary artery disease.

The traditional triad of symptoms in patients with aortic stenosis includes angina, syncope, and heart failure. Lombard and Selzer evaluated the clinical and hemodynamic profiles of 397 patients with severe aortic stenosis, finding that 50.9% of patients had angina. Coexisting coronary disease was present in 60% of patients (mean age, 60 years); however, there was no difference regarding the incidence of angina in this group versus those without coronary disease. These observations suggest that patients manifesting angina may have normal coronary arteries. Marcus et al. demonstrated that reduced coronary reserve to the hypertrophied left ventricle may contribute to the mechanism of angina pectoris. In general, a five-year life expectancy can be predicted once angina develops. Syncope is frequently exertional and may be secondary to exercise-triggered peripheral vasodilation with a fixed cardiac output; atrial or ventricular arrhythmias may also be a mechanism. Once syncope develops, survival is approximately three to four years. Signs of left ventricular failure may also develop, and are associated with a two-year survival. Occult or missed aortic stenosis occasionally presents as intractable heart failure. Although a rare presentation, abrupt loss of all or part of the visual field in one eye has been observed and is attributed to calcium emboli in patients with calcific aortic stenosis.

Physical examination reveals a delayed carotid upstroke with a prominent anacrotic notch at the time of peak turbulence across the valve. There is a prominent, prolonged apical impulse, often with a palpable a-wave. Auscultation reveals an ejection type systolic murmur beginning just after S_1. The murmur is harsh, crescendo-decrescendo and maximal at the second right intercostal space. The intensity and duration of the murmur bear a fair correlation with the severity of aortic stenosis. A high-frequency diastolic murmur of associated aortic regurgitation also may be present. The S_2 may be paradoxically split due to delayed left ventricular emptying. An S_4 is often present in patients in sinus rhythm. A systolic ejection click may be present, which suggests valve mobility and is heard frequently in congenitally biscuspid aortic valves. Differential diagnosis of the murmur of aortic stenosis is described in Table 7.

Since the left ventricle develops concentric hypertrophy in aortic stenosis, the cardiac silhouette may not change on early chest films. Eventually, the chest x-ray reveals a prominent left ventricle and a dilated ascending aorta (due to post-stenotic dilation). The aortic valve itself may be calcified. With decompensation, the left ventricle dilates and pulmonary venous congestion may appear. The electrocardiogram typically reveals left ventricular hypertrophy with secondary repolarization changes and left atrial enlargement. A left-axis deviation may be present and conduction defects (e.g., left bundle branch block, first-degree AV block, etc.) are frequently seen. With severe aortic stenosis, atrial fibrillation may be present.

Two-dimensional and M-mode echocardiography is helpful in the diagnosis of aortic stenosis. Thickened valve leaflets with limited mobility are observed. Valve doming, prominent with any stenotic valve, is also common. Left atrial enlargement and left ventricular hypertrophy, while nonspecific, are supportive echocardiographic features. Doppler echocardiography has become useful in the evaluation of aortic stenosis and in some centers has replaced diagnostic cardiac catheterization unless coronary artery anatomy needs to be defined. The modified Bernoulli equation is used to calculate the maximum instantaneous transvalvular pressure gradient, or "peak gradient" (see Chapter 8). Keep in mind, however, that "peak-to-peak" gradients obtained at cardiac catheterization are usually lower than Doppler-derived peak gradients.

A more recent Doppler echocardiographic technique described by Zoghbi et al. was used to calculate aortic valve area. The valve area was calculated from

Table 7. Differential Diagnosis of Aortic Valve Stenosis	
Disease Entity	Differentiating Features
Aortic valve sclerosis of the elderly, without stenosis (systolic murmur may mimic that of aortic stenosis)	Systolic murmur does not peak late. Carotids do not have delayed upstrokes. No left ventricular hypertrophy by ECG. Echocardiographic visualization of excursion of valve leaflets usually normal or mildly reduced, but valves may not be visualized. No hemodynamically significant aortic valve gradient by cardiac catheterization.
Hypertrophic obstructive cardiomyopathy (IHSS; systolic murmur may be confused with that of aortic stenosis)	Brisk bifid carotid upstrokes. Murmur usually does not radiate into neck. Characteristic change in murmur with various maneuvers. Pseudoinfarct pattern (large septal Q waves) on ECG. Characteristic echocardiographic features.
Mitral regurgitation (systolic murmur may be confused with that of aortic stenosis)	Murmur is holosystolic and radiates to axilla and not carotids. Carotid upstroke may be normal. Dilated left ventricle. Aortic valve normal on echocardiogram unless there is associated aortic valve disease.
Pulmonic stenosis (systolic murmur may be confused with that of aortic stenosis)	Murmur does not radiate into neck; loudest along the left sternal border. Physical exam, chest x-ray film, and ECG may reveal enlarged right ventricle. M-mode echocardiogram reveals right ventricular enlargement and hypertrophy and two-dimensional echocardiography may visualize valve stenosis.

the cross-sectional area of the aortic annulus multiplied by the peak velocity just proximal to the aortic valve, divided by peak aortic jet velocity. This technique resulted in a close correlation with aortic valve area measured at cardiac catheterization (r = 0.94).

Cardiac catheterization reveals a significant gradient between the left ventricle and aorta, as shown in Figure 5. A peak-to-peak gradient >50 mm Hg with a normal cardiac output has been considered severe. Left ventricular systolic and end-diastolic, and left atrial pressures are elevated. Critical aortic stenosis is present when the valve area is less than 0.75 cm^2 in an average-sized adult or 0.4 cm^2/m^2 BSA (normal aortic valve area is 3.0–3.5 cm^2). Coronary angiography is performed to determine if concomitant coronary artery disease is present, particularly in older patients or those with significant risk factors for coronary disease. The incidence of concomitant coronary disease is approximately 35% in all patients with aortic stenosis, and 45% in those older than age 60.

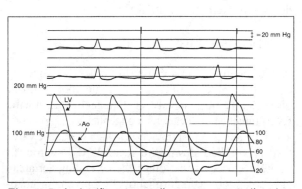

Figure 5. *A significant systolic pressure gradient between the left ventricle (LV) and the central aorta (Ao).*

Therapy

Once a patient becomes symptomatic with evidence of severe obstruction, as described above, surgery generally is indicated. The patient's age per se is not a contraindication to surgical valve replacement. Unless the left ventricular ejection fraction is severely depressed, valve replacement should be strongly considered, since left ventricular function will improve in most instances. There is also evidence that left ventricular hypertrophy will regress over time.

Percutaneous balloon dilatation of the aortic stenosis has been performed to treat nonsurgical candidates, although with less enthusiasm than in mitral stenosis. Using radionuclide ventriculography, McKay, Safian et al. evaluated the effect of aortic balloon valvuloplasty on cardiac performance in critical aortic stenosis. They found considerable variability in responses to valvuloplasty, with some patients showing marked improvement in valvular and ventricular function and others showing little change. These investigators (Safian et al.) reported a success rate of 95% in their series; however, aortic valve area increased by only 50%. Final valve area in most series has been 0.9–1.0 cm², suggesting moderate residual aortic stenosis. In addition, hemodynamic evidence of restenosis occurs in about half of patients by the ninth month after the procedure. Thus, this technique should be used as a palliative procedure and limited to those patients who are not surgical candidates. More information regarding long-term results and benefits with this technique need to be explored.

Medical therapy in aortic stenosis includes endocarditis prophylaxis for dental and surgical procedures and treatment of atrial fibrillation.

AORTIC REGURGITATION

Aortic regurgitation is caused by processes affecting either the valve leaflets or the aortic root. Primary diseases affecting the valve leaflets include rheumatic fever, infective endocarditis, congenital bicuspid valve, and ventricular septal defect (in which the aortic valve leaflet is pulled downward towards the ventricular cavity). Processes that dilate the ascending aorta can also create aortic regurgitation by preventing coaptation of the aortic valve leaflets. They include systemic hypertension, osteogenesis imperfecta, Reiter's syndrome, syphilitic aortitis, ankylosing spondylitis, Marfan's syndrome, cystic medial necrosis, and Ehlers-Danlos syndrome. Aortic regurgitation may be acute, as in acute bacterial endocarditis, aortic dissection, or trauma; or it may be chronic, as in systemic hypertension, rheumatic heart disease, or the collagen vascular diseases (Figure 6).

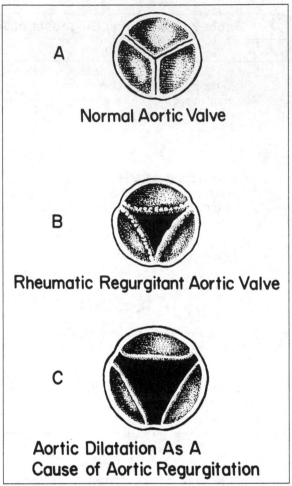

Figure 6. *(a) Normal aortic valve. (b) Rheumatic regurgitant aortic valve. The valve leaflets are fibrotic and shortened. (c) Aortic dilatation as a cause of aortic regurgitation. The valve leaflets are bowed and unable to coapt during diastole. There may be commissural separation as well.*

Diagnosis

In acute aortic regurgitation there is an abrupt increase in left ventricular end-diastolic volume, which results in marked elevations of left ventricular end-diastolic pressure. In chronic aortic regurgitation, the end-diastolic volume increases more gradually, allowing the left ventricle to compensate with gradual dilatation and hypertrophy. Over time the left ventricle further dilates and ultimately fails. During diastole, the rapid runoff of blood volume back into the left ventricle yields a low peripheral diastolic pressure, the mechanism behind many of the physical signs of aortic regurgitation. Low aortic diastolic pressures also reduce coronary perfusion pressure, making angina one of the features of this disease (although it is less common than in patients with aortic stenosis).

With acute aortic regurgitation, patients complain of weakness and severe dyspnea; hypotension may be present. In chronic aortic regurgitation, patients are often asymptomatic for long periods. One of the first symptoms includes an uncomfortable awareness of the heart beat due to increased stroke volume. Other symptoms include exertional dyspnea, orthopnea, paroxysmal nocturnal dyspnea, and palpitations. Angina may also occur. Patients with acute aortic regurgitation are generally tachycardic with marked peripheral vasoconstriction and a normal pulse pressure. The patients appear ill and have signs of decompensated heart failure with pulmonary congestion and edema, S_3 and S_4. The S_1 may be diminished or absent because of premature mitral valve closure. The murmur of acute aortic regurgitation is a short, low-frequency diastolic murmur.

In patients with chronic aortic regurgitation, there is a wide pulse pressure due to elevated systolic pressure created by enhanced stroke volume, and to relatively low diastolic pressure created by the rapid runoff of blood volume back into the left ventricle from the aorta. This situation creates a number of peripheral physical signs. The water-hammer (Corrigan's) pulse, described as a rapid upstroke and collapse, is noted on examination of peripheral pulses. De Musset's sign, referring to head-bobbing with each systole, may be observed. Palpation of the carotid arteries reveals a bisferiens or double-peaked quality of the pulse. Duroziez's sign is the diastolic murmur auscultated when the stethoscope compresses the femoral artery. Quincke's pulse refers to the visible capillary pulsation in the nailbed. Hill's sign, described as an increased popliteal systolic pressure over brachial systolic pressure of ≥ 40 mm Hg, is noted in severe aortic regurgitation. These peripheral signs may be entirely absent if aortic regurgitation is acute or after development of severe left ventricular failure.

In chronic aortic regurgitation, there is inferior and lateral displacement of the left ventricular impulse. The S_1 and A_2 may be diminished. In contrast to acute aortic regurgitation, the diastolic murmur of chronic aortic regurgitation is high-frequency, blowing, and decrescendo beginning just after S_2, and tends to be of longer duration (Table 8). The more severe the chronic aortic regurgitation, the longer the murmur persists in diastole. Auscultation may be facilitated with the patient sitting up and leaning forward, and with the use of the diaphragm of the stethoscope. When the murmur is heard best along the left sternal border, its cause is most likely to be damage to the valve leaflets; if the murmur is heard best along the right sternal border, the cause is most likely aortic root dilation. An Austin Flint murmur is often heard by the astute listener. This is a low-frequency, mid-diastolic apical rumble due to turbulent flow across the mitral valve, which is partially closed by the regurgitant jet.

The chest x-ray is far more helpful in chronic than in acute aortic regurgitation; it reveals an enlarged left ventricle with downward tilting of the apex. There may be calcification of the aortic valve, which is more suggestive of aortic regurgitation combined with stenosis, than of pure aortic regurgitation. Marked dilatation of the aorta may suggest aortic root disease (e.g., Marfan's syndrome). Pulmonary venous congestion may be present. The electrocardiogram generally reveals left ventricular hypertrophy and left atrial enlargement. A diastolic overload pattern may be noted on occasion, manifesting as left ventricular hypertrophy with Q waves anterolaterally. Sinus tachycardia is typical in patients with acute aortic regurgitation.

M-mode and 2D echocardiography, although not completely diagnostic, are useful in alerting the physician to the presence of aortic regurgitation. The M-mode may reveal fine diastolic fluttering of the mitral valve (also the interventricular septum), along with incomplete opening of the valve early in diastole. Early mitral valve closure may also be detected due to the marked elevation of left ventricular diastolic pressure. This finding is typical of acute and severe aortic regurgitation. Over time, left ventricular dilatation and, inevitably, reduction in systolic performance are observed. Doppler echocardiography is the primary noninvasive method used to diagnose the presence of aortic regurgitation. Grayburn et al. assessed the comparative value of pulsed Doppler echocardiography to standard 2D echocardiography and auscultation, and found far greater specificity and sensitivity with pulsed Doppler than with either of the other techniques. Color flow Doppler is especially useful for visualizing the regurgitant jet and may provide clues to the severity of regurgitation (p. *xviii*).

Diastolic mitral regurgitation is a phenomenon described by Downes et al. that marks acute, but not chronic, aortic regurgitation. As noted earlier, pre-

Table 8. Differential Diagnosis of Aortic Valve Regurgitation	
Disease Entity	Differentiating Features
Pulmonary regurgitation (diastolic murmur may be confused with aortic regurgitation)	Murmur of pulmonary insufficiency usually occurs in setting of pulmonary hypertension due to mitral stenosis or right-to-left cardiac shunt. Associated right ventricular enlargement. Absence of peripheral manifestations of aortic regurgitation.
Mitral stenosis (murmur may be confused with aortic regurgitation and Austin Flint murmur)	Murmur is low-pitched diastolic rumble with pre-systolic accentuation. Differentiated from Austin Flint murmur by using amyl nitrite. Austin Flint murmur diminishes with amyl nitrite; murmur of mitral stenosis remains unchanged or increases. Characteristic echocardiographic features of mitral stenosis.
Aortic stenosis (patients with aortic regurgitation may have a prominent aortic systolic murmur due to the increased flow of blood volume across the aortic valve)	With aortic stenosis, there is a delayed carotid upstroke; the murmur tends to peak later in systole; and the echocardiographic features of aortic regurgitation (a hyperdynamic left ventricle and high-frequency vibrations of the anterior leaflet to the mitral valve during diastole) are absent.
Patent ductus arteriosus (murmurs may be confused with those of aortic insufficiency)	Murmur is continued throughout systole and diastole with peak of the murmur at S_2. Systolic ejection murmur accompanying aortic regurgitation usually peaks in midsystole. Left-to-right shunt with radionuclide angiography and cardiac catheterization.

mature mitral valve closure occurs due to the rapid rise of left ventricular diastolic pressure; this may be associated with the appearance of mitral regurgitation into the diastolic phase.

Cardiac catheterization reveals a decreased diastolic systemic pressure and increased left ventricular end-diastolic pressure. There is a rapid diastolic fall on the aortic pressure tracing. Systolic arterial pressure is normal or increased (chronic aortic regurgitation) and pulmonary capillary wedge pressure may be increased. Aortic root angiography is performed on occasion to quantitate the degree of aortic regurgitation (graded from 1+ to 4+). Morphologic abnormalities of the aorta may also be seen, such as dissection, aortic root aneurysm, or calcification of the aortic valve (see also Chapter 9).

Therapy

Immediate surgical intervention is required for acute, hemodynamically unstable aortic regurgitation, since mortality is considerable without it. Intravenous pressors or nitroprusside may be helpful while anticipating surgery.

Asymptomatic patients with mild chronic aortic regurgitation generally need no treatment other than regular follow-up echocardiographic examinations to assess left ventricular function (and chamber dimension), and antibiotic prophylaxis against bacterial endocarditis. For symptomatic patients, diuresis and afterload reduction may be initiated. Symptomatic patients with severe aortic regurgitation, however, should undergo aortic valve replacement.

Some physicians recommend that patients with evidence of left ventricular dysfunction be considered for valve replacement even if symptoms are not yet present. Bonow et al. (1983) evaluated the natural history over 49 months of 77 asymptomatic patients with severe aortic regurgitation and normal resting left ventricular function. Death was rare, and fewer than 4% of patients required valve replacement because of development of symptoms. When aortic valve replacement was delayed until the development of symptoms, survival was excellent and left ventricular size and function improved. The same investigators more recently showed that late (3–7 yrs) after aortic valve replacement, left ventricular dimension decreased further and ejection fraction improved in those patients with a normal ejection fraction preoperatively, but not in those with an abnormal preoperative ejection fraction.

By tradition, radionuclide angiography has been used to assess resting and exercise ejection fraction in determining timing of aortic valve replacement. This information, however, is of no prognostic value with regard to mortality or postoperative left ventricular function.

RIGHT-SIDED VALVULAR HEART DISEASE

TRICUSPID STENOSIS

Undoubtedly the most common cause of tricuspid stenosis is rheumatic heart disease. Typically the tricuspid valve is involved along with the mitral valve. Rarely, congenital tricuspid atresia and large tricuspid valve vegetations or right atrial tumors may obstruct right ventricular inflow, creating functional tricuspid stenosis. Symptoms are generally related to enhanced systemic venous pressure as well as reduced cardiac output owing to the obstruction between right atrium and ventricle. Patients complain of generalized weakness and right upper quadrant discomfort due to hepatic venous congestion.

Physical examination is remarkable for jugular venous distention with a prominent a-wave and slow y descent. There may be an opening snap on auscultation (it may be difficult to distinguish from the opening snap of mitral stenosis). The murmur is a high-frequency diastolic rumbling heard predominantly at the lower left sternal border. Both the opening snap and the murmur are intensified with inspiration. Additionally, in patients in sinus rhythm, there may be presystolic accentuation of the murmur. The liver is enlarged and tender, generally with hepatojugular reflux. Peripheral edema and ascites also may be present. The chest x-ray may demonstrate pleural effusion with right atrial enlargement. The electrocardiogram also displays right atrial enlargement or, on occasion, atrial fibrillation.

Two-dimensional echocardiography reveals doming usually of the anterior tricuspid valve leaflet, with thickening and limited mobility of all leaflets. Flattening of the E-F slope is seen on the M-mode echocardiogram, although, as in mitral stenosis, this is a fairly nonspecific observation. Doppler echocardiography demonstrates an increased transvalvular flow velocity during diastole, just as in mitral stenosis.

An echocardiographic survey of patients with rheumatic heart disease (Guyer et al.) found a 9.5% incidence of tricuspid stenosis in patients by 2D echo and a 26.3% incidence by 2D echo and cardiac catheterization. The sensitivity and specificity of 2D echo were 69% and 96%, respectively. As this study implies, 2D echocardiography is not as helpful in making the diagnosis of tricuspid stenosis as we know Doppler echocardiography to be. The physician should remember that isolated rheumatic tricuspid stenosis is extremely rare, so findings suggestive of concomitant mitral stenosis usually are expected.

If the patient fails intensive medical treatment consisting primarily of sodium restriction and diuresis, surgical intervention should be considered, particularly once the mean diastolic pressure gradient reaches 5 mm Hg with a tricuspid valve area ≤ 2.0 cm^2. (The tricuspid valve is the largest of the four valves, with a normal valve area of approximately 10 cm^2.) Either tricuspid valve replacement or surgical valvuloplasty may be considered. The state of other valve lesions, particularly mitral stenosis, may be the crucial factor in the timing of tricuspid valve intervention. Patients with tricuspid stenosis should receive antibiotic prophylaxis against infective endocarditis.

TRICUSPID REGURGITATION

Tricuspid regurgitation does not often occur due to abnormalities of the valve itself; it usually arises after the development of right ventricular and tricuspid annular dilatation. Any cause of right ventricular or pulmonary artery hypertension with subsequent right chamber dilatation may lead to tricuspid regurgitation. Etiologies creating tricuspid regurgitation from abnormalities of the valve itself include rheumatic heart disease, endocarditis (generally in intravenous drug abusers), Ebstein's anomaly, carcinoid heart disease, prolapse due to myxomatous degeneration, and trauma. Gayet et al. reviewed 12 patients with traumatic tricuspid regurgitation, noting its occurrence with thoracic injuries. They demonstrated the usefulness of echocardiography in making this diagnosis and emphasized the serious underestimation of trauma as a possible cause of tricuspid regurgitation.

Patients with tricuspid regurgitation complain of symptoms of right-sided heart failure, such as peripheral edema, right upper quadrant tenderness (due to hepatic venous congestion), nausea, and vomiting (due to splanchnic congestion). The physical examination reveals distended neck veins with prominent regurgitant systolic v-waves and a rapidly collapsing y descent. A palpable venous systolic thrill and murmur at the base of the neck, described by Amidi et al., may appear in severe tricuspid regurgitation. A right ventricular heave also may be present. If pulmonary hypertension is present, the P_2 will be accentuated. The murmur of tricuspid regurgitation typically is high-frequency, holosystolic, and most prominent along the lower left sternal border. Its enhancement during inspiration may help distinguish it from the murmur of mitral regurgitation. There also may be a right ventricular S_3. The liver may be enlarged and pulsatile, with hepatojugular reflux. Peripheral edema and ascites are often present.

The chest x-ray reveals enlargement of the right atrium and ventricle, often in association with prominence of the superior vena cava and azygous vein. The electrocardiogram displays right atrial enlargement with tall p-waves (p pulmonale), most clearly seen in the inferior leads. There may be a right-axis deviation and prominent anterior forces—evidence of right ventricular hypertrophy. Atrial fibrillation may be present.

Two-dimensional echocardiography reveals a dilated right ventricular chamber with paradoxical motion of the interventricular septum, implying right ventricular volume overload. The right atrium is also enlarged. If tricuspid regurgitation is secondary to abnormalities of the valve itself, the echocardiogram may reveal tricuspid valvular vegetations, nonspecific thickening of the valve, prolapse, or exaggerated valve motion as in the case of Ebstein's anomaly. Doppler echocardiography is extremely sensitive in identifying tricuspid regurgitation. Using the continuous-wave mode, peak velocity of the regurgitant jet can be obtained and pulmonary artery systolic pressure estimated using the simplified Bernoulli equation (see Chapter 8 for further detail). Color flow Doppler is also sensitive for diagnosing tricuspid regurgitation.

Cardiac catheterization typically reveals elevated right atrial and right ventricular end-diastolic pressures. A prominent regurgitant wave with a rapid y descent is observed in the right atrial pressure tracing. Although seldom needed, right ventriculography demonstrates dilated right-sided chambers with regurgitation of dye into the right atrium.

Medical management consisting of sodium restriction, diuretics and digitalis may be sufficient for mild tricuspid regurgitation. Endocarditis prophylaxis should be administered for organic tricuspid disease. Surgical intervention is usually not employed until there is evidence of severe tricuspid regurgitation. If tricuspid regurgitation is due to annular dilation, a technique developed by Carpentier et al., allowing suturing of the annulus to a prosthetic ring, has simplified surgical management considerably. If tricuspid regurgitation is due to primary valvular abnormalities, valve replacement is the usual treatment. However, there has been at least temporary success with excision of the valve in patients with tricuspid regurgitation due to infective endocarditis (intravenous drug abusers).

PULMONIC STENOSIS

Pulmonic stenosis is generally congenital in origin and may be valvular, subvalvular or supravalvular. On rare occasions, valvular pulmonic stenosis may be rheumatic in origin or secondary to plaque collection around the pulmonic valve (or the tricuspid valve) in malignant carcinoid syndrome. Extrinsic compression in the region of the pulmonic valve due to tumors or aneurysm of the sinus of Valsalva may occasionally lead to functional pulmonic stenosis. The normal pulmonic valve area is $2.0 \text{ cm}^2/\text{m}^2$.

Only moderate to severe pulmonic stenosis creates symptoms, which generally include fatigue, exertional dyspnea, lightheadedness, syncope, and, if severe, symptoms of right ventricular failure. The physical examination reveals a prominent jugular venous a-wave with a right ventricular heave. The S_2 is widely split with a soft P_2 component. A right-sided S_3 and S_4 also may be present. The murmur of pulmonic stenosis is a harsh systolic ejection murmur prominent at the upper left sternal border. Late peaking of the murmur implies increased severity of pulmonic stenosis. An ejection click preceding the murmur suggests that the stenosis is valvular rather than sub- or supravalvular. Cyanosis may be present with substantial reductions in cardiac output. With development of right ventricular failure come peripheral edema, ascites, and a tender enlarged liver.

The chest x-ray displays post-stenotic dilatation of the main pulmonary artery and, ultimately, dilatation of the right atrium and ventricle if the pulmonic stenosis is severe. There may be generalized pulmonary oligemia as well. The electrocardiogram demonstrates right atrial enlargement and evidence of right ventricular hypertrophy in advanced pulmonic stenosis. Conduction disturbances, most commonly a right bundle branch block, are not infrequent.

Two-dimensional echocardiography is of limited usefulness in the diagnosis of pulmonic stenosis, as the pulmonic valve is the most difficult to demonstrate echocardiographically. A prominent a-wave may be observed on the M-mode tracing of the pulmonic valve. A reasonably accurate transvalvular gradient can be obtained with Doppler echocardiography; the peak velocity is entered into the simplified Bernoulli equation, as previously described.

Cardiac catheterization may be used to assess the severity of the pulmonic stenosis. If the transvalvular gradient is >50 mm Hg, pulmonic stenosis is considered to be moderate; it is severe if the gradient is >80 mm Hg. Right ventricular end-diastolic pressure and right atrial systolic pressure (the a-wave) may also be increased. Right ventriculography may display doming and thickening of the pulmonic valve leaflets. Cardiac catheterization is also useful in ruling out other concomitant congenital lesions.

Intervention, consisting of either surgical valve replacement or valvulotomy, is usually undertaken once the transvalvular gradient exceeds 50 mm Hg. Kan et al. described success with percutaneous transluminal balloon valvuloplasty for pulmonic stenosis; this lesion was among the first dilated by this technique. All patients with pulmonic stenosis should receive prophylaxis against infective endocarditis.

PULMONIC REGURGITATION

The most common cause of pulmonic valve regurgitation is physiologic, secondary to dilatation of the pulmonary valve ring, as in pulmonary hypertension, or to dilatation of the pulmonary artery. Infective endocarditis may also rarely cause pulmonic regurgitation. Pulmonic regurgitation may be congenital in origin occurring in association with tetralogy of Fallot, ventricular septal defect, or pulmonic valve stenosis.

Patients are generally asymptomatic unless severe pulmonic regurgitation develops with marked right ventricular dilatation and subsequent failure. In these cases, patients complain of generalized fatigue, exertional dyspnea, anorexia, nausea, vomiting, and right upper quadrant discomfort. There may be significant peripheral edema as well. Of note, severe right heart failure may be particularly common in patients with pulmonic regurgitation due to infective endocarditis

(intravenous drug abusers). These patients often develop septic pulmonary emboli with severe pulmonary hypertension.

The physical examination reveals a hyperdynamic right ventricular impulse and occasionally a palpable pulmonary artery in the second left intercostal space. There is a widely split S_2, with prominence of the P_2 if pulmonary hypertension is present. The murmur of pulmonic regurgitation is a low-frequency, decrescendo diastolic murmur most prominent along the upper left sternal border, which is enhanced by inspiration. When the murmur is high-frequency and blowing in quality (Graham Steell murmur), pulmonic regurgitation is most likely secondary to pulmonary hypertension. Other physical findings relate to the development of right ventricular failure. The chest x-ray reveals enlargement of the main pulmonary artery as well as the right ventricle. The electrocardiogram displays evidence of right ventricular hypertrophy.

Two-dimensional echocardiography demonstrates the dilated right ventricle, with hypertrophy if pulmonary hypertension is present. There is generally paradoxical interventricular septal wall motion typical of right ventricular overload states. Tricuspid valve leaflet fluttering during diastole may be observed (similar to that seen on the mitral valve in the setting of aortic regurgitation). Doppler echocardiography is fairly sensitive in identifying pulmonic regurgitation.

Pulmonary regurgitation alone, unless severe, rarely requires specific therapy. However, once evidence of right ventricular failure appears, valve replacement (or correction of the underlying lesion) should be undertaken. Infective endocarditis on the pulmonic valve will require appropriate antibiotic treatment and sometimes valve replacement. Patients with clinically significant pulmonic regurgitation due to structural abnormalities of the valve should have antibiotic prophylaxis against infective endocarditis.

PROSTHETIC HEART VALVES

The selection of a particular prosthetic valve should be done under the direction of the surgeon and cardiologist. There are two general categories of prosthetic valves—mechanical and bioprosthetic.

MECHANICAL VALVES

The Starr-Edwards caged-ball valve with a cloth-covered sewing ring and silastic ball has the advantages of durability, a single orifice, reduced rate of thrombosis (as compared with others), and relative ease of insertion. In addition, the valve functions quietly and has a low incidence of endocarditis. Disadvantages include its large, bulky size, which makes it inappropriate for patients with a small left ventricle or small aortic annulus. In addition, hemolysis occurs in a small percentage of patients.

The standard tilting-disc valve (such as the Bjork-Shiley) consists of a disc occluder closing between two peripheral struts. Its low profile usually results in desirable hemodynamics. Strut fracture and thrombosis are two disadvantages of this valve. A mild amount of valvular regurgitation is inherent in its performance. Omniscience, Omnicarbon, and Medtronic Hall are tilting-disc valves that may have decreased thrombogenicity.

The St. Jude valve consists of two semicircular discs that pivot between open and closed positions. This valve has excellent flow characteristics and is especially useful in children.

All mechanical valves require chronic anticoagulation therapy; usually this is begun a few days after surgery.

BIOPROSTHETIC VALVES

Bioprosthetic valves (Hancock, Carpentier-Edwards, Ionescu-Shiley, etc.), made of either porcine aortic valves or bovine pericardium, were developed primarily in an effort to avoid the need for anticoagulation that exists with the mechanical valves. However, the bioprosthetic valves may be less durable: approximately 20–30% of patients need a second new valve by 10 years after the first implantation. In patients younger than 30-35 years old, the risk of bioprosthetic valve failure is far higher than in patients older than 50 years. Calcification of bioprosthetic valves is also a frequent problem. For this reason, patients with chronic renal failure, secondary hyperparathyroidism, or abnormal calcium metabolism, and children who have active calcium metabolism, should probably receive mechanical prosthetic valves.

Even when bioprosthetic valves are used, anticoagulation may be desirable during the first three months of valve replacement (beginning a few days after surgery). After three months, anticoagulation usually is not needed for bioprosthetic valves in the aortic or the mitral position if patients are in sinus rhythm and there is no evidence of atrial thrombi. However, in patients with atrial fibrillation and a large left atrium,

a history of thromboembolism, or evidence of left atrial thrombus at the time of surgery, anticoagulation should be continued indefinitely.

In young patients, the durability and duration of effectiveness of the valve must be considered. The risk of long-term anticoagulation must be balanced against the probability of reoperation. Mechanical prosthetic valves are relatively contraindicated in young women of child-bearing age, due to the risks of anticoagulation. In an elderly patient, a bioprosthetic valve is generally chosen to avoid anticoagulation; additionally, valve longevity may be less of an issue.

In the tricuspid position, a bioprosthetic valve is generally used, because the risks of thrombosis on the right side of the heart (with its lower pressures) are far greater.

A Veterans Administration randomized trial comparing mechanical and bioprosthetic valves found no significant difference in survival up to eight years after surgery. Differences in valve-related complications were due largely to significant bleeding in patients with a mechanical valve (Hammermeister et al.).

Bibliography

Amidi M, Irwin J, Salerni R, et al: Venous systolic thrill and murmur in the neck: A consequence of severe tricuspid insufficiency. *J Am Coll Cardiol* 7:942, 1986.

Arbulu A, Asfaw I: Tricuspid valvulectomy without prosthetic replacement. Ten years of clinical experience. *J Thorac Cardiovasc Surg* 82:684, 1981.

Bansal R, Shah P: Usefulness of echo-Doppler in management of patients with valvular heart disease. *Curr Probl Cardiol* 14:281, 1989.

Bisno A, Shulman S, Dajani A: The rise and fall (and rise ?) of rheumatic fever. *JAMA* 259:728, 1988.

Block P: Aortic valvoloplasty—a valid alternative? *N Engl J Med* 319:169, 1988.

Block PC: Percutaneous mitral and aortic balloon valvuloplasty. Patient selection and factors determining results. *Cardiovascular Reviews and Reports* 10:44, 1989.

Bonow R, Rosing D, McIntosh C, et al: The natural history of asymptomatic patients with aortic regurgitation and normal left ventricular function. *Circulation* 68:509, 1983.

Bonow R, Dodd J, Maron J, et al: Long-term serial changes in left ventricular function and reversal of ventricular dilatation after valve replacement for chronic aortic regurgitation. *Circulation* 78:1108, 1988.

Bonow R, Picone A, McIntosh C, et al: Survival and functional results after valve replacement for aortic regurgitation from

1976 to 1983: Impact of preoperative left ventricular function. *Circulation* 72:1244, 1985.

Brockmeier L, Adolph R, Gustin B, et al: Calcium emboli to the retinal artery in calcific aortic stenosis. *Am Heart J* 101:32, 1981.

Cabrera E, Baxiola A: A critical reevaluation of systolic and diastolic overload patterns. *Progr Cardiovasc Dis* 2:219, 1959.

Carpentier A: Cardiac valve surgery—The "French correction." *J Thorac Cardiovasc Surg* 86:323, 1983.

Case Records of the Massachusetts General Hospital. Case 19–1989. *N Engl J Med* 320:1260, 1989.

Chopra P, Das Tandon H, Raizada V, et al: Comparative studies of mitral valves in rheumatic heart disease. *Arch Intern Med* 143:661, 1983.

Cobanogu A, Brockman S: Selection of a prosthetic heart valve. Valvular heart disease: Comprehensive evaluation and management. In: *Cardiovascular Clinics*. Philadelphia: F.A. Davis Co.; 1986.

Congeni B, Rizzo C, Congeni J, et al: Outbreak of acute rheumatic fever in Northeastern Ohio. *J Pediatr* 111:176, 1987.

Cosgrove D, Stewart W: Mitral valvuloplasty. *Curr Probl Cardiol* 14:353, 1989.

Currie P, Seward J, Chan K, et al: Continuous wave Doppler determination of right ventricular pressure: A simultaneous Doppler-catheterization study in 127 patients. *J Am Coll Cardiol* 6:750, 1985.

Denny F: T. Duckett Jones and rheumatic fever in 1986. *Circulation* 76:963, 1987.

Desnoyers MR: Balloon valvuloplasty in the treatment of aortic stenosis. *Practical Cardiology* 15:31, 1989.

Devereux R: Diagnosis and prognosis of mitral valve prolapse. *N Engl J Med* 320:1077, 1989.

Downes T, Nomeir A, Hackshaw B, et al: Diastolic mitral regurgitation in acute but not chronic aortic regurgitation: Implications regarding the mechanism of mitral closure. *Am Heart J* 117:1106, 1989.

Galloway A, Colvin S, Baumann F, et al: Current concepts of mitral valve reconstruction for mitral insufficiency. *Circulation* 78:1087, 1988.

Gayet C, Pierre B, Delahaye JP, et al: Traumatic tricuspid insufficiency—an underdiagnosed disease. *Chest* 92:429, 1987.

Gordis L: The virtual disappearance of rheumatic fever in the United States: Lessons in the rise and fall of disease. *Circulation* 72:1155, 1985.

Grayburn P, Smith M, Handshoe R, et al: Detection of aortic insufficiency in standard echocardiography, pulsed Doppler echocardiography, and auscultation—a comparison of accuracies. *Ann Intern Med* 104:599, 1986.

Guyer D, Gillam L, Foale R, et al: Comparison of the echocardiographic and hemodynamic diagnosis of rheumatic tricuspid stenosis. *J Am Coll Cardiol* 3:1135, 1984.

Hammermeister K, Henderson W, Burchfiel C, et al: Comparison of outcome after valve replacement with a bioprosthesis versus a mechanical prosthesis: Initial 5 year results of a randomized trial. *J Am Coll Cardiol* 10:719, 1987.

Hart R, Easton J: Mitral valve prolapse and cerebral infarction. *Stroke* 13:429, 1982.

Hoshino P, Gaasch W: When to intervene in chronic aortic regurgitation. *Arch Intern Med* 146:349, 1986.

Jameison W, Rosado L, Muriro A, et al: Carpentier-Edwards standard porcine bioprosthesis: Primary tissue failure (structural valve deterioration) by age groups. *Ann Thorac Surg* 46:155, 1988.

Kan J, White R, Mitchell S, et al: Percutaneous transluminal balloon valvuloplasty for pulmonary valve stenosis. *Circulation* 69:554, 1984.

Lombard J, Selzer A: Valvular aortic stenosis: A clinical and hemodynamic profile of patients. *Ann Intern Med* 106:292, 1987.

Marcus M, Doty D, Hiratzka L, et al: Decreased coronary reserve. A mechanism for angina pectoris in patients with aortic stenosis and normal coronary arteries. *N Engl J Med* 307:1362, 1982.

Markiewicz W, Stoner J, London E, et al: Mitral valve prolapse in one hundred presumably healthy young females. *Circulation* 53:464, 1976.

McKay R, Safian R, Lock J, et al: Assessment of left ventricular and aortic valve function after aortic balloon valvuloplasty in adult patients with critical aortic stenosis. *Circulation* 75:192, 1987.

McKay R, Lock J, Safian R, et al: Balloon dilation of mitral stenosis in adult patients: Postmortem and percutaneous mitral valvuloplasty studies. *J Am Coll Cardiol* 9:723, 1987.

McKay CR, Kawanishi D, Kotlewski A, et al: Improvement in exercise capacity and exercise hemodynamics 3 months after double-balloon catheter balloon valvuloplasty in the treatment of patients with symptomatic mitral stenosis. *Circulation* 77:1013, 1988.

Miller F: Aortic stenosis: Most cases no longer require invasive hemodynamic study. *J Am Coll Cardiol* 13:551, 1989.

Monrad S, Hess O, Murakami T, et al: Time course of regression of left ventricular hypertrophy after aortic valve replacement. *Circulation* 77:1345, 1988.

Morgan D, Hale R: Occult aortic stenosis as cause of intractable heart failure. *Br Med J* 1:784, 1979.

Nair CK, Sketch MH, Desai R, et al: High prevalence of symptomatic bradyarrhythmias due to atrioventricular node-fascicular and sinus node-atrial disease in patients with mitral anular calcification. *Am Heart J* 103:226, 1982.

Nishimura R, McGoon M, Shub C, et al: Echocardiographically documented mitral valve prolapse: Long-term follow-up of idiopathic mitral valve prolapse in 300 patients: A prospective study. *J Am Coll Cardiol* 11:42, 1988.

Otto C, Pearlman A, Gardner C: Hemodynamic progression of aortic stenosis in adults assessed by Doppler echocardiography. *J Am Coll Cardiol* 13:545, 1989.

Perloff J: *Physical Examination of the Heart and Circulation*. Philadelphia: Saunders; 1982.

Perloff J, Child J: Clinical and epidemiologic issues in mitral valve prolapse: Overview and perspective. *Am Heart J* 113:1324, 1987.

Rahimtoola S: Catheter balloon valvuloplasty of aortic and mitral stenosis in adults: 1987. *Circulation* 75:895, 1987.

Rahimtoola SH: Perspective on valvular heart disease: An update. *J Am Coll Cardiol* 14:1, 1989.

Reis R, Roberts W: Amounts of coronary arterial narrowing by atherosclerotic plaques in clinically isolated mitral valve stenosis: Analysis of 76 necropsy patients older than 30 years. *Am J Cardiol* 57:1119, 1986.

Ross J, Braunwald E: Aortic Stenosis. *Circulation* 36(Suppl IV): IV-61, 1968.

Ross J: Afterload mismatch in aortic and mitral valve disease: Implications for surgical therapy. *J Am Coll Cardiol* 5:811, 1985.

Roth A, Harrison E, Mitani G, et al: Efficacy and safety of medium- and high-dose diltazem alone and in combination with digoxin for control of heart rate at rest and during exercise in patients with chronic atrial fibrillation. *Circulation* 73:316, 1986.

Safian R, Mandell V, Thurer R, et al: Postmortem and intraoperative balloon valvuloplasty of calcific aortic stenosis in elderly patients: Mechanisms of successful dilation. *J Am Coll Cardiol* 9:655, 1987.

Schwarz F, Baumann P, Manthey J, et al: The effect of aortic valve replacement on survival. *Circulation* 66:1105, 1982.

Shoenfeld Y, Eldar M, Bedazovsky B, et al: Aortic stenosis associated with gastrointestinal bleeding. A survey of 612 patients. *Am Heart J* 100:179, 1980.

Skjaerpe T, Hegrenaes L, Hatle L: Noninvasive estimation of valve area in patients with aortic stenosis by Doppler ultrasound and two-dimensional echocardiography. *Circulation* 72:810, 1985.

St. John Sutton MG, St. John Sutton M, Oldershaw P, et al: Valve replacement without preoperative cardiac catheterization. *N Engl J Med* 305:1233, 1981.

Veasy L, et al: Resurgence of acute rheumatic fever in the Intermountain area of the United States. *N Engl J Med* 316:421, 1987.

Wynne J: Mitral valve prolapse. *N Engl J Med* 314:577, 1986.

Yeager M, Yock P, Popp R: Comparison of Doppler-derived pressure gradient to that determined at cardiac catheterization in adults with aortic valve stenosis: Implications for management. *Am J Cardiol* 57:644, 1986.

18 Myocarditis and Cardiomyopathy

Shereif Rezkalla
Robert A. Kloner

MYOCARDITIS

Myocarditis is an inflammatory process involving the heart. There are many causes, including infectious agents, physical agents, chemicals, drugs, and radiation (Table 1).

GENERAL CLINICAL MANIFESTATIONS

Clinical manifestations of myocarditis range from electrocardiographic abnormality in the asymptomatic patient to severe congestive heart failure. Symptoms consist of fatigue, dyspnea, palpitations, chest pain suggestive of pericarditis or myocardial ischemia, and fever. Sinus tachycardia is usually present, and is out of proportion to the degree of fever. The S_1 is soft. Ventricular gallops, a transient apical systolic murmur, and a pericardial friction rub may be heard. In severe cases due to congestive heart failure, pulmonary rales and pulsus alternans may be present. Systemic or pulmonary emboli are complications of myocarditis. The physical findings related to the underlying cause of myocarditis should be sought; for example, the suppurative pharyngeal membrane of diphtheria or skin rashes associated with rickettsial infection. Chest x-ray film is either normal or reveals cardiac enlargement, with or without signs of pulmonary congestion. The electrocardiogram demonstrates ST-T–wave abnormalities, low QRS voltage, conduction disturbances, and various atrial and ventricular arrhythmias. Occasionally, the ECG changes are indistinguishable from acute myocardial infarction.

Echocardiography may demonstrate pericardial effusion and generalized uniform reduction in wall motion; however, regional wall motion abnormalities are not uncommon. Radionuclide ventriculography may detect reduced left ventricular function. A study by Das et al. showed that asymptomatic patients with prior myocarditis may have left ventricular dysfunction during exercise as assessed by radionuclide ventriculography. A preliminary report by Chandraratna et al. suggests that nuclear magnetic resonance imaging may be useful in diagnosis. However, this early report needs to be confirmed.

Although spontaneous recovery from acute myocarditis is common, a certain percentage of patients develop a fulminant illness and progress to severe, end-stage heart failure. In general, therapy is supportive. Adequate rest and oxygenation are important, as exercise and hypoxemia may increase myocardial damage. Congestive heart failure is treated with salt restriction, diuretics, and afterload reducers. Patients with myocarditis tend to be sensitive to digitalis; hence, it must be used with caution. Patients should be monitored for the development of conduction disturbances and arrhythmias. The use of steroids in the acute phase of the disease remains controversial. Antibiotics are used for treating specific myocarditides such as those associated with bacteria, psittacosis, mycoplasma, and tuberculosis. Antitoxin is used for diphtheria myocarditis. If the myocarditis is due to chemicals, drugs, or physical agents, the offending substances or agents must be withdrawn.

SELECTED SPECIFIC MYOCARDITIDES

Viral Myocarditis

Coxsackievirus A and B, echovirus, and influenza virus are the most common viruses causing myocarditis. The disease consists of two phases: the acute phase, characterized by viral replication, during which the virus can be isolated from the myocardium, and

```
┌─────────────────────────────────────────────────────────────────────────┐
│   Table 1. Etiologies of Myocarditis                                      │
├─────────────────────────────────────────────────────────────────────────┤
```

Infectious Agents
Viral: coxsackievirus (especially group B), echovirus, poliovirus, influenza, mumps,
  Epstein-Barr virus, viral hepatitis, rabies, rubella, rubeola, varicella, retrovirus
Bacterial: diphtheria, tuberculosis, salmonella (typhoid fever), streptococcus (rheumatic fe-
  ver or direct streptococcal myocarditis), meningococcus, clostridia (gas gangrene or tet-
  anus), myocarditis associated with bacterial endocarditis, brucellosis
Spirochetal myocarditis: syphilis, leptospirosis (Weil's disease), relapsing fever, Lyme dis-
  ease
Rickettsial myocarditis: typhus, Rocky Mountain spotted fever, Q fever
Chlamydial: psittacosis
Primary atypical pneumonia (myocoplasma)
Fungal: candidiasis, aspergillosis, histoplasmosis, actinomycosis, blastomycosis
Protozoal myocarditis: Trypanosoma cruzi (Chagas' disease), African trypanosomiasis
  (sleeping sickness), malaria, toxoplasmosis, amebiasis
Metazoal myocarditis: schistosomiasis, trichinosis, ascariasis, cysticercosis, echinococcus
Myocardial Damage due to Chemicals, Drugs, Toxins
  Antineoplastic agents: anthracyclines, cyclophosphamide, 5-fluorouracil
  Metal poisoning: lead, mercury, arsenic
  Antiparasitic agents: emetine, chloroquine, antimony compounds
  Catecholamines (e.g., pheochromocytoma)
  Psychotropic drugs: phenothiazines, lithium
  Animal toxins: snake bite, wasp, spider, scorpion stings
  Carbon monoxide
  Phosphorus
Physical Agents
  Radiation, hypothermia, heat stroke
Hypersensitivity Reactions
  Methyldopa, penicillin, sulfonamides, tetracycline, phenylbutazone, serum sickness,
    rejection of cardiac transplant, collagen vascular diseases

which usually represents the first 10 days of the illness; and the late phase, which is characterized by slow deterioration of myocardial function in some patients. It is believed that many cases of idiopathic dilated cardiomyopathy are due to antecedent viral myocarditis. This theory is controversial since there are no longitudinal studies in humans to support it. Recently, Abelmann and colleagues were able to develop a swine model of viral myocarditis, and were able to show that the disease may progress to a dilated cardiomyopathy.

Helpful laboratory tests include isolation of virus from blood, throat, or rectal swabs and determination of antibody titre during the acute and convalescent phases of the disease. A rise in the titres is more suggestive of the disease than the absolute value during the acute phase. Isolation of virus from the heart, although uncommon, is diagnostic for myocarditis. The role of endomyocardial biopsy in the diagnosis is not well established, but it may be helpful in selected cases. In some studies, active inflammation documented on right ventricular biopsy responded to anti-inflammatory drugs. However, routine myocardial biopsy cannot, at this time, be recommended. In a recent review by O'Connell and Mason, recommendations for biopsy were restricted to two indications: patients considered for clinical trials, and patients showing progressive deterioration with such immediate poor prognosis that "any potentially beneficial therapy, even with associated risk, should not be withheld."

Rest is indicated. Nonsteroidal anti-inflammatory drugs should be avoided during the acute phase of myocarditis since they exacerbate the extent of cardiac pathology, and their use should be restricted to symptomatic treatment during the late phase. Beta blockers probably should be avoided during the acute phase as well.

Several clinical reports suggest either a beneficial or a deleterious effect of immunosuppressive therapy on myocarditis. O'Connell et al. studied 35 patients with idiopathic cardiomyopathy presumed to be secondary to myocarditis. Twenty patients had a negative gallium scan and were treated with conventional therapy, and 15 with positive scans were treated with prednisone and azathioprine. Among treated patients, six showed improvement while nine did not. Fenoglio et al. and Daly et al. reported the results of immunosuppressive therapy in a small group of patients, with improvement in some patients; however, due to lack of control groups in these studies, the claimed benefit cannot be distinguished conclusively from spontaneous improvement. A randomized study is in progress to investigate the effect of immunosuppressive therapy on human myocarditis. Currently, however, the role of immunosuppressive therapy in myocarditis is controversial.

A recent report on use of intravenous ribavirin in influenza virus-associated acute myocarditis in three patients revealed that while viral shedding abruptly terminated with therapy, two patients died shortly after treatment, and the third died eight months later (Ray et al.). At present, ribavirin does not appear to be of clear benefit in management of human myocarditis.

Recently, captopril (an ACE inhibitor) was beneficial during both the acute and late phases of the disease in a murine model of myocarditis (Rezkalla et al. 1990); however, human studies are not yet available.

Most patients recover from viral myocarditis within weeks, although electrocardiographic abnormalities often persist for months. Coxsackievirus myocarditis is only occasionally fatal in adults; neonates tend to have a more malignant course than adults.

Acute Rheumatic Fever

See Chapter 17, "Valvular Heart Disease" for discussion of acute rheumatic fever in the etiology of myocarditis.

Diphtheria

Myocardial involvement occurs in approximately 25% of cases of diphtheria and may lead to severe cardiac dysfunction and, in some cases, sudden cardiovascular collapse and death. The myocarditis is due to a toxin produced by the diphtheria bacillus. Clinical manifestations of myocarditis typically appear at the end of the first week of illness and include congestive heart failure, arrhythmias and conduction defects. Treatment includes administration of antitoxin, antibiotics (penicillin G or erythromycin), respiratory support, and supportive therapy for congestive heart failure. Digitalis should be administered cautiously since it may increase atrioventricular block. Transvenous pacemaker therapy is instituted for complete AV block. Ramos et al. reported that the addition of carnitine in a dose of 100 mg/kg/day results in a lower incidence of heart failure and conduction defects and improves survival. Corticosteroid therapy is of no value.

Chagas' Disease (Trypanosomiasis)

Chagas' disease is the most common form of heart disease in Central and South America and is caused by the protozoan *Trypanosoma cruzi*. The protozoan is transmitted to humans through an insect bite. In the acute phase of the illness, patients are usually asymptomatic or experience constitutional symptoms of fever, sweating, muscle pains, vomiting and diarrhea, palpitations, and dyspnea. Tachycardia, signs of congestive heart failure, and hepatomegaly may be present. After a latent phase, 30% of patients progress to the chronic phase of the disease.

Chronic Chagas' disease may be due to an autoimmune mechanism. It is characterized by mononuclear cellular infiltration and fibrosis in the region of the sinoatrial and atrioventricular nodes and His bundle, degeneration of myocardial fibers, and, often, mural thrombi. Clinical manifestations include signs of right-sided and left-sided heart failure, with the former being more predominant. Physical examination reveals a widely split S_2 due to right bundle branch block, and a loud P_2 due to pulmonary hypertension. The murmur of tricuspid regurgitation is common. Ventricular ectopic activity is a frequent finding and some patients develop syncope and sudden death due to ventricular fibrillation even before signs of heart failure have developed. Laboratory evidence of Chagas' disease includes a positive complement-fixation test (Machado-Guerreiro test) or detection of the parasite in the blood of patients during the acute phase of illness. Electrocardiography is a good screening test in areas with a high prevalence of the disease. Electrocardiographic abnormalities include AV and bundle branch block, decreased QRS voltage, prolonged QT interval, T-wave abnormalities, and bradycardia. Echocardiography reveals systolic and diastolic dysfunction; regional wall motion abnormalities are common. Endomyocardial biopsy reveals cellular infiltration, myocardial necrosis, and myocyte hypertrophy.

In general, therapy is supportive. Prevention includes control of the insect vector. Patients with high-degree AV block may require pacemaker therapy. Digoxin and amiodarone should be used with caution, if indicated. Two agents for treating acute Chagas' disease (nifurtimox and benznidazole) have shown promise in decreasing the length of illness and in reducing parasitemia and early mortality. There is no specific therapy for the chronic form of the disease, although in selected subgroups the latter two agents may be effective; however, there is no evidence that they can totally cure the disease. Development of a vaccine is still in experimental stages. Prognosis depends on ventricular function; five-year mortality is 20% in patients with mild left ventricular dysfunction, while in patients with markedly depressed left ventricular function, mortality exceeds 60%.

Trichinosis

Trichinosis is an illness due to infestation with *Trichinella spiralis*. The larva invade skeletal muscle, the tongue, heart, lungs, and other organs, and the most serious complication is myocarditis. Although the parasites invade the heart, they do not encyst in the myocardium. Cardiac damage may be due to inflammation or a hypersensitivity reaction mounted in response to the parasites. The initial clinical manifestations include muscle tenderness, periorbital edema, and eosinophilia. Cardiac symptoms include dyspnea, palpitations and chest pain. These typically occur approximately three weeks after the initial onset of illness. Arrhythmias and congestive heart failure may be present. Electrocardiographic abnormalities are common and include low QRS voltage, prolonged PR interval and QRS duration, and nonspecific T-wave abnormalities. The diagnosis is established by demonstration of larval forms in gastrocnemius muscle biopsies. Eosinophilia and a positive skin test provide supportive evidence of the diagnosis. This myocarditis has been treated successfully with corticosteroids. Thiabendazole is also an efficient mode of therapy.

AIDS Heart Disease

The prevalence of cardiac involvement in patients suffering from acquired immune deficiency syndrome (AIDS) is about 50%. Among patients with AIDS heart disease, mortality due to cardiac complications is about 18%, and is due to either progressive heart failure or lethal ventricular arrhythmias. Four major cardiac manifestations have been described: pericarditis, myocarditis, endocarditis, and cardiac involvement with tumors. Pericarditis may be fibrinous, purulent, or effusive. Myocarditis usually presents as dilated cardiomyopathy. Although retrovirus has been isolated from the myocardium, the most common cause is viruses other than retrovirus, or else idiopathic. Endocarditis is either bacterial or thrombotic nonbacterial. Although malignant lymphoma has been described in the hearts of AIDS patients, the most common tumor found is Kaposi's sarcoma. Two-dimensional echocardiography is helpful in screening patients with cardiac involvement; it may reveal pericardial effusion, decreased myocardial function, or cardiac tumor. Treatment depends on the type of pathology present, but generally it is symptomatic. Pentamidine, a drug used to treat Pneumocystis carinii pneumonia (which may complicate AIDS), should be used with caution in patients with heart disease since it may precipitate ventricular arrhythmias.

Lyme Disease

Lyme disease may be associated with carditis in approximately 10% of cases. Lyme disease is caused by the spirochete *Borrelia burgdorferi*, transmitted by the bite of the *Ixodes dommini* tick. Originally described in Lyme, Connecticut, the disease is endemic to Wisconsin, Minnesota and the Northeastern United States. It usually manifests initially with a characteristic skin lesion (erythema chronicum migrans) and flu-like symptoms. If left untreated, it may progress with neurologic, arthritic and cardiac manifestations. Cardiac involvement is usually a late manifestation, and it may manifest as various degrees of atrioventricular block, myopericarditis and myocardial dysfunction. Atrioventricular block is the most common manifestation, usually requiring temporary pacemaker placement; however, the long-term prognosis with treatment is usually good. Gallium scanning may reveal diffuse myocardial uptake. Myocardial biopsy may show areas of lymphocyte infiltration and myocytic necrosis. Serologic testing is useful in establishing the diagnosis, particularly in the late phase of the disease. Antibiotic therapy with tetracyclines (250 mg four times/day for 10 days), or erythromycin in the same dose, is recommended to all patients. Despite scattered reports of possible benefit from corticosteroids or salicylates, their therapeutic role has not been well established.

CARDIOMYOPATHY

Cardiomyopathy is a disorder in which the prominent feature is a primary involvement of the cardiac muscle. Myocardial dysfunction due to systemic or pulmonary vascular disease, e.g., hypertensive heart disease, or due to structural abnormalities, e.g., valvular or congenital heart disease, is not included in this category.

The annual incidence of cardiomyopathy ranges from 0.7-7.5 cases per 100,000 population, and the prevalence has been reported by William et al. as 8,317 cases per 100,000. Mortality due to cardiomyopathy constitutes about 0.7% of cardiac deaths in the United States, with higher rates among men and blacks.

Cardiomyopathy may be classified on a functional basis as dilated (or congestive), hypertrophic, or restrictive. Alternatively, it may be classified on an etiologic basis, i.e., viral myocarditis, ischemic cardiomyopathy, alcoholic cardiomyopathy, etc.

DILATED CARDIOMYOPATHY

Dilated or congestive cardiomyopathy is characterized by a large, dilated heart with reduced systolic and abnormal diastolic function, frequently associated with the clinical features of congestive heart failure. There are numerous causes (Table 2), but the most common form is idiopathic cardiomyopathy. Although still controversial, considerable evidence suggests that at least some of the cases of dilated cardiomyopathy are a late sequelae of viral myocarditis. All four chambers of the heart are dilated. The degree of hypertrophy of the ventricular wall is disproportionately small in relation to the extent of ventricular dilatation. The clinical manifestations are those of congestive heart failure. They include dyspnea on exertion, orthopnea, fatigue, and paroxysmal nocturnal dyspnea. Peripheral edema, ascites, and hepatomegaly occur later, resulting from right-sided cardiac dysfunction. Systemic and pulmonary emboli may be present.

Diagnosis

Depending on the severity of cardiac dysfunction, physical examination may reveal a narrow pulse pres-

---

Table 2. Etiologies of Dilated (Congestive) Cardiomyopathy

Idiopathic
Peripartum
Post-myocarditis due to infectious agents (viral, parasitic, mycobacterial, Rickettsiae)
Alcoholic
Neuromuscular (muscular dystrophy, myotonic dystrophy)
Connective tissue disorders (systemic lupus erythematosus, rheumatoid disease, polyarteritis)
Beriberi
Glycogen storage diseases
Toxins (cobalt, lead, arsenic)
Doxorubicin hydrochloride, cyclophosphamide, vincristine
Infiltrative: amyloid, hemochromatosis, sarcoid (may have congestive or restrictive features)
Inheritied disorders: Fabry's disease, Gaucher's disease
Metabolic: chronic hypophosphatemia, hypokalemia, hypocalcemia, uremia

---

sure, pulsus alternans, cold clammy skin, and jugular venous distention with prominent a-waves. If tricuspid regurgitation is present, as is frequently the case, prominent regurgitant systolic v-waves are present. The cardiac apical impulse typically is displaced leftward with a left ventricular heave and, in some cases, right ventricular heave. A palpable precordial a-wave may be present. Auscultation may reveal paradoxical splitting of S_2, an S_3 gallop, and, in some cases, an S_4 gallop. The murmurs of mitral and tricuspid regurgitation may be heard. Other signs of left heart failure are common, including pulmonary rales or dullness at the lung bases due to pleural effusion; when right ventricular failure ensues, peripheral edema, ascites, and hepatomegaly are present as well.

Chest x-ray demonstrates diffuse cardiac enlargement, and when hemodynamic deterioration occurs, signs of congestive heart failure are seen, including pulmonary vascular redistribution, interstitial and alveolar edema, and pleural effusions. When right-sided heart failure is present, the azygous vein and superior vena cava are dilated.

The ECG shows a variety of abnormalities. Supraventricular and ventricular ectopy and various con-

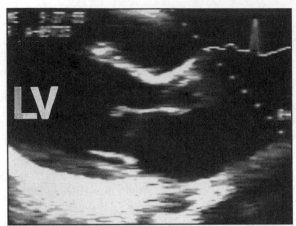

Figure 1. 2D echocardiogram of a patient with dilated cardiomyopathy. The left ventricular (LV) cavity and left atrium are dilated. In real-time, there was global hypokinesis of the LV. Parasternal long-axis view. (Courtesy of Priscilla Peters.)

duction disturbances are common. Left atrial abnormality and either left ventricular hypertrophy or low-voltage QRS may be present. In the absence of a discrete infarction, the ECG may reveal pathologic Q waves and nonspecific ST-T–wave abnormalities. Wilensky and colleagues showed that when serial ECGs from patients with cardiomyopathies were analyzed, progressive prolongation of PR interval and QRS duration were noted.

Two-dimensional echocardiography is virtually diagnostic of cardiomyopathy (Figure 1). Dilated cardiac chambers with generalized poor ventricular function are observed. Mitral valve closure may be delayed and aortic valve closure may occur earlier than normal. Two-dimensional echocardiography is especially useful for detecting a left ventricular thrombus. Doppler echocardiography usually reveals multiple valvular regurgitation. Keren and colleagues studied 17 patients with dilated cardiomyopathy and no evidence of primary valvular disease. Mitral regurgitation was present in all but one patient, with regurgitant fraction ranging between 5% and 53%; regurgitant fraction was >20% in two thirds of the patients.

Radionuclide ventriculography demonstrates increased ventricular volumes and reduced ejection fraction. There is controversy concerning the role of endomyocardial biopsy in patients with idiopathic dilated cardiomyopathy. Apart from its value in detecting early transplant rejection, myocarditis, cardiac

involvement in systemic disease, cardiac tumors, and anthracycline cardiotoxicity, other indications for biopsy are less clear. Even though it may yield a specific diagnosis on a few occasions, it rarely alters therapeutic decisions.

Cardiac catheterization reveals an elevated left ventricular end-diastolic pressure and left atrial pressure, and modest elevation in the pulmonary artery pressure. When right ventricular failure occurs, the right ventricular and right atrial pressures rise as well. The left ventricular end-diastolic pressure is usually higher than that in the right ventricle, and the cardiac index is reduced. Diffuse hypokinetic wall motion, elevated systolic and diastolic volumes, and a reduced ejection fraction are observed during left ventriculography. Mitral regurgitation is frequently detected and, occasionally, mural thrombi are observed.

Therapy

Therapy for patients with dilated cardiomyopathy includes treatment for the underlying disease, if known. Salt restriction and diuretics are indicated as initial therapy. Inotropic drugs that bypass the cyclic AMP system, such as cardiac glycosides, increase isometric tension in cardiomyopathic muscle, whereas agents that increase cyclic AMP, such as phosphodiesterase inhibitors, have a less profound effect. Phosphodiesterase inhibitors have both inotropic and vasodilator effects; amrinone and milrinone may provide short-term improvement in left ventricular function, but chronic use of these drugs has been disappointing. Placebo-controlled long-term trials with oral phosphodiesterase inhibitors have generally not shown beneficial effects on exercise capacity or cardiac function. Infusions of inotropes such as dobutamine for a few days may provide clinical improvement lasting months, possibly by reconditioning the heart. However, this requires careful monitoring of the patient, and has not been shown to improve survival. Newer inotropic agents, such as enoximone and OPC 8212 (Feldman et al.), show some promise; however, controlled randomized trials are needed to evaluate their safety and clinical efficacy.

Although calcium channel blockers may be beneficial in some cases of dilated cardiomyopathy, especially if patients have concomitant hypertension or coronary artery disease, their ultimate role in therapy is not yet clear, and they may occasionally cause significant left ventricular dysfunction, particularly when combined with beta-blocker therapy. In one study by

Figulla et al., 47 patients with dilated cardiomyopathy were assigned to either conventional therapy alone or conventional therapy plus diltiazem in doses ranging from 180–270 mg/day. Patients in the diltiazem group had a significant improvement in both New York Heart Association functional class and mortality.

Despite favorable reports about the efficacy of beta blockers in dilated cardiomyopathy, their role is still controversial. Waagstein et al. recently reported improved functional class, increased ejection fraction, and reduction of left ventricular dilatation, pulmonary wedge pressure, and mitral and tricuspid regurgitation during long-term therapy with metoprolol. The beneficial effect may have been related to an up-regulation of ventricular beta-adrenergic receptors.

Perhaps the mainstay of therapy is vasodilators, because they improve cardiac performance, relieve signs and symptoms of congestive heart failure, and improve survival. The Captopril Multicenter Research Group enrolled 92 patients with chronic congestive heart failure refractory to digitalis and diuretic therapy into a randomized, double-blind trial with either the ACE inhibitor captopril or placebo. The main cause of congestive heart failure was ischemic heart disease. Captopril therapy was well tolerated, and was associated with better exercise tolerance, higher ejection fraction, and better clinical improvement. Hydralazine plus isosorbide dinitrate, and enalapril have been shown to improve survival in patients with heart failure. For further discussion of the role of vasodilators and other agents in heart failure, see Chapter 23.

Arrhythmias may be treated with antiarrhythmic agents, but because many of these agents have negative inotropic effects and may even have proarrhythmic effects, dosages must be carefully titrated and patients monitored frequently during administration of these drugs. There is no clear role for electrophysiologic testing in guiding antiarrhythmic therapy in patients with dilated cardiomyopathy, except perhaps in preparation for implementation of an automatic implantable cardioverter-defibrillator (AICD), which may prove to be the most effective therapy for preventing sudden death in this group of patients. Anticoagulant therapy probably should be administered if there are no contraindications.

In suitable candidates, cardiac transplantation may be considered for better quality of life and improved survival. With current immunosuppressive regimens, the one-year survival rate is 80% and three-year survival rate, 70%—a substantial improvement from medical therapy alone in patients with end-stage dilated cardiomyopathy. (See also Chapter 34.)

Prognosis

Fuster et al. followed 104 patients with a diagnosis of idiopathic dilated cardiomyopathy for up to 20 years. Seventy-seven percent of patients in this study had an accelerated course, with the majority of patients dying within the first two years of diagnosis. Three factors were highly predictive of a poor prognosis: age above 50 years, a cardiothoracic ratio >0.55, and a cardiac index of <3 L/min/m^2.

In a recently published series, Hofmann et al. prospectively followed 110 patients with idiopathic dilated cardiomyopathy for 53 months. Two-year mortality was 34%, and poor left ventricular function was the major predictor of mortality. Furthermore, patients with a low frequency of ventricular pairs/24 hr on ambulatory ECG monitoring were more likely to die from congestive heart failure, while those with a high frequency of pairs were more susceptible to sudden cardiac death.

HYPERTROPHIC CARDIOMYOPATHY

Hypertrophic cardiomyopathy (HCM) refers to inappropriate hypertrophy of the left ventricle, usually in a nondilated ventricle. The hypertrophy often involves the interventricular septum (asymmetric septal hypertrophy, ASH) and may be associated with a left ventricular outflow gradient. The latter condition is known as hypertrophic obstructive cardiomyopathy (HOCM), formerly referred to as idiopathic hypertrophic subaortic stenosis (IHSS).

HCM is characterized by a diastolic abnormality such that left ventricular relaxation is impaired; that is, the left ventricle is noncompliant. This feature impairs left ventricular filling, while systolic left ventricular function may actually demonstrate hypercontractility. While disproportionate ventricular wall thickness usually involves the septum in cases of HCM, it can be limited to the apex or to the upper part of the septum. With HOCM, the anterior mitral leaflet moves forward during systole (systolic anterior motion), and, together with the septal hypertrophy, may cause obstruction to blood flow. The obstruction may occur at rest or after provocative maneuvers that reduce blood volume. Some studies suggest that HOCM is an autosomal dominant disease with incomplete

Table 3. Effect of Various Maneuvers on Systolic Murmurs

	Valsalva	Phenylephrine; Handgrip	Squatting	Amyl Nitrite	Leg Raising
Aortic stenosis	Decrease	Decrease	Increase or Decrease	Increase	Increase
Hypertrophic obstructive cardiomyopathy	Increase	Decrease	Decrease	Increase	Decrease
Ventricular septal defect	Decrease	Increase	No change	Decrease	Increase
Mitral regurgitation	Slight decrease	Increase	No change	Decrease	Increase

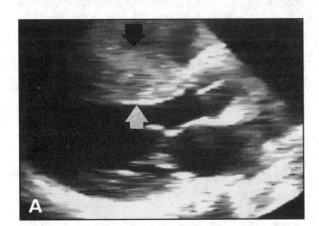

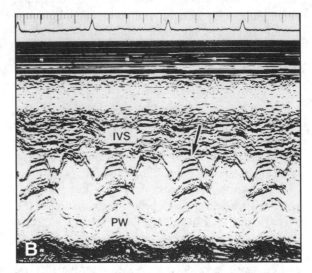

Figure 2. *A. Parasternal long-axis echocardiogram of a patient with hypertrophic cardiomyopathy showing asymmetric septal hypertrophy. The ventricular septum (between arrows) is considerably thicker than the posterior wall. (Courtesy of Priscilla Peters.) B. M-mode echocardiogram at the level of the mitral valve in a patient with hypertrophic cardiomyopathy. Asymmetric hypertrophy of the interventricular septum (IVS) is present. The arrow indicates systolic anterior motion of the mitral valve. PW, posterior wall. (From Wynne J: Hypertrophic cardiomyopathy: A broadened concept of the disease and its management. In: Isselbacher KJ, Adams RD, Braunwald E, Martin JB, Petersdorf RG, Wilson JD, eds: Update III: Harrison's Principles of Internal Medicine. New York: McGraw Hill; 1982, p 129. With permission.)*

penetrance. The incidence of HCM ranges from 2–6% in patients with cardiomyopathy, and is more common in males than females, and in blacks than whites. Occasionally, patients with Pompe's disease, Friedreich's ataxia, or Noonan's syndrome present with cardiac findings indistinguishable from hypertrophic cardiomyopathy.

Symptoms of HCM include dyspnea on exertion, orthopnea, paroxysmal nocturnal dyspnea, palpita-

tions, angina, and syncope. Angina in the absence of concomitant coronary artery disease is probably due to small vessel disease, reduced coronary reserve in the setting of a hypertrophied ventricle, or severely impaired left ventricular diastolic function. Syncope is due either to decreased cerebral perfusion or to emboli from mitral vegetations or ventricular thrombi. The incidence of stroke in HCM is 3%, and of transient ischemic attack (TIA), 4%. The average patient age at presentation of symptoms is the middle 20s; however, a first diagnosis is not uncommon at an older age. It should be pointed out that there is considerable variation from patient to patient in the degree of symptomatology, from totally asymptomatic to severely symptomatic with congestive heart failure. Relatives of patients with documented HCM may have echocardiographic evidence of the disease but often are asymptomatic.

Diagnosis

There are several prominent physical findings in patients with hypertrophic cardiomyopathy. The carotid pulse rises rapidly and typically has a double peak; the jugular venous pulse may reveal a prominent a-wave. The apical impulse is displaced leftward, forceful, and typically consists of a pre-systolic impulse followed by a double systolic impulse. A systolic thrill may be palpable. Auscultation reveals an S_4 gallop and an S_2 that may be split normally, narrowly, or widely. An S_3 may or may not be present. The systolic murmur of HOCM is a harsh, crescendo-decrescendo murmur heard best between the lower left sternal border and the apex. The murmur radiates toward the base of the heart and clavicle but, unlike that of aortic stenosis, does not radiate into the neck. The severity of outflow obstruction and the loudness of the murmur are increased by factors which reduce ventricular volume, increase inotropy or reduce afterload; conversely, the severity of obstruction and the loudness of the murmur are reduced by maneuvers which increase ventricular volume, reduce inotropy, or increase afterload. The murmur increases with Valsalva maneuver, standing, and administration of amyl nitrite or isoproterenol. It decreases with squatting, handgrip, and administration of phenylephrine. The murmur of mitral regurgitation is commonly heard; on rare occasions, the murmur of aortic regurgitation is also heard. The murmur heard in HOCM is probably due to a combination of turbulence in the left ventricular outflow tract and mitral regurgitation. The effects of various maneuvers on systolic murmurs are shown on Table 3.

In patients without an obstructive component of HCM, the physical examination may be relatively unremarkable, except for a left ventricular lift and S_4.

Chest x-ray reveals various degrees of cardiomegaly. Unlike valvular aortic stenosis, post-stenotic aortic dilatation and calcification of the aortic valve are absent, but calcification of the mitral annulus may be

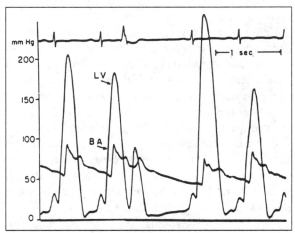

Figure 3. *Simultaneous left ventricular (LV) and brachial artery (BA) pressures in a patient with hypertrophic obstructive cardiomyopathy (HOCM). The contraction following the premature ventricular beat reveals a reduction in brachial artery pressure and an accentuation of the "spike and dome" configuration of the systemic arterial pressure tracing. (From Braunwald E, et al: Idiopathic hypertrophic subaortic stenosis. Circulation 30 [Suppl IV]:78, 1964. Reprinted with permission of the American Heart Association, Inc.)*

present. The ECG reveals left ventricular hypertrophy and ST-T–wave abnormalities. Abnormal Q waves give rise to a pseudoinfarction pattern in 20–50% of patients. These Q waves typically are present in the inferior and/or lateral electrocardiographic leads. Left atrial enlargement may also be present.

The echocardiogram is extremely useful in establishing the diagnosis. The left ventricular walls are hypertrophied, with disproportionate septal thickness (Figure 2A). Systolic anterior motion of the mitral valve may be seen (Figure 2B). The aortic valve leaflets may appear to close partially or to flutter in systole due to the Venturi effect produced by the subvalvular stenosis. Phonocardiography may aid in the interpretation of the effects of various maneuvers on the intensity of the systolic murmur of hypertrophic obstructive cardiomyopathy. Doppler echocardiography may reveal a systolic gradient in the left ventricular outflow tract. Carotid pulse tracings are especially helpful; they may reveal a brisk carotid upstroke in contrast to aortic stenosis, and the wave form often reveals a bisferiens pulse contour. Radionuclide ventriculography allows visualization of the thickened septum and obliteration of the left ventricular cavity. Studies using thallium-201 may reveal the asymmetrically thickened septum.

Holter monitoring has been recommended for patients with hypertrophic cardiomyopathy, since some studies have shown that patients with high grades of ventricular arrhythmia are at high risk for sudden death. Supraventricular arrhythmias are common; atrial fibrillation leads to a loss of atrial contraction with reduced left ventricular filling and clinical deterioration.

Cardiac catheterization studies demonstrate elevated left ventricular end-diastolic pressure and systolic pressure gradient between the body of the left ventricular cavity and the area below the aortic valve (in HOCM). The gradient can be provoked by Valsalva maneuver, amyl nitrite, and isoproterenol. Following a premature beat, the gradient increases with a concomitant fall in aortic pulse pressure (Brockenborough's sign, Figure 3). The systolic arterial wave form may reveal a spike and dome configuration. There is usually a prominent a-wave in the left atrial and left ventricular wave forms, due to diminished left ventricular compliance. Mild pulmonary hypertension is present in 25% of cases. Left ventricular angiography allows visualization of the obstruction, estimation of the degree of hypertrophy and cavity obliteration, and visualization of the systolic anterior motion of the mitral valve. Concomitant coronary artery disease is not uncommon in patients above 50 years of age.

Therapy

The main therapies for hypertrophic cardiomyopathy are beta blockers and calcium channel blockers. Beta blockade reduces the outflow obstruction caused by isoproterenol or by exercise, improves ventricular compliance, and reduces myocardial oxygen demand, thus decreasing the frequency of angina. Verapamil has been shown to reduce the left ventricular outflow gradient, improve exercise capacity, and improve peak left ventricular filling rate. One study showed electrocardiographic evidence of regression of hypertrophy following long-term verapamil therapy. Nifedipine has also been shown to be effective in these patients; like verapamil, it improves left ventricular diastolic abnormalities. In patients who do not respond to medical therapy, surgical intervention in the form of septal myomectomy may be considered. Concomitant mitral valve replacement may also be considered if associated severe mitral valve regurgitation is noted. This procedure improves symptomatology and alleviates significant interventricular gradient, with low operative mortality and a 1.6% annual postoperative mortality rate. The procedure can also be performed in elderly patients (>65 years) with marked symptomatic and hemodynamic improvement and long-term survival.

Pregnant women with HCM may give birth by vaginal delivery unless there is a history of syncope or a severe gradient is documented. Spinal anesthesia should be avoided. General anesthesia along with intravenous propranolol and/or intravenous disopyramide have been used to allow a reduced inotropic state with less obstruction.

Patients with hypertrophic cardiomyopathy should avoid strenuous exercise due to risk of sudden death. Anticoagulation with warfarin should be considered in patients in atrial fibrillation, due to the risk of systemic emboli. All patients should receive prophylactic antibiotics before dental or surgical procedures, because of the risk of endocarditis.

In a large series reported by Goodwin et al., sudden death was associated with a history of syncope, young age at initial diagnosis, and family history of hypertrophic cardiomyopathy and sudden death. Although supraventricular and ventricular arrhythmias play an important role in the genesis of sudden death, they probably are not the only explanation. Antiarrhythmic therapy, particularly with amiodarone, may be beneficial in the management of such arrhythmias. Despite the beneficial effect of propranolol on exercise tolerance, dyspnea, and frequency of chest pain, this drug does not alter the frequency of asymptomatic ventricular arrhythmias, nor the incidence of sudden death. The prognosis of hypertrophic cardiomyopathy is variable. Two thirds of patients with obstructive symptoms remain stable or improve; the remaining one third have a worsening of symptoms. Unfortunately, sudden death may develop in patients regardless of symptoms and does not seem to be prevented by medical or surgical therapy.

RESTRICTIVE CARDIOMYOPATHY

Restrictive cardiomyopathy is characterized by a restriction of ventricular filling during diastole due to reduced ventricular compliance. Systolic function is relatively intact. In the World Health Organization classification, two conditions of unknown cause are listed under restrictive cardiomyopathy: endomyocardial fibrosis and Löffler's endocarditis. The latter starts with eosinophilic infiltration of the heart muscle and

Table 4. Etiologies of Restrictive Cardiomyopathy

Infiltrative
    Sarcoidosis; Amyloidosis
    Hemochromatosis
    Neoplasia
Endocardial fibroelastosis
    Cardiac dilatation with diffuse endocardial hyperplasia. Thickened
    aortic and mitral valve; distorted papillary muscle; primary form af-
    fects infants
Endomyocardial fibrosis
    Fibrous endocardial lesions of the inflow portion of the ventricles;
        may involve AV valves and cause regurgitation. Occurs in tropical
        and subtropical Africa.
Löffler's endocarditis
    Dense endocardial fibrosis with overlying thrombosis; occurs follow-
        ing an arteritis and eosinophilic infiltrate of the myocardium. May
        be related to endomyocardial fibrosis.
Scleroderma
Adipositas cordis (fatty infiltration)
Radiation
Post-myocarditis
Glycogen storage disease
Becker's disease
    Cardiac dilatation with fibrosis of the papillary muscles and suben-
        docardium associated with necrosis and mural thrombosis. Occurs
        in South Africa.

passes through three stages: the necrotic stage, the thrombotic stage, and the fibrotic stage. The fibrotic stage is characterized by endomyocardial fibrosis, with the endocardium showing fibrotic plaques of various sizes and thickness; this condition is indistinguishable from endomyocardial fibrosis. The two conditions, however, are now believed to represent two spectra of the same disease. The etiologies of restrictive heart disease are listed in Table 4.

The clinical symptoms reflect the inability of the ventricle to fill during diastole and to provide an increase in cardiac output when needed. Fatigue, weakness, and poor exercise tolerance with dyspnea on exertion are common. Symptoms of reduced filling of the right ventricle include edema, ascites, right upper quadrant discomfort, and anorexia. Chest pain similar in quality to that caused by myocardial ischemia may be present in a small number of patients.

Diagnosis

Physical examination reveals signs of venous congestion and includes distended neck veins, Kussmaul's sign, edema, ascites, and an enlarged, tender liver. Peripheral arterial pulse pressure is typically narrow; the jugular venous pulse reveals a prominent a-wave with a rapid x and y descent. The cardiac apex is displaced laterally, but in general, cardiomegaly is moderate and not as severe as in patients with dilated cardiomyopathy. Sinus tachycardia and atrial and ventricular arrhythmias may be noted. The heart sounds are often soft and an S_3 and S_4 are common. Murmurs of tricuspid and/or mitral regurgitation may be present. On chest x-ray film, the heart is normal in size or demonstrates mild cardiomegaly. Signs of pulmonary congestion may be present as well, and absence of pericardial calcification may differentiate the condition from constrictive pericardial disease, which has some similarity to restrictive heart disease.

Electrocardiographic features include diffuse low QRS voltage, nonspecific ST-T–wave changes, conduction disturbances, and atrial and ventricular arrhythmias. Echocardiography reveals normal or small ventricular volumes and increased wall thickness, with preserved normal systolic function. Doppler echocar-

Table 5. Differentiating Features of Restrictive Cardiomyopathy versus Constrictive Pericarditis

	Restrictive Cardiomyopathy	Constrictive Pericarditis
Pulmonary capillary wedge pressure (PCW)	PCW > right atrial pressure	PCW = right atrial pressure
Pulmonary artery systolic pressure	Usually >40-50 mm Hg	Usually <40-50 mm Hg
Right vs. left ventricular end-diastolic pressures	Left ventricular > right ventricular end-diastolic pressure	Left ventricular usually = right ventricular end-diastolic pressure
Right ventricular end-diastolic pressure	Usually less than 1/3 of right ventricular systolic pressure	Usually about 1/3 of right ventricular systolic pressure
Cardiac output	Depressed	Often normal or only slightly depressed
Square-root sign in ventricular pressure tracings	More prominent in left ventricular tracing. May diminish with therapy	Sign is equally prominent in right and left ventricular pressure tracing
Right atrial pressure	<15 mm Hg if PCW not markedly elevated	Usually >15 mm Hg

diography reveals shortened deceleration times across atrioventricular valves, which represent the abrupt premature cessation of ventricular filling, as well as abnormal central venous flow velocity reversals with inspiration. Mitral and tricuspid regurgitation are also frequently observed. (See Chapters 7 and 8.)

Technetium-99m pyrophosphate scans may show intense diffuse cardiac uptake, particularly in patients with amyloid disease. In patients with metastatic neoplasms or sarcoid granulomas, thallium-201 studies reveal defects in the myocardial walls. Magnetic resonance imaging reveals enlargement of the atria and inferior vena cava; a prominent signal within the atria in all phases of the cardiac cycle, suggesting impaired ventricular filling; and, possibly, mitral and/or tricuspid regurgitation.

Jugular venous pulse tracings reveal a prominent a-wave, with rapid x and y descents resulting in a characteristic M-shaped tracing. Apexcardiography also reveals a prominent a-wave. There are a number of ancillary tests and findings that aid in the diagnosis of the underlying disorder. These include high serum iron levels with hemochromatosis; hypercalcemia, which occurs in approximately 9% of patients with

sarcoidosis; and rectal biopsy for diagnosing amyloidosis.

Cardiac catheterization is currently the gold standard in diagnosing restrictive cardiomyopathy. There is elevated ventricular end-diastolic pressure (EDP), with left ventricular EDP usually greater than right ventricular EDP. The diastolic portion of the ventricular pressure pulse reveals a dip and plateau configuration, resembling a square root sign. The right atrial pressures are elevated and have an "M" or "W" shape due to rapid x and y descents. Table 5 reviews features that help to differentiate restrictive cardiomyopathy from constrictive pericarditis. Endomyocardial biopsy may be helpful in differentiating restrictive from constrictive disease and in finding a cause for restrictive disease (such as amyloidosis, hemochromatosis, or sarcoidosis).

Therapy

Therapy for symptomatic cardiomyopathy includes low-salt diet, diuretics, and vasodilator therapy. Digitalis is beneficial in some patients but should be used with caution, since patients with restrictive cardiomyopathy, in particular, amyloidosis, may be prone to digitalis toxicity. If patients develop complete heart block, AV sequential pacing is superior to ventricular pacing to allow atrial contraction and enhance ventricular filling. Antiarrhythmic agents are sometimes required, and anticoagulation is indicated to prevent thromboembolic complications. Specific treatment, if available, may be used: sarcoidosis may be treated with steroids, neoplasms with chemotherapy or radiation, and hemochromatosis with repeated phlebotomy and deferoxamine.

SPECIFIC MYOCARDIAL DISEASES

In the following section, we will discuss certain causes of cardiomyopathy that have specific clinical significance.

Ischemic Cardiomyopathies

Ischemic cardiomyopathy refers to severe systolic dysfunction with or without diastolic dysfunction of the myocardium due to severe diffuse coronary artery disease. Dysfunction due to loss of critical mass of the myocardium as a result of a massive infarction, or due to structural complications of myocardial infarction (i.e., ventricular septal defect, mitral regurgitation, or ventricular aneurysm), are not included in this syndrome. Inclusion of this entity under cardiomyopathies is not universally accepted. The pathogenesis of the disease is not well understood. Postmortem studies reveal that severe diffuse coronary disease with multiple sites of scarring might be responsible for ischemic cardiomyopathy. Alternatively, zones of hibernating or stunned myocardium may contribute. Some preliminary data suggest that it might be linked to HLA-DRW6 antigen (Limas and Limas). In addition, remodeling of the left ventricle, which can occur after infarction, may contribute to this entity.

The clinical picture is that of dilated cardiomyopathy, but a restrictive picture is not uncommon. While noninvasive tests (thallium scans, positron emission tomography) may document ongoing ischemia, the presence of significant diffuse coronary disease on angiography helps confirm the diagnosis. Afterload reducers, captopril in particular, are beneficial in the management of such patients. Despite high operative mortality, coronary artery bypass surgery increases long-term survival in selected patients.

Cardiomyopathy Induced by Chemotherapeutic Drugs

Cyclophosphamide, vincristine, vinblastine, cisplatinum and a variety of other chemotherapeutic agents have been implicated in toxic cardiac effects. The agents most commonly associated with cardiotoxicity are anthracyclines (for example, doxorubicin) and 5-fluorouracil.

Anthracycline cardiotoxicity. The incidence of anthracycline cardiotoxicity ranges from 5.3–28% in different series. The common clinical presentation is that of dilated cardiomyopathy, but it may present as restrictive disease, angina pectoris, acute myocardial infarction, or ventricular arrhythmia. The toxicity is dose related, and adoption of a once-a-week, low-dose regimen appears to lower the incidence of the disease. Echocardiography and radionuclide ventriculography support the diagnosis. For a reliable method of early diagnosis, however, exercise radionuclide ventriculography or ventricular biopsy is superior. Preliminary data suggest that prenylamine (Milei et al.) or MM-159 may prevent the cardiotoxicity. Supportive therapy is indicated; in some cases, cardiac function may revert to normal. Calcium channel blockers, especially those with significant negative inotropic effects, should be avoided since they have deleterious effects in animal models.

5-fluorouracil cardiotoxicity. 5-FU cardiotoxicity may present as congestive heart failure, Prinzmetal's angina, or myocardial infarction. In a prospective study of 25 patients receiving 5-FU infusion, patients had a significant increase in the incidence of ST-segment changes suggestive of ischemia during infusion (as compared to baseline recordings). These changes were more common in patients with underlying coronary disease (Rezkalla et al. 1989). The underlying mechanism of cardiotoxicity is not known, and no specific therapy for this condition is established.

Effect of Cocaine on the Heart

Cocaine use has been linked to the development of cardiomyopathy, myocarditis, endocarditis, and various ventricular arrhythmias. The most common clinical presentation is acute myocardial infarction. The link between cocaine and development of cardiomyopathy is supported by the drug's depressant effect on cardiac function in animal models. Arrhythmogenic effects might be related to cocaine's cardiac ischemic effects, or to a direct effect on electrophysiologic properties of cardiac muscle. The mechanism of inducing myocardial ischemia is probably multifactorial. Cocaine has been shown to cause coronary spasm, increase intimal proliferation, and increase platelet aggregation. The incidence of cocaine-induced cardiac effects is not known. In a study of 49 cocaine users presenting to the emergency room for various reasons, significant abnormalities in the surface ECG were found in about 50% (Rezkalla et al. 1990). No specific therapy is known to control cardiac manifestations of cocaine, but beta blockers appear to be beneficial in arrhythmias, and calcium channel blockers and nitrate therapy may ameliorate ischemic effects.

Alcoholic Cardiomyopathy

Excessive alcohol consumption may lead to progressive myocardial dysfunction and dilated cardiomyopathy in susceptible individuals. The mechanism of alcohol-induced cardiac dysfunction is not fully understood, but is believed to be due to direct toxic effects on the myocytes, associated thiamine deficiency, and, occasionally, additives used in the alcohol manufacturing process. The heart increases in weight, with biventricular hypertrophy and dilatation and widespread focal myocardial fibrosis. Sudden death has been reported in alcoholic cardiomyopathy. In a recent series of 752 sudden death patients reported by Vikhert et al., 17% (mostly men, under age 50) had alcoholic cardiomyopathy. Another manifestation of alcohol-induced heart disease is an increased propensity for atrial and ventricular arrhythmias. "Holiday heart" syndrome refers to the occurrence of arrhythmias (especially supraventricular tachyarrhythmias) after alcohol consumption, in the absence of overt cardiomyopathy. Acute alcohol ingestion in otherwise normal individuals may depress myocardial contractility. Cessation of alcohol intake is the only treatment available for alcoholic cardiomyopathy. Following abstinence, patients have shown normalization of chamber dimensions and ventricular function as determined by echocardiography.

Bibliography

Myocarditis

Abelmann WH: Viral myocarditis and its sequelae. *Ann Rev Med* 24:145,1973.
Abelmann WH: Myocarditis. *N Engl J Med* 275:832, 1966.

Acquatella H, Catalioti F, Gomez-Mancebo JR, et al: Long-term control of Chagas' disease in Venezuela: Effects on serologic findings, electrocardiographic abnormalities, and clinical outcome. *Circulation* 76:556, 1987.
Anderson DW, Virmani R, Reilly JM, et al: Prevalent myocarditis at necropsy in the acquired immuno-deficiency syndrome. *J Am Coll Cardiol* 11:792, 1988.
Arvan S, et al. Sudden increase in left ventricular mass secondary to acute myocarditis. *Am Heart J* 116:200, 1988.
Baroldi G, Corallo S, Moroni M, et al: Focal lymphocytic myocarditis in acquired immuno-deficiency syndrome (AIDS). *J Am Coll Cardiol* 12:463, 1988.
Cambridge G, MacArthur CGC, Waterson, AP, et al: Antibodies to coxsackie B viruses in congestive cardiomyopathy. *Br Heart J* 41:692, 1979.
Chandraratna PAN, Bradley WG, Kortman KE, et al: Detection of acute myocarditis using nuclear magnetic resonance imaging. *Am J Med* 83:1144, 1987.
Daly K, Richardson BJ, Olsen EGJ, et al: Acute myocarditis: Role of histologic and virologic examination in the diagnosis and assessment of immunosuppressive treatment. *Br Heart J* 51:30,1984.
Das SK, Brady TJ, Thrall JH, et al: Cardiac function in patients with prior myocarditis. *J Nucl Med* 21:689, 1980.
Fenoglio JJ, Ursell PC, Kellog CF, et al: Diagnosis and classification of myocarditis by endomyocardial biopsy. *N Engl J Med* 308:12, 1983.
Gerzen P, Granath A, Holmgren B, et al: Acute myocarditis: A follow-up study. *Br Heart J* 34:575, 1972.
Gill PS, Chandraratna PAN, Meyer PR, et al: Malignant lymphoma: Cardiac involvement at initial presentation. *J Clin Oncol* 5:216, 1987.
Grey DF, Morse BS, Phillips WF: Trichinosis with neurologic and cardiac involvement: Review of the literature, and report of three cases. *Ann Intern Med* 57:230, 1962.
Helle EP, Koskenvua K, Heikkila J, et al: Myocardial complications of immunizations. *Ann Clin Res* 10:280, 1978.
Levine HD: Virus myocarditis: A critique of the literature from clinical electrocardiographic, and pathologic standpoints. *Am J Med Sci* 277:132, 1979.
Marin-Neto JA, Marzullo P, Sousa AC, et al: Radionuclide angiographic evidence for early predominant right ventricular involvement in patients with Chagas' disease. *Can J Cardiol* 4:231, 1988.
Matsumori A, Tomioka N, Kawai C, et al. Protective effect of recombinant alpha interferon on coxsackievirus B3 myocarditis in mice. *Am Heart J* 115:1229, 1988.
Miklozek CL, Crumpacker CS, Royal HD, et al: Myocarditis presenting as acute myocardial infarction. *Am Heart J* 115:768, 1988.
Monif GRG, Lee CW, Hsiung GD: Isolated myocarditis with recovery of ECHO type 9 virus from the myocardium. *N Engl J Med* 277:1353, 1967.
Morales AR, Vichitbandh P, Chandraung P, et al: Pathologic features of cardiac conduction disturbances in diphtheritic myocarditis. *Arch Pathol Lab Med* 91:1, 1971.
O'Connell JB, Mason JW: Diagnosing and treating active myocarditis. *West J Med* 150:431, 1989.
O'Connell JB, Robinson JA, Henkin RE: Immunosuppressive therapy in patients with congestive cardiomyopathy and myocardial uptake of gallium-67. *Circulation* 64:780,1981.

Pereira-Barretto AC, Mady C, Arteaga-Fernandez E, et al: Right ventricular endomyocardial biopsy in chronic Chagas' disease. *Am Heart J* 111:307, 1986.

Pinamonti B, Alberti E, Cigalotto A, et al: Echocardiographic findings in myocarditis. *Am J Cardiol* 62:285, 1988.

Ramos AC, Elias PR, Barrucand L, et al: The protective effect of carnitine in human diphtheric myocarditis. *Pediatr Res* 18:815, 1984.

Ray CG, Icenogle TB, Minnich LL, Copeland JG, Grogan TM: The use of intravenous ribavirin to treat influenza virus-associated acute myocarditis. *J Infect Dis* 159:829, 1989.

Reilly JM, Cunnion RE, Anderson DW, et al: Frequency of myocarditis, left ventricular dysfunction and ventricular tachycardia in the acquired immune deficiency syndrome. *Am J Cardiol* 62:789, 1988.

Rezkalla S, Khatib G, Khatib R: Coxsackievirus B3 murine myocarditis: Deleterious effects of anti-inflammatory drugs. *J Lab Clin Med* 107:393, 1986.

Rezkalla S, Kloner RA, Khatib R, et al: Effect of metoprolol in acute coxsackievirus B3 murine myocarditis. *J Am Coll Cardiol* 12:412, 1988.

Rezkalla S, Kloner RA, Khaw BA, et al: Detection of experimental myocarditis by monoclonal antimyosin antibody, Fab fragment. *Am Heart J* 117:391, 1989.

Rezkalla S, Kloner RA: Management strategies in viral myocarditis. *Am Heart J* 117:706, 1989.

Rezkalla S, Kloner RA, Khatib G, Khatib R: Beneficial effect of captopril in coxsackie virus B₃ murine myocarditis. *Circulation* 81:1039, 1990.

Rosenbaum MB: Chagastic myocardiopathy. *Prog Cardiovasc Dis* 7:199, 1964.

Sainani GS, Dekate MP, Rao CP: Heart disease caused by coxsackie virus B infection. *Br Heart J* 37:819, 1975.

Salarz SO: An electrocardiographic study of one hundred and fourteen consecutive cases of trichinosis. *Am Heart J* 34:230, 1947.

Silver MA, Macher AM, Reichert CM, et al: Cardiac involvement by Kaposi's sarcoma in acquired immune deficiency syndrome (AIDS). *Am J Cardiol* 53:983, 1984.

Vikerfors T, Stjerna A, Olcen P: Acute myocarditis, serologic diagnosis, clinical findings and follow-up. *Acta Med Scand* 223:45, 1988.

Cardiomyopathy

Abelmann WH, Lorell BH: The challenge of cardiomyopathy. *J Am Coll Cardiol* 13:1219, 1989.

Alcan KE, Robeson W, Graham MC, et al: Early detection of anthracycline induced cardiotoxicity by stress radionuclide cine-angiography in conjunction with Fourier amplitude and phase analysis. *Clin Nucl Med* 10:160, 1985.

Ali MR, Ewer MS, Cangir A, et al: Coronary artery embolism following cancer chemotherapy. *Am J Pediatr Hematol Oncol* 9:200, 1987.

Ali MR, Soto A, Maroongroge D, et al: Electrocardiographic changes after adriamycin chemotherapy. *Cancer* 43:465, 1979.

Appleton CP, Hatle LK, Popp RL: Demonstration of restrictive ventricular physiology by Doppler echocardiography. *J Am Coll Cardiol* 11:757, 1988.

Baandrup U, Florio RA, Rehahn M, et al: Critical analysis of endomyocardial biopsies from patients suspected of having cardiomyopathy. II: Comparison of histology and clinical hemodynamic information. *Br Heart J* 45:487, 1981.

Baandrup U, Florio RA, Roters F, et al. Electronmicroscopic investigation of endomyocardial biopsy samples in hypertrophy and cardiomyopathy: A semiquantitative study in 48 patients. *Circulation* 63:1289, 1981.

Bashour T, Basha HS, Cheng TO: Hypocalcemic cardiomyopathy. *Chest* 78:663, 1980.

Benotti JR, Grossman W, Cohn PF: Clinical profile of restrictive cardiomyopathy. *Circulation* 61:1206, 1980.

Benotti JR, Grossman W, Braunwald E: Effects of amrinone on myocardial energy metabolism and hemodynamics in patients with severe congestive heart failure due to coronary artery disease. *Circulation* 62:28, 1980.

Binkley PF, Lewe RF, Lima JJ, et al: Hemodynamic inotropic response to beta blockers with intrinsic sympathomimetic activity in patients with congestive cardiomyopathy. *Circulation* 74:1390, 1986.

Bjarnason I, Jonsson S, Hardarson T: Mode of inheritance of hypertrophic cardiomyopathy in Iceland: Echocardiographic study. *Br Heart J* 47:122, 1982.

Boccio RV, Chung JH, Harrison DM: Anesthetic management of ceasarean section in a patient with idiopathic hypertrophic subaortic stenosis. *Anesthesiology* 65:663, 1986.

Bonow RO, Rosing DR, Bacharach et al: Effects of verapamil on left ventricular systolic function and diastolic filling in patients with hypertrophic cardiomyopathy. *Circulation* 64:787, 1981.

Bouhour JB, Helias J, deLajartre AY, et al: Detection of myocarditis during the first year after discovery of a dilated cardiomyopathy by endomyocardial biopsy and gallium-67 myocardial scintigraphy. *Eur Heart J* 9:520, 1988.

Braunwald E, Kloner RA: The stunned myocardium: Prolonged post-ischemic ventricular dysfunction. *Circulation* 66:1146, 1982.

Bristow MR, Mason JW, Billingham ME, et al: Dose-effect and structure-function relationships in doxorubicin cardiomyopathy. *Am Heart J* 102:709, 1981.

Brockmeier FK, Rosland GA, Finne PH: Cardiomyopathy induced by anthracycline derivatives. *Acta Paediatr Scand* 73:387, 1984.

Bulkley BH, Weisfeldt ML, Hutchins G: Idiopathic hypertrophic subaortic stenosis: Myocardial disarray with isometric contraction. *N Engl J Med* 296:135, 1971.

Burch GE, Giles TD, Calcolough HL: Ischemic cardiomyopathy. *Am Heart J* 79:291, 1970.

Captopril Multicenter Research Group: A placebo-controlled trial of captopril in refractory chronic congestive heart failure. *J Am Coll Cardiol* 2:755, 1983.

Carroll JD, Gaasch WH, McAdam KP: Amyloid cardiomyopathy: Characterization by a distinctive voltage/mass relation. *Am J Cardiol* 49:9, 1982.

Casanova M, Gamallo C, Quero-Jimenez M: Familial hypertrophic cardiomyopathy with unusual involvement of the right ventricle. *Eur J Cardiol* 9:145, 1979.

Challenor VF, Conway N, Monro JL: The surgical treatment of restrictive cardiomyopathy in pseudoxanthoma elasticum. *Br Heart J* 59:266, 1988.

Chambers HF, Morris DL, Tauber MG, et al: Cocaine use and the risk of endocarditis in intravenous drug users. *Ann Intern Med* 106:833, 1987.

Chandraratna PAN, Aronow WS: Genesis of the systolic murmur of idiopathic hypertrophic subaortic stenosis. *Chest* 83:638, 1983.

Chaudary S, Song SY, Jaski BE: Profound yet reversible heart failure secondary to 5-fluorouracil. *Am J Med* 85:454, 1988.

Cohn J: Vasodilator therapy of dilated cardiomyopathy. *Postgrad Med J* 62:599, 1986.

Collins C, Weiden PL: Cardiotoxicity of 5-fluorouracil. *Cancer Treat Rep* 71:733, 1987.

Colucci WS: Usefulness of calcium antagonists for congestive heart failure. *Am J Cardiol* 59:52B, 1987.

Cooper MM, McIntosh CL, Tucker E, et al: Operations for hypertrophic subaortic stenosis in the aged. *Ann Thorac Surg* 44:370, 1987.

Council on Scientific Affairs: Report on the Positron Emission Tomography Panel. Application of positron tomography in the heart. *JAMA* 259:2438, 1988.

Cutler DJ, Isner JM, Bracey AW: Hemochromatosis heart disease: An unemphasized cause of potentially reversible restrictive cardiomyopathy. *Am J Med* 69:923, 1980.

Dearth J, Osborn R, Wilson E, et al: Anthracycline-induced cardiomyopathy in children: A report of six cases. *Med Pediatr Oncol* 12:54, 1984.

DiBianco R, Shabetai R, Kostok W, et al: Oral milrinone and digoxin in heart failure: Results of a placebo-controlled prospective trial of each agent and the combination (abstr). *Circulation* 76(Suppl IV):256, 1987.

DiPasquale G, Pinelle G, Andrea A: Idiopathic hypertrophic subaortic stenosis and cerebral ischemia. *Stroke* 16:537, 1985.

Eisenberg JD, Sobel BE, Geltman EM: Differentiation of ischemic from nonischemic cardiomyopathy with positron emission tomography. *Am J Cardiol* 59:1410, 1987.

Epstein SE, Henry WL, Clark CE, et al: Asymmetric septal hypertrophy. *Ann Intern Med* 81:650, 1974.

Ewer MS, Ali MK, MacKay B: A comparison of cardiac biopsy grades and ejection fraction estimations in patients receiving adriamycin. *J Clin Oncol* 2:112, 1984.

Feldman AM, Becker LC, Llewellyn MP, et al: Evaluation of a new inotropic agent OPC–8212 in patients with dilated cardiomyopathy and heart failure. *Am Heart J* 116:771, 1988.

Fighali S, Krajcer Z, Leachman RD: Septal myomectomy and mitral valve replacement for idiopathic hypertrophic subaortic stenosis: Short and long-term follow-up. *J Am Coll Cardiol* 3:1127, 1984.

Figulla HR, Rechenberg JV, Wiegand V, et al: Beneficial effects of long-term diltiazem treatment in dilated cardiomyopathy. *J Am Coll Cardiol* 13:653, 1989.

Furlan AJ, Graciun AR, Raju NR, et al: Cerebrovascular complications associated with idiopathic hypertrophic subaortic stenosis. *Stroke* 15:282, 1984.

Fuster V, Gersh BJ, Giuliani ER, et al: The natural history of idiopathic dilated cardiomyopathy. *Am J Cardiol* 47:525, 1981.

Gan TE, Ellims PH, Tong N, et al: Doxorubicin associated delayed ventricular fibrillation in acute promyelocytic leukemia. *Acta Haematol* 69:52, 1983.

Ganz PA, Gold BS, Tandron I, et al: Angina pectoris after doxorubicin and mitomycin therapy. *Cancer Treat Rep* 67:98, 1982.

Gillum RF: Idiopathic cardiomyopathy in the United States 1970–1982. *Am Heart J* 111:752, 1986.

Goldberg SJ, Hutter JJ Jr., Feldman L, et al: Two sensitive echocardiographic techniques for detecting doxorubicin toxicity. *Med Pediatr Oncol* 11:172, 1983.

Gravanis MB, Ansari AA: Idiopathic cardiomyopathies. *Arch Pathol Lab Med* 111:915, 1987.

Greminger P, Eichhorn P, Otto MH: Hemodynamics at rest and during isometric exercise under long-term treatment with captopril in dilated and ischemic cardiomyopathy. *Cardiology* 74:352, 1987.

Hag MM, Legha SS, Choksi J, et al: Doxorubicin induced congestive heart failure in adults. *Cancer* 56:1361, 1985.

Hale SL, Alker KJ, Rezkalla S, et al: Adverse effects of cocaine on cardiovascular dynamics, myocardial blood flow, and coronary artery diameter in an experimental model. *Am Heart J* 118:927, 1989.

Heiss HW, Hasenfuss G, Holubarsch C, et al: Cardiac energetics after intravenous enoximone in idiopathic dilated cardiomyopathy. *Am J Cardiol* 60:53C, 1987.

Herman EH, Ferrans VJ, Bhat HB, et al: Reduction of chronic doxorubicin cardiotoxicity in beagle dogs by bis-morpholinomethyl derivative of razoxane (ICRF-159). *Cancer Chemother Pharmacol* 19:277, 1987.

Hofmann T, Meinertz T, Kasper W, et al: Mode of death in idiopathic dilated cardiomyopathy: A multivariate analysis of prognostic determinants. *Am Heart J* 116:1455, 1988.

Ikram H, Chan H, Bennett SI, et al: Haemodynamic effects of acute beta-adrenergic receptor blockade in congestive cardiomyopathy. *Br Heart J* 42:311, 1979.

Inoue H, Zipes DP: Cocaine-induced supersensitivity and arrhythmogenesis. *J Am Coll Cardiol* 11:867, 1988.

Iskandrian AS, Hakki AH, Kane S: Resting thallium-201 myocardial perfusion patterns in patients with severe left ventricular dysfunction: Differences between patients with primary cardiomyopathy, chronic coronary artery disease or acute myocardial infarction. *Am Heart J* 111:760, 1986.

Isner JM, Estes NA III, Thompson PD, et al: Acute cardiac events temporally related to cocaine abuse. *N Engl J Med* 315:1438, 1986.

Jafri SM, Levine TB, Kloner RA: Recent advances in the medical management of congestive heart failure. *Modern Medicine* 56:50, 1988.

Kereiakes DJ, Parmley WW: Myocarditis and cardiomyopathy. *Am Heart J* 108:1318, 1984.

Keren G, Katz S, Strom J, et al: Non-invasive quantification of mitral regurgitation in dilated cardiomyopathy: Correlation of two Doppler echocardiographic methods. *Am Heart J* 116:758, 1988.

Kino M, Imamitchi H, Morigutchi M, et al: Cardiovascular status in asymptomatic alcoholics with reference to the level of ethanol consumption. *Br Heart J* 46:545, 1981.

Klatsky AL, Friedman GD, Siegelaub AB: Alcohol use and cardiovascular disease: The Kaiser Permanente experience. *Circulation* 64:III-32, 1981.

Kleiman NS, Lehane DE, Geyer CE Jr., et al: Prinzmetal's angina during 5-fluorouracil chemotherapy. *Am J Med* 82:566, 1987.

Klein LW, Horowitz LN: Familial right ventricular dilated cardiomyopathy associated with supraventricular arrhythmias. *Am J Cardiol* 62:482, 1988.

Krikler DM, Davies MJ, Rowland E, et al: Sudden death in hypertrophic cardiomyopathy: Associated accessory atrioventricular pathways. *Br Heart J* 43:245, 1980.

Lorell BH, Paulus WJ, Grossman W, et al: Improved diastolic function and systolic performance in hypertrophic cardiomyopathy after nifedipine. *N Engl J Med* 303:801, 1980.

Lorell BH, Paulus WJ, Grossman W, et al: Modification of abnormal left ventricular diastolic properties by nifedipine in patients with hypertrophic cardiomyopathy. *Circulation* 65:499, 1982.

Limas CJ, Limas C: HLA-DRW6 antigen linkage in chronic congestive heart failure secondary to coronary artery disease (ischemic cardiomyopathy). *Am J Cardiol* 62:816, 1988.

Loubser P, Suh K, Cohen S: Adverse effects of spinal anesthesia in a patient with idiopathic hypertrophic subaortic stenosis. *Anesthesiology* 60:228, 1984.

Majid PA, Ziznick J, Nishizaki S, et al: Favorable effects of pindolol in dilated chemotherapy. *Chest* 90:777, 1986.

Maron BJ, Bonow RO, Seshagiri TN, et al: Hypertrophic cardiomyopathy with ventricular septal hypertrophy localized to the apical region of the left ventricle (apical hypertrophic cardiomyopathy). *Am J Cardiol* 49:838, 1982.

Maron BJ, Savage DD, Wolfson JK, et al: Prognostic significance of 24-hour ambulatory electrocardiographic monitoring in patients with hypertrophic cardiomyopathy: A prospective study. *Am J Cardiol* 48:252, 1981.

Maron BJ, Roberts WC, Epstein SE: Sudden death in hypertrophic cardiomyopathy: A profile of 78 patients. *Circulation* 65:1388, 1982.

Mason JW, O'Connell JB: Clinical merit of endomyocardial biopsy. *Circulation* 79:971, 1989.

Massie B, Bourassa M, DiBianco R, et al: Long-term oral administration of amrinone for congestive heart failure: Lack of efficacy in a multicenter controlled trial. *Circulation* 71:963, 1985.

Matthews EC, Gardin JM, Henry WL, et al: Echocardiographic abnormalities in chronic alcoholics with and without overt congestive heart failure. *Am J Cardiol* 47:570, 1981.

Maze SS, Adolph RJ: Myocarditis: Unresolved issues in diagnosis and treatment. *Clin Cardiol* 13:69, 1990.

McKenna W, Deanfield J, Farugui A, et al: Prognosis in hypertrophic cardiomyopathy: Role of age and clinical electrocardiographic and hemodynamic features. *Am J Cardiol* 47:532, 1981.

Meyer W, Neumann J, Nose M, et al: Inotropic response in CHF: Myocarditis vs. dilated cardiomyopathy. *Am Heart J* 115:1346, 1988.

Milei J, Marantz A, Ale J, et al: Prevention of adriamycin-induced cardiotoxicity by prenylamine: A pilot double-blind study. *Cancer Drug Deliv* 4:129, 1987.

Mortensen SA, Olsen HS, Baandrup U: Chronic anthracycline cardiotoxicity: Hemodynamic and histopathologic manifestations suggesting a restrictive endomyocardial disease. *Br. Heart J* 55:274, 1986.

Nahas G, Trouve R, Demus JR: A calcium channel blocker as antidote to the cardiac effects of cocaine intoxication. *N Engl J Med* 313:519, 1985.

Newman PE: Acute myocardial infarction with angiographically demonstrated normal coronary arteries in the presence of hypertrophic cardiomyopathy. *Chest* 78:893, 1980.

Olsen EGJ: Restrictive cardiomyopathy. *Postgrad Med J* 62:607, 1986.

Pall DS, Marchlinski FF, Buxton AE: Sustained ventricular tachycardia in patients with idiopathic dilated cardiomyopathy: Electrophysiologic testing and lack of response to antiarrhythmic drug therapy. *Circulation* 70:451, 1984.

Pantely GA, Bristow JD: Ischemic cardiomyopathy. *Prog Cardiovasc Dis* 27:95, 1984.

Pasternac A, Noble J, Streulens Y, et al: Pathophysiology of chest pain in patients with cardiomyopathies and normal coronary arteries. *Circulation* 65:778, 1982.

Patel B, Kloner RA, Ensley J, et al: 5-Fluorouracil cardiotoxicity: Left ventricular dysfunction and effects of coronary dilators. *Am J Med Sci* 294:238, 1987.

Praga C, Beretta G, Vigo PL, et al: Adriamycin cardiotoxicity: A survey of 1,273 patients. *Cancer Treat Rep* 63:827, 1979.

Rabkin SW, Otten M, Polimeni PI: Increased mortality with cardiotoxic doses of adriamycin after verapamil pretreatment despite prevention of myocardial calcium accumulation. *Can J Physiol Pharmacol* 61:1050, 1983.

Regan TJ, Haider B: Ethanol abuse and heart disease. *Circulation* 64:III-14, 1981.

Report of the WHO/ISFC Task Force on the Definition and Classification of Cardiomyopathies. *Br Heart J* 44:672, 1980.

Rezkalla S, Kloner RA, Ensley J, et al: Continuous ambulatory electrocardiographic monitoring during 5-fluorouracil therapy. *J Clin Oncol* 7:509, 1989.

Rezkella S, Reddy R, Bhasin S, et al: Electrocardiographic abnormalities in cocaine users: A prospective study. *J Am Coll Cardiol* 15:190A, 1990.

Rosing DR, Kent KM, Maron BJ: Verapamil therapy: A new approach to pharmacologic treatment of hypertrophic cardiomyopathy. *Chest* 78(Suppl I):239, 1980.

Rubin E: Cardiovascular effect of alcohol. *Pharmacol Biochem Behav* 13(Suppl I):37, 1980.

Rubinow A, Skinner M, Cohen AS: Digoxin sensitivity in amyloid cardiomyopathy. *Circulation* 63:1285, 1981.

Saini J, Rich MW, Lyss AP: Reversibility of severe left ventricular dysfunction due to doxorubicin cardiotoxicity. Report of three cases. *Ann Intern Med* 106:814, 1987.

Santos AD, Miller RP, Mathew PK, et al: Echocardiographic characterization of the reversible cardiomyopathy of hypothyroidism. *Am J Med* 68:675, 1980.

Savage DD, Seides SF, Maron BJ, et al: Prevalence of arrhythmias during 24-hour electrocardiographic monitoring and exercise testing in patients with obstructive and nonobstructive hypertrophic cardiomyopathy. *Circulation* 59:866, 1979.

Schoolmaster WL, Simpson AG, Sauerbrunn BJ, et al: Radionuclide angiographic assessment of left ventricular function during exercise in patients with severely reduced ejection fraction. *Am J Cardiol* 47:804, 1981.

Schuster EH, Bulkley BH: Ischemic cardiomyopathy: A clinicopathologic study of fourteen patients. *Am Heart J* 100:506, 1980.

Sechtem U, Higgins CB, Sommerhoff BA, et al: Magnetic resonance imaging of restrictive cardiomyopathy. *Am J Cardiol* 59:480, 1987.

Short EM, Winkle RA, Billingham ME: Myocardial involvement in idiopathic hemochromatosis. Morphological and clinical improvement following venesection. *Am J Med* 70:1275, 1981.

Silverman KJ, Hutchins G, Bulkley B: Cardiac sarcoid: A clinicopathologic study of 84 unselected patients with systemic sarcoidosis. *Circulation* 58:1204, 1978.

Simpson RW, Edwards WD: Pathogenesis of cocaine-induced ischemic heart disease: Autopsy findings in a 21-year old man. *Arch Pathol Lab Med* 110:479, 1986.

Slausky MT, Gurathmey JK, Come PC, et al: Porcine model of myocarditis leading to dilated cardiomyopathy. *J Am Coll Cardiol* 13:253A, 1989.

Spodick DH: Effective management of congestive cardiomyopathy: Relation to ventricular structure and function. *Arch Intern Med* 142:689, 1982.

Steinberg JS, Wasserman AG: Radionuclide ventriculography for evaluation and prevention of doxorubicin cardiotoxicity. *Clin Ther* 7:660, 1985.

Stevenson LW, Bellil D, Grover-McKay M, et al: Effect of afterload reduction on left ventricular volume and mitral regurgitation in severe congestive heart failure secondary to ischemic or idiopathic dilated cardiomyopathy. *Am J Cardiol* 60:654, 1987.

St. John Sutton MG, Tajik AJ, Giuliani ER: Hypertrophic obstructive cardiomyopathy and lentiginosis: A little-known neural ectodermal syndrome. *Am J Cardiol* 47:214, 1981.

Swedberg K, Hjalmarson A, Waagstein F, et al: Adverse effects of beta blockade withdrawal in patients with congestive cardiomyopathy. *Br Heart J* 44:134, 1980.

Unverferth DV, Leier CV, Maguriea RD, et al: Improvement of human myocardial mitochondria after dobutamine: A quantitative ultrastructural study. *J Pharmacol Exp Ther* 215:527, 1980.

Vikhert AM, Tsiplenkova VG, Cherpachenko NM, et al: Alcoholic cardiomyopathy and sudden cardiac death. *J Am Coll Cardiol* 8:3A, 1986.

Virmani R, Tsiplenkova VG, Smialek JE, et al: Cardiovascular effects of cocaine: An autopsy study of 40 patients. *Am Heart J* 115:1068, 1988.

Waagstein F, Caidahl K, Wallentin I, Bergh C-H, Hjalmarson A: Long-term β-blockade in dilated cardiomyopathy. Effects of short- and long-term metoprolol treatment followed by withdrawal and readministration of metroprolol. *Circulation* 80:551, 1989.

Weber KT, Andrews V, Janicki JS: Cardiotonic agents in the management of chronic cardiac failure. *Am Heart J* 103:639, 1982.

Whittaker P, Romano T, Silver MD, Boughner DR: An improved method for detecting and quantifying cardiac muscle disarray in hypertrophic cardiomyopathy. *Am Heart J* 118:341, 1989.

Wiener RS, Lockhart JT, Schwartz RG: Dilated cardiomyopathy and cocaine abuse: Report of two cases *Am J Med* 81:699, 1986.

Wilensky RL, Yudelman P, Cohen AI, et al: Serial electrocardiographic changes in idiopathic dilated cardiomyopathy confirmed at necropsy. *Am J Cardiol* 62:276, 1988.

William DG, Olsen EGL: Prevalence of overt dilated cardiomyopathy in two regions of England. *Br Heart J* 54:153, 1985.

Wizenberg TA, Moz J, Sohn YH, et al: Value of positive myocardial technetium [99m]pyrophosphate scintigraphy in the noninvasive diagnosis of cardiac amyloidosis. *Am Heart J* 103:468, 1982.

Wynne J, Braunwald E: The cardiomyopathies and myocarditis. In: Braunwald E ed. *Heart Disease. A Textook of Cardiovascular Medicine*. Philadelphia: Saunders; 1988, p. 1410.

Zimmerman FH, Gustafson GM, Kemp HG, Jr: Recurrent myocardial infarction associated with cocaine abuse in a young man with normal coronary arteries: Evidence for coronary artery spasm culminating in thrombosis. *J Am Coll Cardiol* 9:964, 1987.

19 Diagnosis and Management of Cardiac Arrhythmias

Thomas B. Graboys

Management of patients presenting with rhythm disorders requires judgment, experience, and integration of the electrocardiographic (ECG) abnormality within the context of each patient's clinical status.

This chapter presents a unified, concise approach to diagnosis and management of arrhythmias.

DIFFERENTIAL DIAGNOSIS OF TACHYARRHYTHMIAS

The differential diagnosis of cardiac arrhythmias is facilitated by a classification based on the width of the QRS interval and the regularity or irregularity of the RR cycle. Thus, when a tachycardia is seen, a logical progression in the differentiation of the rhythm is to determine if the QRS is wide or narrow and the cycling regular or irregular (Table 1). The major differential diagnosis of any wide regular tachycardia would be ventricular tachycardia (VT), supraventricular tachycardia (SVT) with aberration, or preexcitation with antegrade accessory tract conduction.

Wide irregular tachyarrhythmia is probably atrial fibrillation with either aberrancy or fixed or rate-related bundle branch block. Narrow QRS regular tachycardias are classified as sinus, SVT, junctional tachycardia, or atrial flutter. Irregular, narrow complex tachycardias are classified as atrial fibrillation or multifocal atrial tachycardia (MAT).

WIDE, REGULAR TACHYCARDIA

VENTRICULAR TACHYCARDIA

By standard definition, three or more consecutive rapid ventricular beats constitute a salvo of VT. The QRS is wide and, at times, bizarre, particularly if the origin of the tachycardia is far enough from the normal specialized conduction system. Ventricular activity is independent of that within the atrium, resulting in atrioventricular (AV) dissociation (Figure 1). The hallmark on the ECG is partial capture if the sinus

Table 1. Classification of Tachycardias

		QRS Complex		
WIDE (≥0.12 sec)			NARROW (≤0.12 sec)	
Regular	Irregular		Regular	Irregular
VT	AF		ST	AF
SVT (aberration)	(aberration or bundle branch block)		PSVT	MAT
			NPJT	
WPW			AFL	

AF = atrial fibrillation; AFL = atrial flutter; MAT = multifocal atrial tachycardia; NPJT = nonparoxysmal junctional tachycardia; PSVT = paroxysmal supraventricular tachycardia; SVT = supraventricular tachycardia; VT = ventricular tachycardia; ST = sinus tachycardia; WPW = Wolff-Parkinson-White syndrome.

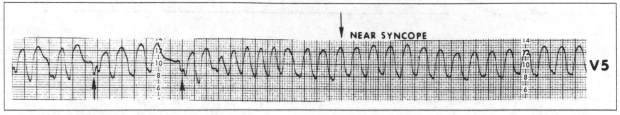

Figure 1. *Ventricular tachycardia with atrioventricular dissociation (arrows).*

mechanism coincides with ventricular depolarization from the VT focus, resulting in a fusion beat. A full 12-lead ECG should be obtained, so as not to base the diagnosis of a tachyarrhythmia on a single lead in which the QRS may be spuriously narrow.

The rate of VT is variable and depends on the clinical circumstances. The form of VT occurring within the setting of an acute myocardial infarction (so-called VT of the vulnerable period) is typically rapid and accelerating, and deteriorates to ventricular fibrillation (VF), often within 30–60 seconds. Paroxysmal VT in the nonischemic setting may have a constant rate of 150 beats/min. Typically, VT salvos have a rate of 150–200 beats/min. Therapy with antiarrhythmic drugs may result in slower nonsustained salvos, with rates of 100–150 beats/min. The rate of VT may exceed 200 beats/min; SVT with aberration should be suspected if the rate exceeds 250 beats/min and the QRS is 120–140 msec.

Slow ventricular foci may represent an idioventricular escape mechanism (60–100 beats/min), VT with 2:1 exit block from the site of tachycardia, or the electrophysiologic effect of antiarrhythmic drugs producing periods of "slow VT." At times, it may be difficult to differentiate electrocardiographically an accelerated idioventricular focus from VT in which the rate has been slowed.

SUPRAVENTRICULAR TACHYCARDIA WITH ABERRANCY

In SVT with aberrancy (Table 2), the rate of the tachycardia is usually 160–220 beats/min, although frequently it exceeds 250 beats/min in the presence of concealed bypass tracts or known preexcitation. The QRS is between 0.11 and 0.13 second. A right bundle branch block pattern is more common, although left ventricular tachycardia may also appear as right-sided intraventricular conduction disturbance. One helpful distinguishing characteristic is that

SVT with aberration usually does not result in a QRS duration >0.13 sec. The presence of P waves preceding each QRS should be sought, utilizing special leads if necessary (Lewis, esophageal, or right atrial). Differentiation from VT may be facilitated if onset of the tachycardia is recorded. The initial premature beat is noted to be narrow, followed by progressive widening of the QRS as rate-related aberrancy ensues.

Carotid sinus massage (CSM) often assists in differentiating SVT with aberration from VT. Carotid sinus massage may interrupt the reentrant mechanism by inducing vagotonia and terminating the tachycardia. If the mechanism is atrial flutter, CSM may slow conduction, converting a 2:1 or 1:1 response transiently to 2:1 or 4:1, resulting in normalization of conduction and confirming the presence of aberration. Rarely, CSM may terminate an episode of VT.

Certain physical findings are helpful in differentiating an aberrant rhythm from VT. Heart sounds are constant in SVT, as opposed to the variable intensity and splitting of both S_1 and S_2 during VT. The presence of cannon a-waves observed in the jugular pulse indicates AV dissociation and a ventricular origin of the tachycardia.

PREEXCITATION SYNDROMES

Preexcitation syndromes are discussed in detail in a later section. Among patients with Wolff-Parkinson-White syndrome (WPW) whose atrial mechanism is fibrillation or flutter, the refractory period of the anomalous pathway may be so short that rapid conduction with rates in excess of 300 beats/min ensues (Figure 2).

WIDE, IRREGULAR TACHYCARDIA

TORSADE DE POINTES

Torsade de pointes (Figure 3) represents chaotic, nonsustained ventricular activity that is invariably asso-

	VT	SVT with Aberration
Table 2. Factors in the Electrocardiographic Diagnosis of Ventricular Tachycardia or Supraventricular Tachycardia with Aberration		
AV dissociation	+	−
Fusion beats	+	−
QRS width	>140 msec	<140 msec
QRS morphology		
RBBB	Monophasic, LAD	Triphasic, normal axis
LBBB	Wide R in lead V$_1$	−
	RAD	−
Regularity	80%	95%
Onset	VPB	APB with ↑ QRS
CSP	− (<2%)	+ (30%)
Rate (beats/min)	150–200	>200

ABP = atrial premature beat; CSP = carotid sinus pressure; LAD = left axis deviation; LBBB = left bundle branch block; RAD = right axis deviation; RBBB = right bundle branch block; SVT = supraventricular tachycardia; VPB = ventricular premature beat; VT = ventricular tachycardia.

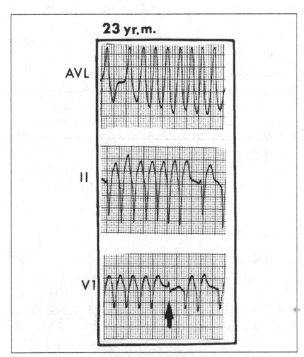

Figure 2. *Atrial fibrillation with rapid ventricular response in a patient with Wolff-Parkinson-White syndrome, indicating antegrade accessory tract conduction.*

ciated with serious symptoms. The ECG hallmark is rapid, bizarre QRS complexes with recurrent alteration of the QRS axis. Mechanisms include antiarrhythmic drugs (the most common being quinidine), phenothiazines, electrolyte disturbances (particularly hypokalemia), hereditary and acquired QT prolongation, AV block, and coronary vasospasm.

ATRIAL FIBRILLATION WITH ABERRANCY OR BUNDLE BRANCH BLOCK

Occasionally, patients with acute onset of atrial fibrillation, particularly in the setting of left ventricular failure, present with a wide-QRS, slightly irregular tachycardia that may be confused with VT. Close scrutiny of the cycle lengths and carotid sinus pressure (CSP) that slows the ventricular response invariably secure the diagnosis.

NARROW, REGULAR TACHYARRHYTHMIAS

SINUS TACHYCARDIA

Sinus tachycardia is defined as acceleration of the normal sinus mechanism beyond 105 beats/min. P waves with the same general morphology as the normal sinus P wave precede each QRS. As the rate increases, the P wave may appear somewhat peaked, and the PR interval may shorten, indicating facilita-

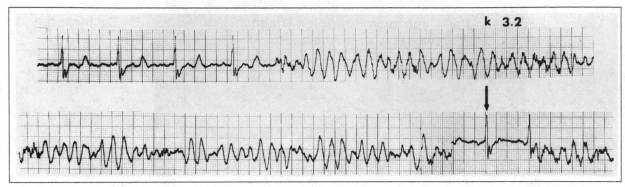

Figure 3. *Torsade de pointes (nonsustained ventricular flutter) in a hypokalemic patient receiving quinidine.*

tion of AV conduction. Rates rarely exceed 160 beats/ min in the adult. However, under unusual circumstances (e.g., thyrotoxicosis), sinus tachycardia may range from 150 to 200 beats/min. The rhythm is typically regular, and the response to CSM is gradual slowing, with prompt resumption of the tachycardia. Carotid sinus massage is particularly helpful if there is either rate-related or underlying bundle branch block. In this circumstance, particularly if the PR interval is somewhat prolonged, the P wave becomes fused with the preceding T wave at rapid rates and the rhythm may appear to be VT. With CSM, slowing unveils the P waves and confirms the presence of a sinus mechanism.

SUPRAVENTRICULAR TACHYCARDIA

When there is a rapid atrial mechanism (150–200 beats/ min), the diagnosis of paroxysmal SVT (PSVT) should be considered (Figures 4 and 5). Recent developments in the techniques of intracardiac recordings have led to better understanding of the pathophysiologic mechanisms of PSVT. The two basic mechanisms are *reentry* and *enhanced automaticity*. Reentrant rhythms involve a complex mechanism, the substrate of which is electrophysiologic inhomogeneity of adjacent cardiac tissue. Reentry accounts for some 90% of episodes of PSVT.

Sixty percent of PSVTs are AV nodal reentrant tachycardia. In about three fourths of patients with AV nodal (junctional) reentrant tachycardia, dual AV nodal pathways are identified in the electrophysiology laboratory. The AV node contains two functionally different pathways, designated alpha and beta. The alpha pathway is slower conducting, but its refractory period is shorter than the faster conducting beta path-

way. Atrial premature beats (APBs) that are sufficiently early block the beta pathway and conduct slowly in the antegrade direction down the alpha pathway. The beta pathway is then available for retrograde conduction, and the appropriate substrate for reentrant tachycardias is established. As with most forms of reentrant SVT, either an APB or ventricular premature beat (VPB) can initiate AV nodal reentrant tachycardias.

If the mechanism of atrial tachycardia is enhanced automaticity, a P wave precedes each QRS. The P wave will be morphologically different from the sinus P wave and it will fire at a constant rate of 160–250 beats/min.

The response to vagal maneuvers such as CSM is variable. If the mechanism is reentry, the reentrant tachycardia may be slowed or terminated. If the mechanism of arrhythmia is based on automaticity, such maneuvers may have no effect or only briefly return the rhythm to sinus.

ATRIAL FLUTTER

Atrial flutter is characterized by coarse, regular, "sawtooth" undulations of the baseline, referred to as F waves. These F waves appear at a rate of approximately 300 beats/min (Figure 6). Atrial flutter is usually associated with 2:1 AV block and a resultant ventricular response of 150 beats/min. Indeed, any regular narrow tachycardia at 150 beats/min should be considered atrial flutter until proved otherwise. Carotid sinus massage is, as noted earlier, most helpful in diagnosis because it induces an increase in AV block, slowing of the ventricular response, and disclosure of the flutter waves. The bulk of data suggest that atrial flutter is due to a reentrant mechanism in-

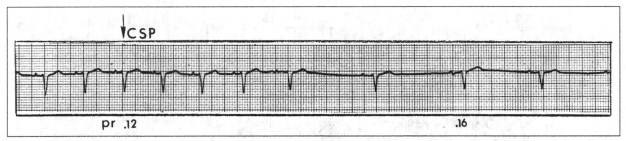

Figure 4. *Slow paroxysmal supraventricular tachycardia (PSVT) at 100 beats/min, which reverted to sinus rhythm with carotid sinus pressure (CSP).*

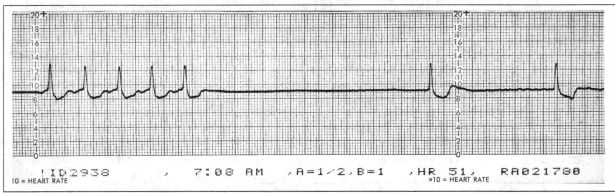

Figure 5. *Spontaneous termination of paroxysmal supraventricular tachycardia with asymptomatic offset pause and junctional escape beat.*

volving pathways in the atrium. This reentrant mechanism results in a predominantly negative deflection of the flutter waves in the inferior leads. A less common type of atrial flutter involves an oppositely directed reentrant circuit, such that the flutter waves are predominantly positive in the inferior leads.

When the frequency of the atrial rate is as low as 250 beats/min, it must be differentiated from SVT; at higher frequencies—400 beats/min—atrial flutter must be differentiated from atrial fibrillation. Pharmacologic interventions may alter the rate of the flutter mechanism. Thus, drugs that prolong the effective refractory period, such as quinidine, procainamide, and disopyramide (class IA drugs), will reduce the flutter rate from 300 to 200–250 beats/min. If the flutter rate is sufficiently slowed, it is possible to intermittently conduct 1:1. Hence, in some patients, administration of class IA agents without concomitant use of drugs to block the AV junction may result in

acceleration of heart rate. Drugs that shorten repolarization, such as digitalis, may enhance the flutter rate, as is often seen during digitalis treatment. About half of patients in atrial flutter convert to atrial fibrillation.

NONPAROXYSMAL JUNCTIONAL TACHYCARDIA (NPJT)

Nonparoxysmal junctional tachycardia, also termed accelerated junctional rhythm, is a manifestation of enhanced automaticity of the AV junction. The average rate is 70–130 beats/min. This arrhythmia may be a manifestation of digitalis toxicity or it may be associated with inferior myocardial infarction. It may be seen in the postoperative cardiac patient or in patients with severe mitral valvular disease. Patients with acute rheumatic fever and rare patients who have no other significant heart disease may manifest NPJT. Antiarrhythmics such as procainamide and quinidine may induce NPJT.

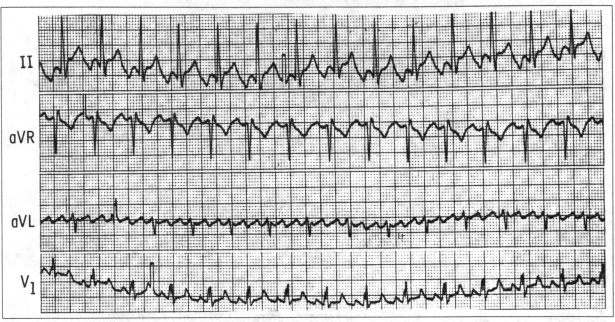

Figure 6. *Atrial flutter with atrial rate of 315 beats/min and 3:1 atrioventricular response.*

NARROW, IRREGULAR TACHYCARDIAS

ATRIAL FIBRILLATION

It has been suggested that both atrial flutter and fibrillation are part of a spectrum of intraatrial reentry. A shift of atrial flutter to fibrillation can be seen when the flutter waves break down into multiple smaller reentrant wavelets. The creation of such wavelets depends on the circulating impulses encountering areas of inhomogeneous refractoriness, resulting in secondary wavelets in multiple areas of reentry. This produces the chaotic, small-amplitude fibrillatory waves seen in atrial fibrillation. Borderline cases are seen and may be described as impure flutter or flutter-fibrillation. Because of the extremely high rate of discharge of the fibrillating atrium (500–600 cycles/min), impulses arriving in the AV junction present a disorganized wave front with insufficient potency to be consistently conducted to the ventricular specialized conduction system (see also Chapter 3).

Although atrial fibrillation may be paroxysmal, it is often a chronic stable rhythm. The critical determinant of the clinical response to atrial fibrillation is the rapidity of the ventricular rate. The average ventricular response to atrial fibrillation among patients not receiving beta blockers or digitalis drugs is 160 beats/min. More rapid ventricular responses are noted in certain clinical conditions. Thus, patients with thyrotoxicosis, preexcitation, or serious myocardial or valvular disease; patients receiving sympathomimetic agents, such as those used to treat chronic obstructive pulmonary disease; patients with alcoholic cardiomyopathy; and patients with certain electrolyte disorders, such as hypokalemia and hypomagnesemia, may exhibit a ventricular rate >160 beats/min (Figure 2). Patients with an intrinsic AV junctional conduction abnormality may exhibit slower ventricular responses. Thus, the patient who is not receiving medication and presents with a ventricular response to atrial fibrillation between 60 and 100 beats/min should be considered to have an intrinsic AV junctional conduction disorder. Occasionally, athletes with extreme vagotonia my present with atrial fibrillation and a slow ventricular response.

MULTIFOCAL ATRIAL TACHYCARDIA

Multifocal atrial tachycardia is defined as a tachyarrhythmia in which the atrial rate is >100 beats/min (Figure 7). There are well-organized discrete P waves of at least three separate morphologies, and there is an irregular variation in the P-P interval. An isoelectric baseline is noted between P waves. This tachycardia is associated with a high mortality rate, primarily due to its association with severe decompensated pulmonary disease, although MAT is often seen among patients receiving bronchodilators. The mechanism must be distinguished from that of other supraventricular rhythm disturbances. Although sinus tachycardia with multifocal APBs usually has a rate greater than 100 beats/min, it can be differentiated from MAT by the predominantly uniform P-P intervals and P-wave morphology except for isolated APBs. The most important differentiation is atrial fibrillation versus MAT. The indistinct morphology of atrial activity and undulating baseline of atrial fibrillation contrast with the discrete P waves and isoelectric baseline seen in MAT. Carotid sinus pressure may transiently decrease the rate of atrial activity in MAT, but this

quickly returns to control levels after release of CSP. At times, patients with MAT also have atrial fibrillation, complicating a unified diagnosis of the dysrhythmia.

THERAPY FOR CARDIAC ARRHYTHMIAS (TABLES 3 AND 4)

VENTRICULAR TACHYCARDIA

Ventricular tachycardia in the acute stage of myocardial infarction (MI) must be treated immediately. Clinical circumstances dictate the acute management. Patients whose condition is hemodynamically unstable during VT and who exhibit a change in mental status should be promptly cardioverted. If the patient loses consciousness, a precordial blow may be successful in reverting VT to sinus rhythm. The small

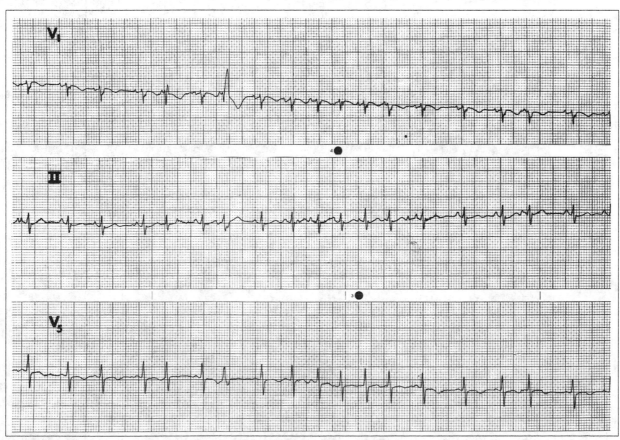

Figure 7. *Multifocal atrial tachycardia (MAT). Note variable rate and P-wave morphology.*

Table 3. Clinical Pharmacology of Antiarrhythmic Drugs

Drug	Indications	Effect on ECG	Dose	Adverse Effects	Therapeutic Plasma Levels
Bretylium	VT-VF		5 mg/kg IV; 5–10 mg/kg q6h	Hypotension; GI (nausea, vomiting); possible aggravation of arrhythmia	
Disopyramide	VEA AEA	QRS, QT, PR prolongation	100–200 mg q6h	Anticholinergic effects; hypotension; heart failure; heart block; tachyarrhythmia	2–8 µg/ml
Lidocaine	VEA	± QT shortening	Loading: 200–300 mg given as 50–100 mg every 5 min with rebolus after 20–40 min prn. Maintenance: 2–4 mg/min	CNS (drowsiness, agitation, seizures); rarely CHF or heart block	1–5 µg/ml
Phenytoin	VEA	± QT shortening	100–300 mg IV given as 50 mg every 5 min (ineffective as oral agent)	CNS (ataxia, nystagmus, drowsiness); hypotension and heart block with rapid IV injection	5–20 µg/ml
Procainamide	VEA AEA	QRS, QT prolongation	500–1,000 mg q4–6 hr (po); 1 g IV load as 100 mg every 3–5 min Maintenance: 2–6 mg/min	Lupus-like syndrome; GI; insomnia; rash; hypotension; aggravation of arrhythmia; blood dyscrasias	3–8 µg/ml
Quinidine	VEA AEA	QRS, QT prolongation	200–600 mg q4–6 hr (po) (average oral dose 300 mg q6h)	Aggravation of arrhythmias ("quinidine syncope"); thrombocytopenia; fever, rash; cinchonism; GI symptoms; digoxin-quinidine interaction (elevation of digoxin levels)	2–7 µg/ml
Beta-adrenergic blocking agents	AEA VEA	PR prolonged	Propranolol (80–160 mg/day): atenolol (50–100 mg/day); nadolol (40–100 mg 1–2 ×/day); metoprol (50–100 mg 2–3 ×/day)	Cardiac (heart block, hypotension, heart failure); asthma; hypoglycemia; lethargy; impotence	
Verapamil	AEA	–	5–15 mg IV; 40–160 mg po q8h	Congestive heart failure, asystole, constipation	

AEA = atrial ectopic activity; CHF = congestive heart failure; CNS = central nervous system; GI = gastrointestinal; VEA = ventricular ectopic activity.

Table 4. Clinical Pharmacology of Newer Antiarrhythmic Drugs

Drug	Indications	IV dose	Oral Dose	Adverse Effects	Comments
Mexiletine	VEA	Loading: 1200 mg/12h Maintenance: 250–500 mg/12h	Loading: 400–600 mg Maintenance: 200–300 mg q8h	GI; neurologic	Lidocaine-like drug. Local anesthetic; half-life, 8–14 hr
Tocainide	VEA	Loading: 0.5–0.75 mg/kg/min for 15 min	Loading: 400–600 mg Maintenance: 400–800 mg q8h	GI; neurologic	Lidocaine-like drug. Half-life, 11 hr in normals; 14–16 hr in patients with high-grade VEA
Amiodarone	AEA (especially in patients with WPW) VEA	IV loading: 300 mg Maintenance: 50 mg/h	Loading: 400–1200 mg/day × 5 d Maintenance: 200–800 mg/day	Constipation; skin rash; may uncover hypo- or hyperthyroidism; nausea; headache; corneal deposits; pulmonary infiltrates	Very long half-life (20–40 days). May increase digoxin level. May worsen existing cardiac conduction disturbances. May prolong Coumadin effect.
Encainide	VT	—	25–50 mg bid or tid	GI, CNS, cardiac (incessant VT)	+ + Negative inotropism. QRS & PR prolongation. Hepatic metabolism to active metabolites (ODE, MODE). Half-life (parent): 3–5 hr. Half-life (metabolites) 8–12 hr
Flecainide	VT SVT WPW	—	100–200 mg bid	GI, CNS, cardiac (incessant VT)	+ + + Negative inotropism QRS, PR prolongation
Propafenone	VT AF	—	150–300 mg tid	GI, CNS, cardiac	+ + Negative inotropism

AEA = atrial ectopic activity; VEA = ventricular ectopic activity; VT = ventricular tachycardia; SVT = supraventricular tachycardia; WPW = Wolff-Parkinson-White; CNS = central nervous system; GI = gastrointestinal; AF = atrial fibrillation.

amount of energy delivered by a precordial thump (1 watt-second) is frequently sufficient to depolarize enough myocardium and initiate a propagated response by electromechanical transduction (see Chapter 36). If VT degenerates to VF, the steep rise in energy requirement for termination of VF renders chest thumping ineffective. The current recommendation is that chest thump be reserved for monitored patients only, the concern being that a thump delivered during the ventricular vulnerable period may result in VF. However, the risk of this event is less than 5%. Lidocaine is the drug of choice for complex forms of VPBs (repetitive, early cycle) and VPBs occurring during acute MI, and is the initial agent used for paroxysmal VT. Second-line agents include intravenous procainamide and bretylium.

Therapy for torsade de pointes requires special mention. Ordinarily, traditional agents are ineffective for this arrhythmia, although lidocaine or phenytoin should certainly be tried. Prevention of torsade de pointes requires shortening of the refractory period. This can be accomplished either by isoproterenol infusion or pacing at rates sufficient to overdrive ectopic activity. Administration of magnesium sulfate has also been useful therapy. The inciting agent (i.e., quinidine) or contributing factors (hypokalemia, hypomagnesemia) should be eliminated.

SUPRAVENTRICULAR TACHYCARDIA

Management of acute SVT is generally directed toward increasing vagal tone with methods such as CSM or the Valsalva maneuver, or evoking the dive reflex by applying ice water to the forehead. If the basis of the arrhythmia is a reentry circuit involving the AV junction, digitalis, beta-adrenergic blocking agents, or verapamil may be effective in restoring normal rhythm. Cardioversion is rarely necessary in PSVT. The acknowledged drug of choice for SVT is verapamil. Intravenous administration terminates most SVT episodes. Oral therapy can be used to prevent recurrences or may be self-administered during an episode.

ATRIAL FLUTTER

Atrial flutter is more difficult to treat pharmacologically. Cardioversion is the treatment of choice. Rapid atrial pacing has also been used to revert flutter. Digitalis glycosides may reduce the ventricular response to atrial flutter, but the response is variable. At times, large doses of digoxin are necessary, presenting a risk

of development of digitalis toxicity, including paroxysmal atrial tachycardia (PAT) with block. If the patient is receiving quinidine concomitantly, differentiation of atrial flutter with a slow flutter mechanism and PAT with block may be difficult. Diminutive atrial complexes in the inferior leads with an isoelectric baseline favors PAT with block. In about half of patients, digitalis converts the rhythm to atrial fibrillation, and in the remainder, sinus rhythm is restored after a brief period of atrial fibrillation. Verapamil rapidly slows the ventricular response while the patient is being readied for cardioversion. Once sinus rhythm is restored, maintenance with quinidine, procainamide, or disopyramide may decrease the risk of recurrence.

ATRIAL FIBRILLATION

Treatment of atrial fibrillation depends on whether the rhythm disturbance is a paroxysmal event in the absence of congestive heart failure, or whether it is a manifestation of decreased left ventricular function. In the former, membrane-stabilizing drugs (quinidine, disopyramide, or procainamide) or cardioversion are effective in reverting atrial fibrillation to sinus rhythm. In the latter, digitalis with other measures to improve left ventricular function restores sinus rhythm.

Management of the patient with paroxysmal (lone) atrial fibrillation may present a complex problem. Typically, the patient has no overt heart disease, normal left atrial size, and fine (<2 mm) fibrillatory waves on the ECG. Many such patients are sensitive to changes in vagal tone; if they are, digitalis may be profibrillatory because of the heterogeneity of cholinergic fibers within the atria. Quindine and disopyramide are useful agents for treating this condition. Procainamide is effective for short-term oral or IV use, but few patients can remain on chronic therapy for longer than three months. Several drugs approved for ventricular arrhythmia are also effective for atrial fibrillation, particularly amiodarone and propafenone.

Verapamil administered either orally or intravenously slows the response to both atrial fibrillation and flutter. Use of this agent for prevention of atrial fibrillation has not yielded impressive results. However, for the patient in whom atrial fibrillation is a fixed rhythm, verapamil may be helpful in maintaining rate control.

The most common cause of atrial fibrillation, particularly in the acute phase of MI, is elevated left ventricular filling pressure. Thus, slowing of the ventricular response is mandatory before sinus rhythm can be established and maintained. Cardioversion offers little advantage in the patient with decompensated cardiac function and atrial fibrillation. Once optimal ventricular function and control of the ventricular response is effected, electrical reversion may be undertaken if necessary. In our experience, oral quinidine or IV procainamide is helpful in stabilizing the atrium before cardioversion and will result in a 10–15% chance of pharmacologic reversion.

MULTIFOCAL ATRIAL TACHYCARDIA

The treatment of MAT is primarily the treatment of the underlying pulmonary disease. Modification of bronchodilator therapy may also reduce the density of MAT. Some success has been reported with verapamil, which may reduce automaticity within the atrium.

"COCKTAIL" THERAPY FOR PAROXYSMAL ARRHYTHMIAS

If the patient's dysrhythmia occurs infrequently—once or twice yearly—and if the patient tolerates the arrhythmia, then the physician might use a therapeutic "cocktail" to revert the arrhythmia. In these situations, the patient does not require chronic antiarrhythmic therapy. Use of a single agent or group of drugs only at the time of the cardiac arrhythmia is the treatment of choice. Thus, for the patient experiencing PSVT, use of verapamil or a beta-adrenergic blocking agent and mild sedatives may be effective in controlling infrequent episodes of tachycardia. Paroxysmal atrial fibrillation may be treated with a "cocktail" of quinidine, a beta-adrenergic blocking agent, and sedative. Atrial flutter usually does not respond to this approach.

PREEXCITATION SYNDROMES AND THERAPY

Preexcitation syndromes (PES) include ECG and clinical conditions resulting from accelerated transmission of impulses from atrium to ventricle via accessory tracts which bypass the normal physiologic delay in the AV junction. Electrocardiographic findings reflect the pathoanatomic tracts. Classic syndromes include WPW and Lown-Ganong-Levine (LGL) syndromes, although a number of variations may be encountered. In patients with WPW, a short or normal PR interval is inscribed; the "slurring" of the QRS is a result of fusion of early ventricular depolarization via the accessory Kent bundle and that which occurs over the normal His-Purkinje system. In LGL syndrome, the ECG hallmark is a short PR interval with normal QRS complex. Conceptually, an anomalous connection circumvents a portion of the AV junction. This tract, described by James, is believed to explain the short PR interval (<0.12 second) and normal QRS in the LGL syndrome.

A rare form of preexcitation involves the fibers of Mahaim. Accessory pathways from either the lower AV junction or His bundle pass directly to the ventricular myocardium. Thus, the PR interval is normal because there is no bypass of the AV junction. The QRS complex exhibits a delta wave that is due to premature depolarization of the ventricle as in the WPW syndrome.

Preexcitation syndromes are common entities. Slightly more men are affected, and about two thirds of patients have no associated evidence of organic heart disease. An array of congenital heart defects are associated with preexcitation syndromes, the most common of which is Ebstein's anomaly of the tricuspid valve.

Most patients with symptomatic preexcitation have SVT. The mechanism is a reciprocating, or reentrant, tachycardia. Usually there is antegrade conduction down the AV node with retrograde conduction from ventricle to atrium by the anomalous pathway. The QRS morphology is regular. In a small proportion of WPW patients, antegrade conduction down the anomalous pathway with retrograde conduction through the AV node or a second accessory pathway occurs. This results in a regular tachycardia, but with a wide and aberrant QRS complex. This tachyarrhythmia is clinically significant in the acute setting because of its ECG similarity to VT.

Atrial fibrillation, which may be seen more often in older WPW patients, can result in rapid depolarization of the ventricle, leading to VF and sudden death. Atrial flutter can be a significant problem when 1:1 conduction occurs over the accessory tract.

Therapy is guided by the clinical circumstances: the patient's symptoms, the rate of the tachyarrhythmia, and the nature of the atrial mechanism (fibrillation, flutter, or reciprocating tachycardia). In an emergency setting, when a patient presents with a bizarre, extremely rapid tachycardia (rates in excess of 250 beats/min), expedient treatment is mandatory.

Intravenous procainamide or lidocaine often block the accessory pathway, reducing the ventricular response and allowing for more definitive therapy. Cardioversion is the therapy of choice if the atrial mechanism is flutter or fibrillation. Quinidine and disopyramide also impede conduction through accessory pathways and are alternatives to IV lidocaine. Digitalis drugs, verapamil, and beta-adrenergic blocking agents are useful if the arrhythmia is a regular reciprocating tachycardia (rates 200 beats/min) with antegrade conduction through the His-Purkinje system. Digitalis drugs and verapamil are contraindicated if the tachyarrhythmia is atrial fibrillation, the concern being that digitalis or verapamil will shorten the refractory period of the accessory pathway in a few patients, promoting enhanced conduction with potential deterioration to ventricular fibrillation. One cannot predict by ECG analysis which patients are susceptible to this problem. It has been suggested that patients with an effective refractory period of the bypass tract of approximately 200 msec (corresponding to a ventricular rate of 300 beats/min) are at highest risk.

SICK SINUS SYNDROME AND THERAPY

Sick sinus syndrome is a heterogeneous entity, both in terms of definition and underlying pathophysiologic mechanisms. The term, coined by Lown in reference to the condition in patients after cardioversion who exhibited bradycardia, sinoatrial arrest, and escape junctional mechanisms, now refers to evidence of sinus node dysfunction producing clinical symptoms; it is also used to describe an asymptomatic patient who has evidence of failure of proper sinoatrial pacemaker function. In effect, sick sinus syndrome represents a generalized disorder of the conduction system of the heart, sinus node dysfunction being only one aspect. Evidence of sinus node dysfunction is observed in diverse populations of patients. The spectrum may range from extreme vagotonia and minor sclerodegenerative changes in the conduction system to bradycardia-tachycardia syndromes, in which the patient experiences ventricular or atrial tachyarrhythmias and becomes symptomatic during prolonged offset pauses. Therapy must be individualized, and insertion of pacemakers should be confined to patients who experience documented symptomatic bradyarrhythmias. One should not assume a priori that patients with asymptomatic offset pauses of as long as 3 seconds after a bout of tachyarrhythmia require permanent pacing. Antiarrhythmic drugs that suppress the tachyarrhythmia may eliminate offset pauses and may not provoke sinoatrial or AV conduction problems in and of themselves. Patients should undergo careful monitoring to establish their response to antiarrhythmic therapy.

CARDIOVERSION AND DEFIBRILLATION

Use of electrical energy for reverting cardiac tachyarrhythmias has become standard practice in the last 25 years because of its safety and reliability (see also Chapter 36). The term *defibrillation* generally applies to depolarization during VF of the entire heart, or a major portion of it, by an unsynchronized electrical discharge. The ensuing cardiac asystole is then terminated by emergence of the cardiac pacemaker with the highest automaticity (usually the sinoatrial node).

Cardioversion is the use of electrical energy to revert specific cardiac arrhythmias. It differs from defibrillation in that the electrical discharge is synchronized with the R wave to avoid triggering VF by accidental discharge during the vulnerable period of the ventricle. The vulnerable period is a span of approximately 30 msec just before inscription of the apex of the T wave on the surface ECG, but may be considerably longer under conditions of ischemia. Discharge of a low-intensity shock will produce VF only when delivered during a vulnerable period. For the sake of simplicity, the R wave has been selected for triggering the electrical discharge. The physiologic basis for cardioversion is that an electrical discharge depolarizes a part of the reentrant pathway that is nonrefractory and interrupts the circus movement.

METHOD OF DEFIBRILLATION

Almost all cardiac arrests are a result of VF. Defibrillation constitutes definitive treatment for this condition, and success is assured only if prompt defibrillation is accomplished. Initial defibrillation of adults should be conducted with a setting between 100–300 watt-seconds. There is no evidence that energies in excess of 400 watt-seconds are needed in humans for defibrillation, provided proper technique is used. Higher energies may result in prolonged periods of asystole or complete heart block, resulting in resumption of VF.

Paddle position for defibrillation and cardioversion is the same. Both anteroposterior and anterolateral electrode positions are used. The anterior electrode is held firmly along the right sternal border at the level of the second and third intercostal spaces while the posterior electrode is placed at the angle of the left scapula. If a lateral paddle is used, it should be placed between the apex and anterior axillary line. The electrodes must be completely covered with conductive gel, particularly along the edges, to reduce the likelihood of skin burns.

METHOD OF CARDIOVERSION

Cardioversion may be done under both elective and nonelective circumstances. The conscious patient with VT who is hemodynamically compromised should be promptly cardioverted after receiving small amounts of IV diazepam or short-acting barbiturates. Alternatively, the patient with atrial fibrillation who is to be electively cardioverted should have the procedure fully explained to allay as much anxiety as possible. Digitalis drugs need not be withheld. Serum levels of digoxin and electrolytes should be determined before the procedure; and, if the patient has had anticoagulation therapy, a recent prothrombin time determination is necessary. Cardioversion may be done at the patient's bedside or in a room equipped for cardiopulmonary resuscitation. There should be a minimum of personnel and activity. A short-acting barbiturate should be administered 1–2 hours before the procedure. This sedation reduces the amount of diazepam given subsequently. At the time of cardioversion, an initial IV dose of 5 mg of diazepam is administered, followed by 2.5-mg increments every 2–3 minutes. Both blood pressure and respiratory rates are monitored before each dose. An average of 15 mg of diazepam is required to achieve adequate sedation, although the range is variable.

The main danger in transthoracic electric discharge is provocation of VF. The current generation of cardioverters incorporates a display that indicates the portion of the QRS to which the circuit is synchronized. The lead that displays the highest R-wave amplitude should be selected for discharge synchronization. Improper synchronization may result when the ECG signal contains artifactual spikes, when there are extremely prominent T waves, and in bundle branch block when the R′ wave is taller than the R wave. The energy levels required to terminate specific arrhythmias are listed in Table 5. During elective cardioversion, energy titration should be used. Low energies may disclose rhythm disturbances in patients with subclinical digitalis toxicity or electro-

Table 5. Average Energy Level Required for Cardioversion	
Rhythm	Energy (watt-second)
VT	10
Atrial flutter	20
Atrial fibrillation	100
SVT	150
SVT = supraventricular tachycardia; VT = ventricular tachycardia.	

lyte disturbance, and they also reduce myocardial damage.

INDICATIONS FOR PACEMAKER INSERTION

Table 6 lists indications for temporary and permanent pacemaker implantation. During acute MI, indications for temporary pacing are the occurrence of complete heart block or advanced AV block in the setting of anterior wall MI. Progressive first- and second-degree AV block in the setting of acute bundle branch block is another indication for temporary pacing. Controversy remains as to the absolute need for pacing in the patient with acute bundle branch block and no evidence of AV conduction disorder whose condition is otherwise stable (see also Chapters 20 and 21).

A permanent pacemaker should be placed only in patients with symptomatic bradyarrhythmia, brady-tachy syndromes, and evidence of Stokes-Adams syncope. Use of pacemaker technology for management of recurrent atrial and ventricular tachyarrhythmias is reserved for only a minority of patients with drug-refractory tachycardia.

Because of the rapidly increasing complexity of types of pacemakers, a code for pacemaker identification (Parsonnet et al.) was developed to describe essential features of each type. The code consists of five letters. The first letter represents the chamber (or chambers) paced (A, atrium; V, ventricle; D, double chamber); the second letter represents the chamber(s) sensed (A, V, D, or O [none]); the third letter represents the mode of response (I, inhibited; T, triggered; D, double [atrial triggered and ventricular inhibited]; O, not applicable). The fourth and fifth

---

Table 6. Indications for Pacing

TEMPORARY
Occurrence of the following events during an
acute myocardial infarction:
   Complete heart block
   Mobitz II atrioventricular block (anterior wall
    infarct)
   Atrioventricular block and acute bifascicular
    block
   Overdrive suppression of ventricular arrhyth-
    mia
PERMANENT
   Complete heart block
   Bradycardia-tachycardia syndrome
   Symptomatic bradyarrhythmia
   Proven efficacy of overdrive suppression

---

letters indicate more sophisticated pacing features, such as programmability or special tachyarrhythmia functions. The bulk of current pacemaker therapy involves the standard ventricular demand pacemaker. The first three letters of the code used to describe this type of device are VVI (ventricular pace, ventricular sensed, and inhibited by natural electrical activity in the ventricular chamber).

In some patients, if there is no competing atrial rhythm, synchronization of atrial and ventricular contraction may improve cardiac performance. Devices capable of this can sense or pace the atrium, and then perform sequential ventricular pacing (VAT, DVI, DDD). If AV conduction is intact, atrial demand pacing may be used (AAI).

STRATEGIES IN THE APPROACH TO SUDDEN CARDIAC DEATH AND INDICATIONS FOR TREATMENT OF VENTRICULAR ARRHYTHMIA

Sudden death from heart disease is the leading cause of death in developed countries. In the past two decades, many advances have been made in the management of the patient with malignant ventricular arrhythmia, as well as in the use of antiarrhythmic drugs for long-term survival. The concept of antiarrhythmic drug aggravation of arrhythmia is now accepted, and accordingly, indications for therapy have been modified.

PROARRHYTHMIA

In addition to the syndrome of torsade de pointes, substantial data underscore the observation that every antiarrhythmic drug has the potential to aggravate the arrhythmia we hope to suppress. This concept of proarrhythmia is manifest either by a significant increase in the density of single ectopic beats; emergence of nonsustained VT when the clinical arrhythmia had only been VPBs; conversion of nonsustained VT to sustained VT; or provocation of cardiac arrest in a patient who had not experienced that event. Proarrhythmia is more likely to occur in the setting of left ventricular dysfunction and if the clinical arrhythmia is either noninfarction VF or sustained VT. As with provocation of torsade de pointes, concomitant diuretic and digitalis therapy enhances the risk of proarrhythmia.

INDICATIONS FOR TREATMENT OF VENTRICULAR ECTOPIC ACTIVITY

The recognition of proarrhythmia as a real entity has reduced the enthusiasm for initiating chronic antiarrhythmic therapy. Although VPBs are associated with an enhanced risk for sudden cardiac death, this finding lacks specificity. The finding of advanced forms of ectopic activity in an asymptomatic, otherwise healthy person is cause for neither alarm nor treatment. Table 7 details indications for treatment of VPBs. Only a few persons with VPBs require chronic antiarrhythmic therapy. For patients who have so-called malignant ventricular arrhythmia, i.e., noninfarction VF or sustained VT, there is no debate as to the need for aggressive therapy. Except for patients who have unusual cardiac conditions such as hypertrophic obstructive cardiomyopathy, hereditary long QT syndrome, or nonsustained VT categorically correlated with symptoms, antiarrhythmic therapy is not associated with an improved survival rate. The Cardiac Arrhythmia Suppression Trial (CAST) showed a 2.5-fold higher incidence of cardiac death or nonfatal cardiac arrest among patients receiving one of the IC drugs (encainide or flecainide), underscoring the concern as to the appropriate use of these agents.

For patients with malignant ventricular arrhythmia, defined as noninfarction-related VF or hemodynamically compromising VT, a systematic approach using electrophysiologic study or noninvasive assessment to antiarrhythmic drug testing and therapy is mandatory because of the risk of recurrence and high annual

Table 7. Indications for the Chronic Treatment of Ventricular Arrhythmias

Primary (noninfarction-related) VF
Sustained symptomatic VT
Mitral valve prolapse in patient with family history of sudden cardiac death and with paroxysms of symptomatic VT
Long QT syndrome with syncope or family history of sudden death
Obstructive cardiomyopathies, particularly with a family history of sudden death
Symptomatic VPBs

VF = ventricular fibrillation; VPBs = ventricular premature beats; VT = ventricular tachycardia.

mortality rate among such patients. Many of these patients can be successfully treated with a combination of antiarrhythmic drugs, significantly improving long-term survival. A few patients with true drug-refractory malignant arrhythmia may be candidates for either surgical resection, using cardiac mapping to define the VT focus, or implantation of an automatic internal cardioverter-defibrillator.

Bibliography

Barold SS, Coumel P: Mechanisms of atrioventricular junctional tachycardia: Role of reentry and concealed accessory bypass tracts. *Am J Cardiol* 39:97, 1977.

Cardiac Arrhythmia Suppression Trial (CAST) Investigators: Preliminary report: Effect of encainide and flecainide on mortality in a randomized trial of arrhythmia suppression after myocardial infarction. *N Engl J Med* 321:406, 1989.

Cranefield PF, Wit AL, Hoffman BF: Genesis of cardiac arrhythmias. *Circulation* 47:190, 1973.

DeSilva RA, Graboys TB, Podrid PJ, et al: Cardioversion and defibrillation. *Am Heart J* 100:881, 1980.

Doering W: Quinidine-digoxin interaction: Pharmacokinetics, underlying mechanism and clinical implications. *N Engl J Med* 301:400, 1979.

Fisch C: Relation of electrolyte disturbances to cardiac arrhythmias. *Circulation* 47:408, 1973.

Godman MJ, Lassers BW, Julain DG: Complete bundle branch block complicating acute myocardial infarction. *N Engl J Med* 282:237, 1970.

Harrison DL, Meffin PJ, Winkle RA: Clinical pharmacokinetics of antiarrhythmic drugs. *Prog Cardiovasc Dis* 20:217, 1978.

Hindman MC, Wagner GS, Jaro M, et al: The clinical significance of bundle branch block complicating acute myocardial infarction: *Circulation* 58:689, 1978.

Josephson ME, Kastor JA: Supraventricular tachycardia: Mechanisms and management. *Ann Intern Med* 87:346, 1977.

Lown B, Graboys TB: Ventricular premature beats and sudden cardiac death. In: McIntosh H, ed. *Baylor Cardiology Series.* Vol 3, 1980, p.1.

Lown B, Podrid PJ, DeSilva RA, et al: *Sudden Cardiac Death: Management of the Patient at Risk.* Vol IV. Chicago: Year Book Medical Publishers; 1980.

Lown B, Graboys TB: Management of patients with malignant ventricular arrhythmias. *Am J Cardiol* 39:910, 1977.

Lown B: Electrical reversion of cardiac arrhythmias. *Br Heart J* 29:469, 1967.

Lown B, Ganong WF, Levine SA: The syndrome of short RR interval, normal QRS complexes and paroxysmal rapid heart action. *Circulation* 5:693, 1952.

Margolis B, DeSilva RA, Lown B: Episodic drug treatment in the management of paroxysmal arrhythmias. *Am J Cardiol* 45:621, 1980.

McAnulty JH, Rahimtoola S, Murphy ES: A prospective study of sudden death in "high risk" bundle branch block. *N Engl J Med* 299:209, 1978.

Minardo JD, Heger JJ, Miles WM, et al: Clinical characteristics of patients with ventricular fibrillation during antiarrhythmic drug therapy. *N Engl J Med* 319:257, 1988.

Moss AF, Davis RJ: Brady-tachy syndrome. *Prog Cardiovasc Dis* 16:439, 1974.

Parsonnet V, Furman S, Smyth NPD: A revised code for pacemaker identification. *PACE* 4:400, 1981.

Podrid P, Lampert S, Graboys TB, et al: Aggravation of arrhythmia by antiarrhythmic drugs—incidence and predictors of occurrence. *Am J Cardiol* 59:38E, 1987.

Rigby WFC, Graboys TB: Current concepts and management of the preexcitation syndromes. *J Cardiovasc Med* 6:277, 1981.

Shine KI, Kastor JA, Yurchak PM: Multifocal atrial tachycardia: Clinical and electrocardiographic features. *N Engl J Med* 179:344, 1968.

Velebit V, Podrid PJ, Lown B, et al: Aggravation and provocation of ventricular arrhythmias by antiarrhythmic drugs. *Circulation* 65:886, 1982.

Wolff L, Parkinson J, White PD: Bundle branch block with short PR interval in healthy young people prone to paroxysmal tachycardia. *Am Heart J* 5:685, 1930.

Zipes DP, Troup PJ: New antiarrhythmic agents. *Am J Cardiol* 41:1005, 1978.

CHAPTER 20

Atrioventricular Conduction Disorders

Peter L. Friedman

Atrioventricular (AV) conduction disturbances represent a frequently encountered problem in contemporary cardiology, often posing both a diagnostic and therapeutic dilemma to the clinician. Whereas the symptomatic patient with complete AV block and a slow idioventricular rhythm clearly requires an artificial pacemaker, the prognostic implications and proper management of lesser degrees of AV block may be less certain or even controversial. This chapter discusses currently available methods for assessing AV conduction, reviews the wide array of chronic AV conduction disturbances one is likely to encounter, and, finally, provides a framework for a rational approach to patients with such problems. AV conduction disturbances occurring in the setting of acute myocardial infarction (MI) are considered in Chapter 15.

PHYSIOLOGY AND PATHOPHYSIOLOGY OF ATRIOVENTRICULAR CONDUCTION

Optimal cardiac performance depends greatly upon an ordered sequence of atrial systole and then, after an appropriate delay, ventricular systole. This ordered sequence of mechanical events, in turn, requires a normally functioning cardiac conduction system, in which pacemaker impulses originating in the sinus node must first depolarize atrial myocardium, then propagate slowly through the AV node, and, finally, be distributed quickly over the His-Purkinje network to the ventricular myocardium.

The function of each link in this electrophysiologic chain is best appreciated by examining the time relationships between P waves and QRS complexes of the surface electrocardiogram (ECG), together with simultaneously recorded intracardiac bipolar electrograms from the high right atrium (near the sinus node), left atrium, and His bundle region (Figure 1). An

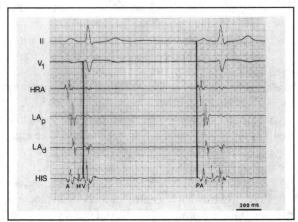

Figure 1. *Simultaneous recordings during sinus rhythm of (top to bottom) surface ECG leads II and V_1 as well as intracardiac bipolar electrograms from the high right atrium (HRA), proximal left atrium (LA_p), distal left atrium (LA_d) and His bundle region (HIS). The dark vertical lines denote onset of the QRS complex (left) and P wave (right). See text for discussion.*

electrode catheter in the His bundle region, because of its strategic position across the AV ring, is in close proximity to both atrial and ventricular myocardium. Consequently, the electrogram recorded from such a lead consists of three deflections: the first of these presents low right atrial muscle depolarization (A in Figure 1) near the origin of the AV node; the second is a rapid deflection signifying His bundle depolarization (H in Figure 1); and the third is a large deflection that represents depolarization of the right ventricular septal myocardium (V in Figure 1). On the surface ECG, the PR interval represents the total time required for transmission of the cardiac impulse from its point of origin in the sinus node to the ventricular myocardium. This interval is actually a sum of conduction times over each different segment of the AV conducting system; namely, conduction time between the sinus and AV nodes, conduction time through the AV node itself, and conduction time from the His bundle to ventricular myocardium. Although specific information about conduction over each of these segments is not apparent from the surface ECG, it is available from simultaneous recordings of the surface ECG and a His bundle electrogram.

The interval between onset of a normal sinus P wave on the surface ECG and depolarization of the low right atrial myocardium (A in the His bundle electrogram) represents intraatrial conduction time from the sinus node to the AV node. This time is referred to as the PA interval, normally requiring from 10–55 msec, and is determined by conduction velocity over the specialized internodal tracts and through atrial myocardium (Figure 1). Because intraatrial conduction normally is quite rapid, the PA interval accounts for only a small part of the PR interval. However, conditions that slow intraatrial conduction velocity (atrial infarction, chronic atrial hypertension, and infiltrative diseases such as amyloidosis or hemochromatosis) all may prolong the PR interval by virtue of prolongation of the PA interval.

Most of the normal delay during AV transmission occurs within the AV node, where cells generate slowly rising, low-amplitude action potentials, and conduction velocity is accordingly slow. AV nodal conduction time, therefore, accounts for a majority of the PR interval. Since the atrial deflection recorded by a His bundle electrode catheter represents depolarization of atrial muscle near the cranial border of the AV node, the AH interval provides an accurate measure of AV nodal conduction time (Figure 1). AV nodal conduction times in normal persons span a wide range, usually 50–140 msec, due largely to variations in sympathetic and parasympathetic tone within the richly innervated AV node. There are many conditions and diseases that can impair AV conduction by interfering with AV nodal conduction. Pharmacologic agents may depress AV nodal conduction via direct electrophysiologic effects on AV nodal cells (verapamil, procainamide) or indirectly, by altering autonomic tone (propranolol, digitalis). Ischemia can also cause AV nodal conduction delay and block. Usually, this is a reflection of compromised flow in the right coronary artery, which is the origin of the AV nodal artery in 90% of patients. Ischemic AV nodal block may be transient, due to hypoxia, parasympathetic reflexes, or various metabolic products liberated by

ischemic myocardium. It may also be permanent, usually reflecting actual infarction of all or part of the AV node. Inflammation of any cause involving the AV node may result in AV nodal delay or block. This is most often seen in acute rheumatic myocarditis, but may also accompany viral myocarditis and occur in association with Lyme disease. Other conditions that can result in impaired AV nodal conduction are infiltrative cardiomyopathies (amyloidosis, sarcoidosis, hemochromatosis), open heart surgery (particularly after replacement of a heavily calcified aortic or mitral valve), and, on rare occasions, primary or metastatic cardiac tumors. Finally, AV nodal block may be congenital.

The terminal portion of the PR in the surface ECG represents conduction through all segments of the AV conducting system distal to the AV node. This includes conduction over the His bundle, down the right and left bundle branches, and through the subendocardial ramifications of the Purkinje network to ventricular myocardium. Total conduction time in this subnodal portion of the AV conduction system is reflected in the HV interval, measured from the H spike in the His bundle electrogram to the earliest point of ventricular depolarization in any intracardiac or surface lead (Figure 1). In the presence of normal conduction distal to the AV node, the HV interval ranges from 35–55 msec. Unlike AV nodal conduction, conduction velocity in the His-Purkinje system does not change appreciably despite wide fluctuations in autonomic tone. However, subnodal conduction can be severely impaired by a variety of conditions or disease states. Perhaps the most common cause of abnormal His-Purkinje conduction is hypertensive cardiovascular disease, which accelerates aging of the cardiac skeleton and may result in fibrosis of the subnodal conduction system. Ischemic heart disease may also lead to disturbances in intraventricular conduction, either because of fibrosis or actual infarction of the His bundle or bundle branches, as well as underlying myocardium. This is most commonly seen in association with anteroseptal MI, since the left anterior descending coronary artery provides most of the blood supply to the His bundle and bundle branches. However, it may also occur with right coronary artery occlusion with resulting compromise of flow in the posterior descending artery. Infiltrative diseases, such as amyloidosis, hemochromatosis, and sarcoidosis may involve the His-Purkinje system, resulting in impaired subnodal conduction. Other common causes include cardiomyopathy, congenital heart disease, trauma associated with cardiac surgery, and most antiarrhythmic drugs, particularly toxic concentrations of agents with local anesthetic properties. Occasionally, impaired His-Purkinje conduction may be due to sclerodegenerative changes in this tissue in the absence of any other cardiac disease (Lev's disease, Lenegre's disease). Infectious causes of impaired His-Purkinje conduction include Chagas' disease and septal abscess formation as a consequence of infective endocarditis. Other uncommon causes of subnodal conduction disturbances are polymyositis, myotonia dystrophica, and Kearns-Sayre syndrome.

DIAGNOSIS AND MANAGEMENT OF AV BLOCK

FIRST-DEGREE BLOCK

First-degree AV block is defined as a PR interval of greater than 0.20 sec and is probably the most commonly encountered manifestation of altered AV conduction. Of course, the single important exception to this definition is prolonged intraatrial conduction time, which, as pointed out above, may result in a prolonged PR interval in the absence of any true disturbance of AV transmission. Usually, first-degree AV block is due to slow conduction through the AV node. Intracardiac recordings in such cases typically reveal a prolonged AH interval, with normal PA and HV intervals.

First-degree AV nodal block may be a manifestation of intrinsic AV node disease or may simply be a reflection of heightened vagal tone or drug effect. In the absence of evidence of higher degrees of block, it requires no therapy. However, prolongation of the PR interval does not always imply slow conduction through the AV node. Figure 2 is an example of a patient with a PR interval of 0.43 sec in whom conduction time through the AV node is normal. Note that in this patient the His bundle electrogram is comprised of two separate deflections separated by an interval of 260 msec, rather than a single, discrete spike. This is referred to as a split His potential and represents extremely slow conduction between the proximal and distal portions of the His bundle. In this particular example, conduction time between the distal His bundle and ventricular myocardium is normal; thus, the PR prolongation is due to first-degree intra-His block. In some patients with prolonged PR intervals, the site of conduction delay occurs in the more peripheral segments of the conducting system and ap-

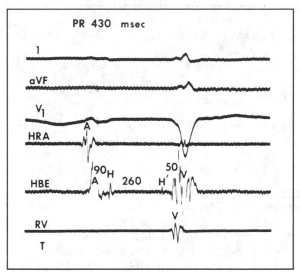

Figure 2. *Simultaneous recordings of (top to bottom) surface ECG leads I, aV$_F$, and V$_I$, as well as intracardiac electrogram from the high right atrium (HRA), His bundle region (HBE), and right ventricular apex (RV). First-degree AV block is present due to prolonged intra-His conduction time (260 msec). (From Josephson and Seides. With permission.)*

pears as a prolonged HV interval, with normal PA and AH intervals. This is referred to as first-degree infra-His block. Unlike first-degree AV nodal block, first-degree intra-His or infra-His blocks are manifestations of serious disease in the conduction system; many patients eventually develop higher degrees of block. In patients with syncope, the presence of first-degree intra-His or infra-His block is an indication for pacemaker therapy. Whether asymptomatic patients with first-degree intra- or infra-His block should receive prophylactic pacemakers is still a matter of conjecture.

SECOND-DEGREE BLOCK

Second-degree AV block is defined as intermittent failure of AV conduction and can be recognized as any of several well-known electrocardiographic patterns. *Type I* second-degree AV block is characterized by Wenckebach periodicity of AV conduction, in which the PR interval lengthens and the RR interval shortens during each cycle until a P wave fails to conduct to the ventricles, resulting in a long RR interval (Figure 3). Occasionally, these long RR intervals may be interrupted by the appearance of junctional escape beats. In its typical form, the PR interval is always shortest

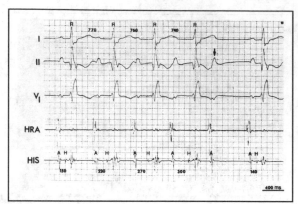

Figure 3. *Simultaneous recordings of surface ECG leads I, II, and V₁, as well as intracardiac electrograms from the high right atrium (HRA) and His bundle region (HIS). Right bundle branch block is present. The surface ECG demonstrates typical 5:4 type I second-degree AV block, with progressive prolongation of the PR interval until the fifth P wave fails to conduct to the ventricle (arrow). In this example, type I second-degree AV block is due to progressive slowing of AV nodal conduction time (AH interval) until conduction through the AV node fails.*

following the dropped QRS, and the greatest increment in PR interval occurs in the second cycle following the blocked P wave. However, this typical pattern may not always occur, and, particularly during long Wenckebach cycles, the PR interval may seem to stabilize for several beats; or, alternatively, the greatest increment in PR interval may occur with other than the second beat after the dropped QRS.

The most common site of type I second-degree AV block is the AV node. His bundle recordings in such cases (Figure 3) reveal progressive lengthening of the AH interval with a constant HV interval, until conduction through the AV node fails. As with first-degree AV nodal block, type I second-degree AV nodal block can occur in a wide variety of circumstances, including congenital or acquired disease of the AV node, digitalis intoxication, and inferior MI. Its presence does not always imply intrinsic disease, since it can occur spontaneously in well-trained endurance athletes and can usually be provoked in normal people by incremental atrial pacing. In some instances, type I second-degree AV block may occur not in the AV node but within the His bundle or in the more distal segments of the conducting system. During type I second-degree intra-His block, one sees a split His potential with progressive prolongation of conduction time between the proximal and distal por-

tions of the His bundle, culminating in failure of transmission to the distal His bundle and, thus, dropout of the QRS. In such cases the AH interval remains constant throughout, even though the ECG reveals Wenckebach periodicity. Type I second-degree infra-His block is also characterized by Wenckebach periodicity, but is due to progressive lengthening of conduction time in the distal conducting system. This appears as progressive prolongation of the HV interval until complete failure of transmission beyond the His bundle to the ventricles occurs, with dropout of the QRS. When evaluating a patient whose ECG reveals Wenckebach periodicity of AV conduction, the occurrence of particularly long Wenckebach cycles, with very little increment in PR interval, or atypical Wenckebach cycles should raise the suspicion of block within or below the His bundle. In such cases, particularly in patients with a history of syncope or presyncope, the diagnosis should be confirmed with a His bundle recording.

Type II second-degree AV block differs from type I in that sudden intermittent failure of AV transmission occurs without any detectable prolongation of conduction time before the dropped beat. The electrocardiographic appearance of this is the sudden failure of a P wave to conduct to the ventricles in the setting of a constant PR interval before and after the blocked beat (Figure 4). Unlike type I second-degree AV block, which can occur within the AV node, within the His bundle, or below the His bundle, type II second-degree AV block occurring within the AV node has never been conclusively demonstrated. Rather, when this type of block occurs, its presence is always a reflection of conduction disease either within or below the bundle of His.

Although type I second-degree AV block is easily distinguishable from type II block in most cases, it is important to note that misdiagnosis may result from only a quick, casual inspection of the surface ECG. When Wenckebach cycles are long in type I block, as described above, the progressive increment in PR interval may be small and easily overlooked, giving the false impression of type II block. Furthermore, the diagnosis of Wenckebach periodicity can be reliably made only in the setting of a constant sinus rate. A sudden increase in sinus rate of only a few beats/minute, for example, can result in block of the first P wave after the rate increase, giving a false impression of type II block. In such cases, careful inspection of a longer rhythm strip after the rate increase will usually make Wenckebach periodicity ap-

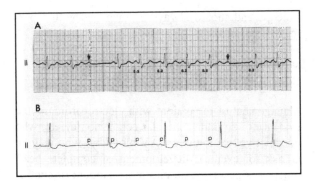

Figure 4. *(A) Lead II of the surface ECG during type II second-degree AV block. The PR interval remains constant preceding and following P waves, which fail to conduct to the ventricles (arrows). (B) Lead II of the surface ECG during complete AV block. There is dissociation between P waves and QRS complexes. Atrial rate is typically faster than the ventricular rate. The normal QRS complex suggests block in the AV node with an escape focus high in the His bundle.*

parent. Similarly, the presence of atrial premature depolarizations makes it difficult to distinguish type I from type II block.

A third type of second-degree AV block is that in which the ratio of P waves to QRS complexes is 2:1, 3:1, or even higher. Obviously, such cases cannot be labeled either type I or type II and, instead, are simply referred to as *high-grade* second-degree AV block. This type of second-degree AV block may occur either in the AV node itself or within or below the His bundle. Occasionally, having a patient exercise may be useful in determining the most likely site of block. The increased sympathetic tone associated with exercise usually improves conduction through the AV node and may thus change the conduction ratio from 2:1 to 1:1. In contrast, block within or below the His bundle is usually exacerbated during rapid heart rates and thus is made worse during exercise. Nevertheless, it is rarely possible to predict the site of block reliably from the surface ECG. Since these distinctions may have important therapeutic implications, symptomatic patients with high-grade second-degree AV block should always undergo electrophysiologic study before pacemaker therapy is advised.

In general, decisions about how best to treat patients with second-degree AV block should be based on the clinical circumstances in which the block occurs, as well as knowledge about the precise site in the conducting system that is diseased. As mentioned previously, type I second-degree AV nodal block usually occurs in association with some transient active problem such as acute rheumatic fever, digitalis intoxication, or acute inferior MI. Although, in such cases, temporary pacing may be required if higher degrees of block occur, the AV conduction disturbance usually disappears as the underlying active process subsides; permanent pacing is seldom, if ever, required. Moreover, in this setting, His bundle recording to document the site of block is not essential. On the other hand, patients who develop type I second-degree block in the absence of some acute intercurrent process, particularly elderly patients with severe coronary artery disease or calcific aortic or mitral disease, should undergo electrophysiologic testing to determine the site of the block. If type I second-degree block in such patients is localized within or below the His bundle, particularly in the setting of prior syncope or presyncope, the likelihood of progression to higher degrees of block is high and permanent pacing should be recommended. Similarly, patients with type II second-degree block or high-grade second-degree block should undergo His bundle studies to confirm the diagnosis before having a permanent pacemaker implanted.

THIRD-DEGREE BLOCK

Third-degree or *complete* AV block is simply defined as complete failure of conduction between the atria and ventricles. In the presence of sinus rhythm, third-degree AV block can readily be distinguished electrocardiographically as dissociation between P waves and QRS complexes, the ventricles being governed by a subatrial pacemaker that is invariably slower than the sinus node (Figure 4B). Occasionally, a supraventricular rhythm other than sinus (atrial fibrillation, for example) may be present. Third-degree AV block, like the lesser degrees of block, may occur at any site in the AV conducting system, such as in the AV node or within or below the His bundle. In some instances, it may be possible to define precisely the site of block electrocardiographically by examination of the ventricular rate and morphology of the QRS complexes. The rate at which subatrial pacemakers depolarize, in general, decreases as one proceeds distally along the His bundle and bundle branches. Thus, third-degree AV block with a ventricular rate greater than 50/min and QRS complexes that are normal in duration is almost certainly due to block in the AV node, with an escape focus high in the His bundle; ventricular rates of 30–40/min, with aberrant QRS complexes, suggest subnodal block with an escape focus in the bundle branches or distal Purkinje system. However, considerable overlap in spontaneous firing rates occurs at different sites of the His-Purkinje system, and bundle branch block patterns may be present even with pacemaker foci located high in the AV junction. Thus, His bundle recording is often necessary to locate the site of block accurately.

The management of patients with third-degree AV nodal block is usually straightforward. If such block occurs in association with a transient active problem, such as acute inferoposterior MI, myocarditis, drug intoxication, or recent cardiac surgery, it will usually resolve spontaneously with time. Such patients are best managed expectantly, without resorting to temporary or permanent pacemakers, provided the junctional escape rate is sufficiently rapid to prevent symptoms or hemodynamic compromise. In some patients, most notably those with congenital complete heart block, the third-degree AV nodal block is fixed rather than transient. Fortunately, most of these patients are asymptomatic, since the rate of the junctional escape pacemaker is adequate to maintain a normal cardiac output; these patients do not require permanent pacemakers. However, occasional patients with congenital third-degree AV nodal block will have a history of syncope, despite an apparently adequate junctional escape rate. In such cases, observing the patient's response to exercise and electrophysiologic testing are important steps in determining the advisability of pacemaker therapy.

Most instances of third-degree AV block are due not to block in the AV node, but rather block within or below the His bundle. In most reported series, third-degree intra-His or infra-His block accounts for nearly 80% of cases of complete heart block. His bundle recordings from patients with third-degree intra-His block typically reveal split His potentials and complete AV dissociation occurring between the proximal and distal His deflections. Alternatively, in cases of third-degree infra-His block, one would instead see a single His spike following each atrial electrogram and dissociated ventricular complexes without a preceding His spike. Functionally, third-degree intra- and infra-His blocks can be considered together. In these cases, the ventricular rate is always slow and unresponsive to autonomic interventions. Typically, patients with such blocks present with a history of

syncope and should always be managed with a permanent pacemaker.

MANAGEMENT OF INTRAVENTRICULAR CONDUCTION DEFECTS

Management of the patient with electrocardiographic evidence of an intraventricular conduction defect, who does not yet exhibit overt AV block but who may be at risk for eventual development of complete heart block, has generated an enormous amount of controversy over the past decade and remains a perplexing issue. In order to understand the prognostic implications of the bundle branch blocks and nonspecific intraventricular conduction defects, an understanding of the functional anatomy of the His-Purkinje system is essential (see also Chapter 10).

The His bundle in the normal human heart originates near the central fibrous body at a point where fibers from the distal end of the AV node coalesce into large longitudinal Purkinje fibers. Anatomically, it forms a discrete bundle that usually courses down the left side of the membranous interventricular septum to the crest of the muscular septum, where it bifurcates into the right and left bundle branches. The right bundle branch is itself a discrete bundle that continues down the right side of the muscular septum to the right ventricular apex, at which point it arborizes into the septal and right ventricular free wall myocardium. In contrast, the left bundle fans out broadly over the left septal surface shortly after its origin. The left bundle branch functions electrophysiologically as though it were composed of two separate divisions, the anterior and posterior fascicles. This knowledge is based upon commonly observed electrocardiographic patterns of left ventricular conduction defects. When conduction delay or block occurs in the anterior fascicle, the result is delayed activation of the upper anterior wall of the left ventricle. This pattern of intraventricular conduction is referred to as *left anterior hemiblock*. The electrocardiographic hallmarks of left anterior hemiblock include a QRS axis in the frontal plane equal to or more negative than $-45°$, small initial R waves in the inferior leads, and then large S waves inferiorly, with dominant R waves in leads I and aV_L. Conduction delay or block in the posterior fascicle of the left bundle branch results in a different electrocardiographic pattern, referred to as *left posterior hemiblock*. The salient electrocardiographic features of left posterior hemiblock include a QRS axis in the frontal plane $\geq +110°$,

Table 1. Prognostic Value of Electrophysiologic Testing to Assess Chronic Bundle Branch Block		
Distribution of HV interval among 313 patients	Group I (<54 msec) Group II (55–69) Group III (>70)	31% 32% 37%
Incidence of development of high-grade AV block during follow-up period (mean three years)	Group I 4% Group II 2% Group III 12%	
Greatest risk for development of high-grade AV block	Infranodal block during atrial pacing. HV interval >100 msec.	

Value of permanent pacemaker implantation
    Reduction of cardiac mortality
    Reduction of sudden death
    Relief of symptoms
	No
	No
	Yes	

(Adapted from Scheinman et al. 1982. See Bibliography.)		

a small initial R wave in lead I, small inferior Q waves, and an initial R wave in lead V_1. This electrocardiographic diagnosis, however, can only be made in the absence of clinical evidence for right ventricular hypertrophy or pulmonary disease. Left posterior hemiblock is less common than left anterior hemiblock, in all likelihood because the posterior fascicle usually has a dual blood supply from both the left anterior descending and posterior descending coronary arteries. It is most commonly seen in the setting of previous extensive myocardial infarction.

In view of the trifascicular nature of the intraventricular conducting system (right bundle branch, left anterior fascicle, and left posterior fascicle) it is clear that as long as one of these major fascicles is able to conduct normally, the risk of developing complete heart block below the His bundle is quite small, even in the presence of bundle branch block or hemiblock involving the remaining two fascicles. In such a situation, one would still expect the HV interval, which is a direct measure of conduction below the bundle of His, to be normal or nearly normal. Thus, in approaching patients with intraventricular conduction defects, there are two important questions that must be considered. First, what is the most effective method for assessing the functional integrity of the apparently uninvolved fascicle or fascicles? And second, if conduction disease can be demonstrated in all three fascicles, does this reliably predict subsequent development of complete heart block?

The answer to the first of these questions is reasonably straightforward. Clinical electrophysiologic studies of various intraventricular conduction defects demonstrate that, in most circumstances, the QRS morphology and length of the PR interval on the surface ECG are of little value in assessing the functional integrity of the His-Purkinje system. For example, in patients who have right bundle branch block associated with either left anterior or left posterior fascicular block, the ECG shows evidence of conduction disease in two out of the three major fascicles. The same is true in patients who have complete left bundle branch block. Unfortunately, the PR interval in such cases is a notoriously poor indicator of disease in the remaining fascicle. In many cases, PR prolongation in patients with electrocardiographic evidence of bifascicular block is due to first-degree AV nodal block, the HV interval being quite normal. In such patients, conduction in the third fascicle clearly is not jeopardized. Conversely, there are some patients who have nonspecific intraventricular conduction defects without complete bundle branch block, hemiblock, or even a prolonged PR interval, in whom the HV interval may be markedly prolonged.

Thus, trifascicular conduction disease can rarely be documented on the basis of a surface ECG; patients with a history of syncope or presyncope and intraventricular conduction defects, who are suspected of having trifascicular disease, should undergo His bundle recording with measurement of the HV interval. There are, however, two important exceptions to this

Table 2. Evaluation and Management of Patients with Intraventricular Conduction Defects

Clinical Presentation	Need for EP Study	Permanent Pacemaker
LBBB		
Asymptomatic	No	No
Symptomatic	Yes	HV >100 msec, subnodal block during atrial pacing
RBBB		
Asymptomatic	No	No
Symptomatic	Yes	HV >100 msec, subnodal block during atrial pacing
RBBB + Hemiblock		
Asymptomatic	No	No
Symptomatic	Yes	HV >100 msec, subnodal block during atrial pacing
Alternating LBBB + RBBB		
Asymptomatic	No	No
Symptomatic	Yes	If other causes excluded
IVCD before cardiac surgery	?	?

IVCD = intraventricular conduction defect; LBBB = left bundle branch block; RBBB = right bundle branch block; EP = electrophysiology; HV = HV interval.

generalization. Patients who have right bundle branch block associated with alternating left anterior and left posterior hemiblock or patients who demonstrate alternating complete right and complete left bundle branch block clearly have significant trifascicular disease and do not require measurement of the HV interval.

Having accepted the concept that, in most circumstances, measurement of the HV interval is a prerequisite for conclusively demonstrating trifascicular conduction disease, the next issue is whether HV prolongation in patients with intraventricular conduction defects is a reliable predictor of eventual complete heart block. Obviously, a related question is whether implantation of a permanent pacemaker in such patients will have a measurable impact on their prognosis. There is still considerable controversy about the correct answers to both of these questions.

In a study of 313 patients with chronic bundle branch block who underwent electrophysiologic study, Scheinman et al. (1982) subdivided the patients into those with normal HV intervals (Group I, Table 1), mildly prolonged HV intervals (Group II, Table 1) and markedly prolonged HV intervals (Group III, Table 1). During a mean follow-up period of three years, progression to complete heart block occurred more frequently in the Group III patients, and was particularly likely to occur if the HV interval was >100 msec or if block below the AV node could be pro-

voked by rapid atrial pacing. Of particular interest was the observation that implantation of a permanent pacemaker had no significant impact on overall cardiac mortality or the incidence of sudden death, although it was effective in relief of symptoms due to bradycardia.

In view of these findings, it seems reasonable to conclude that patients who have symptoms of syncope or presyncope in the absence of neurologic disease to explain their symptoms, and who also have evidence of an intraventricular conduction defect, including complete or incomplete bundle branch block with or without associated hemiblock, should undergo electrophysiologic study. This study includes assessment of sinus node function, measurement of baseline HV interval, and also provocative maneuvers such as rapid and programmed ventricular stimulation to rule out ventricular tachycardia. If HV intervals are prolonged in such patients or if second- or third-degree intra- or infra-His block can be provoked, such patients should probably be treated with a permanent pacemaker (Table 2). Another category of patients who may be candidates for electrophysiologic testing are those with serious underlying heart disease and intraventricular conduction defect who are scheduled for major cardiac surgery. If HV prolongation or provocable high-grade infra-His block is found, serious consideration should be given to implanting permanent epicardial pacing wires at the time of surgery, although the subsequent use of these pacing wires should depend on the patient's postoperative course (Table 2). With regard to patients who have intraventricular conduction defects but who are asymptomatic, it is more difficult to recommend electrophysiologic testing with any conviction. It is probably more prudent simply to follow such patients, relying on the surface ECG and presence or absence of symptoms to determine when further evaluation is warranted.

Bibliography

Denes P, Dhingra RC, Wu D, et al: Sudden death in patients with chronic bifascicular block. *Arch Intern Med* 137:1005, 1977.

Denes P, Levy L, Pick A, et al: The incidence of typical and atypical AV Wenckbach periodicity. *Am Heart J* 89:26, 1975.

Dhingra RC, Denes P, Wu D, et al: Prospective observations in patients with chronic bundle branch block and marked HV prolongation. *Circulation* 53:600, 1976.

Josephson ME, Seides SF: *Clinical Cardiac Electrophysiology.* Philadelphia: Lea and Febiger; 1979.

McAnulty JH, Rahimtoola SH, Murphy ES, et al: A prospective study of sudden death in "high risk" bundle branch block. *N Engl J Med* 299:209, 1978.

Narula OS: *His Bundle Electrocardiography and Clinical Electrophysiology.* Philadelphia: F. A. Davis; 1975.

Narula OS, Narula JT: Junctional pacemakers in man. Response to overdrive suppression with and without parasympathetic blockade. *Circulation* 49:925, 1970.

Rosen KM, Dhingra RC, Loeb HS, et al: Chronic heart block in adults. *Arch Intern Med* 131:663, 1973.

Samet P, El-Sherif N, eds: *Cardiac Pacing.* New York: Grune & Stratton; 1980.

Scheinman MM, Peters RW, Modin G, et al: Prognostic value of infranodal conduction time in patients with chronic bundle branch block. *Circulation* 56:240, 1977.

Scheinman et al: Value of H-Q interval in patients with bundle branch block and the role of prophylactic permanent pacing. *Am J Cardiol* 50:1316, 1982.

21 Pacemaker Therapy

Andrew C. Eisenhauer

When the first pacing system was implanted some 30 years ago, artificial cardiac pacing was largely viewed as a therapy to prevent recurrent syncope and death. Then, committing a patient to a lifetime of cardiac pacing was done with trepidation. Today, cardiac pacing is standard therapy not only for treating manifest syncope but also for controlling near-syncope, exercise intolerance, and chronotropic incompetence.

INDICATIONS

Indications for the implantation of permanent pacing systems have been developed in a consensus conference by a combined committee of the American Heart Association and the American College of Cardiology (Frye et al.). In addition, the Health Care Financing Administration has published guidelines for reimbursement for pacemaker procedures.

Clinically, the reason for implanting a permanent pacing system is generally to prevent symptoms from an inappropriately slow heart rate. As a result, a central requirement for antibradycardia pacing is the presence of a documented symptomatic bradyarrhythmia. When such an event occurs and it is not due to a temporary and remediable cause (such as digitalis excess), permanent pacing is generally indicated. "Prophylactic" permanent pacing is not usually required except in very specific instances such as witnessed development of permanent left bundle branch block in the face of acute myocardial infarction (Tables 1–4).

The clinician contemplating implantation of a permanent pacing system should understand that the notion of a pacemaker is often very distressing to the patient. Patients often place their hopes for resolution of non-bradycardia–related symptoms on permanent pacing. The clinician must clearly define for the patient and the patient's family which symptoms may be expected to be improved by pacing and which symptoms may not.

Despite an extensive evaluation, the clinician is sometimes unable to document bradyarrhythmias as the cause of recurrent syncope, near-syncope, or lightheadedness. Occasionally, a pacing system may be implanted based solely on clinical judgment. This is an uncommon situation, but well within the range of normal clinical practice. By distinction, sinus pauses and periods of sinus bradycardia are very common, particularly in elderly patients and in young, physically active patients. The presence of these findings without associated symptoms should not by itself result in implantation of a pacing system. Except for a possible placebo effect, such implantation does not improve the patient's overall sense of well-being.

Episodic bradyarrhythmias may only be part of a complex disturbance in consciousness (such as vasodepressor syncope). Here, correcting the bradyarrhythmia, although appropriate, may only partially relieve symptoms. Thus, the clinician contemplating pacing should carefully search for a bradyarrhythmia that is correlated with the symptoms to derive the optimal risk/benefit ratio for the patient.

TECHNICAL CONSIDERATIONS

The performance and reliability of a pacing system are determined by the performance and reliability of its weakest component. Thirty years ago, unexpected and unintended component failures were common. Today, most pacing system anomalies are not due to component failure, but to a complex interaction of electrode-tissue interface, pacemaker programming, and the patient's intrinsic cardiac electrophysiology.

A pacing system can be conceptualized as performing two general medical functions: diagnosis and treatment. Diagnostically, a pacemaker must sense

Table 1. Indications for Pacing in Sinus Node Dysfunction	
Class I	**General agreement favors pacing** A. Documented symptomatic bradycardia
Class II	**Divergence of opinion** A. Bradycardia <40 beats/min without documented symptoms
Class III	**Pacing not indicated** A. Asymptomatic sinus bradycardia <40 beats/min due to concurrent drug therapy B. Symptoms suggestive of sinus bradycardia shown not to be associated with slow heart rate

Developed from American College of Cardiology/American Heart Association consensus panel. Modified from Frye et al. See Bibliography.

cardiac activity. If appropriate activity is not sensed, it must supply electrical stimuli to trigger cardiac activity that is lacking. The three areas of pacemaker function are *sensing, analysis* (logic), and *stimulation.* Sensing and stimulation involve not only the basic electronic system, but its interface with the patient.

The "hardware" components that make up a modern pacing system consist of the electrode/lead system and the pulse generator. The pulse generator itself is composed of an energy source and electronic circuit enclosed by a housing that shields the energy supply and circuit from contact with body fluids. Because almost all modern pacemakers are externally adjustable with a specific radiofrequency programming device, the programmer is considered an integral part of the pacing system.

Power Supply

Power is usually supplied by an electrolytic cell or cells arranged in a battery. An electrolytic cell consists of a positive and negative electrode separated by an electrolytic medium. The connection between these two electrodes causes current to flow outside of the cell from the electrochemical reaction. Normal cells contain a certain calculated maximum energy that can be provided over their useful lifetime. The theoretical maximum, however, is greater than the actual maximum because of internal losses. Further, the amount of energy contained in the cell in proportion to its size (energy density) is critical in developing compact pacing devices.

In the early days of pacing, mercury zinc cells were used. They were of relatively low energy density and their internal losses subjected them to unpredictable and sudden failure. Subsequently, a number of cells have been developed using lithium as a cation. In general, these have been successful and have provided high energy densities which, in combination with decreasing pacemaker power requirements, result in very durable devices. During the search for a reliable, durable power source, rechargeable cells, biogalvanic power sources and nuclear energy sources have also been used. Interestingly, nuclear sources are technically successful, but their value has been limited by concern over radiation exposure and component disposal. The availability of very good electrolytic power supplies and failure of other associated components as a limit on pacer longevity have also served to discourage the use of nuclear power sources.

Electronic Circuit

Early electronic circuits of the first implanted devices consisted of little more than a crystal oscillator to provide rhythmic outputs of the stimulating signals. These devices were "fixed-rate devices" that could not sense intrinsic cardiac activity. It quickly became apparent that it was desirable to develop miniature sense amplifiers so that intrinsic cardiac activity could be sensed through the exploring electrode at times when stimulation was not occurring. A device's output could then be suppressed or triggered, depending on the needs of the patient. Before availability of the transistor, no implantable pacemaker could be con-

Table 2. Indications for Pacing in Chronic Acquired Atrio-ventricular Block	
Class I	**General agreement favors pacing** A. Complete heart block accompanied by: Symptomatic bradycardia Congestive heart failure Ventricular ectopy Escape rate <40 beats/min or R-R >3 seconds Mental Confusion B. Second-degree heart block with symptomatic bradycardia C. Atrial fibrillation/flutter with conditions under A, above
Class II	**Divergence of opinion** A. Asymptomatic third-degree AV block: rate >40 beats/min B. Asymptomatic type II second-degree AV block C. Asymptomatic type I second-degree AV block (intra- or infra-His)
Class III	**Pacing not indicated** A. First-degree AV block B. Asymptomatic type I supra-His second-degree AV block
ACC/AHA consensus panel. Modified from Frye et al.	

structed that was small enough and had enough power to be useful. The transistor reduced these shortcomings. Initially, however, the manufacturing, connection and soldering of these devices elicited concerns about reliability. By the late 1970s, with the advent of microcircuitry, solid-state devices could be coupled with these chips, in which transistor-equivalent components number in the thousands. This development offered greater reliability and the possibility of cramming more functions into a smaller space. In modern devices, large-scale integrated circuit technology and microprocessors provide the equivalent of several hundred thousand solid-state components. In fact, current devices can be thought of as small programmable computers that modulate cardiac sensing and stimulation.

Housing

The function of the medium enclosing the components of the pulse generator is simple in concept but difficult to achieve. It must be inert chemically and biologically, and yet confer protection from the hos-

tile environment of the human body. It also must protect the patient from the outward leak of hazardous electrolytes. Early devices utilized silicone or epoxy coatings and were subject to expansion after the encroachment of moisture. Modern devices are triply sealed hermetically, with the electronic circuit and power supply individually isolated in a final sealed "can" constructed of titanium or stainless steel.

Leads

Early pacing systems stimulated the heart through surgically applied epicardial electrodes. The development in 1958 of temporary transvenous pacing and the subsequent refinement of the technique has led to its primacy in cardiac pacing. A transvenous lead consists of a conductor and insulator, and also of an exposed electrode to provide the pacing system/tissue interface. In the unipolar systems, a single electrode at the tip of the lead serves as the cathode and a metallic pacemaker can as an electrically active anode in contact with the tissue fluid. In contrast, bipolar leads are made up of two internal conductors that are

Table 3. Indications for Pacing in Chronic Bi- or Tri-fascicular Block	
Class I	**General agreement favors pacing** A. Intermittent third-degree block with symptomatic bradycardia B. Intermittent Mobitz type II AV block with symptoms
Class II	**Divergence of opinion** A. Intermittent Mobitz type II AV block without symptoms B. "VOODOO" syncope of unknown cause
Class III	**Pacing not indicated** A. Fascicular blocks without AV block or symptoms B. Fascicular blocks, first-degree AV block without symptoms
ACC/AHA consensus panel. Modified from Frye et al.	

Table 4. Considerations that May Influence the Clinical Decision to Implant a Pacing System
Absence of other life-threatening disease
Associated cardiac condition aggravated by bradycardia
Motor vehicle operator
Remote or inaccessible medical attention
Medications that depress conductivity/automaticity
Slowness of basic escape rhythm
Cerebrovascular disease aggravated by bradycardia
Desires of patient and family

insulated one from the other and from the external environment. Each is connected to a separate electrode. The cathode is formed by an electrode at the tip of the lead and the anode by a ring electrode mounted 1–2 cm more proximally. Unipolar leads can generally be manufactured with a smaller diameter and are easier to handle during implantation. The stimulus artifact produced by the output of a unipolar system is large and easily visible electrocardiographically. However, the "antenna effect," created by the wide separation of anode and cathode, renders these systems vulnerable to external interference. Bipolar systems tend to be larger and provide smaller stimulus artifacts, but are far more resistant to external interference at high sensitivities.

MODES OF CARDIAC PACING

The first implanted artificial cardiac pacemakers were simply devices to rhythmically stimulate the heart (Figure 1). Often, the patients in whom they were implanted had little or no intrinsic ventricular activity

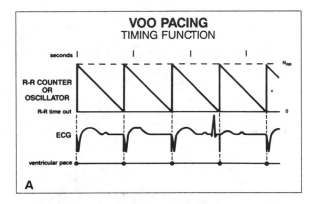

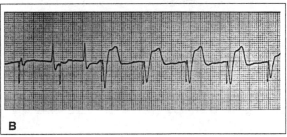

Figure 1. *A. Timing "ladder" diagram for VOO pacing. Pacemaker events are listed on the left. Time is along the horizontal axis. Following a ventricular paced event (the first QRS on the left), the RR counter resets and begins "counting down" a prescribed length of time. At the end of this RR interval or "RR timeout," a second stimulus artifact is placed and the oscillator is reset. Rhythmic stimulus artifacts are produced throughout the remainder of this figure. A native QRS occurs and, appropriately, is not sensed. (Courtesy of Medtronic, Inc.) B. Accompanying ECG strip of a patient with a VOO pacemaker, showing appropriate capture but a complete lack of sensing of ventricular events.*

without cardiac pacing. The sensing of patients' native QRS complexes to avoid potential competition was not a serious problem. In fact, even when patients did have intrinsic cardiac activity, competition between it and artificial pacemaker activity did not usually result in adverse reactions. Insertion of a stimulus into the vulnerable portion of the T wave only rarely resulted in generation of a ventricular tachyarrhythmia. This difficulty was initially solved by developing sensing amplifiers that would trigger a pacemaker output immediately upon sensing a QRS complex. This triggering also provided direct electrocardiographic evidence of appropriate sensing and stimulation by "marking" each of these events with

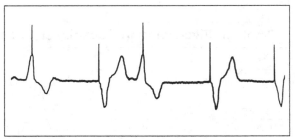

Figure 2. *VVT ECG strip. Every QRS is marked by a stimulus artifact. In this fashion, appropriate sensing is easily demonstrated.*

a stimulus artifact. Additional impulses would be triggered if no QRS complexes were sensed during a time corresponding to the escape rate of the pacemaker (Figure 2). This mode of pacing worked very well, but it did not reduce the frequency of stimulus outputs to conserve energy when intrinsic cardiac activity occurred. As a result, other sensing circuitry was developed to inhibit pulse generator output except after periods of cardiac electrical "silence" (Figure 3). Devices that either suppressed or triggered pacemaker

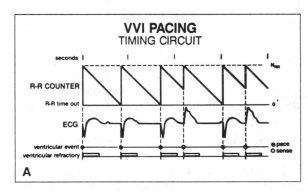

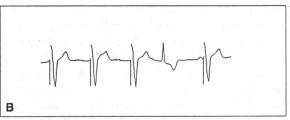

Figure 3. *VVI timing diagram (A) and accompanying ECG strip (B). In the timing diagram, the sensing function is apparent. In the rhythm strip, the fourth QRS from the left is above the pacing rate and resets the RR counter. (Timing diagram courtesy of Medtronic, Inc.)*

Table 5. Five-Position Pacemaker Code					
Position	I	II	III	IV	V
Category	Chamber(s) paced	Chamber(s) sensed	Mode of response(s)	Programmable functions	Special tachyarrhythmia functions
Letters used	**V**-Ventricle	**V**-Ventricle	**T**-Triggered	**P**-Simple programmable (rate and/or output)	**B**-Bursts
	A-Atrium	**A**-Atrium	**I**-Inhibited	**M**-Multi-programmable	**N**-Normal rate competition
	D-Double	**D**-Double	**D**-Double*	**C**-Multi-programmable with telemetry	**S**-Scanning
				R-Rate-modulated	
			O-None		
		O-None	**R**-Reverse†	**O**-None	**E**-External
Manu-facturer's designation only	**S**-Single chamber‡	**S**-Single chamber‡			

* Atrial triggered and ventricular inhibited
† Activated by tachycardia and (usually) bradycardia
‡ Can be used for atrial or ventricular pacing (manufacturer's designation)

output could also, under certain circumstances, be applied to atrial pacing. It soon became necessary to develop a nomenclature for the description of pacemaker function. The Intersociety Commission on Heart Disease Resources (ICHD) developed the first three-position pacemaker code. The first position referred to the chamber paced, the second to the chamber whose activity was sensed, and the third position to the mode of response. The pacemaker that paced and sensed the ventricle and responded to intrinsic cardiac activity by *triggering* a stimulus output is functioning in the VVT mode. In a similar fashion, a ventricular pacemaker whose output was *inhibited* by a native QRS is a device in the VVI mode. The earliest fixed-rate, non-sensing devices were VOO pacemakers. Devices with their single leads placed in the atrium are AOO, AAT and AAI devices (Table 5) (Parsonnet et al. 1981). The ICHD code was later expanded to five positions. The fourth position outlines programmable and rate-modulated functions and the last indicates antitachycardia features.

Even before the first implantation of a permanent pacing system in 1958, some investigators realized that ventricular pacing was not a very physiologic solution to the problem of complete or episodic atrioventricular (AV) block. The normal cardiac impulse arises in the sinoatrial (SA) node and, after the appropriate AV nodal delay (corresponding to the PR interval on surface ECG), travels to the ventricles, producing a QRS complex and subsequent mechanical ventricular systole. Simple ventricular pacing did not mimic normal cardiac activation and did not seem to be the ideal solution to the problem of AV nodal dysfunction. In 1954, Folkman and Watkins developed an apparatus for replacing AV conduction in the canine model of heart block. The apparatus consisted of a sense amplifier that would identify intrinsic atrial activity and, after an appropriate delay, stimulate the ventricle; it was the forerunner of the VAT pacemaker in which ventricular pacing is induced by atrial activity (Figure 4). Although this mode is not used today, the understanding of how it was developed and

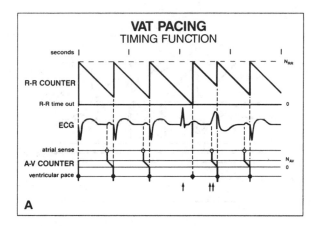

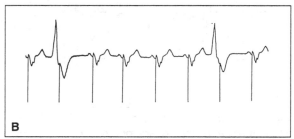

Figure 4. *VAT timing diagram (A) and accompanying ECG strip (B). After the first paced QRS in this diagram, the RR counter is reset (there is no ventricular sensing). A P wave occurs, which initiates another timing cycle (the AV counter), represented at the bottom of the diagram. After this AV delay, a ventricular stimulus is produced that resets the RR counter. This series of events is repeated. After the third QRS, the RR counter is reset again and begins counting down. A premature ventricular complex occurs (first arrow) and it is appropriately not sensed. A ventricular stimulus is produced on the T wave of this PVC, and the RR counter is reset. A hidden P wave occurs (two arrows), triggering another ventricular stimulus artifact, this time in the middle of a PVC. The RR counter is reset once again. Note the atrial refractory period during which atrial sensing cannot occur. The ECG illustrates VAT pacing. (Timing diagram courtesy of Medtronic, Inc.)*

how it behaves is important to the understanding of modes in current use.

VAT Pacing

With development of the VAT mode of atrial-triggered ventricular pacing came the need to develop an electronic analog of conduction system refractoriness.

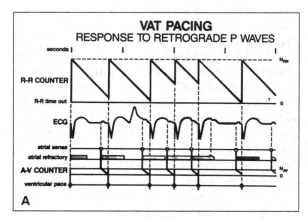

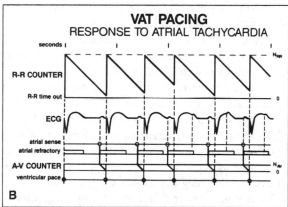

Figure 5. *VAT pacing response to retrograde P waves (A) and to atrial tachycardia (B). In panel A, pacemaker-mediated tachycardia develops (the fourth, fifth, and sixth QRS complexes from the left). The retrograde P wave after the sixth QRS falls within the atrial refractory period and is therefore not sensed. The next event is therefore lower-rate ventricular pacing. In panel B, the atrial rate has accelerated so that only every other P wave falls outside the refractory period, resulting in tracking this fast rate in a 2:1 fashion. (Both panels courtesy of Medtronic, Inc.)*

Just as 1:1 AV conduction at the onset of atrial flutter could be deleterious to a nonpaced patient, so could rapid ventricular pacing triggered by atrial tachyarrhythmias in a patient with a VAT device (Figure 5). Thus, sensing circuitry needs to be "deaf," or refractory, to intrinsic atrial activity that occurs above a selected rate to prevent inappropriate rapid ventricular pacing from the sensing of atrial tachyarrhythmias or wayward extracardiac stimuli.

An additional technical problem was also created by sensing and pacing in multiple chambers. The voltage required to stimulate is orders of magnitude greater than that produced by intrinsic cardiac activity. Thus, the stimulus outputs produced in one chamber could potentially be sensed by an alert sense-amplifier connected to another chamber. For example, a theoretical VAT device could sense atrial activity and produce a stimulus output in the ventricle, and then sense that remote or "far field" stimulus as another atrial event. This would trigger a ventricular stimulus output which itself would be sensed by the atrial channel, inducing a third stimulus output and continuing indefinitely. A potential solution to this problem is to render the sense amplifiers deaf during a stimulus output. This property, referred to as "blanking," prevents self-inhibition or self-triggering, known as "crosstalk."

Initially, VAT pacing was technically difficult. The devices were bulky and transvenous atrial leads were large and difficult to position reliably. Intrinsic ventricular activity was not sensed, so there was often competition with ventricular extrasystoles, junctional beats, or, if heart block was not continual and complete, normally conducted beats. In addition, blanking periods and refractoriness of the atrial channel were so long as to prevent the appropriate tracking of even modest degrees of sinus tachycardia.

Even with the poor reliability of early atrial sensing leads, technical problems with prolonged atrial refractory periods, blanking, and ventricular competition, it became clear that some patients *required* this dual-chamber pacing. In these patients, simple ventricular pacing was intolerable. Some became hypotensive and sensed cannon a-waves in the neck veins and noted very poor exercise tolerance. These patients were suffering from what has become known as the "pacemaker syndrome," involving ventriculoatrial (VA) conduction with retrograde activation of the atria during ventricular pacing. While not all patients with this VA conduction have the pacemaker syndrome, all patients with the syndrome have VA conduction.

DVI Pacing

A potential electronic solution to the problem of the need to maintain AV synchrony but avoiding the difficulties of VAT pacing was to couple an atrial stimulus output with a ventricular pacemaker. In this mode, both chambers are paced but only ventricular activity inhibits pacemaker output. This DVI mode maintains

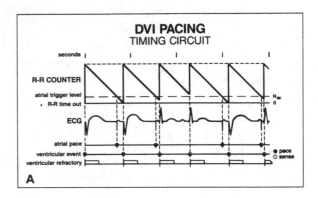

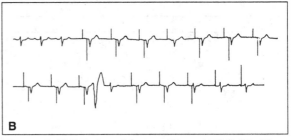

Figure 6. *DVI timing diagram (A) and ECG (B). The ECG shows appropriate lack of atrial sensing. (Timing diagram courtesy of Medtronic, Inc.)*

AV synchrony, but at the expense of being unable to track intrinsic atrial activity (Figure 6). Unlike VAT pacing, it is not an arrangement that produces "replacement" of AV nodal function. It was, however, a good solution to the maintenance of AV synchrony. Just as VAT pacing provides potential competition between ventricular stimulus outputs and intrinsic ventricular activity, DVI pacing can compete with intrinsic atrial activity and may promote atrial fibrillation. An additional electronic problem became evident as DVI pacing developed: How could a device following an atrial stimulus artifact distinguish between appropriate AV conduction and the production of an "early" QRS, a premature ventricular complex (PVC), or extracardiac electronic noise? One would not want the ventricular output to be inappropriately suppressed by crosstalk or noise; nor would one want a stimulus in the vulnerable period of the T wave after a PVC. To solve this problem, early DVI devices were "committed," that is, a ventricular stimulus output was committed to occur following the preceding atrial stimulus, regardless of what happened during the AV delay. Later devices became "partially committed," ignoring everything in the early part of the AV delay but responding with suppression of ventricular output should a ventricular event be sensed in the latter part of the AV interval.

It quickly became apparent that not only was it desirable to maintain AV synchrony in patients with the pacemaker syndrome, but some patients clearly required AV synchrony to maintain active ventricular filling and optimum cardiac output. In some patients, sinus bradycardia at 35 beats/min was preferable hemodynamically to ventricular pacing at 60 beats/min with the loss of AV synchrony. For this reason, "hysteresis" was added to some VVI pacemakers—the pacing rate could be programmed to exceed the escape rate by a selected amount. For example, a VVI device with a programmed rate of 70 beats/min and 20 beats/min of hysteresis would require the heart rate to fall to 50 beats/min or below before it initiated pacing at a rate of 70 beats/min. While theoretically helpful, the electrocardiographic consequences were often confusing to the uninitiated. Further, frequent ineffective PVCs (especially in a bigeminal pattern) could reduce the effective pacing heart rate to below the hysteresis level and produce symptoms from unsupported bradycardia.

DDD Pacing

The benefits of maintenance of AV synchrony became particularly apparent in patients after cardiac surgery. Improved blood pressure and cardiac output could often be related to the maintenance of AV synchrony. However, neither VAT nor DVI devices could *both* track atrial activity and provide AV nodal replacement to maintain AV synchrony under all conditions. Technical developments in lead technology and construction, hybrid and microcircuit design, and surgical techniques made possible the development of devices that function in the DDD mode—sensing and pacing in both chambers. A device that can be programmed to the DDD mode is, in effect, two separate pacing devices interconnected by logic circuitry.

The objective of the DDD mode is to never allow an RR interval to be longer than that corresponding to the programmed lower rate of the pacemaker. Thus, following a ventricular event (either sensed or paced), both atrial and ventricular channels are alert. The next "expected event" would be the appearance of a P wave. This is "expected" with an interval corresponding to that of the lower rate minus the programmed AV delay. For example, if the device is

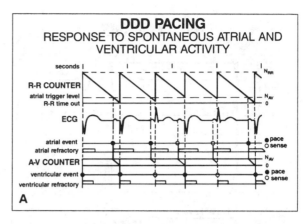

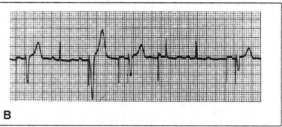

Figure 7. *DDD timing diagram (A) and ECG (B). In the ECG, the first complex illustrates atrioventricular (AV) pacing with fusion between pacemaker stimulus artifact and QRS. The second complex shows spontaneous atrial activity with normal AV conduction. The third complex is P-triggered ventricular pacing. The fourth complex again shows AV pacing with ventricular fusion and the fifth, atrial pacing with normal AV conduction and suppression of ventricular output. Although at first glance, this strip appears confusing, it outlines all the appropriate and normal responses of a system programmed to the DDD mode. (Panel A courtesy of Medtronic, Inc.)*

programmed to a lower rate of 60 beats/min, the corresponding RR interval is 1,000 msec. If that device's AV delay is programmed to 200 msec, then a P wave would be "expected" within the 800 msec after a ventricular event. This period is known as the VA interval, or "VA time out." If a P wave does not occur during this time, the device stimulates the atrium and remains alert for the expected occurrence of a QRS complex within the programmed AV delay. If a QRS does not occur, a ventricular stimulus is emitted triggering one. During the AV delay (with the exception of the blanking period), the ventricular channel remains alert for the occurrence of PVCs. In this fashion, the device senses and paces in both

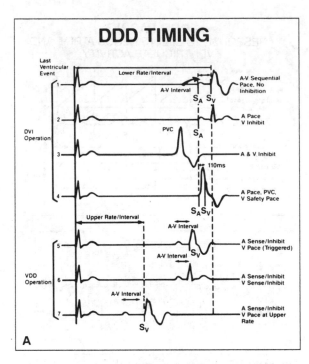

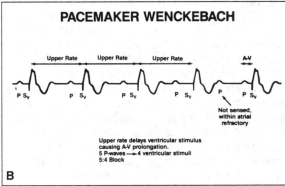

Figure 8. *A. The variety of responses possible for a dual-chamber pacemaker programmed to the DDD mode. B. Pacemaker Wenkebach. (Courtesy of Medtronic, Inc.)*

chambers (Figures 7 and 8). Thus, P-triggered ventricular pacing is permitted, retaining for the patient (if sinus node response is intact) the ability to increase ventricular rate with increasing sinus rates.

Of course, the same potential difficulty exists here as in VAT devices: How can appropriate sinus tachycardia be tracked and inappropriate atrial tachyarrhythmias be rejected? A solution exists in the various upper rate responses designed into dual-chamber pacemakers. When the DDD mode first became available, there were two modes of response, depending on the device. The first involved the development of simple 2:1 AV block. If, following a ventricular event, an atrial event occurred such that triggering a ventricular event would yield ventricular stimulation at a rate above the programmed upper rate of the device, that stimulus would simply be suppressed. This resulted in simple 2:1 AV block. An alternative design was to extend the AV delay such that a ventricular stimulus would be emitted at the upper rate of the pacemaker. This would result in a "pacemaker Wenckebach" (Figure 8B), with a "dropped" beat occurring when a P wave falls within the post-ventricular atrial refractory period. Additional electronic algorithms have been developed to control the upper rate response, such as decreasing the AV delay with increasing heart rate, "rate smoothing," in which the R-R intervals are controlled by an average of the preceding R-R intervals, and others.

Even as dual-chamber pacing was required in some patients with VA conduction and the pacemaker syndrome, it did not abolish all difficulties related to retrograde conduction. Even in the presence of antegrade block, retrograde conduction following a ventricular stimulus may occur. This can produce a retrograde P wave following a QRS complex. This P wave may be electronically similar to a native P wave and indistinguishable from it. If the dual chamber device's atrial channel were alert when a retrograde P wave occurred, it would sense this as another P wave and activate the AV delay while "looking" for a subsequent QRS. If none were to occur, the device would insert one. If this resulted in another retrograde P wave, the cycle could continue indefinitely, producing a "pacemaker-mediated" tachycardia (Figure 9). This could be partially avoided by rendering the atrial channel "deaf" during and immediately after a ventricular event. This period, known as the post-ventricular atrial refractory period (PVARP), was a fixed interval of approximately 250 msec in early devices. It quickly became clear that VA conduction was a transient phenomenon—at times occurring at relatively long intervals and producing P waves outside the early refractory periods. Pacemaker-mediated tachycardia often occurred and was a clinical problem. At present, the PVARP is programmable on all available devices and must be adjusted to prevent sensing of retrograde P waves in patients with VA conduction. Further, algorithms have been developed to interrupt the cycle of tracking of retrograde P waves and prevent continuous high-rate pacing in a pacemaker-mediated tachycardia. The best solution to the

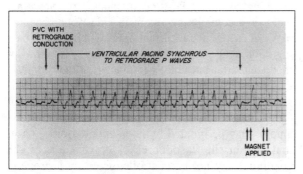

Figure 9. *Pacemaker-mediated tachycardia. Note the initiation by a premature ventricular contraction (PVC) with retrograde conduction and termination by applying a magnet to the pacemaker (disabling its sensing functions) and interrupting the "endless" feedback loop. (Reprinted from Harthorne JW, Eisenhauer AC, Steinhaus DM: Cardiac pacing. In: Eagle KA, Haber E, DeSanctis RW, Austen WG, eds.: The Practice of Cardiology, 2nd ed. Boston: Little Brown; 1989, p. 305. With permission.)*

problem, however, is careful adjustment of the refractory periods based on careful clinical observation and follow-up.

RATE-MODULATED PACING

The ideal candidate for a dual-chamber pacemaker programmed to the DDD mode is a patient with only AV block and a normal sinus node. The dual-chamber device will restore the patient's AV integrity by "replacing" the AV node. The normal heart rate response to exercise will occur with P-wave–triggered ventricular pacing as the patient's sinus rate increases. However, many candidates for cardiac pacing may not present such an ideal picture. Often, the patient with a documented symptomatic bradyarrhythmia has sclerodegenerative conduction system disease, affecting the entire conduction system from the SA node through the His-Purkinje complex. These patients may also have episodic atrial tachyarrhythmias, or sinus bradycardia with inappropriate sinus node responses to exercise. In the case of those with atrial tachyarrhythmias, AV synchrony cannot and should not be maintained. In patients with atrial fibrillation, effective atrial contraction is lost and the maintenance of AV synchrony with pacing is no longer possible.

In the quest to normalize AV conduction and exercise response, engineers and clinicians have at-

tempted to duplicate the sinus node response to exercise. The first of these attempts to become applicable in clinical cardiac pacing was a piezoelectric sensor that reflected body motion. Body motion and motion of the large muscle groups correlates well with exercise. Exercise, in turn, is associated with an increased sinus rate in normal persons. Incorporation of a piezoelectric sensor into a cardiac pacemaker allowed development of a single-chamber device responsive not only to the intrinsic cardiac electrical events, but to body motion as well. Such devices have been shown to be effective in increasing *objective* exercise performance over single-chamber non-rate–modulated pacing. Other sensors, including those that measure central temperature, respiratory rate, and QT interval, have been released for general use in single-chamber pacemakers. Recently, a motion sensor has been added to dual-chamber devices for use in the DDD mode. These "DDDR" devices are becoming widely used in patients in whom maintenance of a rate response and an underlying AV synchrony appears to be clinically important. Rate-modulated pacing will probably continue to grow and develop as additional sensors are developed for use for both single- and dual-chamber pacing.

A challenge is to evaluate the relationship between the improved objective measurements of exercise tolerance and an improved subjective feeling of wellbeing. Further, all rate-modulated devices require careful and individualized programming and follow-up to achieve additional benefits. Historically, most single-chamber pacemakers implanted in the United States are never reprogrammed during their useful life. Rate-modulated pacemakers *must* be programmed based on the results of individual exercise evaluations to achieve maximum benefit. This requires much more careful evaluation and follow-up than has been generally the practice for non-rate–modulated systems.

TROUBLESHOOTING

Successful implantation of a pacing system is not a panacea against the development of other symptoms. Thus, when patients with pacemakers develop other illness or associated symptoms, one is often asked, "Is the pacemaker working?" When faced with this question, it is first appropriate to ask if there is evidence of pacemaker dysfunction, and if so, if there is ECG documentation of it. In addition, the type of pacing system must be identified or determined from records, the patient's pacemaker identification card, chest x-ray, or other information. Finally, a diagnostic session with the patient, the programmer, and an electrocardiograph machine is necessary.

In most pulse generators, isolated electronic malfunction is rare. Most electronic "abnormalities" are an explicable and normal reaction of the pacing system to changing patient conditions, or are the misinterpretation of normal and appropriate function. For example, in a device programmed to the DVI mode, inability to sense atrial activity is normal—not a "failure" of atrial sensing.

However, loss of atrial sensing in dual-chamber devices programmed to the DDD mode is relatively common (especially if the atrial signal was poor at the time of implant). Devices nearing battery depletion, and pulse generators and leads known to be subject to catastrophic premature failure, may produce unusual electronic manifestations. Only rarely does a modern pacing system need to be explored surgically to confirm a diagnosis of pacing system failure. Before surgical exploration is undertaken, the system should be evaluated by a recognized expert.

It is important during analysis of potential pacing system malfunction, that a witnessed ECG anomaly is causative of the symptoms. For example, myopotential triggering or inhibition is very easily and commonly provoked in unipolar pacing systems programmed to high sensitivities. However, this phenomenon is often only of ECG significance—the triggering or inhibition may not be causing any clinical symptoms. Its mere ECG presence does not necessarily indicate a "malfunction." Thus, correlation of clinical symptoms with pacemaker performace is of utmost importance before deciding that an anomaly is of clinical significance.

True pacing system malfunction should always be considered in patients in whom symptoms for which the pacing system was implanted recur, particularly if they recur long after the system has been in place. Recurrent syncope, dizziness, and lightheadedness are potential manifestations. The presence of such symptoms merits a complete pacemaker evaluation. This, of course, begins with obtaining a complete history. Careful attention should be paid to analysis of activities that may elicit symptoms. In particular, for unipolar systems, the use of the upper extremity on the side of the pacemaker implant may cause myopotential inhibition of pacemaker output. This may lead to the recurrence of symptoms of dizziness, lightheadedness or syncope associated with activity such as combing the hair. Postural dizziness, on the other hand, is a common symptom in elderly persons and may not represent a recurrent bradyarrhythmia or pacing failure. The occurrence of episodic symptoms immediately after pacemaker implantation may indicate that the pacing system, despite normal operation, has not relieved the symptom for which it was placed. Symptoms from carotid sinus hypersensitivity, for example, may be blunted by rate support from a pacemaker, but the vasodepressor component of the condition may not be controlled even by a properly functioning dual-chamber system.

Physical examination in a symptomatic pacemaker patient should concentrate first on potential non-pacemaker–related problems that may induce symptoms. For example, aortic stenosis, carotid bruits, carotid sinus vasodepressor effects, atrial myxoma, hypertrophic cardiomyopathy, and other central nervous system disorders should be checked. Postural vital signs should be recorded with the pacing system programmed to allow the patient's underlying rhythm to be dominant and recorded again with pacing. At times, onset of ventricular pacing while the patient is standing results in sufficient hypotension to cause lightheadedness or syncope, whereas onset of pacing with the patient in the supine position does not cause symptoms. The search for myopotential inhibition or triggering with the patient in various positions is also important. In addition, careful inspection of the pulse generator site, tugging on the pulse generator, and pressing on the underlying lead can bring out potential component malfunction such as a loose setscrew or lead fracture. With the exception of component failure, much inappropriate pacemaker function such as the presence of pacemaker-mediated tachycardia, myopotential inhibition, and triggering can be remedied with reprogramming after a diagnostic session.

In some instances, even after a careful history, physical examination and pacemaker evaluation, the relationship of the pacing system to a symptom remains obscure. Under these conditions, it is important to record an ECG during a symptom. If symptoms are frequent (daily), this can be accomplished with continuous ambulatory ECG (Holter) monitoring. If symptoms are less frequent, "continuous-loop" type event recording should be undertaken. Real-time transtelephonic transmission alone is usually inadequate because by the time communication is established, symptoms have often abated.

Every implanted pulse generator eventually develops power source depletion. Each manufacturer has adopted its own indicators for battery depletion. Modern telemetric pacemakers usually have multiple indicators. Most often a rate decrease and/or a pacing pulse-width increase accompany battery depletion. In general, the rate of this decrease is sufficiently shallow to offer six months to one year of reliable pacing even after the manifestations of battery depletion have occurred. Each manufacturer has designated an elective replacement time (ERT) for the pulse generator. In addition, many telemetric pacemakers will transmit information on the battery status. In almost all devices, battery depletion is a predictable, slowly occurring phenomenon. Some battery types, however, are subject to sudden, catastrophic failure, and these devices have largely been recalled.

Pacemaker leads, though much more reliable than in the past, are still the weak link in the chain of pacemaker performance. Lead components can fail either because of insulation failure or because of conductor break. Broken conductors can make intermittent contact and the lead can appear to function perfectly normally at times. When traction is applied and the broken conductor and the ends no longer touch, failure of both sensing and pacing can occur. Most often, conductor fracture results in complete sensing and pacing failure. Careful evaluation of the chest x-ray may reveal the problem. However, a more accurate test is fluoroscopy of the pacing system under conditions which allow the observer to place traction on the pacemaker and/or the lead.

Insulation failure is sometimes more difficult to detect. Lead impedance, where it can be telemetered, may decrease if the failure is incomplete and current is lost to extracardiac sources. This can also result in extracardiac stimulation or myopotential sensing. In the case of lead or insulation failure, pacing system function is unreliable and the lead should be replaced.

Most lead "failures" are actually a failure of the electrode-tissue interface. After implantation, as edema develops around the stimulating electrode, endocardial potentials fall and pacing thresholds rise. In the ventricle, these return to approximately 80% of baseline within about two weeks. Ventricular electrograms are usually so large that failure of ventricular sensing is uncommon. However, during this period of "acute threshold rise," atrial sensing failure is more common. In the acute phase, should atrial sensing failure occur, fluoroscopy should be performed to rule out gross lead dislodgement. If the lead is not dislodged, it is usually best to wait several weeks and re-evaluate the performance periodically to determine if sensing function has returned before repositioning the lead.

The best protection against unanticipated and untreated pacemaker failure is for patients to be followed by a pacemaker clinic that can perform and interpret periodic transtelephonic monitoring and conduct "in-person" testing. Though malfunction of a modern, properly implanted system is uncommon, periodic systematic evaluation of the pacing system by an expert physician, nurse or technician often prevents the rare catastrophe.

The author wishes to thank Sylvia Roberson for her excellent secretarial assistance. The author also wishes to thank J. Warren Harthorne, M.D., not only for permission to use several illustrations, but also for guidance and friendship, and Nancy Stephenson of Medtronic Inc., for permission to use figures. Correct information in this manuscript is largely the result of Dr. Harthorne's teaching; any mistakes are the author's alone.

Bibliography

Alicandri C, Fouad FM, Tarazi RC, et al: Three cases of hypotension and syncope with ventricular pacing: Possible role of atrial reflexes. *Am J Cardiol* 42:137, 1978.

Anderson K, Humen D, Klein GJ, et al: A rate variable pacemaker which automatically adjusts for physical activity (abstr). *PACE* 6:A-12, 1983.

Chardack WM, Gage AA, Greatbatch W: A transistorized, selfcontained, implantable pacemaker for the long term correction of complete heart block. *Surgery* 48:643, 1960.

Elmqvist R, Senning A: An implantable pacemaker for the heart. In: *Proceedings of the Second International Conference on Medical Electronics*. London: Iliffe; 1960, p.253.

Erlebacher JA, Donner RL, Stelzer PE: Hypotension with ventricular pacing: An atrial vasodepressor reflex in human beings. *J Am Coll Cardiol* 4:550, 1984.

Folkman MJ, Watkins E Jr: An artificial conduction system for the management of experimental complete heart block. *Surg Forum* 8:331, 1958.

Frye RL, Collins JJ, DeSanctis RW, et al: Guidelines for permanent cardiac pacemaker implantation. *J Am Coll Cardiol* 4:434, 1984.

Furman S, Robinson G: The use of an intracardiac pacemaker in the correction of total heart block. *Surg Forum* 9:245, 1958.

Harthorne JW: Indications for pacemakers. *Prog Cardiovasc Dis* 23:393, 1981.

Harthorne JW, Eisenhauer AC, Steinhaus DM: Pacemaker mediated tachycardias: An unresolved problem. *PACE* 7:1140, 1984.

Harthorne JW, Eisenhauer AC, Steinhaus DM: Cardiac pacing. In: Eagle KA, Haber E, DeSanctis RW, Austen WG, eds. *The Practice of Cardiology*. Boston: Little, Brown; 1989, p. 287.

Hartzler GO, Maloney JD, Curtis JJ, et al: Hemodynamic benefits of atrioventricular sequential pacing after cardiac surgery. *Am J Cardiol* 40:232, 1977.

Kruse I, Arnman K, Conradson TR, et al: A comparison of the acute and long-term hemodynamic effects of ventricular inhibited and atrial synchronous ventricular inhibited pacing. *Circulation* 65:846, 1982.

Parsonnet V, Furman S, Smyth NPD, et al: Optimal resources for implantable cardiac pacemakers. *Circulation* 68:227A, 1968.

Parsonnet V, Parsonnet M, Manhardt M: Cardiac pacing and pacemakers: VII. Power sources for implantable pacemakers. Part I. *Am Heart J* 94:517, 1977.

Parsonnet V, Furman S, Smyth NPD: A revised code for pacemaker identification. *PACE* 4:400, 1981.

Rickards AF, Donaldson RM, Thalen JJ: The use of QT interval to determine pacing rate: Early clinical experience. *PACE* 6:346, 1983.

Samet P, Bernstein WH, Nathan DA, et al: Atrial contribution to cardiac output in complete heart block. *Am J Cardiol* 16:1, 1965.

Shapland JE, MacCarter D, Tockman B, et al: Physiologic benefits of rate responsiveness. *PACE* 6:329, 1983.

Sutton R, Morley C, Chan SL, et al: Physiologic benefits of atrial synchrony in paced patients. *PACE* 6:327, 1983.

Wirtzfeld A, Stange K, Heinze R, et al: An optical sensor for monitoring mixed venous oxygen saturation for an implantable rate-responsive pacing system (abstr). *PACE* 6:A-12, 1983.

22 Congenital Heart Disease in the Adult

Richard R. Liberthson
Howard Waldman

This chapter focuses on the most common congenital heart lesions seen in the adult. Included are atrial septal defect (ASD), ventricular septal defect (VSD), patent ductus arteriosus (PDA), coarctation of the aorta, pulmonic stenosis, and tetralogy of Fallot. Together they comprise almost all of the adult congenital heart abnormalities. For each entity, the salient anatomic and physiologic features, natural history, clinical manifestations, noninvasive and invasive evaluation, surgical interventions and postoperative management are discussed. Further details and discussion of less common entities are available in more specialized textbooks dealing specifically with congenital heart disease (see Bibliography). Both mitral valve prolapse and bicuspid aortic valve are dealt with in Chapter 17.

ATRIAL SEPTAL DEFECT

Atrial septal defect accounts for approximately 25% of congenital heart lesions seen in the adult. Patients who have eluded earlier diagnosis as well as those who have undergone prior correction of the defect may present to the cardiologist. Women with this disorder outnumber men by three to one.

Anatomy

Size and contour of the defect are variable. Defects are classified as secundum (70%), primum or partial atrioventricular (AV) canal (15%), and sinus venosus types (15%). These classifications are based on the location of the defect within the septum: in the region of the fossa ovalis, the AV junction, or the posterior septum, respectively. This classification system is useful because each type has different associated anomalies: one third of secundum defects have associated mitral valve prolapse, two thirds of primum defects have a cleft anterior mitral valve leaflet, and one half of sinus venosus defects have anomalous drainage of the right pulmonary veins.

Physiology

Regardless of ASD type, the physiology of uncomplicated defects (those with normal pulmonary arteriolar resistance) is the same. Shunting from the left to the right atrium occurs during diastole and is determined by the relative right and left ventricular compliance (the former being greater in the patient with an uncomplicated defect) and by defect size. Pulmonary blood flow is increased. When the defect is small, the shunted volume is small and hemodynamic sequelae are minimal. In larger defects, chronic left-to-right shunting causes right atrial and right ventricular volume overload (Figure 1A). In the patient with an uncomplicated course, the left heart is conspicuously spared and left atrial, left ventricular, and aortic size are normal.

Clinical Course

Symptoms and complications, except for an increased incidence of respiratory tract infections, are uncommon in the infant and small child, and early findings are subtle even in patients with large defects. Adolescents and young adults also have few symptoms. When present, symptoms include fatigue, palpitations, and mild dyspnea. Often, ASD is neither suspected nor diagnosed until adult life. Pregnancy is well tolerated. By the fifth decade, however, exercise intolerance, fatigue, and dyspnea are increasingly

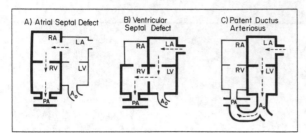

Figure 1. *(A)The pathophysiologic consequences in an uncomplicated ASD revealing right atrial (RA), right ventricular (RV), and pulmonary artery (PA) dilation and preservation of normal left atrial (LA), left ventricular (LV), and aortic (A$_o$) size. (B) Uncomplicated VSD showing LA, LV, RV, and PA enlargement, with preservation of normal RA and A$_o$ size. (C) Uncomplicated patent ductus arteriosus, including LA and LV enlargement, dilation of both the A$_o$ and PA, and preservation of normal RA and RV size.*

common and are nearly universal after age 50 years. By this time, the right atrium and ventricle are dilated and contractility is decreased. After the sixth decade, atrial fibrillation is present in 50% of patients; its onset often heralds progressive symptoms and findings of heart failure. Both primum and secundum ASD may cause mitral regurgitation. In the former, this manifests early in life and is secondary to the associated cleft mitral valve. With secundum defects, it is rare before age 50 years and is secondary to myxomatous and fibrotic degeneration of the mitral valve. Severe pulmonary vascular obstruction with Eisenmenger's physiology is uncommon, occurring in approximately 5% of cases. It is rare before adolescence and after age 50 years. Severe irreversible pulmonary vascular obstruction causes reversal of shunt flow through the ASD from left to right to right to left. Progressive right heart failure, systemic desaturation, erythrocytosis and paradoxical embolus occur; the patient usually dies within 15 years of diagnosis. Both pulmonary and paradoxical systemic embolization occur in the older ASD patient, particularly in those with atrial arrhythmia and heart failure. Infective endocarditis is rare; when it occurs, it usually involves an associated mitral valve lesion or the pulmonic valve. We believe that endocarditis chemoprophylaxis is prudent regardless of prior surgical repair. Lutembacher's syndrome (associated mitral stenosis) is rare. The average age of death of patients with uncorrected ASD is 55 years.

Clinical Findings

Body habitus is usually normal. Patients with Holt-Oram syndrome (congenital hypoplasia of the thumb and radial bones) often have associated ASD. In the absence of severe pulmonary vascular obstruction, patients are acyanotic. The salient clinical findings include an enlarged hyperdynamic right ventricle and a widely and nearly fixed split second heart sound (S$_2$). Even with the patient standing, the S$_2$ does not become single. A grade II/VI basal systolic ejection murmur secondary to increased blood flow across the pulmonic valve is present and increases with inspiration. Thrills are unusual. In older patients, heart failure and atrial fibrillation are common, and an apical holosystolic murmur secondary to mitral incompetence may be present. With severe pulmonary vascular obstruction and shunt reversal, the right ventricle hypertrophies, the pulmonic closure sound becomes loud, splitting narrows, and the pulmonic flow murmur becomes soft. A high-pitched diastolic decrescendo murmur of pulmonary incompetence, a pulmonic ejection sound, a right-sided S$_4$, cyanosis, and clubbing are late findings.

The electrocardiogram (ECG) reveals right ventricular volume overload, showing incomplete right bundle branch block in younger patients and often a complete right bundle block after middle age. Secundum and sinus venosus defects typically have right-axis deviation, although one fourth have a normal frontal-plane QRS axis. Left-axis deviation is rare and suggests associated coronary, myocardial, or mitral valve disease. In contrast, in primum type defects, marked left-axis deviation is the rule. It is secondary to congenital hypoplasia and attenuation of the anterior radiations of the left bundle branch. Atrial fibrillation is common in the elderly patient.

The chest x-ray film shows right atrial and ventricular enlargement, dilation of the main and proximal pulmonary arteries, and increased pulmonary vascular markings (Figure 2). The aorta appears to be small, and with uncomplicated ASD, the left heart is normal sized (Figure 1). If left atrial enlargement is present, mitral incompetence should be suspected.

The two-dimensional echocardiogram delineates the presence, size and location of the ASD, the existence of associated cardiac anomalies, and the extent of secondary findings such as right atrial and right ventricular enlargement. Doppler study estimates the right ventricular and pulmonary artery pressures as well as the interatrial pressure gradient. Paradoxical interven-

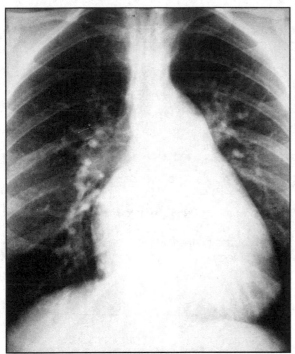

Figure 2. *Posteroanterior chest roentgenogram of a 22-year-old woman with a large secundum atrial septal defect. There is a large right atrium and right ventricle, a dilated pulmonic trunk, and increased pulmonary blood flow. (Reprinted with permission from Liberthson. See Bibliography.)*

tricular septal motion correlates with significant right ventricular volume overload. Use of both color Doppler and an agitated saline intravenous bolus can document the presence of an actual interatrial communication. (See Chapter 8 and p. *xix*.)

Cardiac Catheterization

Catheterization may not be required in children with typical noninvasive findings. In older patients and in those with any questionable findings, catheterization is advisable before surgical repair. Confirmation of the defect is accomplished by catheter passage from the right to the left atrium. Essential data include assessment of right-heart and pulmonary artery pressures, pulmonary arteriolar resistance, and the ratio of pulmonic to systemic blood flow. Table 1 lists formulas used to calculate the magnitude of the shunt. After the fourth decade, coronary angiography and left ventriculography are advisable to identify acquired heart disease. For suspected primum defects

(patients with left-axis deviation on the ECG), biplane left ventriculography is necessary to evaluate an associated cleft mitral valve or interventricular septal defect. Patients with pulmonary hypertension should receive a trial of pulmonary vasodilation therapy to assess reversibility of pulmonary vascular obstruction. Patients with net right-to-left shunting—Eisenmenger's physiology—are inoperable. In contrast, patients with net left-to-right shunting are usually surgical candidates, regardless of the presence of pulmonary hypertension, systemic desaturation, or moderately elevated pulmonary vascular resistance. In these latter patients, the larger the net left-to-right shunt is, the more favorable will be the postoperative result. Transcatheter closure of secundum-type ASDs is possible using double umbrella-type devices, and the specific indications for this approach are now being delineated. Technologic advances now allow for closure of ASDs with diameters of up to 2 cm. This technology warrants consideration in selected circumstances, although surgical repair remains the therapeutic mainstay.

Surgical Intervention

Surgery consists of either suture closure (usually possible in the young patient) or patch closure in older patients, those with large defects, and in those with primum or sinus venosus defects. For best results, surgery should be performed before school age. Thereafter, ASD closure is indicated when the diagnosis is confirmed. The ASD population is predominantly women. The defect should be repaired before marriage and childbearing to avoid the tendency for further delay while raising a young family. Repair before the fourth decade usually results in return of normal heart size and function. Thereafter, although both size and function improve, they rarely become normal. Safe repair may be performed even through the seventh decade. Clinical improvement, even in older patients, may be marked, particularly when associated mitral valve incompetence is relieved. In older patients, chronic anticoagulation therapy is advisable, particularly if heart failure, pulmonary hypertension, or atrial fibrillation is present. We do not advise the use of anticoagulation therapy for young patients or those undergoing primary suture closure. Mitral valve clefts may require plasty revision at the time of ASD closure. Older adults with secundum defects should have intraoperative assessment of the severity of mitral value insufficiency.

Table 1. Calculations of Shunts by Oximetric Analysis

1. Shunts are expressed as:

    Q_p/Q_s: The ratio of pulmonary blood flow (Q_p) to systemic blood flow (Q_s)

    and

    $Q_p - Q_s$: This value is positive if there is a net left-to-right (L→R) shunt, and negative if there is a net right-to-left (R→L) shunt.

2. Calculation of pulmonary blood flow (Q_p) in L/min:

    $$Q_p = \frac{O_2 \text{ consumption (ml/min)}}{PVO_2 \text{ content (ml/L)} - PAO_2 \text{ content (ml/L)}}$$

    where PV = pulmonary venous blood and PA = pulmonary arterial blood.

    If a pulmonary vein has not been entered, systemic arterial O_2 content may be used for PVO_2 if systemic arterial O_2 saturation is 95% or more. If it is <95%, a determination must be made as to whether a R→L shunt is present. If a R→L shunt is present, an assumed value for PVO_2 content is determined as 98% × O_2 capacity. If systemic arterial saturation is <95% and no R→L shunt is present, the observed systemic arterial O_2 content is used.

3. Systemic blood flow (Q_s) in L/min:

    $$Q_s = \frac{O_2 \text{ consumption (ml/min)}}{\text{Systemic arterial } O_2 \text{ content (ml/L)} - \text{mixed venous } O_2 \text{ content (ml/L)}}$$

    where mixed venous O_2 content is average O_2 content of blood in chamber immediately proximal to the shunt. If the shunt is at the level of the right atrium, one commonly used method for estimating mixed venous O_2 content is calculated as:

    $$\frac{3 \text{ SVC } O_2 \text{ content} + 1 \text{ IVC } O_2 \text{ content}}{4}$$

    where SVC = superior vena cava and IVC = inferior vena cava.
    Some institutions use the SVC O_2 content as the mixed venous sample, as this sample gives the maximal shunt size.

4. If bidirectional shunting is present, a more complex formula is used.*

*Grossman and Barry. See Bibliography.

The postoperative course in patients who undergo repair before the fourth decade is typically benign and lifestyle is normal. No restriction is indicated. The course of pregnancy and delivery is normal. Chemoprophylaxis for bacterial endocarditis should be a lifetime commitment, regardless of surgical repair, because of the frequent association with mitral valve prolapse. With pregnancy, prophylaxis for vaginal organisms should be started with the onset of labor and continued for several days after delivery. In the absence of surgical damage to the sinus node or its vascular supply, young patients retain normal rhythm. For those with supraventricular ectopy or atrial fibrillation, digitalis administration is indicated. Patients who have new atrial fibrillation after surgery warrant a trial of electrocardioversion after six weeks; anticoagulation and digitalis treatment should precede this, and quin-idine is often needed to maintain sinus rhythm. After the sixth decade, postoperative arrhythmia is typical. Routine postoperative clinical evaluation is indicated for all patients, particularly for those who undergo repair past middle age. Longevity in those repaired before that time is normal. Thereafter, residual (but improved) heart failure may be present, and pulmonary or systemic embolization may occur. In the older patient, late progressive mitral insufficiency may occur despite ASD closure. In the young patient undergoing repair, the postoperative examination, chest x-ray film, and ECG become normal except for a residual right ventricular conduction defect. In older patients with preoperative heart failure, pulmonary hypertension, and arrhythmia, some right heart enlargement may persist.

Differential Diagnosis

Entities sometimes confused with ASD include persistent patency of the foramen ovale, which occurs in 10–20% of normal autopsies; this finding is of no hemodynamic consequence and has no clinical sequelae unless the pulmonary pressure is elevated. Partial anomalous pulmonary venous drainage with intact atrial septum has similar clinical findings, but rarely causes symptoms or requires correction. Mitral valve stenosis, pectus abnormalities, and pulmonic stenosis may all have similar clinical findings; however, both ultrasound and radionuclide scanning are usually sufficient to differentiate them from ASD.

VENTRICULAR SEPTAL DEFECT

Although VSD occurs in almost 1 in 500 normal births, nearly 50% close spontaneously during childhood; thus, in adults it is less common and accounts for approximately 12% of congenital heart abnormalities seen in adults. Adult patients presenting to the physician include those with small, inconsequential defects, those who have undergone prior palliative or corrective surgical procedures and those with acquired complications. If a patient survives unimpaired to adult age and does not have Eisenmenger's physiology, the VSD is probably small.

Anatomy

Ventricular septal defects are classified according to location within the interventricular septum. Seventy percent are membranous defects and involve the pars membranacea. They are variably sized and shaped and often close spontaneously. Muscular defects occur within the muscular portion of the septum, toward the apex, and mid- and posterior regions. Multiple defects may be present and also often close spontaneously. In both of these circumstances, associated cardiac defects are uncommon. AV canal type defects involve the posterobasal septum, are usually large and are associated with mitral and tricuspid valve clefts, as well as a primum type ASD. These are common in patients with Down's syndrome. Supracristal (subaortic) defects are uncommon (5%). They are usually small; however, their strategic location beneath the aortic annulus may undermine aortic leaflet support and may cause progressive aortic incompetence.

Physiology

The hemodynamic consequences of VSD vary with defect size. When small, they are minimal. With uncomplicated VSD (those with normal right ventricular pressure and normal pulmonary artery resistance), shunting occurs from the left ventricle to the right ventricle. If the defect is larger; both ventricles enlarge and pulmonary blood flow increases. Left atrial return is increased, causing left atrial enlargement. When left-to-right shunt flow is very large, heart failure may be present. The right atrium is normal sized in uncomplicated VSD (Figure 1B). With large defects, pulmonary hypertension and pulmonary vascular obstruction may develop, which leads to pulmonary artery and right ventricular hypertension, decreased left-to-right shunting, and eventually right-to-left shunting (Eisenmenger's syndrome).

Clinical Course

The clinical course of patients with VSD is variable because of the variability in defect size, the common occurrence of spontaneous defect closure, development of complications in the unoperated patient, and the now common practice of early surgical intervention for those with large defects.

Patients with small defects have a history of a loud murmur present from early infancy, but they are asymptomatic. Complications do not develop except for bacterial endocarditis.

Overt clinical heart failure occurs in the infant with large VSD and may be fatal. Chronic left-heart volume overload may cause dyspnea and both symptoms and findings of heart failure may be late sequelae in adult life.

In patients who had large shunts, often with heart failure, during infancy, pulmonary vascular obstruction and Eisenmenger's syndrome may develop. In these patients, the chronic effects of increased pulmonary artery pressure and flow cause pulmonary arteriole narrowing, pulmonary artery and right ventricular hypertension, and reversal of interventricular shunt flow from the previous left-to-right direction to right-to-left. Systemic desaturation, cyanosis (which is often increased with exertion), and erythrocytosis develop. Late right-heart failure and hemoptysis and systemic embolization may occur. Because of right-to-left shunting, iatrogenic systemic embolization may occur secondary to careless intravenous technique. Bacterial endocarditis occurs regardless of

VSD size or earlier repair and usually involves the right ventricular outflow tract. In approximately 5% of patients with VSD, progressive hypertrophy of the right ventricular infundibulum develops and obstructs pulmonary blood flow, causes right ventricular hypertension and hypertrophy, and may cause right-to-left interventricular shunting (see "pink tetralogy," under Tetralogy of Fallot section). Patients with supracristal defects may have aortic insufficiency, which is progressive and becomes severe. Patients with atrioventricular canal defects often have heart failure during infancy, and Eisenmenger's syndrome may develop (see Chapter 28).

Clinical Findings

Body habitus in VSD is normal except in patients with Down's syndrome, who have characteristic features. The patient with uncomplicated VSD has a systolic thrill at the left sternal border, an enlarged hyperdynamic left ventricle, and a loud holosystolic murmur heard best at the left sternal border on expiration and with isometric maneuvers. In general, the louder the murmur, the smaller the defect. This murmur begins with the S_1 and ends with S_2. With muscular defects, the murmur may end before the S_2 if the defect closes with ventricular contraction. Pulmonary vascular obstruction causes this murmur to diminish in intensity. In these patients, right ventricular hypertrophy, a loud pulmonic closure sound, an ejection sound, and late cyanosis develop. With late right ventricular failure, pulmonary and tricuspid incompetence occur. Patients with aortic incompetence have a high-pitched diastolic decrescendo murmur. With canal defects, mitral or tricuspid incompetence murmurs may be present.

The ECG is helpful in diagnosing the type of defect and the presence of complications. With small defects, the ECG is normal. Larger defects cause a right ventricular conduction defect and both left atrial and left ventricular enlargement. Uncomplicated defects have a normal frontal-plane QRS axis. The QRS axis is an accurate indicator of right ventricular pressure in older children and adults. A normal axis (between $-30°$ and $+90°$) usually rules out right ventricular hypertension, thus making pulmonary vascular obstruction or right ventricular infundibular obstruction unlikely; right-axis deviation suggests their presence. As with primum type ASD, patients with canal type VSD have marked left-axis deviation (more negative than $-30°$) regardless of pulmonary artery pressure.

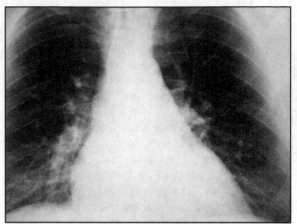

Figure 3. *Posteroanterior chest roentgenogram of a 30-year-old man with a large ventricular septal defect. There is biventricular and left atrial enlargement, a dilated pulmonic trunk, and increased pulmonary blood flow.*

In the patient with a small, uncomplicated VSD, the chest x-ray film is normal. With larger defects, characteristic findings (Figure 3) include increased pulmonary vascular markings, left atrial and left ventricular enlargement, a small aortic shadow and, sometimes, right ventricular enlargement. The right atrium is normal-sized (Figure 1B).

Two-dimensional echocardiography and Doppler examination are diagnostic; they delineate the presence, size, and location of VSDs, and the presence of associated cardiac lesions and secondary problems including right ventricular or pulmonary artery hypertension. Color flow Doppler is particularly useful in delineating shunt flow, especially for small residual communications after surgery or for small muscular defects associated with larger VSDs. Ultrasound study permits identification of associated great artery abnormalities such as transposition, double outlet right ventricle, and truncus arteriosus, and differentiation of the defect from single ventricle (see Chapter 8).

Cardiac Catheterization

In general, asymptomatic patients with small defects, normal-sized hearts, normal ECGs (including a normal axis), and no evidence for associated valvular abnormalities do not require catheterization. Catheterization is necessary before surgical intervention. Its objectives include assessment of left-to-right shunt size, pulmonary artery pressure and resistance, and right ventricular pressure. Angiographic delineation of the defect and any associated lesions is necessary. Eisenmenger's syndrome (net right-to-left shunting) must be identified because affected patients are not surgical candidates. Because catheterization in these latter patients carries increased risk, it should be undertaken cautiously and only after careful noninvasive assessment, and should be performed only by those experienced with this problem. Patients with pulmonary hypertension should receive a trial of pulmonary vasodilator therapy during catheterization to determine whether obstruction is reversible.

Surgical Intervention

Asymptomatic patients with small defects, normal heart size, normal ECG, and no associated valvular defects do not require surgery. Endocarditis chemoprophylaxis is recommended in all patients with VSD. Palliative banding of the pulmonary artery is infrequently performed today but was common in early years, and patients who have had this procedure may still be seen. This procedure was performed in those with large VSDs to prevent development of pulmonary vascular obstruction by protecting the pulmonary circulation from increased flow and pressure. However, it caused right ventricular hypertension, often with right-to-left shunting through the VSD and its associated complications. The late sequelae of pulmonary banding include cyanosis, erythrocytosis, and systemic embolization. Pulmonary bands sometimes distort the pulmonary arteries as well. Patients who have undergone prior banding require catheterization to delineate pulmonary artery anatomy and the VSD before VSD closure and band removal.

Corrective surgery consists of either suture or prosthetic patch closure of the VSD. It is indicated for patients who have symptoms, cardiomegaly, elevated pulmonary pressure (including elevated pulmonary resistance, provided there is still net left-to-right shunting), and for those with significant left-to-right shunting (greater than 2:1). Patients with associated infundibular stenosis should undergo VSD closure and often also require infundibulectomy. Young patients with supracristal VSD who do not have aortic incompetence or who have only mild incompetence often benefit from VSD closure, which buttresses the aortic annulus, thus preventing progressive insufficiency. This sometimes obviates the need for aortic valve replacement. Surgery is indicated for infants with medically refractory heart failure. Patients with severe pulmo-

nary vascular obstruction and net right-to-left shunts are not surgical candidates.

After successful VSD closure, postoperative problems are minimal and a normal lifestyle is usual. Patients may have a residual VSD that was not appreciated at the time of repair or may have incomplete patch closure, but only when left-to-right shunting is large do these require repair. The late course of patients with a buttressed aortic valve in supracristal defects or of the palliated AV valvular incompetence in canal defects is not known, and these patients require close follow-up.

Patients with Eisenmenger's syndrome usually die within 15 years from the time of diagnosis. They are not candidates for VSD closure. They are at increased risk for arrhythmic death when subjected to any form of surgery or to general anesthesia. These patients are also at increased risk with physical exertion or exposure to high altitude. Pregnancy carries an increased risk of death and should be prevented — often not an easy matter. Birth control pills hasten the progression of the pulmonary vascular obstruction and are contraindicated. Intrauterine devices carry a risk of bacterial endocarditis and should not be used. The procedure of tubal ligation itself is a risk. Bacterial endocarditis chemoprophylaxis is essential. Cautious phlebotomy with replacement of excessive volume loss with volume expanders may be helpful for those with severe erythrocytosis and hematocrit >65%. In patients with heart failure, medical treatment may improve symptoms.

Differential Diagnosis

The differential diagnosis of VSD includes single ventricle with small outlet chamber and VSD associated with abnormality of the great artery position including complete transposition, double outlet right ventricle, and truncus arteriosus. Although similar clinically to patients with large VSD, patients with these abnormalities also often have cyanosis. Ultrasound examination differentiates these patients from those with simple VSD.

PATENT DUCTUS ARTERIOSUS

Although PDA is an obligatory component of the normal fetal circulation, persistent patency beyond early infancy is abnormal. Patent ductus arteriosus is present in 10% of adults with congenital heart abnormalities. Both unoperated patients and those with previously corrected PDA may present to the physician. PDA is particularly common in infants whose mothers had rubella infection during their first trimester of pregnancy, in premature infants, in infants with lung disease, and in infants born at high altitude. It is more common in women than in men.

Pathophysiology

The anatomic spectrum of PDA includes a wide range of duct caliber, length, and shape. The ligamentum arteriosus is the fibrotic remnant of the obliterated ductus. The physiologic consequences vary, depending on the cross-sectional area of the ductus lumen. In patients with uncomplicated ductus (those with normal pulmonary arteriolar resistance), flow of blood is from the aorta to the pulmonary circulation (left to right). Large ducts allow large volume pulmonary blood flow, which causes increased pulmonary artery pressure, increased left atrial return, left ventricular enlargement, and enlargement of the aorta proximal to the ductus (Figure 1C). The right atrium and ventricle are normal in size.

Clinical Course

The natural history depends on ductus size. Many ducts close spontaneously during early infancy. Thereafter, an annual spontaneous closure rate of 0.6% has been reported. Patients with a small ductus are asymptomatic. Heart failure occurs in infants with large ductus and may be fatal. Adults with large ductus have both symptoms and findings of heart failure. In patients with large ductus, pulmonary vascular obstruction may develop early in life. In these patients, the late sequelae of Eisenmenger's physiology (right-to-left shunting) include cyanosis and right-sided heart failure. Regardless of ductus size, infective endocarditis may occur. It typically involves the pulmonary side of the ductus. There may be infected pulmonary embolization. Rarely, in elderly patients ductal calcification, aneurysmal dilation, and dissection may develop. These may be preceded by hoarseness secondary to left vocal cord paralysis due to left recurrent laryngeal nerve compression.

Clinical Findings

Body habitus is normal except in those with the congenital rubella syndrome, who have cataracts and are deaf and retarded. Patients with uncomplicated ducts of large size have hyperdynamic arterial pulses, wide pulse pressure, and an enlarged hyperdynamic left ventricle. These findings are absent in those with small ductus. Regardless of ductus size, a loud continuous machinery-like murmur is typically present, heard best in the left infraclavicular area. It obliterates the heart sounds in this region. With severe pulmonary vascular obstruction, the diastolic murmur shortens and becomes softer and pulmonic closure intensity increases. When reversal of shunt direction occurs in patients with PDA, the lower extremities receive the desaturated pulmonary artery blood flow, and cyanosis and clubbing of the toes develop. In contrast, the upper extremities still receive fully oxygenated blood flow from the ascending aorta; therefore, the fingers are pink and are not clubbed. The differential cyanotic distribution is diagnostic of PDA with Eisenmenger's physiology.

The electrocardiogram reveals left ventricular and left atrial enlargement when shunt flow is large. It is normal with a small ductus.

If the ductus is small, the chest x-ray film appears normal; if the ductus is large, the x-ray may be diagnostic (Figure 4). Pulmonary plethora, dilation of the proximal pulmonary artery and of the ascending aorta, a prominent aortic knob (in contrast to those with intracardiac shunts, who have a small aortic knob), and left atrial and left ventricular enlargement are seen. The right heart is conspicuously normal-sized in uncomplicated PDA (Figure 1C). In older adults the ductus is calcified.

Two-dimensional echocardiography and Doppler study allow direct imaging of the ductus. Doppler study allows assessment of shunt magnitude and color Doppler mapping is useful for delineation of the small and tortuous ductus. Associated cardiac lesions and secondary findings are readily identified. Magnetic resonance imaging can also accurately delineate the presence and size of a PDA.

Catheterization confirms the presence of a PDA and is generally performed in patients being assessed for correction. Its objectives include assessment of shunt size and pulmonary pressure and resistance. The catheter should be passed through the ductus to confirm its existence and to differentiate ductus from other great artery shunts, such as aorticopulmonary window, and from coronary arteriovenous fistula. Angiographic delineation of the ductal anatomy is useful in the older adult to alert the surgeon to aneurysms or atypical anatomy. Patients with elevated pulmonary artery pressure should have a trial of pulmonary

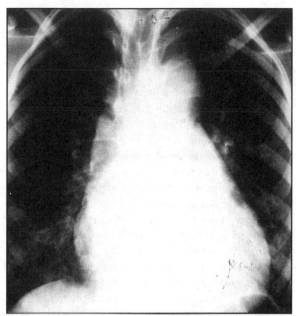

Figure 4. *Posteroanterior chest roentgenogram of a 19-year-old woman with a large patent ductus arteriosus and pulmonary artery hypertension. There is cardiomegaly with left atrial and left ventricular enlargement, and enlarged pulmonic trunk and aortic knob, and increased blood flow. (Reprinted with permission from Liberthson.)*

vasodilation to identify reversible pulmonary vascular obstruction. Patients with net left-to-right shunting should undergo surgery; those with net right-to-left shunting are not surgical candidates.

Transcatheter methods of closing a PDA with a Teflon plug have been performed since 1967, with few complications. More recently, a double-umbrella prosthesis has been used to close PDA.

Surgical Intervention

Surgical intervention for PDA consists of double ligation of the ductus with or without division to insure obliteration. It does not require heart-lung bypass. It is performed through a left posterior thoracotomy. In children, all ducts should be closed. The optimal age for elective ligation is one year. Emergency surgery is indicated for infants with medically refractory heart failure. Elective ligation is indicated thereafter at the time of confirmed diagnosis. Older adults with aneurysmal dilation or calcification of the ductus warrant appropriate surgical precautions, including the avail-

ability of cardiac bypass, as dissection and rupture may occur.

Postoperatively, the patient typically has no further difficulties. Very rarely, recanalization of an improperly ligated and undivided ductus occurs. Patients with large ductus and those who undergo repair after early childhood should receive postoperative bacterial endocarditis chemoprophylaxis because of the presence of residual endothelial irregularity, which may be a nidus for infection.

It is not established whether the asymptomatic young adult with small PDA and normal heart size, normal pulmonary artery pressure, and normal pulmonary resistance must have duct closure. Aneurysmal dilation and dissection are rare. We generally advise elective closure; however, close interim observation may be an acceptable alternative. Infective endocarditis precautions are mandatory.

Indomethacin may stimulate "medical" closure of PDA in the newborn but is of no value in older children or adults. It acts by inhibition of prostaglandin activity, which functions to sustain ductal patency.

Differential Diagnosis

An innocent venous hum is often confused with PDA. Appropriate clinical maneuvers, including auscultation with the patient lying flat or cervical venous occlusion readily differentiate these conditions. More critical is identification of patients with aorticopulmonary window at catheterization, because this condition requires heart-lung bypass surgery and median sternotomy. Patients with VSD and aortic incompetence have some similar clinical findings, but can usually be differentiated both clinically and noninvasively. Sinus of Valsalva and coronary arteriovenous fistulas may resemble PDA clinically; but in both, the murmur is typically louder over the heart than beneath the left clavicle. Angiography is the confirmatory procedure in both. Angiography is also required to differentiate patients with pulmonary or systemic arteriovenous fistulas, in whom findings on physical examination may closely resemble those of PDA.

COARCTATION OF THE AORTA

Coarctation accounts for 15% of congenital heart abnormalities in adults. Increasing numbers of patients with coarctation are being identified in hypertension screening programs and by careful scrutiny of hypertensive patients. Often coarctation is not diagnosed until adult life. Both undiagnosed patients and those who have undergone prior repair are seen. Men with this condition outnumber women by two to one. This discussion concerns adult type, or periductal, coarctation.

Pathophysiology

Coarctation is a fibrotic narrowing of the aortic lumen in the region of the insertion of the ductus or ligamentum arteriosus. The caliber, configuration, and extent of narrowing varies, as does its relationship to the origin of the left subclavian artery and insertion of the ductus. In some patients, the left subclavian artery arises distally to the coarctation. At least one third of patients have an associated bicuspid aortic valve. Infants who have early symptoms usually have significant associated VSD, PDA, or aortic stenosis.

Physiologically, coarctation causes obstruction to left ventricular outflow. The left ventricle and the proximal aorta and its proximally arising branches (the carotid and the subclavian arteries) have elevated blood pressure and strong pulse relative to the distal aorta and lower limbs, which have lower blood pressure and delayed arterial pulse. Concentric left ventricular hypertrophy occurs, although in late adult life there may be heart failure and left ventricular dilation. With significant coarctation narrowing, blood flow to the lower body comes in part from collateral arterial circulation, which arises from the subclavian arteries. The internal mammary and posterior intercostal arteries carry most of this flow and are enlarged. The more severe the coarctation, the more extensive the collateral development.

Clinical Course

Symptoms are minimal or absent in the young patient and, when present, are secondary to hypertension, which occurs in nearly all patients regardless of age. Headache, epistaxis, forceful carotid pulsations, and lower extremity claudication with exertion occur. Infants who have significant associated defects may have heart failure, which may be fatal, but with isolated coarctation this is uncommon. Heart failure is rare after infancy and before the fourth decade, but thereafter occurs in two thirds of patients. About 8% of patients have a cerebral vascular accident; it is rare in infants and uncommon in children, but occurs in 20% of older adults. It is attributed to both chronic

hypertension and to the incidence of congenital berry aneurysm of the circle of Willis associated with coarctation. Cerebral vascular accident is less common after correction, but may still occur. Infective endocarditis occurs in 5% of patients, including some who have had repair. It may involve the coarctation or the surgical resection site, or associated lesions, notably a congenitally bicuspid aortic valve, which is present in approximately 25% of patients. Significant stenosis of the bicuspid aortic valve is uncommon until late in life, when calcification and fibrosis develop. Significant obstruction may develop regardless of prior coarctation repair, and late aortic valve replacement may be necessary. Aortic dissection at or near the site of the coarctation is rare. Rarely, coarctation may complicate pregnancy. Both severe hypertension and toxemia are more common in these pregnant women, and aortic dissection is a risk. In the absence of earlier repair, survival beyond age 50 years is unusual.

Clinical Findings

Body habitus is usually normal, although some patients have underdeveloped lower extremities and hypertrophy of their arms and upper body. With Turner's syndrome, coarctation is common and these patients have a typical Turner's appearance. The clinical findings in patients with coarctation are diagnostic. Upper extremity hypertension is nearly always present. The upper extremity pulses are more forceful than the lower extremity pulses, which are typically weak and delayed or absent. All pulses should be checked, as aberrant subclavian artery origin distal to the coarctation occurs. In patients with extensive collaterals, femoral pulses may be surprisingly strong, but careful comparison with the carotid or brachial pulses reveals a relative difference. Extensive collaterals are evident by both palpation and auscultation over the chest wall. Unlike the normal person, whose blood pressures in the lower extremities are slightly higher than in their upper extremities, in the patient with coarctation, the leg pressures are lower than those in the arms. Left ventricular hypertrophy is present. An ejection sound, which derives from an associated bicuspid aortic valve or from the dilated ascending aorta, may be present. A soft systolic ejection murmur, secondary to a bicuspid valve, may also be present; and a systolic murmur over the left upper back, originating from the coarctation, is typical. Findings of heart failure are common in older patients.

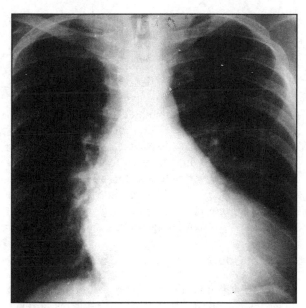

Figure 5. *A posteroanterior chest roentgenogram of a 64-year-old woman with coarctation of the aorta. The heart is enlarged owing to left ventricular hypertrophy. The aortic knob shadow is small. The left subclavian artery is enlarged, and there is post-coarctation dilation, causing a "figure 3" sign. There is prominent rib notching. (Reprinted with permission from Liberthson.)*

Electrocardiographic findings are nonspecific. The left ventricle is the dominant chamber; however, frank left ventricular hypertrophy and strain are often absent until the third or fourth decade. In younger patients, a right ventricular conduction abnormality is common.

The chest x-ray film is often diagnostic (Figure 5). The coarctation itself is demarcated by an indentation bordered proximally by the dilated left subclavian artery and distally by a poststenotic aortic dilation "figure 3" sign. The ascending aorta is dilated. Notching of the posterior inferior ribs develops by adolescence and increases with age. Notching may resolve after correction. Heart size is normal, except in those with heart failure who have left ventricular and left atrial enlargement. Calcification of an associated bicuspid valve may be a late finding. Two-dimensional echocardiography and Doppler study provide diagnostic confirmation and often complete preoperative assessment of coarctation. The morphologic location and severity of obstruction are readily determined in infants and children but is somewhat more difficult to evaluate in adults. Doppler ultrasound helps to local-

ize the site and severity of the coarctation, although those with a large PDA may have no pressure gradient. Ultrasound is particularly useful for those with residual or recurrent postoperative coarctation. Magnetic resonance imaging is also of value in delineating the anatomy of coarctation and residual or recoarctation after surgery.

Cardiac Catheterization

Catheterization should be performed before repair. Its objectives are delineation of the specific coarctation anatomy and anatomy of the arch vessels; assessment of the presence of adequate collateral circulation to permit safe aortic cross-clamping, without risk of spinal cord ischemia; and identification of associated cardiac lesions, particularly aortic stenosis, VSD, and PDA. In older patients, evaluation to rule out acquired coronary and myocardial disease is advisable. Determination of the pressure gradient across the coarctation is not essential and has limited value because the severity of the coarctation varies directly with the degree of collateral development that tends to decrease the transcoarctation gradient.

Percutaneous balloon angioplasty to dilate residual stenosis or restenosis after earlier surgical repair may be an alternative to surgical revision. For previously unoperated coarctation, dilation carries some risk of late aneurysm development; thus its role for these patients is not yet determined.

Surgical Intervention

Surgery consists of coarctectomy and either primary aortic re-anastomosis (sometimes using a proximal left subclavian flap and distal subclavian ligation) or insertion of a tubular prosthetic graft. Optimally, elective repair should be performed before school age to avoid residual hypertension. Thereafter, surgery is still indicated at the time of diagnosis regardless of age. Even older adults who have long-standing hypertension should undergo correction, because 50% still become normotensive postoperatively and the remainder have more manageable pressures. Older patients with heart failure also benefit from correction.

Postoperative problems include residual coarctation, which is rare except in those who undergo correction during infancy. Residual hypertension with a blood pressure gradient >20 mm Hg systolic between the arms and legs is an indication for recatheterization and reoperation or balloon dilation. Children who undergo repair before school age rarely have post-operative hypertension, and have a normal lifestyle free of restriction. Thirty percent to 50% of those repaired after childhood do have hypertension, al-though it is usually mild and often does not require antihypertensive medication. In those with an asso-ciated bicuspid aortic valve, late stenosis must be watched for. Chemoprophylaxis for infective endo-carditis should be a lifetime commitment regardless of prior repair.

Differential Diagnosis

The clinical findings in acquired aortic obstruction secondary to arteritis, notably Takayasu's disease, may closely resemble those of coarctation, although the two are readily differentiated by angiography. Aortic dissection and traumatic para-aortic hematoma or tu-mor may have similar findings. Preoperative differ-entiation of the above greatly alters management. Pseudocoarctation has radiologic features similar to those of coarctation but does not have its clinical se-quelae because there is neither aortic obstruction nor hypertension. It does not warrant correction. So-called fetal coarctation is sometimes confused semantically with adult-type coarctation. The difference is great, however, in that the former is a variant of the hy-poplastic left-heart syndrome and has associated hy-poplastic left ventricle and ascending aorta, and often aortic and mitral stenosis or atresia. The right heart perfuses the systemic circulation via a large patent ductus. Affected infants usually die within weeks of birth, although extensive staged surgical revision (Norwood procedure) or cardiac transplantation may offer "guarded" hope.

PULMONIC STENOSIS

Pulmonic stenosis accounts for approximately 10% of congenital heart abnormalities in adults. Both unop-erated and postoperative patients may present to the physician.

Pathophysiology

In most cases, pulmonic stenosis is valvular and sec-ondary to a partially fused, bicuspid or tricuspid valve. These valves have a domed, "fish-mouth" appear-ance. Because of the chronic pressure load imposed on the right ventricle, that chamber hypertrophies.

Sometimes there is selective hypertrophy of the in-fundibulum beneath the pulmonic valve, which con-tributes to the overall right ventricular outflow tract obstruction.

The physiologic consequences of pulmonic steno-sis vary with its severity. When severe, there is right ventricular hypertrophy with decreased right ventric-ular compliance and elevation of end-diastolic pres-sure. Pulmonic stenosis is classified as mild, moderate and severe, according to the pressure gradient be-tween the right ventricle and the pulmonary artery. These gradients are <40 mm Hg in mild stenosis, between 40 mm Hg and 70 mm Hg in moderate ste-nosis, and >70 mm Hg in severe stenosis.

Clinical Course

Patients with mild and moderate pulmonic stenosis have few or no symptoms, and lifestyle is normal. The condition may not be diagnosed until adult life, but often the patient has a long-standing history of a loud, asymptomatic murmur. Complications, even late in life, are few. Some patients with moderate stenosis have progressive fatigue and dyspnea late in life. Se-vere stenosis may cause heart failure and cyanosis (owing to right-to-left shunting through a patent fo-ramen ovale) during infancy. Fatigue and dyspnea occur in children and adults with severe cyanosis, but overt clinical heart failure and atrial arrhythmia are not common. With severe stenosis, chest pain can mimic angina pectoris. It is attributed to the excessive demand placed on coronary flow by the hypertrophied right ventricle. Right ventricular ischemia and infarc-tion occur but are rare. Infective endocarditis is also rare. With severe stenosis and chronic heart failure, "cardiac" cirrhosis of the liver may develop second-ary to passive congestion. Paroxysmal dyspnea is un-common but is an ominous finding that sometimes heralds sudden death with severe stenosis.

Clinical Findings

Body habitus is normal and patients are acyanotic unless they have an associated patent foramen ovale or ASD, which permits right-to-left shunting and, therefore, systemic desaturation. With valvular ste-nosis, there is an ejection sound. Its position relative to the S_1 correlates inversely with the severity of ste-nosis. When very close or merged with the S_1, ste-nosis is severe. The ejection sound is louder during expiration than inspiration, unlike other right heart auscultatory phenomena. Patients have a systolic ejection murmur heard best at the upper left sternum that is loudest with inspiration. Its intensity and duration correlate directly with the severity of stenosis. Very loud and long murmurs that reach to the S_2 indicate severe stenosis. The later the peaking of the murmur, the more severe the stenosis. Pulmonic valve closure intensity correlates inversely with the severity of stenosis. The more severe the stenosis, the softer the pulmonic closure intensity. In addition, the more stenotic the valve, the more delayed the pulmonic closure sound from aortic closure. Patients with moderate or severe stenosis have palpable right ventricular hypertrophy and, typically, a systolic thrill at the upper left sternal border. A prominent jugular venous a-wave and a right ventricular S_4 are present with severe stenosis.

The electrocardiogram shows right atrial and right ventricular hypertrophy and right-axis deviation in moderate and severe stenosis; the ECG is normal in patients with mild gradients.

The chest x-ray film is often diagnostic. Patients with moderate or severe stenosis have right ventricular and right atrial enlargement. Patients with valvular stenosis have characteristic post-stenotic dilation of the main and left pulmonary arteries (Figure 6). Post-stenotic dilation does not correlate with severity of stenosis. Pulmonary blood flow is normal.

Cardiac ultrasound examination delineates the location and severity of pulmonic stenosis and the presence and significance of associated anomalies and secondary complications. It also permits estimation of the size of the stenotic valve annulus in those undergoing percutaneous balloon angioplasty.

Cardiac Catheterization

Patients with mild stenosis and no symptoms do not require catheterization, in contrast to those with cardiomegaly or symptoms or clinical findings suggesting moderate or severe stenosis. Catheterization is always indicated before surgical intervention. Its objectives include assessment of right ventricular pressure, both absolute and relative to systemic pressure, and determination of the right ventricular outflow tract gradient. Detailed angiographic delineation of the right ventricular outflow tract is essential.

For both children and adults with moderate or severe valvular stenosis, percutaneous balloon pul-

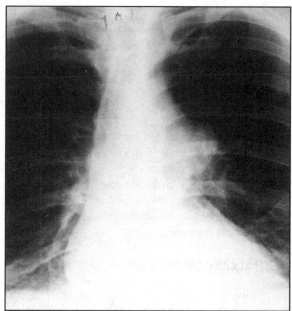

Figure 6. *Posteroanterior chest roentgenogram from a 48-year-old man with valvular pulmonic stenosis. There is prominent poststenotic dilation of the main and left pulmonary artery. (Reprinted with permission from Liberthson.)*

monic valvuloplasty offers results comparable to those achieved surgically; thus it is an attractive therapeutic alternative.

Surgical Intervention

Patients with mild stenosis do not require surgery. Those with cardiomegaly, symptoms, and severe stenosis should have surgical revision.

For most patients, pulmonic valve surgery consists of plasty revision to open the valvular commissures and relieve obstruction. Pulmonic valve replacement is rarely necessary. Some patients require resection of hypertrophied and obstructing infundibular muscle, and some require an outflow tract patch if the pulmonary annulus is hypoplastic.

The postoperative course after successful relief of obstruction is excellent, and patients become asymptomatic. A soft residual systolic murmur and sometimes a pulmonic diastolic murmur may be present. Residual stenosis occurs, but usually is limited to those with unicuspid or annular stenosis. It may necessitate reoperation if severe. Pulmonary valve incompetence is common but generally well tolerated. In the older adult who has fibrosis secondary to chronic right ventricular hypertrophy, right ventricular dysfunction with fatigue, dyspnea, and, sometimes, ventricular arrhythmia may persist.

Differential Diagnosis

Patients with the "straight back syndrome," pectus deformity of the sternum, small ASD, and idiopathic dilation of the pulmonic artery have some findings on physical examination that resemble those of mild pulmonic stenosis. These conditions are rarely confused with more significant stenosis, however. They can be differentiated noninvasively.

TETRALOGY OF FALLOT

Ten percent of adults with congenital heart disease have tetralogy of Fallot. It is the most common cyanotic cardiac lesion seen after infancy and accounts for more than 50% of cyanotic heart disease in adults. Internists infrequently see an unoperated patient, but more often see patients who have had either prior palliative surgery or definitive corrective procedures.

Anatomy

By definition, tetralogy has four anatomic components: (1) Right ventricular obstruction is secondary to both infundibular and pulmonic valvular stenosis. Both are of variable severity. Some patients have complete atresia of the right ventricular outflow tract. The pulmonary arteries themselves may also be small and sometimes hypoplastic, which may prevent surgical correction. (2) The VSD is membranous and large and approximates the size of the aortic annulus. (3) Aortic overriding across the ventricular defect is of variable degree and may approach 50% in those with severe pulmonic stenosis. (4) The right ventricle is hypertrophied secondary to its chronic pressure load; patchy interstitial fibrosis occurs in older adults.

Physiology

Tetralogy has two essential physiologic components: the right ventricular outflow tract obstruction causes decreased pulmonary blood flow, and the large VSD allows blood to flow from the right ventricle to the systemic circulation (right-to-left shunting). Systemic desaturation is variable, depending on the severity of right ventricular obstruction. When severe, desaturation is marked. In order to survive without surgical intervention, patients with severe pulmonic stenosis or atresia must develop collateral blood flow from the systemic to the pulmonary circulation. In older patients, these natural collateral channels are extensive. When right ventricular obstruction is mild, right-to-left shunting is minimal and patients may be acyanotic ("pink tetralogy").

Clinical Course

Cyanosis is typically present from early infancy and is progressive and worsened by exertion. A history of "tet spells" during the first years of life is sometimes given. Spells typically occur in hot weather, follow exertion or feeding, and are characterized by irritability, dyspnea, hyperventilation, cyanosis, and, sometimes, syncope and seizure. Some patients have late residua of these spells, including seizure disorders and cerebral vascular accident. Spells are rare after age two years. Squatting is learned from infancy and is often incorporated into a child's activities. More socially acceptable squatting postures, such as crossing the legs when sitting, are sometimes adopted by adults. Squatting increases systemic resistance and, therefore, decreases right-to-left blood flow across the ventricular defect and forces more blood to the lungs. Patients with chronic right-to-left shunting and systemic desaturation compensate by increased erythropoietin secretion, and erythrocytosis develops. When the erythrocytosis becomes excessive (hematocrit >65%), however, dyspnea, fatigue and in situ thrombosis may occur. Patients who have not undergone surgical intervention may have a history of repeated phlebotomy. With long-standing erythrocytosis, uric acid elevation and symptomatic gout may be present. Chronic right-to-left shunting subjects both unoperated patients and those who have had only palliative surgical procedures to the risk of systemic embolizations. These may occur with careless intravenous technique. Cerebral abscess is another sequela of chronic right-to-left shunting, and must be suspected in patients with neurologic symptoms or findings. Bacterial endocarditis occurs in patients with uncorrected tetralogy and in those with palliated and corrected tetralogy. It usually involves the right ventricular outflow tract or the overriding aortic valve, but it may occur at the site of palliative shunt insertion. Chemoprophylaxis is, therefore, a lifetime obligation. In the adult, ventricular tachyarrhythmia is an ominous finding and may herald sudden death. The risk of mortality is increased in pregnant women with uncorrected tetralogy, and the incidence of fetal death is also greatly increased.

Clinical Findings

The salient findings in unoperated patients include generalized cyanosis and digital clubbing. Body habitus is normal, although kyphoscoliosis occurs in 20%. Those who have had a prior palliative procedure have a thoracotomy scar. Corrective procedures are performed via a median sternotomy. In the adult who has not had prior surgery, continuous collateral bruits are heard throughout the chest. Those with a functioning palliative shunt will have a continuous bruit beneath their thoracotomy scar.

The cardiac examination in patients with palliative shunts and those who have not had prior surgery is the same because both still have the anatomic components of tetralogy. Successfully palliated patients differ only in having less cyanosis, because their pulmonary blood flow has been augmented: often they have no digital clubbing. However, previously palliated patients may outgrow or close their shunts and develop progressive cyanosis. In both uncorrected and palliated patients, there is palpable right ventricular hypertrophy, and a palpable systolic thrill secondary to pulmonic stenosis. The S_1 is normal; the S_2 is single and often loud; it corresponds to aortic closure. Patients with very mild tetralogy (''pink tet'') may have an audible pulmonic closure sound, which is otherwise atypical in tetralogy. An ejection sound is common and arises from the overriding aortic valve and is best heard on expiration. A systolic ejection murmur secondary to right ventricular outflow tract obstruction is typical. The length, intensity, and contour of this murmur help the clinician to assess the severity of pulmonic stenosis. Long, loud, late-peaking murmurs indicate less severe right ventricular obstruction than do short, soft, early-peaking murmurs. With pulmonary atresia, no outflow tract murmur is present.

The ECG reveals right ventricular hypertrophy and right-axis deviation in patients with either uncorrected or palliated tetralogy.

The chest x-ray film is often diagnostic. In the young patient, pulmonary vascular markings are diminished. However, with age and proliferation of collateral circulation, pulmonary vascular markings may actually be increased (Figure 7). Functioning pallia-

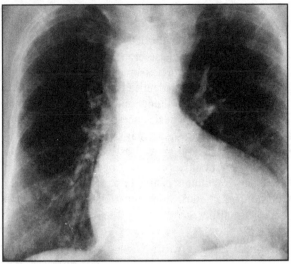

Figure 7. *Posteroanterior chest roentgenogram from a 59-year-old woman with tetralogy of Fallot and extensive systemic-to-pulmonary collateral vasculature with secondary rib notching. The cardiac silhouette has a distinctive ''boot'' shape secondary to the upturned apex, secondary to right ventricular hypertrophy and the concave pulmonary artery segment. There is a right aortic arch. (Reprinted with permission from Liberthson.)*

tive shunts also cause increased pulmonary markings and enlargement of the pulmonary branch into which they enter. In unoperated patients and in those with palliative shunts, the cardiac silhouette is typical. There is an upturned apex, secondary to right ventricular enlargement, and a concave left basal region caused by the small main pulmonary artery. This combination gives the heart a boot shape. Approximately 25% of patients with tetralogy have a right-sided aortic arch.

Ultrasound examination delineates the morphology of the right ventricular obstruction, the VSD, the overriding aorta, and the hypertrophied right ventricle. It also differentiates tetralogy from more complex entities, including single ventricle and variants of transposition of the great arteries.

Cardiac Catheterization

Catheterization is required before surgical intervention. Its objectives include detailed angiographic study of the right ventricular obstruction, including assessment of the caliber of the pulmonary arteries; assessment of the VSD and exclusion of multiple or atypical septal defects; and evaluation of the coronary arteries to identify the approximately 5% of patients who have anomalous origin of major left coronary branches from the right coronary. These branches cross the anterior right ventricle and can be damaged at the time of right ventriculotomy if not identified. In patients who have had prior palliative shunts, pulmonary artery anatomy, pressure, and resistance must be assessed because long-standing shunts may cause severe pulmonary vascular obstruction as well as kinking and hypoplasia of a pulmonary branch. Angiographic study of these surgical shunts is also important before surgical revision. Catheterization must also exclude more complex entities.

Surgical Intervention

Surgery for tetralogy of Fallot began with the palliative procedures involving creation of a shunt between the systemic and pulmonary circulations to increase pulmonary blood flow and to alleviate systemic desaturation. The Blalock-Taussig shunt involves ligation of the distal subclavian artery and insertion of its proximal end into the ipsilateral pulmonary artery. Complications with this procedure are rare, and excellent long-term alleviation of desaturation is typical. Both pulse and blood pressure in the ipsilateral arm are sacrificed, but arm function and development are usually normal. The Potts shunt involves creation of a surgical window between the left pulmonary artery and the descending aorta. It also achieves excellent long-term palliation of desaturation. However, in about one fourth of patients, early heart failure owing to excessive pulmonary flow or late pulmonary vascular obstruction develops. Patients with these shunts require assessment of pulmonary artery pressure and resistance at the time of catheterization. When the latter is high, corrective surgery may be precluded. The Waterston shunt is a surgical window between the ascending aorta and the right pulmonary artery. It also provides excellent palliation. However, its complications include hypoplasia and stenosis of the right pulmonary artery secondary to kinking; early heart failure if the shunt is too large; and, occasionally, pulmonary vascular obstruction. Regardless of shunt type, patients may outgrow them, or they may kink or close, and recurrent and progressive cyanosis occurs. If so, catheterization and further surgery are indicated. Despite their success in relieving cyanosis, shunts do not alter the intracardiac pathology of tetralogy; therefore, the chronic sequelae of right-to-left shunting and right ventricular hypertension remain. For these reasons, patients with palliative shunts should still have definitive surgical repair and shunt closure.

Correction of tetralogy consists of surgical relief of right ventricular obstruction (which may require the use of a patch across the outflow tract), and patch closure of the VSD such that left ventricular outflow is directed to the overriding aorta. When the outflow tract requires a patch to enlarge it, patients have residual pulmonic incompetence. Most centers perform elective total correction during infancy or early childhood. Infants who have tet spells require either emergency palliation or definitive repair. In all other cases, surgery should be performed when the diagnosis is confirmed. After the fifth decade, risks of total correction increase because of right ventricular dysfunction secondary to chronic hypertrophy and fibrosis.

After successful tetralogy repair, patients become acyanotic, clubbing resolves over a period of years, exercise tolerance markedly improves, and lifestyle becomes normal. Some patients have residual problems and all require continued surveillance. Problems include an incompletely closed VSD and residual right ventricular obstruction, which, when severe (gradient >50 mm Hg), requires reoperation. In the former, when shunt size exceeds 2:1, repeat operation is appropriate. Patients with right ventricular outflow tract patches have pulmonic incompetence, but this is usually well tolerated. If an anomalous coronary artery was damaged at the time of repair, patients may have anterior wall myocardial infarction. Ventricular ectopy usually arises from the right ventricle and may be secondary to fibrosis or to aneurysm or infarction in those patients with a damaged anomalous coronary artery. It is an ominous finding and requires intensive antiarrhythmic treatment; invasive electrophysiologic study may help in the selection of an antiarrhythmic regimen. When ventricular ectopy is associated with significant residual right ventricular obstruction, VSD, or severe pulmonic incompetence, patients may require reoperation. Right bundle branch block and left anterior hemiblock occur in 10% of patients after repair, but rarely lead to more advanced degrees of heart block. Syncope in these patients is uncommon.

Differential Diagnosis

Patients with pulmonic stenosis and VSD who also have variants of transposition of the great arteries, as well as those who have single ventricle rather than a

VSD alone, may be impossible to differentiate clinically from those with tetralogy of Fallot. Both ultrasound and angiography are important in identifying these patients. The latter is essential because in some, reparative surgery is precluded and in others its risk may be great.

Bibliography

Grossman W, Barry WH: Cardiac catheterization. In: Braunwald E, ed. *Heart Disease*. Philadelphia: WB Saunders; 1988, p. 242.

Liberthson RR: *Congenital Heart Disease Diagnosis and Management in Children and Adults*. Boston: Little, Brown; 1989.

Perloff J: *The Clinical Recognition of Congenital Heart Disease* (3rd ed.). Philadelphia: WB Saunders; 1987.

Roberts WC: *Adult Congenital Heart Disease*. Philadelphia: FA Davis; 1987.

23 Heart Failure

Robert A. Kloner
Victor J. Dzau

DEFINITION AND MECHANISMS OF HEART FAILURE

Heart failure affects approximately 3 million Americans, developing in about 400,000 each year. It is especially common in the elderly. This clinical syndrome results from an abnormality of cardiac function such that the heart cannot pump blood at a volume adequate to meet the metabolic needs of the tissues of the body (forward failure), or it cannot distend sufficiently during diastole, leading to congestion (backward failure). The syndrome is associated with an increase in atrial pressures, reduced exercise tolerance, ventricular arrhythmias, and shortened life expectancy (Cohn; Parmley). The abnormality in cardiac function may be due to an abnormality in the myocardial cells themselves (myocardial failure) or to some other structural abnormality, such as valvular stenosis impairing ventricular ejection.

Myocardial failure may be due to a quantitative loss of functioning myofibers, as in heart failure associated with a large myocardial infarction (MI), or to a generalized qualitative abnormality in myocyte function, as occurs with congestive cardiomyopathy. The precise mechanism of abnormal myocyte function in myocardial failure is controversial. One possible mechanism is a reduction in myofibrillar ATPase, seen in the hearts of patients and experimental animals with congestive heart failure. Reduced myocardial contractility is associated with a change in myosin isozyme from myosin V_1 (a myosin with increased ATPase activity) to myosin V_3 (which has reduced ATPase activity). Another possible mechanism comes from animal studies that suggest that sarcoplasmic reticulum is defective in its ability to pump calcium. Normally, the sarcoplasmic reticulum takes up intracellular calcium during the relaxation phase of the cardiac cycle. During electrical depolarization, extracellular calcium enters the cell and intracellular calcium is released from the sarcoplasmic reticulum. The calcium interacts with the contractile apparatus, resulting in a contraction. Experimental studies suggest that in myocardial failure, the sarcoplasmic reticulum is defective in its ability to take up calcium during relaxation. As a result, little calcium is available for release to the contractile apparatus during systole. In myocardial failure, the mitochondria may become the main site of uptake of calcium and source of calcium for contraction. Because release of calcium from the mitochondria is a slow process, only limited amounts of calcium may be available to activate the contractile mechanism. Cardiac tissue from patients with heart failure who were undergoing cardiac transplantation also show reduced rates of calcium uptake by the sarcoplasmic reticulum, as well as reduced rates of release.

Other possible explanations for myocardial failure include reduced coronary blood flow and myocardial oxygen consumption per unit of tissue and alterations of mitochondrial function. Depletion of myocardial norepinephrine stores and decline in norepinephrine production have been observed in myocardial failure. Although regional norepinephrine stores do not play a role in the intrinsic contractile state of the myocardium, the adrenergic nervous system is an important compensatory mechanism for the failing heart. The depleted norepinephrine levels may impede this compensatory mechanism. Decreased beta receptors have been described in heart failure, although their importance remains controversial. Myocardial hypertrophy with excess collagen deposition may also contribute to heart failure and has been implicated as a cause of diastolic dysfunction.

359

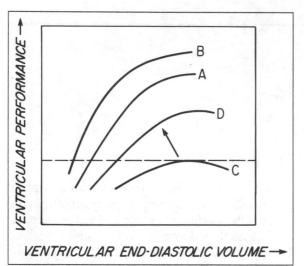

Figure 1. *Starling curves showing ventricular end-diastolic volume plotted on the horizontal axis and ventricular performance on the vertical axis. The horizontal axis could also be ventricular end-diastolic pressure, and the vertical axis could be stroke volume or stroke work. Curve A represents the normal curve; curve B a curve of increased contractile state; curve C that of reduced contractile state; and curve D the curve of a failing heart after digitalis treatment.*

COMPENSATORY MECHANISMS IN HEART FAILURE

The heart relies on several compensatory mechanisms for maintenance of its pumping ability in the setting of myocardial failure or an excessive hemodynamic burden (such as systemic hypertension, aortic regurgitation, or stenosis). The first is the Frank-Starling mechanism, in which the force of contraction or extent of shortening depends on the initial muscle length. When the muscle and, therefore, sarcomere length is increased by an increase in preload to provide optimal overlap between the actin (thin) and myosin (thick) filaments, cardiac performance is enhanced.

Figure 1 shows a typical Frank-Starling curve. As ventricular end-diastolic volume or preload increases, so does ventricular performance. Braunwald (1988b) described factors that result in changes along a given curve (changes in preload resulting in different degrees of stretching of the myocardium) and changes that shift the curve (alterations of the contractile state of the myocardium). Factors that alter ventricular end-

diastolic volume and, hence, result in movement along a given Frank-Starling curve include total blood volume; body position; intrathoracic and intrapericardial pressure; venous tone; the pumping action of skeletal muscle that returns blood to the heart; and the atrial contribution to ventricular filling. Factors that shift the Frank-Starling curve upward and to the left (increase in the contractile state of the myocardium as shown in curve B) include sympathetic nerve stimulation; circulating catecholamines; positive inotropic agents such as digitalis; and the force-frequency relationship (an increase in heart rate resulting in an increase in contractility). Factors that shift the Frank-Starling curve down and to the right (depressed contractile state of the myocardium; curve C) include anoxia, hypercapnia, acidosis, pharmacologic depressants (such as quinidine and local anesthetic agents), loss of myocardium, and intrinsic myocardial depression.

Patients with myocardial failure function along this depressed (curve C) Frank-Starling curve. To maintain the same ventricular performance as in a normal heart, they must have a higher ventricular end-diastolic volume. If the metabolic demands of the body increase, requiring increased cardiac performance, this occurs in such patients at the expense of a higher ventricular end-diastolic volume (and increased left ventricular filling pressure), which may in turn result in the symptoms of dyspnea or even pulmonary edema (Figure 2).

Neurohumoral systems are activated in heart failure. The effects include activation of the sympathetic nervous system with increased plasma catecholamine levels, activation of the renin-angiotensin-aldosterone system, and increased production of arginine vasopressin (antidiuretic hormone). Although the changes in these systems are meant to be compensatory—to defend against traumatic loss of blood volume and dehydration—and are capable of restoring blood pressure, they may have adverse effects in patients with heart failure (Figure 2). Sympathetic stimulation, renin release, and arginine vasopressin act to increase systemic vascular resistance and promote salt and water retention. The increase in cardiac afterload can ultimately depress cardiac performance and the increase in volume may worsen congestive symptoms. Increase in heart rate due to sympathetic stimulation may precipitate arrhythmias as well as ischemia.

Levels of atrial natriuretic peptide (ANP) are elevated in patients with heart failure. Atrial natriuretic

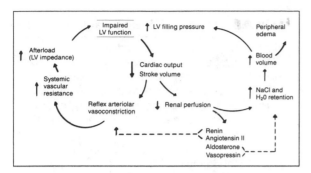

Figure 2. *Two interrelated vicious cycles in congestive heart failure. Left: Impairment of left ventricular (LV) function leads to a decrease in cardiac output. This leads to a reflex increase in systemic vascular resistance by the neurohumoral mechanisms. This increases the effective afterload of the left ventricle and further reduces stroke volume. Right: A reduction in cardiac output and arterial pressure leads to a decrease in renal perfusion. This activates the renin-angiotensin-aldosterone system. Overall, there is retention of salt (NaCl) and water (H₂O), leading to a further increase in filling pressure and to peripheral edema. These cycles, therefore, can feed back on each other to worsen the heart failure state. (Reprinted from McCall and O'Rourke. With permission of the American Heart Assn. See Bibliography.)*

peptides are located within secretory granules within the atria and are released upon increased atrial pressure or volume. In animal and human studies, infusion of atrial extracts has been shown to induce natriuresis, diuresis, and vasodilation. Saito et al. showed that infusion of ANP in patients with congestive heart failure reduced pulmonary capillary wedge pressure, improved stroke volume, and reduced systemic vascular resistance. The effect of ANP on diuresis was blunted compared with that in normal patients. Presumably, release of ANP is a compensatory mechanism in heart failure; whether exogenous administration of ANP in patients with heart failure will have an important therapeutic role remains to be determined.

Long-term compensatory mechanisms of the heart with valvular or myocardial abnormalities include myocardial hypertrophy and dilatation. In the initial stages of heart failure, the compensatory mechanisms may sustain the circulatory needs of the body. Eventually, however, as myocardial failure progresses, the compensatory mechanisms can no longer maintain the

pump function of the heart and the clinical syndrome of heart failure emerges.

THE CLINICAL SYNDROME OF HEART FAILURE

FORWARD VERSUS BACKWARD HEART FAILURE

The clinical syndrome of heart failure has been hypothesized to arise from either backward or forward cardiac failure, or both. *Backward failure* refers to blood damming up behind one or both ventricles, because the ventricle cannot discharge its contents. Symptoms result from an increase in systemic venous pressure with right ventricular failure, resulting in transudation of fluid into the interstitium of the liver, mesentery, and subcutaneous tissue; or from an increase in pulmonary venous pressure with left ventricular failure, resulting in transudation of fluid into the interstitium of the lung. The *forward failure* hypothesis refers to inability of the heart to pump an adequate amount of blood into the arterial tree, resulting in symptoms of underperfusion of the vital organs. Reduced perfusion to the kidneys results in increased sodium and water retention, leading to an increase in extracellular fluid level and tissue congestion. The renal mechanisms for increased water retention are complex; they include reduced renal water excretion due to decreased renal blood flow with reduced glomerular filtration rate, enhancement of the renin-angiotensin-aldosterone system, and enhanced antidiuretic hormone release. Reduced forward output to the brain results in mental confusion, and to the skeletal muscles in exercise intolerance and weakness.

In most patients with chronic heart failure, both backward and forward failure result in symptoms.

RIGHT- VERSUS LEFT-SIDED HEART FAILURE

Right ventricular failure, associated with blood "damming up" in the systemic venous circuit, includes symptoms and signs of edema, congestive hepatomegaly, ascites, and, eventually, signs of low forward output, including weakness and mental confusion. Symptoms and signs of left ventricular failure are due to blood "damming up" behind the left ventricle and to pulmonary congestion. Long-standing left ventricular failure may eventually result in signs of right ventricular failure, with generalized accumulation of fluid. Experimental studies show that failure of one ventricle induced by a hemodynamic stress eventually results in biochemical changes (depletion of norepinephrine and abnormalities in the activity of actinomyosin ATPase) of the other ventricle. This may be secondary to the fact that muscle bundles composing one ventricle are in continuity with those of the other ventricle.

LOW- VERSUS HIGH-OUTPUT CARDIAC FAILURE

Heart failure causing low cardiac output is the most common form of heart failure and is usually due to an ischemic, valvular, hypertensive, congenital, or cardiomyopathic process. Heart failure also may result from several high-output states such as beriberi, Paget's disease, thyrotoxicosis, arteriovenous fistula, and anemia. Low-output failure is characterized by reduced stroke volume, peripheral vasoconstriction with cold and pale extremities, reduced pulse pressure, and widened arteriovenous oxygen difference; high-output failure is characterized by a widened pulse pressure and peripheral vasodilatation, with warm and flushed extremities. High-output states are associated with reduced arteriovenous oxygen difference. Arteriovenous oxygen difference does not decrease much in patients with high-output states once congestive heart failure develops.

CAUSES OF HEART FAILURE

The general underlying causes of heart failure are outlined in Table 1. It is important to realize that 50% of episodes of clinical heart failure are secondary to a precipitating cause. Thus, in treating heart failure, both the underlying and precipitating causes must be recognized. The most common underlying causes of heart failure (in the United States) are coronary artery disease, hypertension, cardiomyopathy, and valvular heart disease.

THE CONCEPT OF DIASTOLIC HEART FAILURE

Heart failure is usually associated with an abnormality of systolic function (reduced ability to expel blood from the ventricular cavities); it also may occur with

Table 1. Causes of Heart Failure

Primary abnormality of myocardial cells
  Cardiomyopathy and myocarditis
Secondary abnormality of myocardial cells
  Due to prolonged exposure to a hemodynamic burden (i.e., aortic regurgitation, hypertensive heart disease, primary or secondary pulmonary hypertension)
  Due to reduced O_2 delivery (ischemia)
Structural abnormalities
  Valvular heart disease
  Congenital heart disease
  Pericardial disease
  Coronary artery disease (ischemia, myocardial infarction, left ventricular aneurysm)
  Intracavity outflow obstruction
High-output states
Precipitating causes
  Increased salt intake
  Inappropriate reduction of a drug regimen
  Excess exertion or emotion
  Arrhythmias
  Systemic infection
  Onset of high-output states: anemia, hyperthyroidism, pregnancy
  Pulmonary embolism
  Increased fluid load
  Renal failure
  Myocardial ischemia
  Cardiac depressants (e.g., disopyramide)

an abnormality of diastolic function despite normal systolic function (reduced ability of the left ventricle to accept or fill with blood). When the ventricles fail to relax adequately to accept blood, ventricular diastolic pressures increase, causing atrial pressures to increase and leading to systemic or pulmonary congestion. Thus, some patients with heart failure may have normal or near-normal ejection fractions but still have the symptoms and signs of congestion. Transient diastolic heart failure may be seen in patients with coronary artery disease who, during ischemia, have a reduction in left ventricular compliance, an increase in left ventricular filling pressures, and subsequent dyspnea. It is also seen in patients with hypertrophic cardiomyopathy, restrictive cardiomyopathies such as amyloid, and replacement of myocytes by scar tissue, as occurs with myocardial infarction.

SYMPTOMS OF LEFT-SIDED HEART FAILURE

The major clinical symptoms of left ventricular heart failure include exertional dyspnea, orthopnea, paroxysmal nocturnal dyspnea, dyspnea at rest, exercise intolerance, weakness, fatigue, nocturia, and mental confusion.

Dyspnea is the sensation of breathlessness, difficulty in breathing, or increased awareness of breathing that occurs with elevation in left atrial pressure resulting from pulmonary capillary hypertension. It is associated with a restrictive ventilatory defect due to the replacement of air with fluid or blood in the lungs. The work of breathing is increased in order to distend the stiffened lungs. In the early phases of left ventricular heart failure, the dyspnea occurs only with exertion; with increasing heart failure, the level of exertion resulting in dyspnea diminishes until, in severe heart failure, dyspnea occurs at rest. Orthopnea is dyspnea that occurs while the patient is recumbent and is relieved by standing or sitting. It is caused by redistribution of fluid from the dependent parts of the circulation to the thorax, where the depressed left ventricle cannot pump the additional volume of delivered blood. Orthopnea results from pulmonary venous and capillary congestion. The severity of the orthopnea can often be determined by asking the patient how many pillows he or she sleeps on.

Paroxysmal nocturnal dyspnea, an extreme form of orthopnea, occurs when a patient wakes from sleep with a sense of severe breathlessness and suffocation. It is often associated with bronchospasm and, hence, has been called "cardiac asthma." Paroxysmal nocturnal dyspnea usually occurs at night and often is unrelieved by sitting upright. A pathophysiologic feature of this condition is interstitial pulmonary edema.

Pulmonary edema associated with heart failure occurs when left atrial pressure is markedly elevated with subsequent transudation of fluid into the alveoli. It is the severest form of breathlessness associated with heart failure. In acute pulmonary edema, patients are severely short of breath at rest, with associated agitation or dizziness. Pulmonary edema, which is considered a medical emergency, can be caused by any etiology of heart failure (Table 1). Several noncardiac causes of pulmonary edema (increased capillary "leakage" without elevation of atrial pressures) should be considered (Table 2).

Differentiating between dyspnea due to cardiac disease and dyspnea due to pulmonary disease may be difficult, especially when they coexist. Table 3 presents some differentiating features.

Other symptoms of left-sided heart failure reflecting reduced forward output include fatigue, weakness, and, in severe cases, mental confusion.

The New York Heart Association (NYHA) devised a functional classification of heart disease that grades the severity of heart failure according to the amount of exertion required to cause symptoms. Although the classification is based on subjective findings, it is useful in following the course of patients during their disease, assessing results of therapy, and comparing groups of patients.

Class I.   No limitation of physical activity. No dyspnea, fatigue, or palpitations with ordinary physical activity.

Class II. Slight limitation of physical activity. These patients have fatigue, palpitations, and dyspnea with ordinary physical activity, but are comfortable at rest.

Class III. Marked limitation of activity. Less than ordinary physical activity results in symptoms but patients are comfortable at rest.

Class IV. Symptoms are present at rest and any physical exertion exacerbates the symptoms.

SYMPTOMS OF RIGHT-SIDED HEART FAILURE

The common specific etiologies of right-sided heart failure are listed in Table 4. A rare form of cardiomyopathy affects primarily the right ventricle and is called arrhythmogenic right ventricular dysplasia. This entity is associated with arrhythmias, right-sided heart failure and sudden death in young patients.

Symptoms of predominantly right-sided heart failure are those of systemic venous congestion, including dependent edema; right upper quadrant pain due to stretching of the hepatic capsule from liver engorgement; anorexia, nausea, and bloating due to congestion of the mesentery and liver; and fatigue as forward output diminishes. Pulmonary symptoms are uncommon unless concomitant left-sided heart failure is present.

SIGNS OF HEART FAILURE

The general appearance of patients in left-sided heart failure depends on the severity of the heart failure.

Table 2. Noncardiac Causes of Pulmonary Edema
Decreased plasma oncotic pressure: hypoalbuminemia due to renal, hepatic disease, nutritional cause, or protein-losing enteropathy
Altered alveolar-capillary membrane permeability (often referred to as adult respiratory distress syndrome [ARDS])
Pneumonia: viral, bacterial, parasite, aspiration
Inhaled toxins: smoke, nitrogen dioxide, phosgene
Circulating toxins: bacterial endotoxins, snake venom
Radiation pneumonitis
Endogenous vasoactive substances: kinins, histamines
Disseminated intravascular coagulation
Uremia
Immunologic reactions: hypersensitivity pneumonitis
Associated with drowning
Lymphatic insufficiency: carcinomatosis, fibrosing lymphangitis
Unknown or not well understood
Narcotic overdose: heroin
High altitude pulmonary edema
Neurogenic: subarachnoid hemorrhage, central nervous system trauma
Eclampsia
Post-cardiopulmonary bypass
Post-cardioversion
Post-anesthesia

With mild failure, patients may appear entirely comfortable sitting at rest and do not appear breathless or in any distress until they undertake physical activity or lie flat. With severe failure, patients at rest may appear to be in severe distress, tachypneic, pale, and with cool extremities. They may be cyanotic.

Examination of the lungs in patients with mild left heart failure reveals moist rales at the bases; with severe failure and pulmonary edema, rales may be heard over the entire lung fields and may be associated with blood-tinged sputum. Dullness on percussion at the lung bases may reflect a pleural effusion.

If heart failure is secondary to left ventricular failure, evidence of dilatation and/or hypertrophy of that chamber may be present, including displacement of the apical impulse downward and toward the axilla (dilatation) and a left ventricular heave, which is a localized sustained outward motion of the ventricle during systole (left ventricular hypertrophy). With right ventricular enlargement, the right heart border may be percussed to the right of the sternum and a right ventricular heave may be felt as a diffuse lift over the lower portion of the sternum.

The S_1 is often normal; the P_2 may be accentuated with the development of left ventricular failure and pulmonary hypertension. A protodiastolic, or S_3 gallop, heard 0.13-0.16 second after the S_2, is a common sign of congestive heart failure. This sound occurs in association with increased ventricular volumes and is caused by a rapid deceleration of ventricular inflow occurring just after the early filling phase of the ventricle. Reduced ventricular distensibility may contribute to the gallop sound.

Fourth heart sounds (pre-systolic gallop) may be heard when congestive heart failure is associated with conditions in which the atrium contracts forcibly into a noncompliant ventricle and occurs with ventricular hypertrophy. Gallops emanating from the left ventricle are best heard at the apex with the patient in the left lateral decubitus position; gallops emanating from the right ventricle are best heard at the lower left sternal border and, typically, increase with inspiration. Gallops are best heard using the bell of the stethoscope. Murmurs due to mitral regurgitation or tricuspid regurgitation secondary to ventricular dilatation are not uncommon in heart failure.

Tachycardia is another common manifestation of heart failure and is a compensatory mechanism whereby the heart attempts to maintain cardiac output in the setting of reduced stroke volume. Pulsus alternans is

Table 3. Differentiation of Cardiac versus Pulmonary Dyspnea

Cardiac Dyspnea	Pulmonary Dyspnea
Onset of dyspnea more sudden	Dyspnea tends to occur more gradually (except with infectious bronchitis, pneumonitis, pneumothorax, asthma)
Dyspnea usually not associated with sputum production	Dyspnea at night often associated with sputum production and relieved by coughing up sputum
No history of pulmonary disease	History of chronic obstructive lung disease; smoking history; noxious inhalants
No history of smoking	
No evidence of lung disease on chest x-ray film	Chest x-ray evidence of lung disease
Restrictive ventilatory defect by pulmonary function tests	Obstructive or restrictive ventilatory defect by pulmonary function tests
Arm-to-tongue circulation time usually increased (>16 sec)*	Arm-to-tongue circulation time more likely to be normal

*The circulation time may be a useful test to perform when trying to distinguish pulmonary from cardiac dyspnea and low-output from high-output heart failure. Three to five ml of Decholin is injected rapidly intravenously and the time until the patient senses a bitter taste is measured. Normal values are 9-16 seconds. In patients with low-output heart failure, values are >16; in patients with high-output failure, circulation time is normal or reduced; in patients without heart failure, values are normal.

characterized by a regular rhythm in which there is an alternation of strong and weak contractions as detected by palpation of the pulse or by sphygmomanometry. This phenomenon occurs secondary to alternating stroke volume due to incomplete recovery of contractile cells on every other beat. Cheyne-Stokes respiration occurs in patients with advanced cardiac failure and is characterized by alternating periods of apnea and hyperpnea. This condition is due to a reduced sensitivity of the respiratory center to CO_2, and prolonged circulation time from lung to brain associated with left ventricular failure. When congestive failure is severe and long-standing, cardiac cachexia may occur with anorexia and weight loss.

Signs of right ventricular failure include jugular venous distention, hepatojugular reflux, hepatomegaly, right upper quadrant tenderness, edema, and ascites. When severe congestion of the viscera occurs, a protein-losing enteropathy may exacerbate development of ascites by a reduction in plasma oncotic pressure. With development of tricuspid regurgitation, a systolic regurgitant v-wave may be seen and palpated in the jugular veins.

LABORATORY EXAMINATION IN CONGESTIVE HEART FAILURE

A typical chest x-ray feature of congestive heart failure includes cardiomegaly with a cardiothoracic ratio of >0.5–0.6. The appearance of the lung fields serves as an estimate of the pulmonary capillary pressure. Normally the apices of the lung are less well perfused than the bases. With pulmonary capillary pressures of 15-20 mm Hg, apical and basal perfusions equalize; with pulmonary capillary pressures of 20-25 mm Hg, upper lobe pulmonary veins become more prominent than those in the lower lobe. With pulmonary capillary pressures >25 mm Hg, interstitial pulmonary edema and Kerley B lines (interlobular edema) occur, and with pressures >25-30 mm Hg, alveolar edema and pleural effusions may be seen (see Chapter 4).

The electrocardiogram (ECG) may help define the underlying etiology (especially ischemia) of the heart failure and confirm the presence of ventricular hypertrophy (see Chapter 3).

Echocardiography is useful in assessing the severity and etiology of heart failure and may aid in serial

Table 4. Specific Causes of Right-Sided Heart Failure
Mitral stenosis with pulmonary hypertension
Cor pulmonale due to chronic obstructive lung disease
Pulmonary valve stenosis
Pulmonary hypertension due to other causes
Congenital heart disease
Primary pulmonary hypertension
Collagen vascular disease
Tricuspid valve regurgitation (causes right ventricular [RV] failure)
Tricuspid valve stenosis; obstruction of flow into RV without RV myocardial failure
Right ventricular myocardial infarction
Chronic left-sided congestive heart failure due to valvular or ischemic disease
Arrhythmogenic RV dysplasia

evaluation of the effect of therapy. Surgically correctable valvular disease must first be excluded. Global or diffuse left ventricular dysfunction suggests a cardiomyopathic process. Regional wall motion abnormalities are suggestive of coronary artery disease. Radionuclide ventriculography is another useful non-invasive technique for assessing ventricular function. Serial ejection fractions may be followed and areas of abnormal ventricular wall motion detected. Serial exercise testing and exercise radionuclide ventriculography may be used to follow the response of patients with chronic heart failure to treatment regimens. Coronary angiography may be undertaken to diagnose significant coronary artery disease, which may be treated with angioplasty or surgical therapy. Cardiac catheterization is also useful in identifying other underlying causes of heart failure but is rarely needed to make the diagnosis of heart failure. Catheterization may be helpful in assessing the effect of pharmacologic interventions such as vasodilators or experimental inotropic agents in patients whose heart failure is refractory to other forms of medical therapy.

Several blood chemistry tests may be abnormal in patients with congestive heart failure, including elevated liver enzyme levels (SGOT, SGPT) and bilirubin secondary to hepatic congestion. Urinalysis may reveal proteinuria and high urine specific gravity. With reduced renal flow, the BUN becomes elevated. With chronic cor pulmonale, polycythemia may occur. Serum electrolytes are usually normal in most cases of mild to moderate congestive heart failure before treatment. With severe heart failure, diuretic therapy, salt restriction, and reduced ability to excrete free water result in dilutional hyponatremia.

Hypokalemia may result from thiazide or loop diuretics. Hyperkalemia may result from spironolactone administration, especially in the presence of a nonsteroidal anti-inflammatory drug or an angiotensin converting enzyme (ACE) inhibitor. It may occur in severe heart failure with markedly reduced renal blood flow or underlying diabetic nephropathy.

PROGNOSIS

The five-year mortality rate for heart failure is generally high: 60% for men and 45% for women. Patients with class IV heart failure do worse, with a one-year survival rate of only 50%. Ventricular arrhythmias are common in patients with congestive heart failure. Sudden death accounts for 33-47% of deaths in patients with severe heart failure. Only recently have certain vasodilator agents been shown to improve survival in patients with heart failure (see later).

THERAPY OF CONGESTIVE HEART FAILURE

MANAGEMENT OF ACUTE CARDIOGENIC PULMONARY EDEMA

The major aim of the management of acute cardiogenic pulmonary edema is to improve oxygenation and reduce pulmonary capillary pressure. Oxygen should be administered by nasal prongs or face mask at high flow rate (except with chronic obstructive lung disease and CO_2 retention). At least one large bore (No. 18 or larger) intravenous catheter should be placed for access to the circulation. The patient should be sitting upright, which increases venous pooling, reduces central venous pressure, and improves pulmonary perfusion-ventilation matching. Arterial blood gas levels before oxygen administration should be determined and a 12-lead ECG should be immediately recorded. Other nonpharmacologic interventions include applying tourniquets in rotation or in three of four extremities, and phlebotomy. The value of the former has not been clearly established and the latter is usually reserved for dire emergencies.

Intravenous morphine is immediately administered in acute pulmonary edema. Morphine reduces both preload and afterload. It also reduces the sympathetic overdrive and anxiety, which can worsen pulmonary edema in these patients. Morphine (3-10 mg) is administered slowly. Signs of respiratory depression must be sought. Naloxone or nalorphine hydrochloride (morphine antagonists) should be available. Relative contraindications to morphine include severe pulmonary disease, severe kyphoscoliosis, liver failure, and myxedema. Aminophylline given parenterally (250-500 mg IV over 15–20 minutes) improves ventilation. More important is the use of intravenous furosemide for diuresis. Furosemide (10-40 mg) induces veno- and arteriolar dilatation and also causes diuresis 10-30 minutes after IV administration; the peak effect is in 60 minutes. Digitalis is useful, especially if atrial tachyarrhythmia with rapid ventricular response is present. If the patient has a systolic blood pressure >95 mm Hg, sublingual or IV nitroglycerin may be administered in order to reduce ventricular preload. Intravenous nitroprusside is also used as vasodilator therapy in patients with acute pulmonary edema. However, some studies suggest that in acute ischemic syndromes it may cause a coronary steal phenomenon.

Precipitating causes of pulmonary edema (such as myocardial ischemia, arrhythmia, infection, anemia, thyrotoxicosis, and fluid overload) should be treated. Response to therapy is gauged by symptoms, physical examination, chest x-ray, and special tests such as echocardiography, rest and exercise radionuclide ventriculography, treadmill exercise tests, and, in some cases, acute drug testing during the time of cardiac catheterization.

TREATMENT OF CHRONIC HEART FAILURE

The therapeutic approach to heart failure, as recently described by Parmley, is summarized in Table 5.

The first step is to determine the origin of the heart failure and whether it can be corrected. Patients in whom heart failure is due to aortic stenosis may benefit from surgical correction; patients in heart failure with mitral stenosis may benefit from surgical correction or percutaneous balloon valvuloplasty. Patients with heart failure due to alcoholic cardiomyopathy benefit from abstinence from alcohol. If severe coronary artery disease with recurrent ischemia is the cause of heart failure, then angioplasty or surgical therapy may be important. Treatment of hypertension benefits patients with hypertensive heart disease. Precipitating causes of heart failure should be identified and treated. Several general treatment measures are useful. Salt restriction, reduction of stressful physical exertion, avoidance of emotional stress, and weight loss by the obese patient are all important.

Patients with class II-III heart failure require pharmacologic therapy in addition to the general treatment measurements described above. There are three broad categories of pharmacologic therapy for congestive heart failure: inotropic agents, diuretics, and vasodilators. There are no hard and fast rules for which agent(s) to use first. Patients with congestive symptoms, pulmonary edema, and systemic edema will benefit from diuretics. Patients with early symptoms of left ventricular dysfunction may benefit from the use of an ACE inhibitor, resulting in less long-term cardiac dysfunction and left ventricular dilatation. Patients with more severe heart failure should also receive digoxin. Initially, one class of drugs should be used, and drugs from one of the other classes may be added. Patients with very severe heart failure (class IV) may require the more potent inotropic agents such as dopamine, dobutamine, or phosphodiesterase inhibitors (for which hospitalization is necessary). In patients with predominant diastolic abnormalities of the heart, as may occur in some patients with hypertrophic cardiomyopathies, calcium antagonists may improve left ventricular relaxation. Patients with very severe heart failure who are appropriate candidates can be considered for special measures such as cardiac transplantation, left ventricular assist devices, and the artificial heart. Certain vasodilators (combination of hydralazine plus isosorbide dinitrate, ACE inhibitors) have been shown to improve the survival

Table 5. Therapeutic Approach to Congestive Heart Failure
Determine the etiology
Evaluate relative importance of diastolic dysfunction
Surgical correction where possible
Nonpharmacologic treatment
Reduce salt intake; avoid salt excess
Reduce physical and emotional stress
Pharmacologic approach
Either diuretic, digoxin or vasodilator as first-line therapy
Add second and third drugs as necessary
Vasodilators are generally used because they can prolong life
ACE inhibitors
Combination of hydralazine and isosorbide dinitrate
Add potent inotropic agents if the above are ineffective
Intermittent dobutamine
Phosphodiesterase inhibitors
For dilated cardiomyopathy, consider low-dose metoprolol
Consider heart transplant for appropriate patients with end-stage heart failure
(From Parmley. With permission of the American College of Cardiology. See Bibliography).

rate in patients with moderate to severe heart failure. This observation raises the as yet unanswered question of whether all patients should receive vasodilator therapy.

DIGITALIS

Digitalis, a class of steroid or steroid glycosides, has a positive inotropic effect on the heart. Its mechanism of action is still not completely understood. Evidence suggests that digitalis exerts its inotropic effect by inhibiting $Na-K^+$-ATPase, increasing intracellular sodium concentration, which leads to increases in calcium influx via the $Na-Ca^{++}$ exchange mechanism. Increase in cytosolic calcium results in activation of contractile elements. Digitalis also affects the electrophysiologic properties of the heart (Table 6). It exerts both direct and neurally mediated effects, resulting in slowing of conduction velocity and an increase in effective refractory period of the atrioventricular (AV) node; and it increases the excitability and automaticity of Purkinje fibers. The conduction velocities of the atrium and ventricle increase and their effective refractory periods decrease with digitalis administration.

Digoxin is the most widely used digitalis compound in the United States. Eighty percent of oral digoxin is absorbed. It is excreted predominantly by the kidney. Renal excretion is proportional to the glomerular filtration rate, although digoxin also may be secreted by the tubule. Enterohepatic recycling of digoxin is relatively insignificant. In persons with normal renal function, one third of body stores are lost daily and the average half-life of the drug is 36 hours. The loading dose of digoxin depends on the patient's lean body weight (0.0075 mg/lb lean body weight). Thus, an average oral loading dose is 1.25–1.5 mg, which can be given as three or four divided doses at 6-8–hour intervals over 24 hours. The IV loading dose is usually 0.75 mg in three or four divided doses over 24 hours. Therapeutic digoxin levels can be achieved in five to seven days of "maintenance" dosing without a loading dose, because steady state can be reached in four or five half-lives. The maintenance dose in a patient with normal renal function is usually 0.25 mg/day, in order to replace the 37% loss and maintain steady-state blood levels. In patients with renal impairment, the maintenance dose must be adjusted. The loading dose is unchanged but the maintenance dose can be estimated as follows:

Table 6. Electrophysiologic Properties of Digitalis	
Pacemaker automaticity	
SA node	→ ↓ (↑ after atropine or toxic doses)
Purkinje fibers	↑
Excitability	
Atrium	→[a]
Ventricle	Variable[a]
Purkinje fibers	↑[a]
Membrane responsiveness	
Atrium	Variable[a] (↓ after atropine)
Ventricle	↓ (toxic doses)
Purkinje fibers	↓ (toxic doses)
Conduction velocity	
Atrium, ventricle	↑ (slight)[a]
AV node	↓
Purkinje fibers	↓
Effective refractory period	
Atrium	↓ (↑ after atropine)
Ventricle	↓
AV node	↑
Purkinje fibers	↑[a]

Arrows indicate direction, not magnitude, of the changes indicated: ↑ = increased; ↓ = decreased; → = no significant change. [a] Decreased with high toxic doses of digitalis.
From Moe GK, Farah AE: Digitalis and allied cardiac glycosides. In: Goodman LS, Gilman A, eds. *The Pharmacological Basis of Therapeutics*, 5th ed. New York: Macmillan; 1975; p. 661.

$$\text{Maintenance dose (mg)} = \% \text{ daily loss} \times \text{loading dose (mg)}$$

$$\% \text{ daily loss in men} = 11.6 + \frac{20}{\text{serum creatinine}}$$

$$\% \text{ daily loss in women} = 12.6 + \frac{16}{\text{serum creatinine}}$$

Use of Digitalis in Congestive Heart Failure

Digitalis increases contracility and reduces ventricular end-diastolic pressure of the dysfunctioning heart. Digitalis shifts the ventricular function curve of the failing heart upward and to the left (curve D), indicating that the drug increases the force of systolic ejection and, thus, contractility (Figure 1). End-systolic volume is reduced and end-diastolic pressure declines. Thus, the same stroke work can be delivered from a markedly reduced filling pressure. Digitalis also increases the contractile state of the normal ventricle. However, this is not always translated into increased cardiac output in normal persons because digitalis may induce peripheral vasoconstriction in the normal circulation, resulting in increased impedance to ventricular ejection. In contrast, digitalis results in an overall reduction of systemic vascular resistance in patients with heart failure, due to improved cardiac output and a secondary decrease in peripheral resistance.

While digitalis is unquestionably useful in patients who have heart failure plus atrial fibrillation with a rapid ventricular response, there has been debate about the drug's efficacy in treating heart failure patients in normal sinus rhythm. Overall, the weight of evidence is in favor of a salutary effect of digoxin especially in patients with severe heart failure. Recent studies do suggest that if digoxin is withdrawn from the treatment regimen of patients in heart failure, their heart failure worsens (Arnold et al. 1980; Dobbs et al.). A recent multicenter study compared the effects of digoxin, captopril, and placebo in patients with heart failure in sinus rhythm. Digoxin caused greater improvement in left ventricular ejection fraction than the other drugs. Lee et al. demonstrated that digoxin reduced the severity of heart failure in more than half of patients. Those patients who benefited most with digoxin had more chronic and severe heart failure, dilated left ventricles, reduced ejection fraction, and third heart sounds.

The positive inotropic effect of digitalis increases myocardial oxygen consumption in the normal ventricle. In heart failure, however, myocardial oxygen consumption decreases because heart size and wall tension are reduced. Thus, digitalis can be beneficial in chronic ischemic heart disease with ventricular dysfunction.

In acute MI without congestive failure, digitalis is contraindicated because it increases myocardial oxygen consumption and may increase myocardial ischemia. However, digitalis may be of great value in acute MI complicated by atrial tachyarrhythmia, especially atrial fibrillation. In mild heart failure due to MI, diuretics alone or with vasodilators are the preferred treatment. However, digitalis may be helpful in patients with cardiomegaly and frank heart failure in the setting of acute MI.

Cor Pulmonale and Digitalis

Digitalis is of no value to patients with chronic obstructive pulmonary disease without heart failure. In patients with right ventricular failure due to cor pulmonale, measures that improve hypoxemia and reduce pulmonary vascular resistance constitute the primary mode of therapy. Digitalis can be used as an adjunct, since it may decrease right ventricular end-diastolic pressure and increase stroke volume. However, in the setting of hypoxemia, sensitivity to digitalis toxicity is increased, probably due to increased cardiac and plasma catecholamine levels.

Mitral Stenosis and Digitalis

Digitalis is of no benefit to patients with mitral stenosis in normal sinus rhythm, except those with right ventricular failure. However, it is useful in patients with mitral valve disease in atrial fibrillation, since control of ventricular response improves diastolic filling and cardiac output. In patients with mitral stenosis

and right ventricular failure, digitalis can be helpful in improving right ventricular contractility and thus improving overall cardiac function.

Hypertrophic Obstructive Cardiomyopathy and Digitalis

Digitalis is of little value and may even be detrimental in hypertrophic obstructive cardiomyopathy. Increased contractility may result in increased obstruction to ventricular outflow. The only setting in which digitalis may be helpful in hypertrophic obstructive cardiomyopathy is end-stage disease, when cardiac dilatation and frank congestive heart failure have developed.

Wolff-Parkinson-White Syndrome and Digitalis

In the presence of Wolff-Parkinson-White syndrome, atrial fibrillation may develop, with conduction down the accessory pathways at very fast rates. Digitalis can be hazardous in this setting because it can shorten the refractory period of the accessory pathway, resulting in rapid increases in ventricular responses and increased sensitivity to ventricular fibrillation.

Digitalis Levels

Serum digoxin levels can be measured by radioimmunoassay. In adults, the therapeutic serum digoxin level is 0.5–2 ng/ml. In this range, most patients have evidence of clinical response without toxicity. The mean serum digoxin level in patients receiving 0.25 mg/day is 1.25 ± 0.4 ng/ml. The serum digoxin level of patients with clinical evidence of toxicity is usually >2 ng/ml. However, 10% of patients without toxicity have serum digoxin concentrations of 2-4 ng/ml, although 10% of patients with toxicity have serum digoxin levels <2 ng/ml. In this group of patients, electrolyte abnormalities, hypoxemia, or increased automatic activity is usually present.

Determination of serum digoxin levels is indicated in patients in whom the status of digitalis treatment is uncertain, particularly in patients with severe congestive heart failure; in patients with gastrointestinal disease or after surgery, in whom absorption may be a problem; in patients with clinical suspicion of digitalis toxicity without overt ECG manifesta-

Table 7. Conditions Predisposing to Digitalis Toxicity
Renal insufficiency
Electrolyte disturbances (hypokalemia, hypercalcemia, hypomagnesemia)
Severe heart disease (NYHA class III or IV)
Acute MI
High-output state
Advanced age
Thyroid disease, especially hypothyroidism
Hypoxic states, acute or chronic pulmonary disease
Multiple drug therapy (especially institution of quinidine)
Hypertrophic obstructive cardiomyopathy, WPW syndrome, and amyloid heart disease
Sinoatrial and AV block.

tions; in those who may be noncompliant to therapy; and for follow-up of therapy for digitalis toxicity.

Digitalis Toxicity

It is estimated that 8-25% of hospitalized patients receiving digitalis have drug toxicity. Conditions that predispose to digitalis toxicity are shown in Table 7. The manifestations of toxicity are classified as noncardiac and cardiac. Noncardiac manifestations include anorexia; nausea and vomiting; fatigue; restlessness, agitation or drowsiness; psychosis; and visual complaints including hazy vision, yellow halos, and scotomata. The toxic effects of digitalis on cardiac rhythm are listed below:

Depression of conduction: second-degree atrioventricular (AV) block of Wenckebach type, third-degree AV block with junctional or ventricular escape, sinoatrial or AV junctional exit block.

Increased automaticity of subsidiary or ectopic pacemakers: ventricular ectopic beats, ventricular bigeminy or tachycardia, nonparoxysmal AV junctional tachycardia.

Combination of above: paroxysmal atrial tachycardia with AV block, AV dissociation with simultaneous atrial and AV junctional tachycardia (bidirectional tachycardia), atrial fibrillation with regularization of ventricular response due to accelerated AV junctional or ventricular pacemaker focus.

Atrial fibrillation or flutter, supraventricular premature beats, sinus tachy- or bradycardia, and multifocal atrial tachycardia are usually not manifestations of digitalis toxicity.

Treatment of Digitalis Toxicity

Digitalis-induced ectopic arrhythmias (ectopic atrial, junctional, or ventricular) can be effectively treated with phenytoin or lidocaine. Phenytoin is first given as a loading dose (100 mg slowly infused intravenously every 5 minutes until control of arrhythmia or onset of phenytoin toxicity) followed by a maintenance dose of 400-600 mg/day. Phenytoin may also improve sinoatrial block and AV conduction, making it an ideal drug for treatment of digitalis intoxication. Lidocaine is administered as usual (100 mg loading dose and 1-3 mg/min continuously as maintenance dose). Quinidine and procainamide are also useful. However, both drugs carry the risk of cardiac toxicity, especially in eliciting ventricular arrhythmia. Propranolol, although effective in suppressing ectopic arrhythmia, can depress sinoatrial and AV pacemakers, as well as AV conduction, and could result in severe bradycardia or asystole.

Atropine can be effective in treating sinus bradycardia, AV block, or sinoatrial exit block. However, temporary transvenous pacing is occasionally required in patients with sinoatrial block, sinus arrest, or second- or third-degree block with extremely slow ventricular rate.

In advanced life-threatening digitalis toxicity, digoxin-specific antibody Fab fragments have proved successful and are commercially available.

Table 8. Drug Interactions with Digitalis	
Cholestyramine, neomycin, nonabsorbable antacids, and Kaopectate	Decreases oral absorption
Diuretic	Decreases glomerular filtration rate Hypokalemia Hypomagnesemia Hypercalcemia (thiazide)
Anesthesia	Increases sympathetic activity Arrhythmogenic
Quinidine	Decreases tubular secretion of digoxin Displaces digoxin from tissue
Verapamil, amiloride, spironolactone, triamterene	Decrease tubular secretion of digoxin

Potassium replacement is generally indicated for digitalis toxic patients with hypokalemia and ectopic arrhythmias. However, it is contraindicated if hyperkalemia or conduction abnormalities are present because elevated serum potassium levels can further depress AV conduction. Direct-current cardioversion should be avoided because digitalis toxicity increases the likelihood of ventricular fibrillation after electrical cardioversion, but cardioversion should not be withheld if all other measures have failed.

Drug Interactions

Drugs can alter the serum digoxin concentration by interfering with absorption, excretion, and volume of distribution. Certain drugs can also increase the activity of the myocardium to digitalis effect and toxicity (Table 8).

Quinidine-digoxin interaction. Several studies show that serum digoxin concentrations increase by 0.5 ng/ml or more in approximately 90% of patients when standard doses of quinidine are added to a stable chronic regimen of digoxin. The serum digoxin level on the average doubles (range from zero to sixfold), when a new steady state is reached with quinidine treatment. The increase in serum digoxin level can be seen on the first day and reaches a plateau after approximately five days, when quinidine is added without a loading dose. With a loading dose, the serum digoxin level reaches a steady state within three days.

The exact mechanism of interaction is unclear. Evidence suggests that quinidine reduces the renal clearance of digoxin by up to 40-50%. This may be due to quinidine effects on tubular secretion of digoxin. A decrease in non-renal rate of excretion has also been noted. Investigators demonstrated that quinidine reduces the volume of distribution of digoxin by displacing digoxin from tissue compartments to plasma; others suggest that some of the increase in cardiac effect of digoxin occurring during quinidine treatment is mediated in the central nervous system.

Whether frank digitalis toxicity is more likely to occur as a result of this interaction is subject to debate. Retrospective data analysis indicated a 17-41% incidence. However, no prospective study involving a large number of patients has been performed. We recommend that the digoxin maintenance dose be reduced to half when quinidine is to be added. Serum digoxin levels should be monitored and the digoxin dose readjusted to achieve therapeutic nontoxic levels. Other investigators advocate careful follow-up without adjustment of digoxin doses. Alternatively, antiarrhythmic agents other than quinidine or other

Table 9. Commonly Used Diuretics in Heart Failure

Drug	Site of Action	Total Daily Dose in CHF	Frequency	Complications
Acetazolamide	Proximal tubule	250-375 mg	qod or qd × 2 days, skip day 3	Metabolic acidosis
Thiazides	Distal tubule			
Hydrochlorothiazide		50-200 mg	qd to bid	Hyponatremia, hypokalemia, metabolic alkalosis, hyperuricemia, glucose intolerance, lipid abnormalities, hypercalcemia, reduced GFR, allergy, thrombocytopenia, agranulocytosis, leukopenia, anemia, sexual dysfunction
Chlorothiazide		500-1500 mg	qd to bid	
Indapamide	Distal tubule (Direct vasodilator)	2.5-5 mg	qd	As above, but hypokalemia and lipid abnormalities less common
Phthalimidine derivatives	Distal tubule			
Chlorthalidone		50-200 mg	qd	Similar to thiazides, but hypokalemia may be profound
Metolazone		2.5-10 mg	qd	
Loop diuretics	Loop of Henle			
Furosemide		40-320 mg	qd to bid	Hyponatremia, hypokalemia, metabolic alkalosis, hyperuricemia, glucose intolerance, interstitial nephritis, ototoxicity, thrombocytopenia, agranulocytosis, leukopenia, anemia
Ethacrynic acid		50-400 mg	qd to bid	
Bumetanide		0.5-10 mg	qd bid-tid qod	
Potassium-sparing diuretics	Distal tubule			
Spironolactone		25-200 mg	qd to tid	Hyperkalemia, mental confusion, nausea, and gynecomastia (spironolactone only)
Triamterene		100-300 mg	qd to bid	
Amiloride		5-20 mg	qd	

digitalis preparations can be used. Several type I antiarrhythmic agents do not cause changes in serum digoxin concentrations (Bigger).

DIURETICS

Sixty percent to 75% of the filtered sodium load is reabsorbed in the proximal tubule of the nephron, 20% in the ascending limb of the loop of Henle, and the rest in the distal tubule and collecting duct. In congestive heart failure, the filtered sodium load is decreased. Furthermore, the proximal tubular sodium reabsorption is increased due to a decrease in peritubular hydrostatic pressure.

Diuretics increase urine flow and sodium excretion by acting at various sites along the nephron to interrupt sodium and water reabsorption. Reduction of sodium and water retention results in reduced ventricular preload and improves congestive symptoms. A reduction in ventricular volume at the onset of ejection may also decrease afterload and improve ventricular function. Furthermore, thiazides and furosemide may also have direct vasodilating effects. Diuretics may be classified by their site of action. Table 9 is a list of commonly used diuretics and their site of action, common oral dosage, and side effects.

Special Considerations in the Use of Diuretics

1. Carbonic anhydrase inhibitors, e.g., acetazolamide, act primarily at the proximal tubule. Acetazolamide increases sodium bicarbonate excretion and thus may lead to the development of metabolic acidosis. It reduces glomerular filtration rate. Tolerance to the drug can develop within a few days. When given to patients with liver impairment, it may cause drowsiness and confusion.
2. Thiazide diuretics act in the distal tubule and tend to reduce glomerular filtration rate. They are ineffective in patients with glomerular filtration rates <30 ml/min. Metabolic alkalosis may occur as a result of hypokalemia or volume contraction. The activity of these agents is not affected by alkalosis or acidosis. Thiazide diuretics may increase cholesterol and triglyceride levels. However, the agent indapamide has no effect on cholesterol levels.
3. Like chlorothiazide, metolazone exerts its action on the distal tubule. However, it does not reduce glomerular filtration rate or renal blood flow. Thus, it may be effective in patients with impaired renal function.
4. Spironolactone, triamterene, and amiloride act on the distal tubule. These agents reduce potassium excretion and may lead to metabolic acidosis and hyperkalemia due to reduced potassium-hydrogen exchange.
5. The effectiveness of loop diuretics is not affected by reduced glomerular filtration rates. These agents inhibit chloride transport in the ascending limb. Metabolic alkalosis may be a complication of therapy with these drugs. Their effectiveness is not inhibited by metabolic alkalosis or acidosis.
6. Hyponatremia may be a complication of diuretic therapy. Furosemide, ethacrynic acid, and thiazides reduce free water excretion; antidiuretic hormone and thirst may be increased in patients with congestive heart failure. The combination of these factors can result in hyponatremia. Treatment consists of withholding diuretics if tolerated, restricting fluid intake, and improving cardiac function.
7. Patients with severe heart failure may be refractory to treatment with oral thiazides or furosemide due to poor gastrointestinal absorption secondary to bowel edema. These patients often respond well to a course of IV furosemide or ethacrynic acid. Combinations of oral diuretics can also be used. Combined use of a loop diuretic (furosemide) with a distal tubular agent (e.g., thiazide or spironolactone) may be effective in patients refractory to a single diuretic regimen. We have found the regimen of furosemide and hydrochlorothiazide or metolazone to be particularly effective. However, hypokalemia and hyponatremia frequently complicate this regimen.
8. Use of an ACE inhibitor may enhance the effect of diuretics and increase natriuresis. On the other hand, nonsteroidal anti-inflammatory drugs (NSAIDs) may attenuate the effect of diuretics. Both ACE inhibitors and NSAIDs may induce hyperkalemia if used in the setting of renal failure or when used concomitantly with potassium-sparing diuretics.

VASODILATOR THERAPY

Therapy of heart failure is directed at reducing the workload of the heart and manipulating factors that control cardiac performance. Major determinants of cardiac performance are heart rate, wall tension (in-

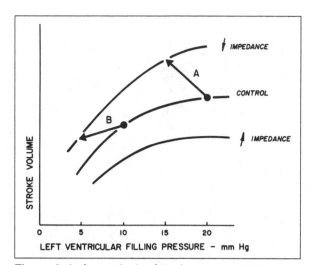

Figure 3. *Left ventricular function curves plotting stroke volume as a function of left ventricular filling pressure. The control curve is in the middle. With a vasodilator drug such as nitroprusside, there would be a decrease in impedance, which would shift the curve up and to the left. Note that if a patient on the control curve were given a vasodilator at an initial filling pressure of 20 mm Hg, the reduction of filling pressure would be accompanied by an increase in stroke volume (line A). However, if the same patient began at a filling pressure of 10 mm Hg, with a decrease of filling pressure to 5 mm Hg, there would be a decrease in stroke volume (line B). Thus, the effects of a vasodilator (such as nitroprusside) depend on the left ventricular filling pressure. (Reproduced with permission from Grune & Stratton. From Chatterjee K, Parmley WW: The role of vasodilator therapy in heart failure.* Prog Cardiovasc Dis 19:301, 1977.)

cluding preload and afterload), and contractility. These factors determine, to a great degree, how the heart can meet the metabolic demands of the body as well as the metabolic cost of this cardiac work. In patients with congestive heart failure, special attention must be paid to the state of preload and afterload. Preload refers to left ventricular fiber length at the end of diastole and, in essence, is left ventricular end-diastolic pressure (LVEDP), which is governed by venous return. In patients with advanced congestive heart failure, LVEDP is elevated. This results in an increase in hydrostatic pressure and transudation of fluid in the plumonary capillaries, with symptoms of pulmonary congestion. Afterload refers to the tension that is generated in the left ventricular wall to open

the aortic valve and discharge the stroke volume into the systemic circulation. Afterload is determined by arterial pressure, ventricular volume at the onset of ejection, systemic vascular resistance (SVR), and aortic impedance. In advanced congestive heart failure, SVR is elevated as a compensatory mechanism to maintain systemic blood pressure. The increase in arteriolar tone is maintained by increased neurohumoral activities, such as the sympathetic and renin angiotensin systems. The increase in SVR results in increased impedance to left ventricular ejection. The vicious cycle leads to a new steady state when cardiac output will be lower and SVR higher than is optimal for the patient.

How a venodilator affects cardiac performance depends on the initial level of left ventricular filling pressure (LVFP). In patients with heart failure who undergo maximal diuresis to near-normal LVFP, administration of a venodilator can result in decreases in stroke volume and cardiac output. On the other hand, if one starts at a high LVFP, a reduction in filling pressure will occur along the flat portion of the ventricular function curve and will not produce a marked reduction in ventricular performance, but will relieve pulmonary venous congestion (Figure 3).

Arteriolar dilators increase cardiac output primarily by reducing SVR. This reduction in impedance and instantaneous wall stress results in augmentation of myocardial fiber shortening with an increase in stroke volume output; hence, blood pressure may only fall slightly or not at all.

Vasodilators diminish left ventricular wall tension during systole (ventricular afterload) by two principal mechanisms. First, these agents reduce SVR and decrease aortic impedance to left ventricular ejection, allowing a greater stroke volume and cardiac output. Second, peripheral vasodilator drugs may also cause venodilatation, resulting in peripheral pooling of blood and reduced venous return. Consequently, LVFP and LVEDP (preload) are reduced and pulmonary congestion is relieved. In addition, myocardial oxygen consumption is reduced by the decrease in ventricular wall tension during contraction due to peripheral vasodilator-induced decrease in ventricular volume and aortic impedance.

Choice of Vasodilators

Arteriolar dilators (e.g., hydralazine) are of particular value to patients with low forward cardiac output and declining perfusion of vital organs as a result of in-

Table 10. Commonly Used Vasodilators in Heart Failure

Drug	Site of Action	Route of Administration	Usual Initial Dose	Maximal Dose	Complications
Nitroprusside	Arteriolar and venous	IV	10-25 µg/min IV	Up to 300 µg/min IV	Thiocyanate toxicity, methemoglobinemia
Trimethaphan	Arteriolar and venous	IV	1-15 mg/min IV		Postural hypotension, bowel and bladder atony, respiratory depression
Nitrates					
Nitroglycerin	Venous	Sublingual (SL)	0.4 mg SL		Headache, postural hypotension, methemoglobinemia
		IV	5-10 µg/min IV	500 µg/min IV	
		Cutaneous ointment	1/2-1" q 6 hr	2-3" q 3-6 hr	
		Patch	5-10 mg/24 hr		
Isosorbide dinitrate		Oral or SL	2.5-10 mg q 2 hr (SL); 10-40 mg qid (oral)		Headache, postural hypotension
Hydralazine	Arteriolar	Oral	10 mg tid to qid	200-300 mg/day	Headache, positive ANA, SLE-like syndrome (10-20% if dose >400 mg/day), drug fever, skin rash
Prazosin	Arteriolar and venous	Oral	1 mg tid	24 mg/day	Postural hypotension, fluid retention, polyarthralgia
Captopril	Arteriolar and venous ACE inhibitor	Oral	6.25-25 mg tid	450 mg/day	Skin rash, proteinuria, renal failure, taste disturbance, agranulocytosis, nonproductive cough, hypotension
Enalapril	Arteriolar and venous ACE inhibitor	Oral	2.5 mg qd-10 mg bid	30 mg/day	Hypotension, renal failure, angioedema, laryngeal edema, cough
Lisinopril	Arteriolar and venous ACE inhibitor	Oral	10-20 mg qd	80 mg/day	Hypotension, proteinuria, renal insufficiency, rash, cough
Minoxidil	Arteriolar	Oral	2.5 mg qd to bid	40 mg/day	Hirsutism, sodium retention, pericardial effusion, question of pulmonary hypertension
Nifedipine	Arteriolar and venous (calcium blocker)	Oral	10 mg tid	120 mg/day	Hypotension, tachycardia, palpitation, flushing, headache, ankle edema

tense vasoconstriction. In patients with volume overload due to mitral or aortic regurgitation, afterload reduction decreases the magnitude of regurgitation and improves left ventricular forward stroke volume.

Venodilators (e.g., nitrates) decrease preload and pulmonary venous pressure. They are useful for patients in whom the primary manifestation of the heart failure is pulmonary congestion due to increased LVFP. They should be used with caution in patients who have received excessive diuresis, since this may precipitate hypotension.

Balanced vasodilators (e.g., α_1 blockers and ACE inhibitors) act on both arterial and venous sides. They can reduce LVFP and relieve pulmonary congestion as well as decrease SVR and increase cardiac output. Since most patients with heart failure have symptoms of both low-output and pulmonary congestion, they respond well to combined veno- plus arteriolar dilation. Agents with veno- and arteriolar dilating properties (i.e., "mixed" vasodilators such as the ACE inhibitors) are preferred in these patients. Alternatively, the combination of pure venodilator and arteriolar dilators such as isosorbide dinitrate and hydralazine can be used. Table 10 is a list of commonly used vasodilators in heart failure, their doses, site of action, and complications.

Special Considerations in Choice of Vasodilators

Blood pressure. Acute or chronic elevation of systemic blood pressure further increases aortic impedance and can aggravate heart failure in an already compromised heart. The presence of hypertension is a clear indication for aggressive vasodilator therapy. In patients with heart failure who have a history of long-standing hypertension, but in whom blood pressure is normal or only slightly elevated, further reduction in blood pressure by vasodilators can lead to improvement of cardiac hemodynamics.

Patients with hypertension may have heart failure symptoms without frank ventricular dilation. These patients usually have concentric hypertrophy with a small or normal ventricular cavity size and reduced ventricular compliance during diastole. This subset of patients may be particularly responsive to calcium entry blockers such as nifedipine, which can improve diastolic relaxation as well as reduce SVR.

Special attention should be paid to the effects of acute vasodilation on renal function in patients with long-standing hypertension. Many of these patients have varying degrees of nephrosclerosis; a precipitous drop in perfusion pressure may worsen renal function.

End-organ perfusion. Vasoconstriction in congestive heart failure results in reduction and redistribution of blood flow to various organs. Renal, splanchnic, and cutaneous blood flow are particularly reduced, because these organs are greatly influenced by circulating angiotensin and the sympathetic nervous system. Vasodilators can affect the distribution of cardiac output. Hydralazine and ACE inhibitors increase renal blood flow with or without increasing glomerular filtration rate. Used properly, these agents may improve renal function and potentiate renal response to furosemide. During ACE inhibitor therapy; glomerular filtration rate may decrease and azotemia may develop in some patients, usually those who have undergone excessive diuresis and those in whom glomerular filtration rate is dependent on angiotensin-induced efferent arteriolar constriction. Prazosin has no effect on renal flow, but increases hepatic blood flow and may be particularly effective in patients with hepatic and splanchnic hypoperfusion. All of these agents improve exercise tolerance.

Etiology of congestive heart failure. Vasodilator therapy should be initiated cautiously in patients with ischemic cardiomyopathy. Reflex tachycardia with vasodilator treatment is generally not a problem in patients with chronic heart failure, since the myocardial norepinephrine stores are depleted and the baroreceptor reflex is blunted in these patients. In patients with coronary artery disease, ACE inhibitors such as captopril have been shown to improve exercise tolerance times. However, in patients with acute heart failure, nonspecific vasodilators may induce tachycardia and increase myocardial oxygen consumption. Excessive hypotension may precipitate angina and worsen cardiac function in both acute and chronic heart failure.

Transient decreases in systemic blood pressure to 75 mm Hg systolic and 50 mm Hg diastolic are generally well tolerated in patients whose heart failure is not a result of coronary artery disease.

Drug tolerance. Attenuation of response to vasodilators, reported with almost all vasodilators, presents a significant problem in the therapy of heart failure. Attenuation of drug effect may reflect progression of the primary myocardial disease; it may also be due to primary or secondary activation of neurohumoral mechanisms, alterations of receptor density and responsiveness, or changes in drug metabolism. Attenuation of the prazosin vasodilator effect in heart failure has been well documented. Prazosin tolerance is associated with increases in plasma norepinephrine concentration and plasma renin activity.

Beta-adrenergic receptor agonists, including dobutamine, pirbuterol, and salbutamol, are effective in reducing systemic vascular resistance and increasing cardiac output. However, a significant degree of hemodynamic and clinical attenuation occurs during long-term treatment. The clinical attenuation seen with these agents may be related to "down-regulation" of beta-adrenergic receptors in the myocardium and blood vessels. Similarly, tolerance to hydralazine may be a result of receptor adaptation or alterations in drug metabolism. In contrast, there appears to be little evidence of tolerance to ACE inhibitors in the therapy of heart failure. Angiotensin converting enzyme inhibitors appear to blunt the baroreceptor reflex and prevent secondary rises in plasma catcholamines in patients with heart failure. Indeed, tachycardia is not observed with these drugs despite the decrease in arterial blood pressure. Furthermore, plasma norepinephrine and epinephrine levels remain unchanged after captopril therapy in patients with advanced heart failure. Thus, the sustained effectiveness of captopril may be related to its blockade of neurohumoral mechanisms.

Packer observed that patients refractory to one vasodilator may respond to another vasodilator that acts by a different mechanism. Thus, alternating the use of several vasodilators and the combined use of two vasodilators may reduce the incidence of clinical tolerance.

Angiotensin Converting Enzyme Inhibitors

The ACE inhibitors interrupt the renin-angiotensin-aldosterone system, which contributes to systemic vasoconstriction. Angiotensin converting enzyme inhibitors are rapidly becoming the most widely used vasodilators for the treatment of heart failure. They have been shown consistently to diminish heart failure in patients who do not respond to diuretics or digoxin. These drugs have been shown to improve heart failure symptoms and NYHA functional class, prolong exercise tolerance time, reduce the number of hospitalizations, reduce left ventricular dilation, improve cardiac hemodynamics, correct hyponatremia, and, in some studies, reduce the incidence of ventricular arrhythmias. In the CONSENSUS trial, patients with severe heart failure already treated with

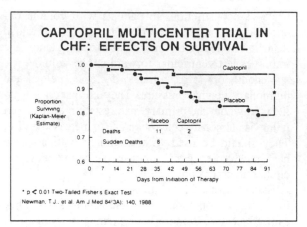

Figure 4. *Survival curves for captopril and placebo patients with moderate to severe heart failure (intention-to-treat analysis). (From Newmann et al. See Bibliography).*

digitalis and diuretics who then received enalapril had a significantly lower (31%) mortality at one year than did patients not given enalapril. Captopril has been shown to improve survival in patients with moderate to severe heart failure (Newmann et al.; Figure 4).

The ACE inhibitors appear to be beneficial in patients with mild to moderate as well as severe heart failure and are now used by some physicians as first-line therapy. While tachyphylaxis has been described for the effects of some vasodilators in heart failure, this is not the case with the ACE inhibitors. Potassium levels may increase while patients are treated with ACE inhibitors; thus, these agents, in general, should not be given with potassium-sparing diuretics, and potassium levels should be closely monitored in patients receiving potassium supplements. Although ACE inhibitors are well tolerated, the most frequent side effect is hypotension. This effect can be minimized by starting therapy with low doses and reducing diuretic therapy to prevent hypovolemia at the time that ACE inhibitors are administered.

Drug Interactions

Nonsteroidal anti-inflammatory drugs (NSAIDs) inhibit prostaglandin synthetase activity. Since vasodilator prostaglandins E_2 and I_2 modulate SVR and renal perfusion, the use of NSAIDs may reduce renal blood flow and glomerular filtration rate in patients with heart failure. These agents may also attenuate the effects of diuretics and vasodilators. Indomethacin has been shown to attenuate the effect of furosemide, whereas aspirin blocks the effect of spironolactone. Indomethacin reduces the vasodilating effect of captopril. Finally, in patients with prerenal azotemia, NSAIDs may precipitate renal failure.

The Effect of Drug Therapy on Survival

Certain vasodilators or combinations of vasodilators have been shown to improve the survival of patients with heart failure. The first such study to show this was the Veterans Administration Vasodilator Heart Failure Trial (V-HeFT) (Cohn et al.). Patients with moderate heart failure received either placebo, prazosin, or a hydralazine–isosorbide dinitrate combination. At 12 months, mortality was 28% lower in the hydralazine-isosorbide dinitrate group than in placebo; prazosin alone did not reduce mortality. As described earlier, the CONSENSUS trial also showed that patients receiving the ACE inhibitor enalapril had a reduction in mortality. In patients with moderate to severe heart failure, captopril improved overall survival (Figure 4). The incidence of sudden death was eight patients in the placebo group versus one in the captopril group (Newmann et al.). A pooled analysis by Furberg and Yusuf suggested that ACE inhibitors improved survival in patients with heart failure, whereas other vasodilators alone did not appear to have this benefit. The demonstration that pharmacologic therapy improves survival in patients with heart failure is a major advance.

NON-DIGITALIS INOTROPIC AGENTS

Dopamine and Dobutamine

Dopamine is an endogenous catecholamine capable of stimulating dopaminergic, alpha-adrenergic, and beta-adrenergic receptors. A systemic infusion of dopamine at 2-5 μg/kg body weight/min induces peripheral vasodilation, and increases renal blood flow, coronary flow, and myocardial contractility with little change in heart rate. The vasodilatory effect of dopamine is mediated by vascular dopaminergic receptors. Dopamine also acts directly on beta$_1$-adrenergic receptors and releases norepinephrine from nerve terminals, resulting in increased cardiac contractility. In doses of >5-10 μg/kg/min, systemic vasoconstriction occurs, leading to increased blood pressure and decreased renal blood flow. This is due to the activation of alpha-adrenergic receptors by dopamine. In this dose range, increased beta$_1$ stimulation also increases heart rate, myocardial oxygen consumption, and coronary resistance.

Dobutamine is a synthetic sympathomimetic amine capable of stimulating beta$_1$, beta$_2$, and alpha adrenoreceptors. Its effect on beta$_1$ is greater than on beta$_2$, and its effect on alpha$_1$ is greater than on alpha$_2$. In low doses (2-5 μg/kg/min), it causes slight vasoconstriction and stimulates increased myocardial contractility. Larger doses (5-10 μg/kg/min) induce a biphasic vasoconstriction-vasodilator response, mediated by alpha$_1$ and beta$_1$ receptors, respectively. Dobutamine does not directly affect renal blood flow, but causes a redistribution of cardiac output in favor of coronary and skeletal muscle circulation. Dobutamine may have less marked arrhythmogenic and chronotropic effects than dopamine.

Dopamine and dobutamine may be used in patients with advanced acute and chronic decompensated heart failure. Addition of a parenteral vasodilator such as nitroprusside to dopamine or dobutamine can further augment cardiac output by reducing afterload. In combination, these agents enhance diuretic activity of furosemide, and have been very successful in treating patients with heart failure.

Intravenous infusions of dobutamine for 72 hours may be associated with several weeks of sustained clinical benefit. This sustained benefit may be related to reconditioning the myocytes, and improvements in cardiac ultrastructure have been reported. While this agent may be useful for intermittent in-hospital therapy with cardiac monitoring, its use outside the hospital has not been proved. One clinical study in which a portable infusion device was used to deliver IV dobutamine to ambulatory patients was discontinued due to excessive mortality.

Orally Active Beta Agonists

Several orally active beta agonists have been used to treat patients with heart failure. Levodopa administered orally is converted to dopamine and has been shown to improve hemodynamics acutely. Ibopamine and dopexamine also have beneficial acute effects. However, long-term beneficial effects of these agents have not been documented. Pirbuterol stimulates beta$_1$ and beta$_2$ adrenergic receptors and thus has both positive inotropic as well as vasodilator properties. Although it improved hemodynamics acutely in patients with heart failure, tolerance developed over the course of one month. Prenalterol increased cardiac inotropy but was associated with an increase in ventricular arrhythmias in some patients. Whether any of these potent inotropic agents have long-term beneficial effects is questionable due to the development of tolerance, arrhythmias, and increase in oxygen consumption with their long-term use.

Phosphodiesterase Inhibitors

Phosphodiesterase inhibitors result in an increase in cyclic adenosine monophosphate, which enhances contractility and also causes vasodilation. Amrinone is the prototype of this group of drugs and its cogener milrinone has recently been approved. Both are used intravenously to treat patients with refractory heart failure. They improve cardiac output and reduce filling pressures. Amrinone is administered as an IV bolus of 0.75 mg/kg followed by an infusion of 5–10 μg/kg/min for use in short-term management of severe heart failure. Long-term oral amrinone therapy failed to improve exercise capacity or cardiac function. Side effects included thrombocytopenia, ventricular arrhythmias, hypotension, gastrointestinal complaints, fever, and hepatotoxicity.

Milrinone also is indicated for short-term IV administration in patients with severe congestive heart failure. The recommended dose is 10–30 mg/day. It is more potent than amrinone and does not have the thrombocytopenic side effect; but it also has been disappointing in long-term trials. In a recent double blind trial, DiBianco et al. compared patients with moderately severe heart failure receiving either oral milrinone, digoxin, or digoxin plus milrinone over a twelve-week period. They observed that both digoxin and milrinone increased exercise tolerance. However, milrinone or a combination of milrinone plus digoxin had no advantage over treatment with digoxin alone. Within the first two weeks of therapy, clinical deterioration was more common in patients taking milrinone. Digitalis, but not milrinone, increased ejection fraction. There was a trend toward decreased survival and increased risk of ventricular arrhythmias in patients receiving milrinone.

Although phosphodiesterase inhibitors may be useful for short-term IV treatment of refractory heart failure, they will probably not be used as chronic therapy because of risk of arrhythmias and a possible worsening of mortality risk (Packer et al. 1984).

Beta-Blocking Agents

It may seem paradoxical that beta-blocking drugs, which have a negative inotropic effect, might play a role in the management of heart failure. Some studies suggest that careful titration of cardioselective beta blockers results in clinical improvement in patients with dilated cardiomyopathy. Fowler et al. showed that such therapy in patients awaiting cardiac transplantation actually increased ejection fraction and resulted in clinical improvement in 60% of patients. Twenty-six percent of these patients were removed from the cardiac transplantation list. Other studies have suggested improved exercise tolerance and a trend toward improved survival. Proposed mechanisms for these beneficial effects include restoration of down-regulated beta-adrenergic receptors, increased sensitivity of the beta receptors, and blockade of the cardiotoxic effects of catecholamines.

If cardioselective beta blockers are administered to patients with heart failure, very low doses should be used initially and patients should be carefully monitored for signs of worsening heart failure. Whether such therapy will attain wide acceptance is unknown at this time.

OTHER THERAPIES

Other adjunctive therapies for heart failure include antiarrhythmic drugs. However, many antiarrhythmic agents may lead to proarrhythmic as well as negative inotropic effects. Therefore, until further clinical trials are available, the physician must use his best judgment, on a case-by-case basis, as to whether antiarrhythmic therapy should be instituted. As mentioned above, ACE inhibitors have been observed to reduce ventricular arrhythmias in patients with heart failure.

If patients fail the above measures, they may be considered for heart transplantation (see Chapter 34). Left ventricular assist devices may be a useful form of short-term therapy in patients with heart failure. Investigative work is under way to develop permanent left ventricular assist devices. Although some patients have received the total artificial heart, problems with thrombus formation and hemorrhage due to the necessary anticoagulation therapy indicate that it is not a viable long-term solution. The artificial heart had been used as a bridge to heart transplantation.

INPATIENT VERSUS OUTPATIENT MANAGEMENT

Mild to moderate congestive heart failure can be successfully treated with outpatient management once a cause and precipitating factors have been worked up. Diet, restriction of salt intake, modification of physical activity, and treatment with digitalis, diuretics, or vasodilators may be instituted; and patients should be seen at least two weeks after therapy has been started. Follow-up examination should include complete cardiovascular examination, including weight; and electrolytes, BUN, Cr, and periodic noninvasive cardiac workup such as echocardiography. Initial management of severe heart failure, acute or chronic, should be instituted in the hospital.

Bibliography

Abelmann WH, Lorell BH: The challenge of cardiomyopathy. *J Am Coll Cardiol* 13:1219, 1989.

Anderson JL, Lutz JR, Gilbert EM, et al: A randomized trial of low-dose beta-blockade therapy for idiopathic dilated cardiomyopathy. *Am J Cardiol* 55:471, 1985.

Arnold SB, Byrd RC, Meister W, et al: Long-term digitalis therapy improves left ventricular function in heart failure. *N Engl J Med* 303:433, 1980.

Arnold SB, Williams RL, Ports TA, et al: Attenuation of prazosin effect on cardiac output in chronic heart failure. *Ann Intern Med* 91:345, 1979.

Bigger TJ: The quinidine-digoxin interaction. *Mod Concepts Cardiovasc Dis* 51:73, 1982.

Beller GA, Smith TW, Abelman WH, et al: Digitalis intoxication: Prospective clinical study with serum level correlations *N Engl J Med* 284:989, 1971.

Braunwald E: Clinical manifestations of heart failure. In: Braunwald E, ed. *Heart Disease. A Textbook of Cardiovascular Medicine.* 3rd edition. Philadelphia: Saunders; 1988, p. 471. (a)

Braunwald E: Determinants and assessment of cardiac function. *N Engl J Med* 296:86, 1977.

Braunwald E: Pathophysiology of heart failure. In: Braunwald E, ed. *Heart Disease. A Textbook of Cardiovascular Medicine.* 3rd edition. Philadelphia: Saunders; 1988, p. 426. (b)

Captopril-Digoxin Multicenter Research Group. Comparative effects of captopril and digoxin in patients with mild to moderate heart failure. *JAMA* 259:539, 1988.

Captopril Multicenter Research Group: A cooperative multicenter study of captopril in congestive heart failure: Hemodynamic effects and long-term responses. *Am Heart J* 110:439, 1985.

Cohn JN: Current therapy of the failing heart. *Circulation* 78:1099, 1988.

Cohn JN, Archibald DG, Ziesche S, et al: Effect of vasodilator therapy on mortality in chronic congestive heart failure. *N Engl J Med* 314:1547, 1986.

Colucci WS, Alexander W, Williams GH, et al: Decreased lymphocyte beta adrenergic receptor density in patients with heart failure and tolerance to the beta adrenergic agonist pirbuterol. *N Engl J Med* 305:185, 1982.

Colucci WS, Wynne J, Holman BL, et al: Chronic therapy of heart failure with prazosin: A randomized double-blind trial. *Am J Cardiol* 45:337, 1980.

Colucci WS, Wright RE, Braunwald E: New positive inotropic agents in the treatment of congestive heart failure. *N Engl J Med* 314:349, 1986.

CONSENSUS Trial Study Group. Effects of enalapril on mortality in severe congestive heart failure. *N Engl J Med* 316:1429, 1987.

DiBianco R, Shabetai R, Kostuk W, et al: A comparison of oral milrinone, digoxin, and their combination in the treatment of patients with chronic heart failure. *N Engl J Med* 320:677, 1989.

Dies F, Krell MJ, Whitlow P, et al: Intermittent dobutamine in ambulatory outpatients with chronic cardiac failure (abstract). *Circulation* 74(II):38, 1986.

Dietz R, Haass M, Kubler W: Atrial natriuretic factor. Its possible role in hypertension and congestive heart failure. *Am J Hypertension* 2:295, 1986.

Dobbs SM, Kenyon WL, Dobbs RJ: Maintenance digoxin after an episode of heart failure: Placebo controlled trial in outpatients. *Br Med J* 1:749, 1977.

Doherty JE: How and when to use the digitalis serum levels. *JAMA* 239:2594, 1978.

Dzau VJ, Colucci WS, Williams GH, et al: Sustained effectiveness of converting enzyme inhibition in patients with severe congestive heart failure. *N Engl J Med* 302:1373, 1980.

Dzau VJ: Angiotensin converting enzyme inhibition in the treatment of hypertension and congestive heart failure. Update IV. In: Isselbacher KJ, et al., eds. *Harrison's Principles of Internal Medicine.* New York: McGraw-Hill; 1983, p. 137.

Engelmeier SR, O'Connell JB, Walsh R, et al: Improvement in symptoms and exercise tolerance by metoprolol in patients with dilated cardiomyopathy: A double-blind randomized, placebo-controlled trial. *Circulation* 72:536, 1985.

Fisher ML, Plotnick GD, Peters RW, Carliner NH: Beta-blockers in congestive cardiomyopathy. Conceptual advance or contraindication? *Am J Med* 80(Suppl 2B):59, 1986.

Forrester JS, Waters DD: Hospital treatment of congestive heart failure: Management according to hemodynamic profile. *Am J Med* 65:173, 1978.

Fowler WB, Bristow MR, Laser JA et al: Beta blocker therapy in severe heart failure: Improvement related to beta-1-adrenergic receptor up regulation? *Circulation* 70(Suppl II):112, 1984.

Francis GS: Neurohumoral mechanisms involved in congestive heart failure. *Am J Cardiol* 55:15A, 1985.

Francis GS, Goldsmith SR, Levine TB, et al: The neurohumoral axis in congestive heart failure. *Ann Intern Med* 101:370, 1984.

Furberg CO, Yusuf S: Effect of vasodilators on survival in chronic congestive heart failure. *Am J Cardiol* 55:1110, 1985.

Goldberg LI: Dopamine: Clinical uses of an endogeneous catecholamine. *N Engl J Med* 291:707, 1974.

Jafri SM, Levine TB, Kloner RA: Recent advances in the medical management of congestive heart failure. *Modern Med* 56:50, 1988.

Johnston DL, Humen DP, Kostuk WJ: Amrinone therapy in patients with heart failure. Lack of improvement in functional capacity and left ventricular function at rest and during exercise. *Chest* 86:395, 1984.

Katz AM: Changing strategies in the management of heart failure. *J Am Coll Cardiol* 13:513, 1989.

Lee DC, Johnson RA, Bingham JB: Heart failure in out-patients: A randomized trial of digoxin vs. placebo. *N Engl J Med* 306:699, 1982.

Leier CV, Heban PT, Huss P, et al: Comparative systemic and regional hemodynamic effects of dopamine and dobutamine in patients with cardiomyopathic cardiac failure. *Circulation* 56:918, 1977.

Liang C-S, Sherman LG, Doherty JU, et al: Sustained improvement of cardiac function in patients with congestive heart failure after short-term infusion of dobutamine. *Circulation* 69:113, 1984.

Magorien RD, Triffon DW, Desch CE, et al: Prazosin and hydralazine in congestive heart failure: Regional hemodynamic effects in relation to dose. *Ann Intern Med* 95:5, 1981.

Massie B, Ports T, Chatterjee K, et al: Long-term vasodilator therapy for heart failure. *Circulation* 63:269, 1981.

Massie BM: New trends in the use of angiotensin converting enzyme inhibitors in chronic heart failure. *Am J Med* 84(Suppl 4A):36, 1988.

McCall D, O'Rourke R: Congestive heart failure. *Mod Concepts Cardiovasc Dis* 52:55, 1985.

Miller RR, Awan NA, Joye JA, et al: Combined dopamine and nitroprusside therapy in congestive heart failure. *Circulation* 55:881, 1977.

Newmann TJ, Maskin CS, Dennick LG, et al: Effects of captopril on survival in patients with heart failure. *Am J Med* 84:3A, 1988.

Packer M: Neurohumoral interactions and adaptations in congestive heart failure. *Circulation* 77:721, 1988.

Packer M, Kessler PD, Lee WH: Calcium-channel blockade in the management of severe chronic congestive heart failure: A bridge too far. *Circulation* 75(Suppl V):V-56, 1987.

Packer M, Medina N, Yushak M: Hemodynamic and clinical limitations of long-term inotropic therapy with amrinone in patients with severe chronic heart failure. *Circulation* 470:1038, 1984.

Parmley WW: Pathophysiology and current therapy of congestive heart failure. *J Am Coll Cardiol* 13:771, 1989.

Patak RV, Mookerjee BK, Bentzel CJ, et al: Antagonism of effects of furosemide by indomethacin in normal and hypertensive man. *Prostaglandins* 10:649, 1975.

Pfeffer MA, Lamas GA, Vaughan DE, et al: Effect of captopril on progressive ventricular dilatation after anterior myocardial infarction. *N Engl J Med* 319:80, 1988.

Raine AEG, Erne P, Burgisser E, et al: Atrial natriuretic peptide and atrial pressure in patients with congestive heart failure. *N Engl J Med* 315:533, 1986.

Rajfer SL, Anton AH, Rossen JD, et al: Beneficial hemodynamic effects of oral levodopa in heart failure: Relation to the generation of dopamine. *N Engl J Med* 310:1357, 1984.

Reinock HJ, Stein JH: Mechanisms of action and clinical use of diuretics. In: Brenner BM, Rector FC, eds. *The Kidney*, ed 2. Philadelphia: Saunders; 1981, p. 1097.

Saito Y, Nakao K, Nishimura K, et al: Clinical application of atrial natriuretic polypeptide in patients with congestive heart failure: Beneficial effects on left ventricular function. *Circulation* 76:115, 1987.

Sanders MR, Kostis JB, Frishman WH: The use of inotropic agents in acute and chronic heart failure. *Med Clin North Am* 73:283, 1989.

Smith TW, Butler VP, Haber E, et al: Treatment of life-threatening digitalis intoxication and digoxin-specific Fab antibody fragments: Experience in 26 cases. *N Engl J Med* 307:1357, 1982.

Sonnenblick EH, Frishman WH, LeJemtel TH: Dobutamine: A new synthetic cardioactive sympathetic amine. *N Engl J Med* 300:17, 1979.

Unverferth DV, Magorien RD, Lewis RP, Leier CV: Long-term benefit of dobutamine in patients with congestive cardiomyopathy. *Am Heart J* 100:622, 1980.

Wellens HJJ: The electrocardiogram in digitalis intoxication. In: Yu N, Goodwin JF, eds. *Progress in Cardiology*. Philadelphia: Lea & Febiger; vol 5, 1976, p. 271.

Wenger NK, Franciosa JA, Weber KT: Heart failure. *J Am Coll Cardiol* 10:73A, 1987.

Yancy CW, Firth BG: Congestive heart failure. *Disease-a-Month* 34:469, 1988.

24 Pericardial Diseases

CHAPTER

Haim Hammerman
Robert A. Kloner

The mode of presentation of pericardial disease depends on both the etiology and the type or stage of pericardial inflammatory reaction. Thus, pericardial diseases are classified by etiology and according to stage. The etiologies of pericardial disease are classified as infectious, neoplastic, metabolic, autoimmune-related, traumatic, and idiopathic (Table 1). The stages of inflammatory reactions include acute, subacute, and chronic, with or without effusion and constriction (Table 2).

Clinically, pericardial involvement may manifest as an acute disease, with or without evidence of pericardial effusion or tamponade. Sometimes it presents as a subacute constrictive disease, or effusive constrictive process. Chronic pericarditis can manifest as (1) relapses of acute attack, (2) chronic pericardial effusion, or (3) chronic constrictive pericarditis.

ACUTE PERICARDITIS

Common etiologies of acute pericarditis include viral, post-myocardial infarction (MI), uremic, idiopathic, and autoimmune-related diseases. Acute pericarditis is a clinical entity characterized by three major features: chest pain, friction rub, and fever. The pain of pericarditis characteristically is sharp or stabbing, variable in intensity, persistent, and aggravated by respiration, coughing, and movement. The pain is usually precordial, sometimes substernal, and occasionally radiates to the neck, arms, and back. It may be relieved by leaning forward or sitting and exacerbated by lying down. Some patients have acute pericarditis without pain; in others, the pain mimics that of ischemic disease.

The most characteristic physical sign is a precordial friction rub. This is a scratchy noise, caused by friction between the pericardial layers, and may have three components: presystolic, systolic, and proto-diastolic. All three components are not always heard in any one patient. The quality of the rub typically changes with patient position and often is transitory. The rub is best heard during expiration, with the patient leaning forward. Although a pericardial friction rub is pathognomonic for pericarditis, it is found in only 60–70% of patients with acute pericarditis. It may be difficult to distinguish the rub from a murmur when only one component of the rub is heard. Therefore, every attempt must be made to repeat the auscultatory examination in order to detect other components or a change in the friction rub. Absence of a friction rub does not rule out pericardial effusion. Other common signs of acute pericarditis are fever and tachycardia. Associated symptoms and signs of systemic disease should be sought. Patients should be evaluated for clinical signs of cardiac compression (e.g., tamponade).

Laboratory findings depend on the etiology of the disease. In cases of viral, immune-related, infectious, or idiopathic pericarditis, sedimentation rate and leukocyte count may be elevated. The electrocardiogram (ECG) shows sinus tachycardia and diffuse ST-segment elevation in multiple leads in the early stages (see Chapter 3). This ST elevation is different from that in acute myocardial infarction (MI), in which it is localized and accompanied by Q-wave formation. Sometimes, only T-wave changes are detected. A decrease in QRS amplitude is seen in patients with pericardial effusion, and atrial arrhythmias occasionally are detected. Chest x-ray film may be normal or, with pericardial effusion, the heart shadow may be enlarged (see Chapter 4).

Management of acute pericarditis includes: (1) observation for development of pericardial effusion and signs of tamponade (monitor heart rate, arterial and

Table 1. Etiologic Classification of Pericardial Disease

Infectious
  Viral (Coxsackie B, A; echo; influenza; infectious mononucleosis)
  Bacterial (pneumococci, staphylococci, meningococci, gonococci)
  Tuberculous
  Fungal (histoplasmosis, aspergillosis)
  Parasitic
  Acquired immunodeficiency syndrome (AIDS)
Pericarditis associated with acute MI
Neoplastic
  Primary (mesothelioma)
  Secondary (lung, breast, melanoma, lymphoma, leukemia)
Metabolic
  Uremia
  Myxedema
  Cholesterol
Autoimmune related
  Connective tissue diseases (systemic lupus erythematosus, rheumatoid arthritis, scleroderma, poly-
    arteritis nodosa, Takayasu's disease, Wegener's granulomatosis)
  Post–cardiac injury (late post–myocardial infarction syndrome–Dressler's syndrome; postcardiotomy
    syndrome; post-trauma syndrome)
  Drug induced (procainamide; hydralazine; penicillin; isonicotinic acid hydrazide; phenylbutazone;
    minoxidil; high-dose cyclophosphamide in children)
Trauma
  Penetrating chest injury
  Closed chest injury
  After thoracic surgical procedures
  After cardiac catheterization and pacemaker insertion
  Rupture of heart or great vessels
Aortic dissection and rupture of heart
Radiation
Miscellaneous
  Sarcoidosis
  Amyloidosis
  Acute pancreatitis
  Chylopericardium
  Familial Mediterranean fever
  Familial pericarditis
Idiopathic

venous pressure); (2) determining and treating the underlying etiology; and (3) analgesics and anti-inflammatory agents for viral or idiopathic pericarditis. Most patients with viral or idiopathic pericarditis recover rapidly with the help of symptomatic therapy, such as aspirin, for a few days. Indomethacin is often used, but probably has little advantage over aspirin. Glucocorticosteroids are more potent, but should be used only in severe cases that do not respond to nonsteroidal anti-inflammatory agents. Chronic recurrent or relapsing pericarditis may follow acute pericarditis. This syndrome often develops in patients who have been treated with glucocorticosteroids and later had the dose reduced. Management of this relapsing syndrome includes very slow reduction of the glucocorticosteroid dose. Pericardiectomy should be considered in relapsing cases that require long periods (more than a year) of steroid therapy.

Table 2. Stages of Inflammatory Reaction in Pericarditis

Acute pericarditis
  Noneffusive (fibrinous)
  Effusive
Subacute pericarditis
  Effusive constrictive
  Constrictive
Chronic pericarditis
  Effusive
  Constrictive
  Adhesive

ACUTE PERICARDITIS WITH PERICARDIAL EFFUSION

Pericardial effusion (accumulation of fluid in the pericardial space) can occur in the acute phase of pericarditis and develop either rapidly or slowly and insidiously. Pericardial effusion may or may not be associated with compression of the heart. If fluid has accumulated to a point of causing increased intrapericardial pressure, compression of the heart can develop. The rate at which the fluid accumulates is important, because slow accumulation allows the pericardium to stretch over time; with rapid accumulation this compensatory mechanism does not have time to develop. The primary effect of accumulation of fluid in the pericardial space is eventual restriction of diastolic filling. The influence on systolic contraction is negligible. Systemic arteriolar contraction, salt and water retention, and increased venous tone act initially as compensatory mechanisms to preserve cardiac output (see section on cardiac tamponade). Thus, the clinical picture of compensated pericardial effusion with compression is increased systemic venous pressure. In cases of cardiac tamponade, there is failure of the compensatory mechanisms with a drop in cardiac output. Pericardial effusion can present as a wide range of clinical syndromes, from an asymptomatic undetected effusion without hemodynamic compromise to dramatic life-threatening tamponade. The two main factors governing presentation are the amount of fluid and rate of accumulation. Extent of prior inflammation or thickening of the pericardium affects its capability to stretch and, hence, the amount of fluid required for tamponade.

Clinical findings of pericardial effusion include the pain of associated pericarditis (sometimes the pain may become less sharp in quality once fluid accumulates), shortness of breath, orthopnea, cough, tachycardia, elevated central venous pressure, hepatic enlargement, a weak apical cardiac impulse, and faint heart sounds. The friction rub of pericarditis may disappear. In large effusions there may be an area of dullness to percussion and bronchial breathing at the angle of the left scapula, probably caused by lung compression (Ewart's sign).

Electrocardiographic findings are similar to those noted above. In large effusions, typically, QRS amplitude is decreased.

The chest x-ray film reveals an enlarged cardiac silhouette (Chapter 4) with clear lungs. Epicardial fat lines may be seen within the cardiac shadow. Fluoroscopy shows diminished cardiac pulsations. Echocardiography is an accurate and convenient noninvasive tool for diagnosing pericardial effusion (see Chapter 7). Both M-mode and two-dimensional echocardiograms show fluid accumulation and pericardial thickening. In general, the amount of fluid can be semiquantitated by M-mode echocardiography. In small to moderate effusions, fluid appears as an echo-free space posterior to the left ventricle. In the absence of adhesions, fluid also appears anteriorly in moderate to large effusions. Very large effusions often extend behind the lower left atrium. Exaggerated heart movements ("swinging heart") are seen with large effusions and are often associated with an echocardiographic appearance simulating mitral and tricuspid prolapse ("pseudoprolapse"). Two-dimensional echocardiography provides a better idea as to the quantitation of fluid, especially if a large volume has accumulated or if the fluid is loculated (Figures 1 and 2). Serial echocardiography is valuable in following the course of pericardial effusions. Radionuclide scans and intravenous injection of CO_2 with contrast angiocardiography may be used to detect effusion in cases in which echocardiography is unsatisfactory.

CARDIAC TAMPONADE

Cardiac tamponade is an accumulation of fluid in the pericardium in an amount sufficient to cause serious restriction of diastolic filling, with failure of compensatory mechanisms. Development of tamponade is related to distensibility of the pericardium and the speed of fluid accumulation. It is not proportional to

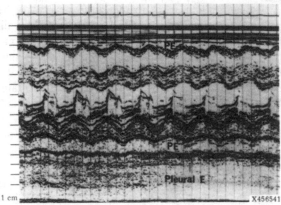

Figure 1. *M-mode echocardiogram from a patient with pericardial and pleural effusions (E). The pericardial effusion (PE) can be seen both anteriorly and posteriorly. (Reproduced with permission from Feigenbaum. See Bibliography.)*

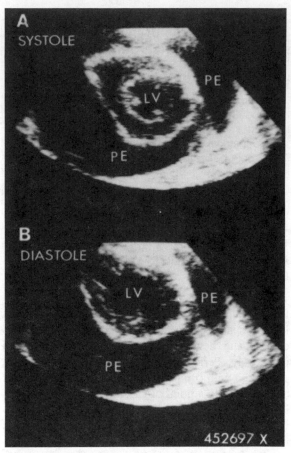

Figure 2. *Short-axis two-dimensional echocardiogram from a patient with a large pericardial effusion (PE) demonstrating the shift in cardiac position from systole to diastole. LV=left ventricle. (Reproduced with permission from Feigenbaum.)*

the amount of fluid present, since massive effusions may be present without tamponade, and relatively small amounts of fluid collecting quickly may produce severe compression and tamponade. Circulation cannot be sustained for long once pericardial pressure exceeds venous pressure. Any cause of pericardial effusion can induce cardiac tamponade. Frequent causes are neoplasms, radiation, trauma, bleeding after cardiac surgery, pyogenic infections, tuberculosis, and uremia (Table 3). Tamponade occasionally occurs during acute viral or idiopathic pericarditis and in patients treated with anticoagulants during the course of acute pericarditis.

The clinical manifestations are the result of a fall in cardiac output and elevated venous pressure. Patients complain of lightheadedness and dizziness as forward output decreases, as well as other symptoms of pericardial effusion discussed above. Physical examination reveals jugular venous distention, tachycardia, systemic hypotension, narrow pulse pressure, paradoxical pulse and, in some cases, tender and enlarged liver. When tamponade is severe, there is evidence of shock state with signs of organ hypoperfusion.

Paradoxical pulse, defined as an abnormally large (>10 mm Hg) drop in arterial systolic pressure with inspiration, is a valuable sign of cardiac tamponade. This physical sign can be detected by palpation of the pulse. During inspiration the amplitude of the pulse drops markedly. The degree of paradoxical pulse can be estimated by measuring blood pressure during the respiratory cycle. It should be measured during normal respiration, since deep breathing as well as artificial respiration exaggerate paradoxical pulse. In cases of severe hypotension, this sign is difficult to appreciate. Paradoxical pulse can be accurately determined by means of direct arterial pressure measurements. In patients with chronic constrictive pericarditis, paradoxical pulse is often minimal or absent. Although this finding is consistently found in tamponade, it is not pathognomonic of it; it is seen in acute and chronic obstructive lung diseases, severe myocardial failure, hemorrhagic shock, and in some forms of restrictive cardiomyopathies. Kussmaul's sign (rise in central venous pressure with inspiration) occasionally occurs in cardiac tamponade, but it is more common in patients with constrictive pericarditis; it also occurs in some patients with tricuspid valve disease. Typically,

Table 3. Common Causes of Tamponade
Neoplastic disease
Idiopathic pericarditis
Uremia
Trauma
Infection (tuberculous, pyogenic)
Rupture of heart or great vessels
Anticoagulant therapy (during pericardial disease)
Iatrogenic (after thoracic surgery, catheterization, pacemaker)
Radiation

the x and y descents of the jugular venous pulse are approximately equal, or the x descent is predominant. Auscultation typically reveals tachycardia; the heart sounds may be faint with or without a pericardial friction rub.

The ECG shows features similar to those described for effusion. Electrical alternans (alternation of the QRS amplitude on every other beat) appears in severe cases of tamponade.

The chest x-ray film may show either a normal or large heart shadow, with clear lung fields. Symmetric enlargement of the heart shadow occurs when more than 200–300 ml of fluid accumulates. Fluoroscopy reveals diminished cardiac pulsations.

Echocardiography establishes the presence of pericardial fluid and allows a reasonably accurate estimation of the size of the effusion (Figures 1 and 2). Detection of abnormal diastolic right ventricular wall motion may be a sensitive indicator of a hemodynamically significant pericardial effusion. There is posterior motion of the anterior right ventricular wall that represents true collapse of the right ventricle in early diastole. Echocardiographic findings of a pericardial effusion—an inspiratory increase in right ventricular dimensions and right atrial and ventricular diastolic collapse—strongly suggest cardiac tamponade. In various studies, the sensitivity and specificity of right ventricular collapse for tamponade are 79–92% and 90–100%, respectively. Patients with pulsus paradoxus and severe cardiac tamponade have a marked increase in respiratory variation in transvalvular flow velocities, flow velocity integrals and left ventricular ejection and isovolumic relaxation times. These changes were seen also in some patients with pericardial effusion but without overt hemodynamic compromise.

However, tamponade is diagnosed primarily on the basis of clinical findings and characteristic hemodynamic features rather than echocardiography. In cases of life-threatening tamponade, echocardiography should not be performed if it will delay the decision to perform pericardiocentesis. The clinical features of right ventricular infarction sometimes mimic tamponade. Detection of fluid by echocardiography with no evidence of right ventricular enlargement or abnormal right ventricular contractility favor the latter diagnosis.

Cardiac catheterization is not required when the diagnosis is certain, but it is important in equivocal cases or when an element of pericardial constriction is suspected. Characteristically, venous pressure is elevated with normal inspiratory decline (Kussmaul's sign usually absent). Prominent y descent, which is characteristic of constrictive pericarditis (described later), is absent in tamponade. Paradoxical pulse can be recorded from a systemic artery or from left ventricular pressures, and, in extreme cases, pulsus alternans (alternation of systolic pressure amplitude every other beat) can be recorded. Typically, both right and left ventricular diastolic pressures equal intrapericardial pressure. Right atrial pressure is elevated above normal, and right atrial pressure, right ventricular end-diastolic pressure, pulmonary artery diastolic pressure, and pulmonary capillary wedge pressure are within 5 mm Hg of each other. After pericardial aspiration, pericardial and right atrial pressures fall, right ventricular diastolic pressure comes down to a normal level, and cardiac output increases.

Patients with acute pericarditis should be observed carefully for development of pericardial effusion with tamponade. In the presence of pericardial effusion, heart rate and arterial and central venous pressures should be monitored continuously and serial echocardiograms recorded to detect any change in the amount of pericardial fluid. In case of cardiac tamponade, the definitive emergency treatment is removal of pericardial fluid by pericardiocentesis or surgical drainage. Medical support is often necessary to stabilize the patient's condition while preparations are made for the definitive procedures. Intravenous fluids are administered in order to help restore left ventricular filling volumes. Despite venous congestion, significant volumes should be administered (up to 300–500 ml/15 min). Inotropic support may be beneficial in improving cardiac output. Isoproterenol is infused initially at a rate of 2–4 µg/min and the rate is increased up to 20 µg/min until improvement or appearance of arrhythmias. Dobutamine may be infused starting at a rate of 1–2 μg/kg/min and the rate is increased to 15 μg/kg/min. Expansion of blood volume combined with nitroprusside has been shown to increase cardiac output and improve blood pressure in numerous studies of animals with tamponade. However, in humans, the hemodynamic benefits of volume expansion alone or combined with nitroprusside are very limited. Medical support is not an alternative mode of treatment and should not cause a delay in performing pericardiocentesis or surgical drainage.

PERICARDIOCENTESIS

Pericardiocentesis—needle aspiration of the pericardial sac—has been used successfully in the management of pericardial effusion and tamponade. Pericardiocentesis is performed for two major reasons: therapeutically, for relief of tamponade as an emergency procedure or, in cases of large effusion, for relief of symptoms; and to obtain fluid for diagnostic purposes. Pericardiocentesis is associated with potentially dangerous complications (e.g., ventricular laceration or puncture, coronary artery laceration, ventricular arrhythmias, MI, and even cardiac arrest), and should be performed by those experienced in this procedure. Some believe that pericardiocentesis should be performed only for emergency relief of cardiac tamponade, and recommend surgical drainage in elective cases.

Optimally, pericardiocentesis is performed in the cardiac catheterization laboratory under ECG and fluoroscopic control. However, it can be performed at the bedside with proper monitoring. In general, a needle is inserted 2–4 cm below the junction of the subxiphoid process and the left costal margin at an angle of 20–30°, so that it passes underneath the sternum into the pericardial sac. A chest lead of the ECG is connected to the needle and monitored throughout the insertion. When the needle touches the myocardium, ST elevation is detected. The location of the needle can also be determined by fluoroscopy (sometimes with the aid of a contrast agent injection), by echocardiography, by measuring pressure contour from the needle, or by identifying the type of fluid aspirated. Aspirated bloody fluid should be compared to venous blood for its hemoglobin content in order to determine whether a cardiac chamber was punctured. Bloody pericardial fluid tends not to clot, in contrast to blood aspirated accidentally from a cardiac chamber. The pericardiocentesis tends to be low risk when there is a large anterior pericardial effusion, determined by echocardiography. Intrapericardial pressures should be measured before and after aspiration of fluid. In tamponade, this pressure exceeds or equals central venous pressure, and in some cases it may exceed 20 mm Hg. Intrapericardial pressure drops after removal of fluid. Some pericardial needles have a plastic cannula over them; after successful entry into the pericardial space, the needle is removed, leaving the cannula for drainage. Some cardiologists prefer to exchange the needle for a catheter, and this may be accomplished by passing a guide wire through the needle and then passing a small multihole catheter over the guide wire into the pericardial sac. This catheter can be left for continuous drainage for a short period or for intrapericardial drug administration.

Open surgical drainage is an alternative treatment for cardiac tamponade. Subxiphoid pericardiotomy under local anesthesia can be performed in acutely ill patients for relief of tamponade. Surgical drainage is indicated in cases of repeated accumulation of pericardial effusion.

The pericardial fluid should be analyzed for color, turbidity, cell counts, cultures, chemistries, and cytology. However, in a number of diseases (viral pericarditis, collagen-vascular diseases, uremia) the pericardial fluid has no pathognomonic features. The quality of fluid inspected visually may be of some diagnostic yield. Serosanguineous or sanguineous effusion is found after cardiac surgery, trauma, pericarditis after acute MI treated with anticoagulants, neoplastic pericarditis, and rupture of the heart and great vessels. Serous effusion is commonly found in viral pericarditis, radiation pericarditis, heart failure, tuberculous pericarditis, collagen diseases, and hypoalbuminemia. Chylous effusion may follow cardiac surgery with injury to lymph vessels or when neoplasm interferes with lymph drainage. Cholesterol effusion is found in cases of myxedema.

The fluid should be characterized as a transudate (protein <3 g/100 ml) or an exudate (protein >3g/100 ml). Transudates occur in heart failure, hypoalbuminemia, Dressler's syndrome, postpericardiotomy syndrome, drug-induced pericarditis, some cases of collagen diseases, and radiation pericarditis. Exudates are more likely to occur in infection, neoplasms, uremia, chylous pericarditis, and collagen diseases. Cholesterol content is elevated in cases of myxedema. Glucose content of the fluid is low in bacterial pericarditis.

Other tests that should be performed include blood cell count and differential; gram stain; Ziehl-Neelsen stain; cultures for aerobic and anaerobic bacteria; cultures for tuberculosis; and, when suspected, fungal cultures. Positive cytologic findings have been reported in 50–75% of patients with neoplastic involvement of the pericardium, depending on the number of samples examined. Pericardiocentesis can provide positive culture diagnosis in 15% of cases of tuberculosis and in almost all cases of pyogenic pericarditis.

As mentioned previously, pericardiocentesis is not without hazards; therefore, it, as well as surgical exploration, should be performed only when indicated, namely, in tamponade or high pressure pericardial effusion, suspicion of pyogenic pericarditis, and the need to obtain fluid for diagnosis.

CHRONIC PERICARDITIS

Chronic pericarditis may be associated with relapses of acute pericarditis, chronic pericardial effusion or constriction, or adhesion to surrounding structures. Chronic pericardial effusion can follow any cause of pericarditis, presenting as a wide variety of clinical pictures depending on the degree of compression of the heart and the manifestations of the underlying disease. In some patients chronic asymptomatic pericardial effusion develops that does not progress to compression or cardiac constriction.

CHRONIC CONSTRICTIVE PERICARDITIS

This condition occurs when the healing of acute pericarditis is followed by formation of scar tissue surrounding the heart, compressing its chambers and restricting diastolic filling. Constrictive pericarditis may follow idiopathic pericarditis, tuberculosis, pyogenic infection, radiation, uremia, neoplasm, trauma, and viral and connective tissue diseases. Often the etiology of pericarditis cannot be determined in late stages of constrictive pericarditis. The fundamental pathophysiologic abnormality characteristic of constrictive pericarditis is restriction of diastolic filling due to limitation imposed by the fibrous scarred pericardium. Stroke volume is diminished and ventricular end-diastolic pressures as well as mean atrial pressure and systemic and pulmonary vein pressures are equally elevated. Sometimes pericardial fibrosis is associated with myocardial fibrosis, which leads to ventricular contraction abnormality.

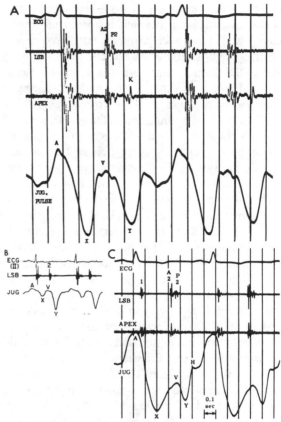

Figure 3. *Jugular pulses in three examples of pericardial constriction. In example A, both x and y descents are deep. A pericardial "knock" (K) coincides with the y trough. Example B shows a deep y descent but a shallow x descent. A few sound vibrations are located in early diastole at the expected time of the knock. Example C displays a deep x descent with a relatively short y descent. All three examples display early v-wave peaking (around the time of S₂), an early y trough (less than 0.2 second after A₂), and an early, prominent H wave. These features are characteristic of pericardial constriction. (From Tavel. Reproduced with permission from Year Book Medical Publishers.)*

Clinical manifestations include shortness of breath, orthopnea, and fatigue due to limited cardiac output reserve, and elevated systemic jugular venous pressure. Kussmaul's sign may be present. The jugular venous pulse has a characteristic wave form. The peak of the v-wave is early, and there is a deep y descent. This is followed by an early diastolic rise, terminating in an early H wave and a plateau (Figure 3). Paradoxical pulse is observed in some cases. Signs of congestive hepatomegaly, splenomegaly, and ascites may be found; dependent edema is less common than ascites. Constrictive pericarditis is a frequently missed diagnosis. Patients with chronic constrictive pericarditis may be erroneously diagnosed as having cirrhosis of the liver; others are suspected of having gastrointestinal malignancy and undergo a lengthy clinical workup. These diagnostic errors can be avoided simply by careful examination of the venous pressure, which is elevated in constrictive pericarditis. The precordial pulse is either imperceptible or appears to retract during systole. Heart sounds typically are faint. A diastolic pericardial knock, which is an early, high pitched sound (0.06–0.12 second after aortic closure), may be heard and is related to the phase of early diastolic filling of the heart. It coincides with the y trough described for the venous pulse. Studies have related this sound to the sudden halt of ventricular filling in constrictive pericarditis. This sound, like Kussmaul's sign, occurs frequently in constrictive pericarditis but rarely in cardiac tamponade.

Hancock (1980) suggested that there are two forms of constriction, one elastic and the other more rigid. These two forms are believed to cause different patterns of diagnostic signs. The elastic form is similar to cardiac tamponade and is associated with prominent paradoxical pulse and systolic descent in venous tracings. The rigid type has a less prominent paradoxical pulse and a more conspicuous diastolic descent in the venous pressure tracing, often associated with a pericardial knock.

Electrocardiographic abnormalities in about 25% of patients include low QRS amplitude, T-wave changes, notched P waves, and atrial fibrillation. Chest x-ray film shows a normal or slightly enlarged cardiac shadow, with clear lung fields. Pericardial calcification may be seen (see Chapter 4). Computed tomography as well as magnetic resonance imaging are valuable in identifying pericardial thickening and other findings consistent with constrictive pericarditis, including dilatation of large systemic veins and narrowing of the right ventricle. Pericardial thickening on echocardiography in the absence of effusion is a nonspecific finding and is not diagnostic of constriction. Abnormal left ventricular filling, as reflected by a sharp posterior motion of the posterior wall in early diastole followed by a flat segment, can be seen in constriction, with prominent early diastolic anterior motion of the ventricular septum. Two-dimensional echocardiography may show small ventricles with enlarged atria, dilatation of the inferior vena cava, and

bulging of the interventricular and interatrial septa into the left side of the heart in inspiration. Patients with constrictive pericarditis can be differentiated from those with restrictive cardiomyopathy by comparing respiratory changes in transvalvular flow velocities. Patients with constrictive pericarditis show respiratory variation in left ventricular isovolumic relaxation time and in peak mitral flow velocity in early diastole. These changes disappear after surgery and are not present in patients with restrictive cardiomyopathy or in normal subjects.

Cardiac catheterization reveals that ventricular end-diastolic pressures are elevated. Right ventricular pressure shows a consistent steep early diastolic dip, followed by a plateau ("square-root sign"). The end-diastolic pressure of the right ventricle is higher or equal to one-third of its systolic pressure. The wave form and amplitude of left ventricular diastolic pressure is identical to that of the right ventricle. Pulmonary arterial diastolic pressure is equal to end-diastolic pressure in the ventricles. Severe constriction is associated with filling pressures of 20–25 mm Hg (Figure 4). The right atrial pressure pulse has an M-shaped pattern. The typical venous M-shaped pattern and ventricular square root sign are characteristic of constriction and differentiate it from tamponade. Cardiac catheterization helps differentiate constrictive pericarditis from restrictive cardiomyopathy. Transvenous endomyocardial biopsy may be of value when differential diagnosis between restrictive myocardial or constrictive pericardial disease is necessary.

Pericardial resection is the treatment of choice in symptomatic cases. Operative mortality is about 5%. Long-term results are satisfactory, especially in radical resection of the pericardium; however, hemodynamic improvement may be gradual. In cases with no improvement, one should look for either myocardial involvement or inadequate pericardial resection. Recurrence of constriction is rare.

SUBACUTE EFFUSIVE-CONSTRICTIVE PERICARDITIS

In this condition, constrictive pericarditis coexists with pericardial effusion and tamponade. The constriction is by the visceral pericardium rather than by the parietal pericardium. Causes of effusive-constrictive pericarditis include tuberculosis, recurrent relapses of idiopathic pericarditis, trauma, radiation effects, uremia, and connective tissue diseases. Physical findings

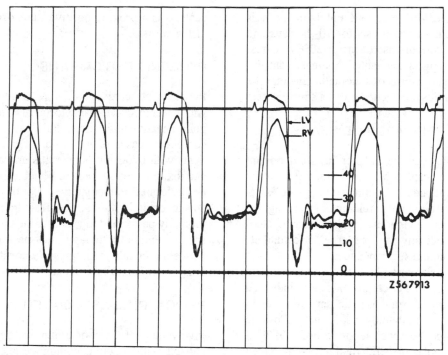

Figure 4. *Simultaneous left ventricular and right ventricular pressure recordings from a patient with constrictive pericarditis. The classic "square root" sign of the ventricular pressures during diastole can be noted. (Reproduced with permission from Feigenbaum.)*

include paradoxical pulse and elevated venous pressure with prominent x descent. An S_3 or diastolic knock may be present. The ECG reveals low or borderline QRS amplitude with T-wave changes. Chest x-ray film reveals a large heart and echocardiography often reveals effusion and pericardial thickening. After removal of fluid by pericardiocentesis, venous pressure typically remains elevated due to remaining constriction. The intracavitary pressure tracings shift from those typical of tamponade before pericardiocentesis (x = y descent or x > y descent, no square root sign) to those typical of constriction after pericardiocentesis (y > x descent, square root sign). This condition may progress to chronic constrictive pericarditis. Surgical excision of the pericardium is indicated in severe cases.

ADHESIVE PERICARDITIS

In this condition, there are adhesions between pericardium and structures in the mediastinum. Adhesive pericarditis usually does not interfere with cardiac function.

FEATURES OF SPECIFIC FORMS OF PERICARDIAL DISEASE

VIRAL OR ACUTE BENIGN FORM OF PERICARDITIS

Viral pericarditis is common and can be caused by a wide range of viruses (Coxsackie B or A, influenza, echo, herpes simplex, mumps, chicken pox, and adenovirus). It can cause a variety of inflammatory reactions (serous, fibrinous, hemorrhagic, or suppurative), probably depending on the virus. Sometimes acute pericarditis is related to or associated with a viral infection by history. Viral cultures are not always helpful; fourfold or greater increases in convalescent serum titer are usual, but because most infections are benign, this variable is not tested. When viral etiology cannot be established but is presumed, the illness is referred to by some physicians as *acute benign pericarditis*. This condition is more frequent in young adults. Pain is usually accompanied by fever; pneumonitis and pleuritis are common. There is evidence of pericardial effusion, but tamponade is unusual. The acute disease lasts for 10–14 days and relapses of the acute disease occur in 20% of cases. No specific therapy is available. Analgesic anti-inflammatory drugs (aspirin or indomethacin) may be used; corticosteroids are needed only in severe cases.

NEOPLASTIC PERICARDIAL DISEASE

Metastatic tumors (also see Chapter 26) are important because they are responsible for serious pericardial effusion and tamponade. Common malignancies affecting the pericardium are carcinoma of the lung and breast, melanoma, lymphoma, and leukemia. Neoplasms characteristically produce large pericardial effusions and, sometimes, tamponade.

Pericardial metastases can be detected in some cases by echocardiography. Pericardiocentesis is indicated to relieve tamponade, symptomatic pericardial effusion, and for obtaining cytologic specimens. Positive cytologic findings have been reported in 50–75% of patients with neoplastic pericardial effusion. Open pericardial biopsy taken from suspected foci in the pericardium can be of diagnostic value in up to 90% of the cases with neoplastic involvement. In recurrent pericardial effusion or tamponade, intrapericardial chemotherapy administration or operation should be considered.

RADIATION PERICARDITIS

Radiation pericarditis may occur early after radiation therapy or many years after exposure. This entity must be diagnosed in patients with neoplastic diseases and differentiated from metastatic involvement of the pericardium because radiation pericarditis has a better prognosis. Sometimes they can be differentiated by cytologic or histologic examination of the fluid and pericardium. Although acute pericarditis and effusion may follow radiation exposure to the heart, effusive constrictive pericarditis is more common.

TUBERCULOUS PERICARDITIS

The incidence of tuberculous pericarditis is decreasing in developed countries. It must be diagnosed in the acute stage, since antituberculous drugs are effective. This condition tends to be associated with large pericardial effusions and, if not treated, progresses to an effusive-constrictive phase and eventually to chronic constrictive pericarditis. Pericardio-

centesis can provide positive diagnosis in only 15% of the cases.

PYOGENIC PERICARDITIS

Pyogenic pericarditis is a rare condition associated with pneumococcal, staphylococcal, streptococcal, and gram-negative infections. Purulent pericarditis may complicate cases of systemic fungal infections. Patients with pyogenic pericarditis are very ill, febrile, and toxic. If it is suspected, pericardiocentesis should be performed immediately to confirm the diagnosis and to obtain cultures. Surgical drainage should be promptly performed to evacuate the purulent fluid and specific antibiotic therapy must be started. Pyogenic pericarditis tends to progress to constrictive pericarditis despite antibiotic therapy.

PERICARDITIS ASSOCIATED WITH AIDS

Involvement of the pericardium has been described in patients with acquired immunodeficiency syndrome. Most of the patients with pericardial disease have concomitant involvement of the myocardium. The pericarditis is usually nonspecific by etiology, associated with Kaposi's sarcoma or due to pathogens such as *Mycobacterium tuberculosis* and *Cryptococcus*. Often, the pericardial disease is associated with pericardial effusion. Pericardiocentesis may yield a clear serosanguineous fluid.

UREMIC PERICARDITIS

Uremic pericarditis is associated with advanced chronic renal failure and is a serious complication because it may be associated with tamponade. Intense hemodialysis is indicated for treatment of uncomplicated uremic pericarditis and results in resolution of pericarditis in 40–60% of patients. Serial physical examination, chest x-rays, and echocardiograms are useful for follow-up of chronic dialysis therapy in renal patients and for identifying patients with fluid accumulation. Resolution of uremic pericarditis complicated by tamponade is accomplished in most cases by intense hemodialysis in association with pericardiocentesis. Surgical pericardial excision is recommended in patients with recurrent episodes of pericarditis. Treatment of intractable uremic pericardial effusion by local steroid (triamcinolone hexacetonide) administration into the pericardial sac has been described in a few patients (Popli et al.). Frequently, mild degrees of pericardial effusion are associated with fluid overload, congestive heart failure, and left ventricular dysfunction, which often occurs in chronic renal disease. Cardiac catheterization may be needed to establish whether tamponade is a dominant component in these cases.

TRAUMATIC HEMOPERICARDIUM

Traumatic hemopericardium can result from penetrating wounds of the heart or as a result of closed chest trauma caused by the steering wheel in automobile accidents. Hemopericardium due to closed chest trauma may be difficult to recognize because it may develop slowly. Cardiac tamponade may develop after cardiac operations early or late in the patient's course and, rarely, after cardiac catheterization and pacemaker insertion.

POST-CARDIAC INJURY SYNDROME

Post-cardiac injury syndrome occurs as an inflammatory reaction after either pericardial injury induced in the course of a cardiac operation or trauma to the heart or after the first 14 days of an MI. Prominent clinical features include fever, pericarditis, and sometimes pneumonitis and pleuritis. The post-cardiac injury syndrome may occur several days to months after the injury or infarction. Pericarditis may be accompanied by pericardial effusion. The clinical picture mimics acute viral pericarditis, but it is believed to be a hypersensitivity immune reaction after myocardial injury. Patients are generally managed by analgesic anti-inflammatory drugs; in severe disabling or recurring cases, corticosteroids may be effective.

PERICARDIAL EFFUSION ASSOCIATED WITH CONGESTIVE HEART FAILURE

Effusion may accompany heart failure without evidence of pericarditis. In general, pericardial effusion due to heart failure does not lead to tamponade. In one study, cardiac disease associated with congestive heart failure was found to be the most common cause of pericardial effusion in patients referred for echocardiography. Parameters of left heart function are markedly abnormal in patients with congestive heart failure and pericardial effusion.

Bibliography

Acierno LJ: Cardiac complications in acquired immunodeficiency syndrome (AIDS): A review. *J Am Coll Cardiol* 13:1144, 1989.

Alcan KE, Zabetakis PM, Mariho ND, et al: Management of acute cardiac tamponade by subxiphoid pericardiotomy. *JAMA* 247:1143, 1982.

Applefeld MM, Slawson RG, Hall-Craigs M, et al: Delayed pericardial disease after radiotherapy. *Am J Cardiol* 47:210, 1981.

Appleton CP, Hatle LK, Popp RL: Cardiac tamponade and pericardial effusion: Respiratory variation in transvalvular flow velocities studied by Doppler echocardiography. *J Am Coll Cardiol* 11:1020, 1988.

Armstrong WF, Schilt BF, Helper DJ, et al: Diastolic collapse of the right ventricle with cardiac tamponade. An echocardiographic study. *Circulation* 65:1491, 1982.

Chandraratna PA, Aronow WS: Detection of pericardial metastases by cross-sectional echocardiography. *Circulation* 63:197, 1981.

Culliford AT, Lipton M, Spencer FC: Operation for chronic constrictive pericarditis: Do the surgical approach and degree of pericardial resection influence the outcome significantly? *Ann Thorac Surg* 29:146, 1980.

Felner JM: Pericardial disease. In: Hurst JW, ed. *The Heart*. New York: McGraw-Hill; 1978, p.473.

Feigenbaum H: Pericardial disease. In: Feigenbaum H, ed. *Echocardiography*. Philadelphia: Lea and Febiger; 1976, p. 419, and 1986, p. 548.

Fowler NO: The significance of echocardiographic-Doppler studies in cardiac tamponade. *J Am Coll Cardiol* 11:1031, 1988.

Fowler NO: The recognition and management of pericardial disease. In: Hurst JW, ed. *The Heart*. New York: McGraw-Hill; 1978; p. 1640.

Fowler NO: Pericardial diseases. In: Fowler NO, ed. *Cardiac Diagnosis and Treatment*. New York: Harper & Row; 1980, p. 976.

Hancock EW: Cardiac tamponade. *Med Clin North Am* 63:223, 1979.

Hancock EW: Subacute effusive-constrictive pericarditis. *Circulation* 43:183, 1971.

Hancock EW: On the elastic and rigid forms of constrictive pericarditis. *Am Heart J* 100:917, 1980.

Hatle LK, Appleton CP, Popp RL: Differentiation of restrictive cardiomyopathy by Doppler echocardiography. *Circulation* 79:357, 1989.

Kamar S, Lesch M: Pericarditis in renal disease. *Prog Cardiovasc Dis* 22:357,1980.

Kerber RE, Gascho JA, Litchfield R, et al: Hemodynamic effects of volume expansion and nitroprusside compared with pericardiocentesis in patients with acute cardiac tamponade. *N Engl J Med* 307:929, 1982.

Kessler KM, Rodriguez D, Rahim A, et al: Echocardiographic observations regarding pericardial effusions associated with cardiac disease. *Chest* 78;736, 1980.

Kirkorian JG, Hancock EW: Pericardiocentesis. *Am J Med* 65:808, 1978.

Lewis BS: Real time two-dimensional echocardiography in constrictive pericarditis. *Am J Cardiol* 49:1789, 1982.

Lorell B, Leinbach RC, Pohost GM, et al: Right ventricular infarction: Clinical diagnosis and differentiation from cardiac tamponade and pericardial constriction. *Am J Cardiol* 43:465, 1979.

Martins JB, Manuel WJ, Marcus ML: Comparative effects of catecholamines in cardiac tamponade: Experimental and clinical studies. *Am J Cardiol* 46:59, 1980.

Popli S, Ing TS, Daugirdas JT, et al: Treatment of uremic pericardial effusion by local steroid instillation via subxiphoid pericardiotomy. *J Dial* 4:83, 1980.

Posner MR, Cohen GI, Skarin AT: Pericardial disease in patients with cancer: The differentiation of malignant from idiopathic and radiation-induced pericarditis. *Am J Med* 71:407, 1981.

Shabetai R: The pericardium: An essay on some recent developments. *Am J Cardiol* 42:1036, 1978.

Spodick DH: The normal and diseased pericardium: Current concepts of pericardial physiology, diagnosis and treatment. *J Am Coll Cardiol* 1:240, 1983.

Tavel ME: The jugular pulse tracing: Its clinical application. In: Tavel ME, ed. *Clinical Phonocardiography and External Pulse Recording*, 3rd ed. Chicago: Year Book Medical Publishers; 1978, p. 250.

Tyberg TI, Goodyear AV, Langon RA: Genesis of pericardial knock in constrictive pericarditis. *Am J Cardiol* 46:570, 1980.

Walsh TJ, Baughman KL, Gardner TJ, et al: Constrictive epicarditis as a cause of delayed or absent response to pericardiectomy: A clinicopathological study. *J Thorac Cardiovasc Surg* 83:126, 1982.

Wong B, Murphy J, Chang EJ, et al: The risk of pericardiocentesis. *Am J Cardiol* 44:1110, 1979.

25 Infective Endocarditis

CHAPTER

Leonard S. Lilly

Infections of the heart valves and endocardium remain an important cause of cardiovascular morbidity and mortality despite increased clinical awareness and potent antibiotic therapies. Although endocarditis may develop in otherwise normal hearts, it is more likely to occur when previous cardiac structural abnormalities exist, and may present as an indolent "subacute" form (SBE) or as a more fulminant "acute" syndrome (ABE) depending on the invasiveness of the associated organism.

ETIOLOGY

Many bacterial species have been implicated in infective endocarditis; however, streptococcal and staphylococcal species account for more than 80% of infections on native valves (Table 1). The organisms that cause SBE, primarily streptococcal species found within the body's normal flora, tend to be of low invasiveness, generally establishing infection only when previous cardiac structural abnormalities are present. More aggressive organisms, responsible for the fulminant ABE, often infect healthy cardiac valves; such bacteria are not generally part of the normal flora, and include *Staph aureus, Neisseria gonorrhoeae*, gram-negative bacilli, and fungal species. These agents, which most commonly afflict hospitalized patients and intravenous drug addicts, gain access to the circulation through diverse sites, including the oral cavity and respiratory tract, the gastrointestinal and genitourinary systems, skin infections and burns, or via indwelling intravenous catheters.

PATHOGENESIS

SBE develops in the setting of an underlying cardiovascular structural abnormality (Table 2A), in which a pressure gradient between two cardiac chambers generates turbulent blood flow, which disturbs the surface of the abnormal valve or adjacent endocardium within the lower pressure chamber; a sterile platelet-fibrin thrombus then forms at the site of the endothelial disturbance. Subsequent infection develops when a transient bacteremia delivers the offending infectious agent to the sterile platelet-fibrin mesh, where adhesion and multiplication of organisms leads to vegetation formation. Cardiac lesions that do not generate pressure gradients and turbulent blood flow do not predispose to SBE (Table 2B).

The pathogenesis of the ABE is less complex, in that the organisms involved are highly invasive. Upon gaining access to the circulation, they are required in only small numbers to adhere to endocardium and incite infection, even upon previously healthy cardiac structures.

CLINICAL FEATURES

The presentation of SBE is often subtle: low-grade fever, accompanied by nonspecific malaise, anorexia and weight loss, generalized weakness, headache, monoarticular arthralgias, and myalgias. A careful history may reveal the portal of bacterial entry, such as recent dental work. The symptoms may mimic an upper respiratory tract infection, and if oral antibiotics are mistakenly prescribed, later blood cultures may be rendered falsely negative. Although these generalized symptoms may last for months, the diagnosis is usually suspected sufficiently early that "classic" cutaneous and ocular features of endocarditis (Table 3) only occasionally develop.

The onset of ABE is more explosive: sudden illness is heralded by rigors and high fever, sometimes in association with widely disseminated metastatic infections involving multiple organ systems, especially if *Staph aureus* is involved.

Table 1. Etiologies of Infective Endocarditis

Organism	Frequency (%)
Streptococci	50
Staphylococci	25-35
Gram-negative bacilli	7
"Culture-negative"	5-15
Fungi, rickettsia, chlamydia and uncommon bacteria	5

Heart murmurs are found in more than 90% of patients with SBE, usually reflecting the predisposing valvular lesion. In ABE, murmurs on presentation are less common but may develop if valvular destruction ensues. Other common physical findings in both forms of endocarditis include pallor, splenomegaly, and, if congestive heart failure has developed, pulmonary rales and an S_3 on cardiac examination.

Particularly in ABE, fragments of valvular vegetation may dislodge and embolize, most commonly to the brain, kidneys, spleen, mesentery and coronary arteries, with subsequent metastatic infection or infarction of the involved organ. Large emboli, especially in association with fungal endocarditis, may lodge in major arterial branches and result in the sudden loss of a peripheral pulse. Septic pulmonary emboli may result from right-sided heart valve endocarditis, particularly common in intravenous drug abusers (see following).

One third of patients manifest neurologic complications during the course of endocarditis, including headache, confusion, and seizures. Focal neurologic abnormalities, such as hemiplegia or hemisensory loss, may result from cerebral emboli and may be the initial presentation of endocarditis. Particularly in ABE, pyogenic organisms may lead to brain abscess formation or purulent meningitis. Intracerebral "mycotic" aneurysms develop from immune complex deposition within the arterial wall, or secondary to embolic occlusion of the vasa vasorum, and should be suspected in a patient with endocarditis who describes severe localized headache; intracerebral or subarachnoid hemorrhage may follow.

Potentially lethal cardiac complications may punctuate the course of both SBE and ABE. Local extension of infection may disrupt the valve leaflets, chordae tendineae, or supporting structures, resulting in progressive valvular regurgitation and congestive heart

Table 2A. Cardiac Conditions Predisposing to Endocarditis

Rheumatic valvular disease

Other acquired valvular lesions
    Calcific aortic stenosis
    Aortic regurgitation
    Mitral regurgitation
    Mitral valve prolapse (if murmur detected, or more than "trace" mitral regurgitation by Doppler)

Hypertrophic obstructive cardiomyopathy ("IHSS")

Congenital heart disease, including:
    Ventricular septal defect
    Patent ductus arteriosus
    Tetralogy of Fallot
    Aortic coarctation
    Bicuspid aortic valve
    Pulmonic stenosis

Surgically implanted intravascular hardware, including:
    Prosthetic heart valves
    Pulmonary-systemic vascular shunts
    Ventriculo-atrial shunts for hydrocephalus

Previous episode of endocarditis

Table 2B. Cardiac Conditions Not Predisposing to Endocarditis

Isolated ostium secundum atrial septal defect

Previous coronary artery bypass graft surgery

More than six months following:
    Ligation and division of patent ductus arteriosus
    Surgical repair of atrial septal defect, without prosthetic patch

failure, the major cause of death in endocarditis. Myocardial abscess formation may extend into the cardiac conduction tissues with resulting AV nodal or ventricular conduction blocks and arrhythmias. A myocardial abscess may rupture through the interventricular septum or into the pericardial sac with resulting cardiac tamponade. In addition, in cases of aortic valve endocarditis, mycotic aneurysms at the sinuses of Valsalva may rupture into the right ventricle or right atrium, creating an acute left-to-right shunt.

Table 3. Cutaneous and Ocular Findings in Endocarditis (now uncommon)

Petechiae	Located in conjunctivae, oral cavity, skin
Subungual hemorrhages	Linear splinter-like lesions that do not extend to the distal nail bed
Osler's nodes	Erythematous, painful nodules in pulp spaces of terminal phalanges, thenar and hypothenar eminences
Janeway lesions	Erythematous, nontender macules on palms and soles
Roth's spots	White retinal dots surrounded by hemorrhage

INFECTIVE ENDOCARDITIS IN INTRAVENOUS DRUG ABUSERS

Bacteremia in IV drug addicts results from cellulitis at an IV injection site or from microbial contamination of the injected material. More than 50% of cases of endocarditis in this population are due to *Staph aureus*; other commonly involved organisms include *Candida* species and gram-negative rods, including *Pseudomonas* and *Serratia* species. Unlike the general population, streptococcal infections account for less than 20% of endocarditis infections in this group. The majority of endocarditis lesions in IV drug abusers develop at previously normal intracardiac sites, and the clinical presentation is that of an acute fulminant infection. Metastatic abscess formation is common, due to the pyogenic organisms involved. Tricuspid valve endocarditis, which afflicts 50–60% of this group of patients, commonly results in septic pulmonary emboli, reflected by multiple patchy infiltrates on chest x-ray.

PROSTHETIC VALVE ENDOCARDITIS

After heart valve replacement, 3% of patients develop endocarditis in the first postoperative year; infections occur with equal frequency in mechanical and biological prostheses. Within the first two months after surgery, valvular infection generally results from intraoperative contamination or bacterial seeding from pneumonia, urinary tract infection, or mediastinitis. The predominant organism involved is *Staph epidermidis*, and there is a high frequency of *Staph aureus*, gram-negative rods, diphtheroids, and fungal species. A late form of prosthetic endocarditis, which arises after the first several postoperative months, generally involves the same organisms responsible for endocarditis on native valves, except that *Staph epider-*

midis is again unusually common, accounting for more than 20% of such infections.

Unlike infections of native heart valves, which usually remain confined to the leaflets, endocarditis of prosthetic valves frequently extends into perivalvular structures and causes detachment of the sewing ring, paravalvular regurgitation, and congestive heart failure. Local abscess formation at the valve ring occurs in approximately 40% of prosthetic valvular infections; this may be detected by progressive abnormalities of AV nodal or ventricular conduction as seen on the electrocardiogram. Less commonly, valvular stenosis may result from vegetation encroachment on the prosthetic orifice.

LABORATORY FINDINGS

The diagnosis of endocarditis is confirmed, and appropriate antibiotic therapy selected, by demonstration of the responsible organism by blood culture. As bacteremia is continuous in endocarditis, if a single blood culture demonstrates the organism, all are likely to be positive. To minimize confusion by contaminants, at least three sets of blood cultures should be drawn before initiating antibiotics. In SBE, in which immediate therapy is not as crucial as in ABE, blood cultures can be obtained over a period of 12–24 hours. In suspected ABE, however, therapy must not be delayed, and all blood culture sets should be drawn immediately from separate venous sites, followed by initiation of empiric antibiotic therapy. Aerobic and anaerobic cultures should be held for three weeks to insure identification of slowly growing organisms.

Approximately 10% of patients with infective endocarditis have negative blood cultures, and the diagnosis rests on clinical and/or echocardiographic findings as well as the response to empiric therapy. Causes of negative blood cultures include recent antibiotic therapy (within two weeks of blood cultures), fastidious growth requirements (especially *Legionella, Brucella, Hemophilus, Chlamydia, Rickettsia* and fungal organisms), and technical difficulties, such as inappropriate incubation. Antibiotic removal binding resins should be used to aid organism growth in patients on recent antibiotic treatment. Serologic tests can help identify endocarditis due to *Chlamydia, Brucella* and *Legionella* species.

Other laboratory abnormalities are often detected. Normochromic normocytic anemia is common, particularly in SBE. The white blood cell count may be normal in SBE, but is usually elevated in ABE with a shift towards less mature forms. The erythrocyte sedimentation rate is elevated unless congestive heart failure coexists. Nonspecific immunoglobulin abnormalities are often detected, including the presence of rheumatoid factor in 25–50% of patients, and circulating immune complexes in 90%. The latter has been implicated as a cause of arthralgias, skin lesions and acute glomerulonephritis. Microscopic hematuria and proteinuria have been reported in up to 50% of patients due to glomerulonephritis, renal emboli, or metastatic renal abscess.

Echocardiography is helpful but overemphasized in the diagnosis of endocarditis; the sensitivity of this technique is approximately 80%, so that a normal study does not exclude the diagnosis. Echocardiography is more useful in documenting the *complications* of endocarditis: flail valvular leaflets, ruptured chordae tendineae, acute valvular regurgitation, and evidence of perivalvular myocardial abscess. The size of vegetations can be measured, which in some studies has correlated with the development of future embolic events or progressive CHF. Prosthetic valvular vegetations may be visualized by echocardiography if they are large, but small lesions may be obscured by the mechanical prosthetic echoes. Standard or transesophageal pulsed and color flow Doppler recordings, in conjunction with echocardiography, have become valuable for the identification and quantification of regurgitant valvular lesions, and to assess valvular stenosis due to orifice encroachment by vegetations (see Chapter 7 and Chapter 8).

THERAPY

Before the antibiotic era, infective endocarditis was almost always fatal. Antimicrobial and surgical therapies have greatly reduced mortality, but to achieve a cure, appropriate intravenous therapy must be administered in high dosage for prolonged periods, usually four to six weeks, in order to eradicate microorganisms deep within the vegetation which are protected from normal host defenses. Bactericidal antibiotics must be used, and although dosages have not been standardized, Table 4 lists a compilation of currently recommended regimens.

The initiation of antibiotic therapy in suspected SBE can generally await blood culture results. However, in ABE, early appropriate therapy is crucial to prevent life-threatening complications; while awaiting cultures, a gram stain of the peripheral blood buffy coat smear may help identify the responsible organism. If the patient is an intravenous drug abuser, or if there is a strong suspicion of staphylococcal sepsis, a penicillinase-resistant penicillin or cephalosporin should be used (Table 4). If urinary or gastrointestinal sepsis is suspected, initial antibiotics should cover gram-negative bacilli. When the suspected infecting organism remains occult, an empiric regimen of IV ampicillin (2 g q4h), nafcillin (2 g q4h) and gentamicin (1.5 mg/kg q8h) is recommended until blood culture results become known. Once the responsible organism has been identified and sensitivities determined, the antibiotic dosage should be adjusted such that a 1:8 dilution of the patient's serum, drawn just prior to a dosage of antibiotic, is bactericidal for the infecting organism in culture.

With the exception of enterococci, most streptococcal species are exquisitely sensitive to penicillin. For patients who have previously suffered penicillin-induced anaphylaxis or hives, vancomycin should be used. For low-grade, delayed, or uncertain penicillin allergy, cephalosporins may be used cautiously. As *Strep bovis* bacteremia is often associated with malignancies of the gastrointestinal tract, its presence should prompt GI investigation.

An increasingly common cause of endocarditis, *Staph epidermidis*, is often difficult to eradicate, particularly on prosthetic valves; vancomycin is the preferred therapy (with the addition of rifampin and gentamicin in the case of prosthetic valve infection).

Antimicrobial therapy of fungal endocarditis yields generally disappointing results, especially if the infection is associated with prosthetic valves. Amphotericin B is the most potent antifungicidal agent, but is poorly tolerated due to toxicity to the kidney and bone marrow. Flucytosine, an oral fungistatic drug, may be useful in addition to amphotericin B when

Table 4. Antibiotic Therapy for Most Common Forms of Endocarditis

Organism	Therapy	Alternate Therapy	Duration (weeks)
Viridans streptococci Non-enterococcal group D strep	Penicillin G 20 million U/ day (divided into q4h dosage)	Vancomycin 15 mg/kg IV q12h or Cefazolin 2 g IV q8h	4
Enterococci	Penicillin G 20 million U/ day (divided into q4h dosage) plus Gentamicin 1 mg/kg IV q8h	Vancomycin 15 mg/kg IV q12h plus Gentamicin 1 mg/kg IV q8h	4-6
Staph aureus Methicillin-sensitive	Oxacillin or nafcillin 2 g IV q4h	Vancomycin 15 mg/kg IV q12h or Cefazolin 2 g IV q8h	4-6
Staph aureus Methicillin-resistant	Vancomycin 15 mg/kg IV q12h		4-6
Staph epidermidis Methicillin-sensitive	Oxacillin or nafcillin 2 g IV q4h	Vancomycin 15 mg/kg IV q12h or Cefazolin 2 g IV q8h	4-6
Staph epidermidis Methicillin-resistant Native valve Prosthetic valve	Vancomycin 7.5 mg IV q6h Vancomycin 7.5 mg IV q6h plus Rifampin 300 mg po q8h plus Gentamicin 1 mg/kg IV q8H for first 2 weeks		4-6 6

the organism has demonstrated sensitivity. However, bulky vegetations often form, with local myocardial invasion and peripheral embolization to large arteries, requiring early surgical removal of the infected valve.

Absolute indications for surgical intervention and valvular replacement in endocarditis include: ① progressive or refractory congestive heart failure due to valvular dysfunction; ② persistent bacteremia after several days of antibiotic therapy; ③ recurrent major peripheral emboli, with vegetation visualized on echocardiogram; ④ myocardial abscess formation, suggested by otherwise unexplained ECG conduction defects, or by echocardiography; ⑤ ruptured sinus of Valsalva aneurysm; and ⑥ fungal endocarditis.

The response of prosthetic valve endocarditis to antibiotic therapy is often poor, especially if non-streptococcal species are involved. The overall mortality rate is 30–60%, and is least favorable in the group with "early" prosthetic involvement. Surgical replacement of the infected prosthesis should be done

Table 5. Procedures Warranting Endocarditis Prophylaxis

Dental manipulations that produce gingival bleeding

Rigid bronchoscopy and surgery of the upper respiratory tract

Genitourinary procedures, including:
Indwelling bladder catheter
Cystoscopy
Prostatectomy
Vaginal delivery (if peripartum infection present)

Gastrointestinal surgery, including cholecystectomy

moval of the infected prosthesis. Anticoagulation therapy should be continued in patients with mechanical prostheses; however, there is a risk of intracranial bleeding if cerebral embolization or mycotic aneurysm rupture should ensue. Therefore, the prothrombin time should be kept at approximately 1.5 times control.

The importance of daily examination of the patient with endocarditis for new heart murmurs, evidence of heart failure or peripheral emboli, and frequent electrocardiograms to identify conduction disturbances, cannot be overemphasized.

PROPHYLAXIS

Patients with a predisposition to endocarditis (Table 2A) should receive prophylactic antibiotic therapy for "dirty" procedures likely to result in substantial bacteremias, examples of which are listed in Table 5. The prophylactic antibiotic regimens recommended by the American Heart Association are listed in Table 6; these will likely be updated soon to recommend more simple oral regimens for low-risk patients undergoing minor procedures. The following proce-

on an emergent basis if progressive congestive heart failure is demonstrated, or systemic embolization or continued bacteremia is observed despite antibiotic therapy. Ideally, surgical replacement should be preceded by at least several days of antibiotics, which should then be continued for a full course after re-

Table 6. Recommendations for Endocarditis Prophylaxis

Type of Procedure	Therapy	Alternate (penicillin allergy)
Dental or upper respiratory tract	Oral: Penicillin V 2 g 1 hr before procedure; 1 g 6 hr later Parenteral: Penicillin G 2 million U IV or IM 30-60 min before procedure; 1 million U 6 hr later Maximal protection (prosthetic valves): Ampicillin 1-2 g IV/IM plus gentamicin 1.5 mg/kg IV/IM 30 min before procedure; eight hours later, repeat this regimen, or use penicillin V 1 g po 6 hr later	Oral: Erythromycin 1 g 1 hr before procedure; 500 mg 6 hr later Parenteral: Vancomycin 1 g IV over 1 hr before procedure; repeat dosage not necessary
Gastrointestinal and genitourinary	Ampicillin 2 g IV/IM plus gentamicin 1.5 mg/kg IV/IM 30-60 min before procedure; repeat once, 8 hr later Low-risk procedures (see text): Amoxicillin 3 g po 1 hr before procedure; 1.5 g po 6 hr later	Vancomycin 1 g IV over 1 hr plus gentamicin 1.5 mg/kg IV/IM 30-60 min before procedure; repeat once, 8 hr later

dures generally do not require antibiotic prophylaxis unless a prosthetic valve is present: uncomplicated vaginal delivery (if there is no evidence of pelvic infection), D&C of the uterus, "in and out" bladder catheterization with sterile urine, barium enema, sigmoidoscopy, fiberoptic gastroscopy without biopsy, percutaneous liver biopsy, and diagnostic cardiac catheterization.

The diagnosis and therapy of bacterial endocarditis remain substantial challenges warranting a high degree of clinical suspicion and vigilant attention to the patient in order to prevent life-threatening complications and to effect a cure.

Bibliography

Alsip SG, Blackstone EH, and Kirklin JW: Indications for cardiac surgery in patients with active endocarditis. *Am J Med* 78(6B):138, 1985.

Bayer AS: Staphylococcal bacteremia and endocarditis. State of the art. *Arch Int Med* 142:1169, 1982.

Brandenburg, RO, Giuliani ER, Wilson WR, et al: Infective endocarditis—a 25-year overview of diagnosis and therapy. *J Am Coll Cardiol* 1:280, 1983.

Buda AJ, Zotz RJ, LeMire MS, et al: Prognostic significance of vegetations detected by two-dimensional echocardiography in infective endocarditis. *Am Heart J* 112:1291, 1986.

Calderwood SB, Swinski LA, Karchmer AW, et al: Prosthetic valve endocarditis: Analysis of factors affecting outcome of therapy. *J Thorac Cardiovasc Surg* 92:776, 1986.

Cowgill LD, Addonizio VP, Hopeman AR, et al: Prosthetic valve endocarditis. *Current Probl Cardiol* 11:618, 1986.

Durack DT: Current issues in prevention of infective endocarditis. *Am J Med* 78:149, 1985.

Hickey SW, Wilcken DEL: Mitral valve prolapse and bacterial endocarditis: When is antibiotic prophylaxis necessary? *Am Heart J* 109:431, 1985.

Ivert TSA, Dismukes WE, Cobbs CG, et al: Prosthetic valve endocarditis. *Circulation* 69:223, 1984.

Karchmer AW, Archer GL, and Dismukes WE: Staphylococcus epidermidis causing prosthetic valve endocarditis: Microbiologic and clinical observations as guides to therapy. *Ann Intern Med* 98:447, 1984.

Kaye D: Prophylaxis for infective endocarditis: An update. *Ann Intern Med* 104:419, 1986.

Klein RS, Recco RA, Catalano MT, et al: Association of Streptococcus bovis with carcinoma of the colon. *N Engl J Med* 297:800, 1977.

O'Brien JT, Geiser EA: Infective endocarditis and echocardiography. *Am Heart J* 108:386, 1984.

Schulman ST et al: Prevention of bacterial endocarditis: A statement for health professionals by the Committee on Rheumatic Fever and Infective Endocarditis of the Council on Cardiovascular Disease in the Young. *Circulation* 70:1123A, 1984.

Van Scoy RE: Culture-negative endocarditis. *Mayo Clin Proc* 57:149, 1982.

Weinstein L, Schlesinger JJ: Pathoanatomic, pathophysiologic and clinical correlations in endocarditis. *N Engl J Med* 291:832, 1122, 1974.

CHAPTER 26

Cardiac Tumors

Robert A. Kloner

PRIMARY CARDIAC TUMORS

The incidence of primary cardiac tumors is quite low (less than 0.002% to 0.28% of the general population). Approximately 75% of all primary cardiac tumors are histologically benign; the most common are myxomas, followed by lipomas, papillary fibroelastomas, rhabdomyomas, and fibromas. Twenty-five percent of primary cardiac tumors are malignant, the most common being rhabdomyosarcomas and angiosarcomas.

BENIGN PRIMARY TUMORS

Left Atrial Myxomas

Myxomas are the most common primary tumor of the heart and account for 30–50% of all cardiac tumors. Although there has been some debate in the past as to whether these tumors actually represent neoplasms or just well-organized thrombi, studies in which tissue from myxomas was grown in culture showed that the cells had neoplastic properties. These tumors in general are considered benign, but occasionally exhibit malignant behavior. Myxomas tend to arise in the atria—in the left atrium three to four times more often than in the right atrium. Occasionally they are multiple and arise in several cardiac chambers. A small percentage of patients with cardiac myxomas have a complex of features including pituitary adenomas with gigantism or acromegaly, myxoid fibroadenoma of the breast, testicular tumors, and primary pigmented nodular adrenocortical disease with or without Cushing's syndrome. It is important to identify this group of patients since they tend to have cardiac myxomas at a young age, a familial occurrence, and an increased incidence of multiple and recurrent cardiac myxomas.

Left atrial myxomas typically are pedunculated and mobile and prolapse through the mitral valve orifice, resulting in obstruction to flow through the valve, or mitral regurgitation. The symptoms, due to the obstruction and regurgitation, may mimic those of rheumatic mitral valve disease and include dyspnea, orthopnea, paroxysmal nocturnal dyspnea, fatigue, cough, chest pain, and occasionally syncope. If the tumor becomes lodged in the mitral orifice, acute circulatory failure may occur. Unlike mitral stenosis, the onset of these symptoms is often sudden and may vary with the position of the patient; atrial fibrillation is not common. Tumor emboli are common with atrial myxomas (20–45% of patients with myxoma) due to their friability and intracavitary location. Left atrial myxomas result in systemic emboli, while right atrial myxomas cause pulmonary emboli and pulmonary hypertension. If the emboli affect a peripheral vessel, a histologic diagnosis of myxoma can be made by recovering the systemic embolic material. Systemic symptoms may occur in patients with myxoma; these include fever, weight loss, general malaise, arthralgia, and pallor. It has been postulated that these symptoms result from an immunologic mechanism, from products secreted by the tumor, or tumor necrosis. These systemic symptoms plus those of embolization may mimic endocarditis. The presence of splenomegaly favors endocarditis rather than myxoma.

The physical examination of patients with left atrial myxoma reveals a loud S_1 and S_4, and an early diastolic sound called a "tumor plop," which occurs when the tumor strikes the endocardial wall or when its motion is suddenly halted. This tumor plop usually occurs later and is lower in frequency than an opening snap; it occurs earlier and is higher in frequency than an S_3. A low-pitched diastolic rumble due to obstruction of flow through the mitral orifice may mimic the murmur of rheumatic mitral stenosis; a holosystolic murmur at the apex due to mitral regurgitation has also been described. These murmurs typically vary in intensity with the patient's position. Friction rubs due to contact of the tumor with the atrial and ventricular endocardium are occasionally present.

Examination of the lungs may reveal rales due to pulmonary congestion, and examination of the extremities may show clubbing. Laboratory studies usually demonstrate anemia, elevated sedimentation rate, hypergammaglobulinemia, leukocytosis, thrombocytosis, or thrombocytopenia. Chest x-ray findings in patients with left atrial myxoma include an enlarged left atrium, pulmonary congestion, and, in 10% of cases, calcification within the intracardiac tumor (see Chapter 4). The electrocardiogram may show atrial arrhythmias (atrial fibrillation or flutter), right ventricular hypertrophy, and abnormal p-waves. Two-dimensional echocardiography has been extremely useful for assessing the presence of cardiac tumors. It is superior to M-mode echocardiography for visualization of all cardiac chambers and assessment of size, shape and attachment sites of the myxoma. Left atrial myxomas can be visualized as a mass of echoes in the left atrium during systole. Since myxomas are commonly pedunculated, they prolapse into the left ventricle during diastole, resulting in a mass of echoes behind the anterior leaflet of the mitral valve (see Chapter 7).

Radionuclide imaging of the tumors by gated blood pool scanning (resulting in a filling defect), computer-assisted tomography, and magnetic resonance imaging is helpful if the echocardiogram is nondiagnostic. Cardiac catheterization should be considered if noninvasive evaluation is not adequate to visualize tumor location and all cardiac chambers, if malignant cardiac tumor is suspected, or if coexisting cardiac disease might affect the surgical procedure. Angiography (performed by filming the levo-phase of a pulmonary arteriogram, in order to avoid dislodging tumor fragments) reveals a mobile left atrial filling defect which may prolapse into the left ventricle during diastole. An atrial ball-valve thrombus may look like a myxoma on angiography, but is usually associated with thrombus in the atrial appendage.

There have been cases of left atrial myxoma associated with arterial aneurysms demonstrating intraluminal tumor, consistent with tumor emboli and peripheral tumor growth. Even after resection of the primary myxoma, benign myxomatous emboli may continue to grow in the periphery (also documented in brain and bone), simulating malignant behavior.

Right Atrial Myxomas

Right atrial myxomas produce symptoms of right-sided heart failure including peripheral edema, fatigue, ascites, and abdominal discomfort due to obstruction of tricuspid valve flow or tricuspid regurgitation. Tricuspid regurgitation is due to actual valve trauma from the tumor or interference with normal tricuspid closure. Cyanosis, dizziness, and syncope may be related to body position. Tumor emboli to the pulmonary arteries may result in pulmonary hypertension. Physical examination reveals jugular venous distension with a prominent a-wave in the jugular venous pulse, hepatomegaly, ascites, peripheral edema, and the murmurs of tricuspid stenosis or tricuspid regurgitation. Friction rubs, clubbing, cyanosis, and signs of superior vena caval obstruction may be present. These findings often mimic those of constrictive pericarditis, rheumatic tricuspid disease, Ebstein's anomaly, and right-sided endocarditis. Typical laboratory abnormalities include elevated sedimentation rate, leukocytosis, and hypergammaglobulinemia. If a right-to-left shunt has developed through a patent foramen ovale due to elevated right atrial pressure, polycythemia may occur. ECG abnormalities include large p-waves, low voltage, and right bundle branch block; chest x-ray may show right atrial enlargement and intracardiac tumor calcification. The right atrial tumor may be visualized by echocardiography and angiography; superior vena caval injection is suggested for angiography in order to avoid tumor dislodgement.

The treatment of both left and right atrial myxomas is surgical excision. Complete cure has been documented in long-term follow-up. Recurrence or development of a second cardiac myxoma occurs in about 1–5% of cases. Many surgeons prefer wide resection of the atrial septum surrounding the attachment of the tumor because recurrence is possible if resection is incomplete. This may necessitate repair of an atrial defect with a Dacron patch.

Rhabdomyomas

These tumors are found mainly in infants and children. They involve the ventricular walls, affecting right and left sides equally. Rhabdomyomas are not true neoplasms but represent hamartomas, and their histology is characterized by a lack of mitotic figures and glycogen-laden immature myocardial cells. Children with rhabdomyomas may have symptoms related to obstruction of a cardiac chamber or valve orifice, may present as stillborn infants or die shortly after birth with severe intracavitary obstruction, or be asymptomatic. Rhabdomyomas commonly occur in association with tuberous sclerosis. Clinical features include symptoms and signs of left- and/or right-sided congestive heart failure, systolic and diastolic murmurs, syncope, cyanosis, and occasionally sudden death. Left-axis deviation, left ventricular hypertrophy, and left bundle branch block may be present on electrocardiography. Treatment is surgical excision.

Fibromas

Fibromas are another benign tumor that most commonly affect infants and children and occur within the ventricular myocardium. Fibromas may be asymptomatic or result in obstruction to intracardiac flow, abnormalities in ventricular contraction, or conduction disturbances. A whorled pattern of intracardiac calcification may be present on chest x-ray.

Lipomas

Lipomas may be located within the subendocardium, subepicardium, or intramural myocardium. They may be asymptomatic or produce atrioventricular (AV) or intraventricular conduction abnormalities and arrhythmias or impair ventricular contraction.

Mesotheliomas

Mesotheliomas occur predominantly in women and tend to be located in the area of the AV node. These slow-growing cystic tumors may result in complete heart block, syncope, and sudden death.

There are a number of benign pericardial tumors, including teratomas and leiomyomas, most of which are asymptomatic.

MALIGNANT PRIMARY TUMORS

Malignant tumors comprise approximately 25% of all primary tumors of the heart and in most cases are sarcomas. The most common of these include angiosarcoma, rhabdomyosarcoma, and fibrosarcoma. The development of these tumors is more common in adults and can involve either atrium or ventricle, but is more common on the right side of the heart. Clinical features include those of progressive right-sided and/or left-sided heart failure, arrhythmias, pericar-

dial effusion, chest pain, and cardiac tamponade. These tumors may be rapidly growing, invading the myocardium, intracardiac chambers and pericardial space, and often they metastasize. They may obstruct either the superior vena cava, resulting in edema of the face and upper extremities, or the inferior vena cava, causing mesenteric, hepatic, and lower extremity edema. Most patients have a progressively downhill course and die within weeks to a few years once symptoms are present.

In general, various forms of radiation therapy, chemotherapy, and surgery are palliative and have failed to alter the poor prognosis of cardiac sarcomas.

METASTATIC TUMORS TO THE HEART

Metastatic tumors to the heart are more common than primary cardiac tumors. Cardiac metastases occur with many types of tumors (carcinomas more commonly than sarcomas). Malignant melanoma involves the heart in more than 50% of cases and cardiac metastases occur in about 33% of cases of bronchogenic carcinoma and carcinoma of the breast. Microscopic cardiac infiltration is present in about half of cases of leukemia and about one sixth of cases of lymphoma, especially reticulum cell sarcoma. Cardiac metastases occur most frequently in patients over the age of 50, with an equal gender incidence. Metastatic tumors to the heart have been described in up to 6% of unselected autopsies and 2–21% of patients dying with malignancy. Cardiac metastases, in general, are encountered with widespread systemic tumor dissemination—only rarely are metastases limited to the heart or pericardium.

Metastatic tumors are believed to reach the heart by hematogenous or lymphatic spread or by direct invasion. Lymphatic spread is particularly frequent with carcinoma of the bronchus and breast. Intracavitary metastatic tumors are disseminated via the great veins. Thus, metastases from carcinoma of the kidney, testis, and thyroid invade the right atrium via the vena cava and may mimic myxoma; metastases from bronchogenic carcinoma may enter the left atrium via the pulmonary veins. Metastases to valvular tissue or the endocardium are unusual, since these structures are avascular. When they do occur, it is probably by direct extension. Endocardial and valve metastases may be polypoid and form emboli mimicking myxomas and endocarditis. They can result in valvular stenosis or regurgitation. Pericardial metastases occur more frequently than myocardial metastases and are common in patients with carcinoma of the breast or lung (by lymphatic spread) or mediastinal lymphoma (by direct extension) and in leukemia by hematogenous spread. Pericardial effusions and tamponade or a constrictive pericarditis may occur. Finally, intramural metastases may be present in either left or right ventricle. Intramural metastases usually do not affect cardiac function in most cases. Myocardial infarction has resulted from metastatic tumor encircling or compressing the epicardial coronary arteries.

Kaposi's sarcoma metastatic to the heart has been described in patients with acquired immunodeficiency syndrome (AIDS). Silver et al. reported five patients with AIDS who had focal deposits of Kaposi's sarcoma at autopsy; in each patient the dermal lesion of Kaposi's sarcoma was the initial manifestation of AIDS. None of the patients had symptoms of cardiac disease, and ECGs were normal. The Kaposi's sarcoma involved the subepicardial adipose tissue adjacent to the coronary arteries, but without evidence of compression of the coronary arteries. However, Steigman et al. recently reported a case of fatal cardiac tamponade due to epicardial Kaposi's sarcoma in a patient with AIDS. In this study, there was also a nodule of Kaposi's sarcoma involving the endocardial surface of a papillary muscle.

Besides Kaposi's sarcoma, primary non-Hodgkin's lymphoma of the heart has been described in patients with AIDS (Guarner et al.). In a report of two cases of cardiac lymphoma in AIDS patients associated with myocardial and pericardial involvement and arrhythmias, the pattern and distribution of tumor suggested *de novo* origin of the lymphoma in the heart (Balasubramanyam et al.).

Cardiac symptoms occur in less than 10% of patients with cardiac metastases proven by autopsy. The metastases usually are not a major factor contributing to the death of the patient. Symptoms depend more on the location than the size of the tumor; for example, metastases from a hypernephroma may infiltrate the AV node, resulting in complete heart block. Metastatic tumor to the heart should be suspected when a patient with metastatic disease develops cardiac dysfunction without apparent cause. Common signs and symptoms include those of pericardial involvement including chest pain, a persistent pericardial rub, evidence of cardiac tamponade or pericardial constriction, and rapid increase of heart size. It is important to distinguish malignant from nonmalignant pericardial involvement, which can coexist in patients

with cancer. Kralstein and Frishman noted that cough, facial swelling, and pericardial tamponade are associated with malignant pericardial disease. Fever, rub, and clinical improvement on nonsteroidal anti-inflammatory agents are more suggestive of idiopathic pericarditis. Other common clinical manifestations of cardiac metastases include development of heart block, arrhythmias, changing cardiac murmurs, evidence of obstruction to the great vein orifices, and intractable and unexplained cardiac failure. This latter feature may be due to lymphatic obstruction by the tumor, with severe myocardial interstitial edema and secondary pressure on the myofibers resulting in cardiac decompensation.

Electrocardiographic abnormalities are common and include ST-T–wave changes, which sometimes mimic myocardial infarction (especially when the cardiac metastases produce necrosis); arrhythmias including supraventricular tachyarrhythmias (especially when the metastases involve the atria); AV block and bundle branch block (due to tumor infiltration of the conducting system); abnormal P waves; and reduced QRS amplitude in cases both with and without pericardial effusion. The arrhythmias often do not respond to digitalis or any other standard therapy. Two-dimensional echocardiography, computer-assisted tomography, and magnetic resonance imaging have been shown to be useful for assessing the presence of cardiac tumors and malignant pericardial involvement. Pericardiocentesis will be needed to treat tamponade but also may be needed to help diagnose malignant infusion. Bloody pericardial fluid with protein content >3 mg/dl and specific gravity >1.016 in the absence of myocardial infarction is suggestive of malignant effusion. Positive cytology may be found in 50–70% of patients. Pericardial biopsy may be needed in cases in which the clinical presentation suggests malignant effusion but in which the pericardial fluid is negative for malignancy.

Rarely, malignant or metastatic cardiac tumors may be amenable to surgery. Palliative radiation therapy and systemic chemotherapy may afford symptomatic relief, but radiation to the chest may produce myocardial fibrosis and damage to the conduction system. Radiation has caused regression of pericardial effusion, but pericardiocentesis is required in cases of tamponade. As noted, the pericardial fluid may then be examined for cytology. Recurrent effusions resulting in tamponade or the presence of pericardial constriction may require pericardiectomy.

Bibliography

Allen DC, Alderdice JM, Morton P, Mollan RAB, Morris TCM Pathology of the heart and conduction system in lymphoma and leukemia. *J Clin Pathol* 40:746, 1987.

Attum AA, Johnson GS, Masri Z, Girardet R, Lansing AM: Malignant clinical behavior of cardiac myxomas and "myxoid imitators." *Ann Thorac Surg* 44:217, 1987.

Balasubramanyam A, Waxman M, Kazal HL, Lee MH. Malignant lymphoma of the heart in acquired immune deficiency syndrome. *Chest* 90:243, 1986.

Bulkley BH, Hutchins GM: Atrial myxomas: A fifty year review. *Am Heart J* 97:639, 1979.

Burday MJ, Lombardi AC. Cardiac tumors. *Am Fam Physician* 37:301, 1988.

Colucci WS, Braunwald E: Primary tumors of the heart. In: Braunwald E ed: *Heart Disease: A Textbook of Cardiovascular Medicine*. Philadelphia: Saunders; 1988, p. 1470–1483.

Come PC, Riley MF, Markis JE, et al: Limitations of echocardiographic techniques in evaluation of left atrial masses. *Am J Cardiol* 48:947, 1981.

Constantino A, West TE, Gupta M, Loghmanee F. Primary cardiac lymphoma in a patient with acquired immune deficiency syndrome. *Cancer* 60:2801, 1987.

Donaldson RM, Emanuel RW, Earl CJ: The role of two-dimensional echocardiography in the detection of potentially embolic intracardiac masses in patients with cerebral ischemia. *J Neurol Neurosurg Psychiatry* 44:803, 1981.

Farah MG: Familial atrial myxoma. *Ann Intern Med* 83:358, 1975.

Fyke FE, Seward JB, Edwards WD, et al: Primary cardiac tumors: Experience with 30 consecutive patients since the introduction of two-dimensional echocardiography. *J Am Coll Cardiol* 5:1465, 1985.

Gill PS, Chandraratna AN, Meyer PR, Levine AM: Malignant lymphoma: Cardiac involvement at mitral presentation. *J Clin Oncol* 5:216, 1987.

Glancy DL, Roberts WC: The heart in malignant melanoma: A study of 70 autopsy cases *Am J Cardiol* 21:255, 1968.

Godwin JD, Axel L, Adams JR, et al: Computed tomography: A new method for diagnosing tumor of the heart. *Circulation* 63:448, 1981.

Goodwin JF: Symposium on cardiac tumors. Introduction: The spectrum of cardiac tumors. *Am J Cardiol* 21:328, 1968.

Guarner J, Brynes RK, Chan WC, Birdsong G, Hertzler G: Primary non-Hodgkins lymphoma of the heart in two patients with acquired immunodeficiency syndrome. *Arch Pathol Lab Med* 111:254, 1987.

Harvey WP: Clinical aspects of cardiac tumors. *Am J Cardiol* 21:328, 1968.

Huggins TJ, Huggins MJ, Schnapf DJ, et al: Left atrial myxoma: Computed tomography as a diagnostic modality. *J Comput Assist Tomogr* 4:253, 1980.

Kralstein J, Frishman W. Malignant pericardial diseases: Diagnosis and treatment. *Am Heart J* 113:785, 1987.

Kutalek SP, Panidis IP, Kother MN, et al: Metastatic tumors of the heart detected by two-dimensional echocardiography. *Am Heart J* 109:343, 1985.

Lappe DL, Bulkley BH, Weiss JL: Two dimensional echocardiographic diagnosis of left atrial myxoma. *Chest* 74:55, 1978.

Larrieu AJ, Jamieson WR, Tyers GF: Primary cardiac tumors: Experience with 25 cases. *J Thorac Cardiovasc Surg* 83:339, 1982.

Lubell DL, Goldfarb CR: Metastatic cardiac tumor demonstrated by 201 thallium scan. *Chest* 78:98, 1980.

Markel ML, Waller BF, Armstrong WF. Cardiac myxoma: A review. *Medicine* 66:114, 1987.

McAllister HA Jr: Primary tumors and cysts of the heart and pericardium. In: Harvey WP, ed: *Current Problems in Cardiology*, 1979.

McCarthy PM, Piehler JM, Schaff HV, et al: The significance of multiple, recurrent, and "complex" cardiac myxoma. *Thorac Cardiovasc Surg* 91:389, 1986.

O'Dea D, Kay R, Blake J, et al: Electrocardiographic pseudo-myocardial infarct pattern in malignant cardiac disease. *Cancer* 63:958, 1989.

Panidis IP, Kotler MN, Mintz GS, Ross J: Clinical and echocardiographic features of right atrial masses. *Am Heart J* 107:745, 1984.

Parmley LF, Salley RK, Williams JP, Head GB: The clinical spectrum of cardiac fibroma with diagnostic and surgical considerations: Noninvasive imaging enhances management. *Ann Thorac Surg* 45:455, 1988.

Pizzarello RA, Goldberg SM, Goldman MA, et al: Tumor of the heart diagnosed by magnetic resonance imaging. *J Am Coll Cardiol* 5:989, 1985.

Pohost GM, Pastore JO, McKusick KA, et al: Detection of left atrial myxoma by gated radionuclide cardiac imaging. *Circulation* 55:88, 1977.

Poole GV, Meredith JW, Breyer RH, Mills SA: Surgical implications in malignant cardiac disease *Ann Thorac Surg* 36:484, 1983.

Roberts WC, Bodey GP, Wentlake PT: The heart in acute leukemia: A study of 420 autopsy cases. *Am J Cardiol* 21:388, 1968.

Seibert KA, Rettenmier CW, Waller BF, et al: Osteogenic sarcoma metastatic to the heart. *Am J Med* 73:136, 1982.

Selzer A, Sakai FJ, Popper RW: Protean clinical manifestations of primary tumors of the heart. *Am J Med* 59:9, 1972.

Silver MA, Macher AM, Reichert CM, et al: Cardiac involvement by Kaposi's sarcoma in acquired immune deficiency syndrome (AIDS). *Am J Cardiol* 53:983, 1984.

St. John Sutton MG, Mercier LA, Giuliani ER, et al: Atrial myxomas: A review of clinical experience in 40 patients. *Mayo Clinic Proc* 55:371, 1980.

Steigman CK, Anderson DW, Macher AM, Sennesh JD, Virmani R: Fatal cardiac tamponade in acquired immunodeficiency syndrome with epicardial Kaposi's sarcoma. *Am Heart J* 116:1105, 1988.

Tway KP, Shah AA, Rahimtoola SH: Multiple bilateral myxomas demonstrated by two-dimensional echocardiography. *Am J Med* 71:896, 1981.

Vidaillet HJ Jr., Seward JB, Fyke FE, Su WPD, Tajik HJ: "Syndrome myxoma": A subset of patients with cardiac myxoma associated with pigmented skin lesions and peripheral and endocrine neoplasm. *Br Heart J* 57:247, 1987.

Weinberg BA, Conces DJ, Waller BF. Cardiac manifestations of noncardiac tumors. Part I. Direct Effects. *Clin Cardiol* 12:289, 1989.

Wolverson MK, Grider RD, Sundaram M, et al: Demonstration of unsuspected malignant disease of the pericardium by computed tomography. *CT* 4:330, 1980.

27

CHAPTER

Evaluation and Management of Hypertension

Allen J. Naftilan
Victor J. Dzau

DEFINITION AND PREVALENCE OF HYPERTENSION

Since systemic arterial pressure fluctuates throughout the day and the blood pressure in the general population falls in a Gaussian distribution, the limits of normal blood pressure cannot be precisely defined. There is no evidence for a threshold level beyond which cardiovascular risk increases precipitously, but numerous clinical trials indicate the levels at which treatment of blood pressure decreases risk. The Joint National Committee on the Detection, Evaluation and Treatment of High Blood Pressure (JNC IV) proposes the levels listed in Table 1.

Data from the National Health and Nutrition Examination Survey (NHANES II) indicate that approximately 58 million Americans are at an increased risk for morbidity and premature death due to high blood pressure (Subcommittee, 1985). The prevalence is higher in blacks than in whites (38% vs. 29%), and

increases with age. According to NHANES II, slightly more than half (53.9%) of all hypertensives are aware that they have high blood pressure. Of these, 60–67% (depending on race, age, and sex) are taking medication. Thus, only 33.1% of all hypertensive patients sampled by the NHANES II study are receiving antihypertensive therapy, and only about half of these patients have their blood pressure adequately controlled.

PHYSIOLOGY

The major determinants of blood pressure are cardiac output and systemic vascular resistance, both of which are controlled by various neurohumoral mechanisms and the kidney. The autonomic nervous system and the renin-angiotensin system are involved in short-term regulation of blood pressure in humans, but the kidney exerts long-term control by regulation of sodium and extracellular fluid volume. Early in the de-

Table 1. Definitions of Hypertension*

Classification	Blood Pressure Levels
Normotension	Systolic <140 mm Hg
	Diastolic <85 mm Hg
High-normal blood pressure	Diastolic = 85–89 mm Hg
Mild hypertension	Diastolic = 90–104 mm Hg
Moderate hypertension	Diastolic = 105–114 mm Hg
Severe hypertension	Diastolic ≥115 mm Hg
Borderline isolated systolic hypertension	Systolic = 140–159 mm Hg
Isolated systolic hypertension	Systolic ≥160 mm Hg

* Classification based on the average of two or more readings on two or more occasions. Based on JNC IV. (See text.)

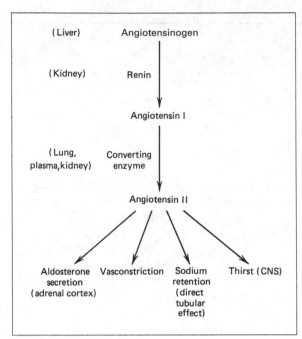

Figure 1. *Schematic of renin-angiotensin-aldosterone system.*

velopment of hypertension, elevated blood pressure can result from any circulatory disturbance that increases cardiac output or total peripheral vascular resistance or both. Initially in essential hypertension, the cardiac output is elevated (Lund-Johansen). Some investigators believe that this increase in cardiac output results in an increase in peripheral resistance, which maintains or even perpetuates the hypertension. Patients with more established long-standing essential hypertension tend to have normal cardiac output and increased peripheral vascular resistance, findings that support this theory (Julius et al.; Korner). In patients with a long history of hypertension, cardiac output may be decreased; in these cases, the increase in blood pressure is entirely the result of an increase in peripheral vascular resistance.

The development of specific pharmacologic inhibitors of the renin-angiotensin system is an important advance in hypertension therapy. Renin is a proteolytic enzyme released by the juxtaglomerular cells in the afferent arterioles of the kidney (Dzau and Pratt) (Figure 1). Renin cleaves its substrate in plasma, angiotensinogen, an α_2-globulin synthesized by the liver. Angiotensin I, a decapeptide that is a product of the renin and angiotensinogen reaction, is physiologically

inactive and is converted to the octapeptide angiotensin II by angiotensin converting enzyme.

Angiotensin II is a potent vasoconstrictor and the primary stimulus for aldosterone secretion from the adrenal cortex. Along with the peripheral renin-angiotensin system, there are locally active renin-angiotensin systems in the kidney, heart and blood vessel wall (Dzau 1986). These local systems may be as important or more important than the peripheral system in several physiologic functions.

The autonomic nervous system may also be important in the initiation and maintenance of hypertension. Patients with hypertension have exaggerated pressor responses to stress, which may be due to abnormal sympathetic and parasympathetic control mechanisms (Jorgensen and Houston; Bianchetti et al.).

EVALUATION OF THE HYPERTENSIVE PATIENT

Evaluation of the hypertensive patient should include a careful history and physical examination as well as screening laboratory tests, with the following goals:

1. Proper documentation of hypertension
2. Assessment of cardiovascular risk factors
3. Search for evidence of end-organ damage
4. Decision regarding when to perform a workup for secondary hypertension

Along with a general physical examination, with particular attention to the cardiovascular and peripheral vascular system (Table 2), the most critical part of the initial evaluation is accurate determination of blood pressure. During the initial visit, blood pressure should be measured in both the supine and upright positions. At least three blood pressure measurements should be taken, at least 5 minutes apart. Proper cuff size is critical. The cuff should be approximately two-thirds the width of the arm, or 15 cm in an average adult. A cuff that is too short can falsely elevate the readings (Linfors et al.; Manning et al.; Frohlich et al.). A rolled sleeve should not constrict the arm, as this can also affect blood pressure. The cuff should be inflated to 20–30 mm Hg above the systolic pressure. The systolic pressure is the point where the Korotkoff sounds are first heard with every heart beat. Usually, the diastolic pressure is best recorded at the level where the heart sounds disappear, Korotkoff phase V (Finnie et al.) In patients with high cardiac output and in children, blood pressure should be measured at the point where the sounds become muffled, Korotkoff phase IV (Frohlich et al.; Finnie et al.).

With few exceptions, blood pressure level should be determined from more than one office visit before deciding on a treatment plan. Home blood pressure recordings are also useful in determining if treatment is necessary. Recently, automatic portable home 24-hour blood pressure monitors have become available (Kleinert et al.; Pickering et al. 1985). Despite this, "casual" blood pressure levels remain important predictors of cardiovascular complications. Indeed, all of the major epidemiologic studies on hypertension and cardiovascular risk use office–casual blood pressure determinations.

Twenty-four-hour blood pressure monitoring is becoming increasingly utilized. The damage caused by hypertension is generally believed to be a function of the time at which the circulation is exposed to elevated pressures; if this is so, ambulatory 24-hour blood pressure monitors may be better than office measurements in assessing the need for antihypertensive treatment. Several prospective studies have correlated 24-hour ambulatory pressures versus casual pressures in the clinic with clinical evidence of target organ damage (Pickering and Devereux; Sokolow et al.). One study of more than 1,000 patients followed for an average of five years showed a significant correlation between ambulatory and office blood pressures, but found that ambulatory pressures were an average of 10-15 mm Hg lower than office pressures (Perloff et al.). Patients who had elevated ambulatory pressures were at greater risk for cardiovascular damage, suggesting that ambulatory measurement may be a good discriminator between high- and low-risk groups within a given level of office blood pressure, especially in mildly hypertensive patients. These and other studies must be further analyzed before the role of ambulatory blood pressure monitoring is clear.

The physical examination should include a careful search for evidence of end-organ damage and atherosclerotic vascular disease, i.e., left ventricular (LV) hypertrophy, congestive heart failure, cardiomegaly, evidence of abdominal bruits, and careful examination of the femoral pulses for a pulse delay. Special attention should be given to the ophthalmoscopic examination, looking for arteriolar narrowing, hemorrhages, exudates, and, possibly, papilledema, especially in the severely hypertensive patient. During neurologic examination, evidence of remote stroke would prompt more rigorous control of blood pressure.

Table 2. Clinical Evaluation of the Hypertensive Patient

History
- Age, sex, duration of hypertension, response to therapy
- Symptoms of headaches, TIA, CVA, CHF, angina, PVD
- Symptoms of episodic headaches, palpitations, perspiration (pheochromocytoma), muscular weakness, cramps and polyuria (primary aldosteronism), headache and lower extremity claudication (coarctation of aorta)
- Family history of hypertension: history of smoking, diet, exercise, and other risk factors (diabetes, gout)
- Medication: birth control pills, amphetamines (diet and cold capsules, nasal sprays), cocaine abuse, large quantities of licorice, adrenal steroid, thyroid hormones

Physical
- Vital signs including postural BP; arm and leg BP; weight
- Funduscopic examination for retinopathy
- Cardiac and chest examination for heart size, murmurs and gallops
- Abdominal examination for masses, bruits
- Peripheral vascular examination
- Neurologic examination
- Check for evidence of gout, hyperlipidemia, thyroid disorder, Cushing's syndrome; signs of neurofibromatosis, cafe au lait spots

Laboratory (initial)
- Serum potassium and sodium; creatinine or BUN; FBS, cholesterol; ECG; urinalysis
- Additional: CBC, uric acid

TIA = transient ischemic attack; CVA = cerebrovascular accident; CHF = congestive heart failure; PVD = peripheral vascular disease; FBS = fasting blood sugar; CBC = complete blood count; BP = blood pressure.

The laboratory examinations should evaluate end-organ function, evidence of secondary hypertension, and concomitant risk factors (Table 3). They should include a hematocrit, urinalysis, electrolytes, BUN, and creatinine to evaluate renal function; blood glucose level; serum uric acid; and total cholesterol and triglyceride levels (Gifford et al.). If serum total cholesterol is >200 mg/dl, a 12-hour fasting serum cho-

Table 3. Baseline Laboratory Tests for Evaluation of Hypertension	
Tests	Information
Complete blood count	Baseline (stress erythrocytosis)
Serum potassium concentration	Pretreatment baseline (diuretic therapy)
	Screening for primary or secondary aldosteronism (etiology)
Serum creatinine	End-organ function (complication)
	Renal hypertension (etiology)
Fasting blood sugar	Risk factor
Serum cholesterol	Risk factor
Serum uric acid	Baseline (diuretic therapy)
	Indicator of nephrosclerosis (complication)
Electrocardiogram	Risk factor
Urinalysis	Renal hypertension (etiology)
	End-organ function (complications)

Modified from Slater EE, Harber E: Hypertension. In: Johnson RA, Haber E, Austen WG, eds. *The Practice of Cardiology*. Little, Brown and Co.: Boston; 1989.

lesterol, high-density lipoprotein (HDL) cholesterol, and triglyceride (TG) determination should be performed. Based on the formula, low-density lipoprotein (LDL) cholesterol = Total cholesterol − HDL chol −TG/5, the atherogenic potential may be predicted.

A chest x-ray is of little value in the routine examination of a hypertensive patient because it has a very low predictive value for cardiac hypertrophy. If a patient has a history of known pulmonary disease or has smoked cigarettes for a long time, a chest x-ray may be useful for evaluating pulmonary pathologic conditions. An electrocardiogram (ECG) is recommended as a baseline and also to detect LV hypertrophy. The role of echocardiography is unclear. It is clear that echocardiography is more sensitive and specific than the ECG for evaluating a patient for LV hypertrophy (Table 4) (Woythaler et al.; Casale et al. 1985; Devereux et al.). Several studies suggest that LV hypertrophy may be a good predictor of future cardiovascular risk (Casale et al. 1986; Levy et al.). However, routine echocardiography in all hypertensive patients is not suggested. Echocardiography may be useful in the patient with long-standing hypertension and evidence of congestive heart failure to rule out hypertrophic cardiomyopathy as a cause of heart failure, rather than poor LV function. Echocardiography is also useful for the patient with borderline hypertension; evidence of mild diastolic

dysfunction or LV hypertrophy indicates a need for treatment because these conditions suggest a higher risk of cardiovascular events.

The role of random plasma renin activity (PRA) determinations in the initial assessment of a hypertensive patient should be noted. Essential hypertension may be classified as high, normal and low renin, and it has been suggested that these classifications may be used to predict cardiovascular complications and guide therapy (Helmer; Brunner et al.). However, the current consensus is that PRA is not a useful screen and is not recommended in the initial assessment of the uncomplicated essential hypertensive patient (Birkenhager et al.; Kaplan).

An important and difficult decision in the initial evaluation is whom to evaluate for secondary causes of hypertension. Screening for secondary hypertension should be reserved for selected patients who show one of the following features (Gifford et al.): 1) onset of hypertension at an age younger than 30 years; 2) a rapid onset later in life, sometime after age 50, and no history of essential hypertension; 3) a negative family history for hypertension, and diastolic blood pressure >110 mm Hg; 4) refractoriness to antihypertensive therapy; 5) presence of features indicative of secondary causes upon initial screening: hypokalemia (defined as a serum potassium level <3.5 mEq/L in a patient not taking oral diuretics or <3 mEq/L in a patient receiving diuretics); evidence of an ab-

Table 4. Left Ventricular Hypertrophy: Electrocardiographic versus Echocardiographic Assessment			
	Sensitivity (%)	Specificity (%)	Accuracy (%)
ECG Criteria			
$SV_1 + RV_5$ or $RV_6 > 35$	33	94	67
RE point score >4	30	93	65
RE point score >5	19	96	61
Sokolow-Lyons voltage	21	95	65
R $aV_L > 11$	7	98	58
$R_1 + S_3 > 25$	8	97	58
Echo Criteria			
M-mode: LV mass	93	95	94
Penn-cube method	100	86	90

RE = Romhilt-Estes

$$\text{Sensitivity (\%)} = \frac{\text{true positives correctly diagnosed}}{\text{total true positives}} \times 100$$

$$\text{Specificity (\%)} = \frac{\text{true negatives correctly diagnosed}}{\text{total true negatives}} \times 100$$

$$\text{Accuracy (\%)} = \frac{\text{positives + negatives correctly diagnosed}}{\text{total tested}} \times 100$$

dominal bruit on physical examination; history of variable blood pressures with sweating, tachycardia, palpitations and tremor of the upper extremities, which suggest pheochromocytoma; and use of oral contraceptives by a young woman.

SECONDARY FORMS OF HYPERTENSION

The screening tests for specific forms of hypertension are listed in Table 5.

RENOVASCULAR HYPERTENSION

Renovascular hypertension accounts for about 2% of hypertension in adults. Renal artery stenosis usually occurs as a result of atherosclerosis or fibromuscular disease. Atherosclerosis is more frequently seen in older patients, usually with evidence of diffuse arteriosclerotic disease. Fibromuscular disease is more common in young patients, predominantly women. The hypertension is usually of recent onset. The family history is often negative; an abdominal bruit is present in 50-60% of patients with renovascular hypertension. Hypokalemia is seen in 20% of patients and reflects secondary hyperaldosteronism.

Plasma Renin Activity

Random PRA measurement is of little value. Only 50-60% of patients with renovascular hypertension have elevated peripheral plasma activity. Basal PRA levels overlap substantially between patients with essential hypertension and those with renal artery stenosis. The stimulated PRA has been used as a screening test by several investigators. This test is performed by sodium restriction (10 mEq sodium for three days) plus 2-4 hours of upright posture, or the simpler intravenous furosemide test (40 mg IV followed by 1/2 h of upright posture on an unrestricted diet). A PRA level >10 ng/ml/hr is suggestive of surgically correctable renovascular hypertension. The stimulated PRA does, however, have a high incidence of false-positive results.

Intravenous Pyelogram and Digital Subtraction Angiography

Rapid-sequence "hypertensive" intravenous pyelography (IVP) is used to assess renal morphology and renal blood flow. This technique, first introduced by Maxwell et al. in 1964, is performed by injecting an

Table 5. Screening Tests for Specific Forms of Hypertension	
Diagnosis	Screening Test
Renovascular hypertension	DSA, captopril renography Hypertensive IVP
Primary aldosteronism	Stimulated PRA 24-hour urine potassium excretion
Cushing's syndrome	Overnight dexamethasone suppression
Pheochromocytoma	24-hour urine metanephrine, VMA, and catecholamines
Renal hypertension	Urinalysis, BUN, creatinine, IVP, ultrasound, urine culture
Coarctation of aorta	Chest x-ray
Hyperparathyroidism	Serum calcium and phosphorus levels
Hyperthyroidism	Serum T4 and thyroglobulin levels

DSA = digital subtraction angiography; PRA = plasma renin activity; VMA = vanillylmandelic acid; IVP = intravenous pyelogram.

opaque radiocontrast medium; films are taken at 20 seconds and at 1, 2, 3, 4, 5, 10, 15 and 25 minutes. Findings suggestive of obstruction of the main renal artery are: 1) delayed appearance of the opaque medium in the callaces of the involved kidney; 2) increased density or delayed excretion of the contrast in the delay films; 3) decreased pole-to-pole diameter of the kidney (disparity of renal size >1.5 cm); and 4) ureteral notching from enlarged collateral vessels, which is a very important sign of functional stenosis. The IVP yields a sensitivity and specificity of 85–90%; these are significantly decreased if segmental or bilateral disease is present. In addition, in most centers rapid-sequence IVPs yield a 15% false-positive rate and a 20–25% false-negative rate. The National Heart, Lung, and Blood Institute's cooperative study on renovascular hypertension clearly indicates that rapid-sequence IVP is not helpful in predicting the prognosis from surgery in patients with renal artery stenosis; 40–85% of patients with a normal IVP respond favorably to surgery. Thus, rapid-sequence IVP is no longer routinely used in many centers.

Digital subtraction angiography (DSA) is a safe and informative procedure. The procedure involves injecting contrast material into the brachiocephalic vein or the superior vena cava, or directly into the renal arteries. The image is then digitized by a computer to remove overlying bone, soft tissue and gas shadows. Digital subtraction angiography does require patient cooperation to minimize motion artifact. It has limited spatial resolution, and renal vessels may be obscured by overlapping mesenteric vessels. Finally, images may be nondiagnostic in patients with impaired renal and cardiac function.

Overall, DSA yields a sensitivity and specificity of 87.6% and 89.5%, respectively, but 7.4% of all renal DSAs are uninterpretable. In experienced centers, the DSA may replace rapid-sequence IVP as the initial screening test.

Saralasin or Captopril Test

Two pharmacologic tests, the saralasin test and the captopril test, are used to screen for renovascular hypertension. Saralasin is an angiotensin II antagonist with weak agonist properties. At high levels of circulating angiotensin II, saralasin competitively inhibits binding of angiotensin II to the vascular receptor, diminishing arterial pressure. At low levels of circulating angiotensin II, because of its weak agonist properties, saralasin can mildly increase arterial pressure.

The saralasin infusion test was first described by Hollenberg and Williams. They reported that in 70% of patients with unilateral renal disease, diastolic blood pressure decreased by at least 10 mm Hg in response to this test. Pooling of published data yields an 86% true-positive (determined by improvement or cure six months after surgery) and a 14% false-positive rate (Dzau et al.; Horne et al.). It is important to note that patients with bilateral renal artery stenosis do not respond to this test.

The test consists of intravenous infusion of sara-lasin in 5% dextrose at a constant rate of 0.10–1.0 μg/kg/min for 45 minutes. A positive response is defined as a sustained decrease in diastolic pressure of at least 10 mm Hg. Plasma renin activity is also measured 30 minutes after the infusion, and a precipitous rise in PRA may clarify an ambiguous decrease in diastolic blood pressure. The test is most meaningful when it is administered after four days of sodium restriction (10 mEq diet), with or without the administration of furosemide (40-80 mg). Although early reports suggested high sensitivity and specificity, recent evaluations dispute these findings, and the recommendation that the test be used as a routine screening procedure has been challenged.

The captopril test was first reported by Case and Laragh, who examined the responses to both intravenous saralasin and converting enzyme inhibition with teprotide in 47 untreated patients with surgically correctable renovascular hypertension. They found that an exaggerated increase in PRA was a much better indicator of surgery-correctable renovascular hypertension than was an exaggerated decrease in blood pressure. The stimulated PRA value was also a much better predictor than baseline PRA, and vigorous pretest stimulation of the renin-angiotensin system, mostly by salt restriction, diminished discrimination between patients with renovascular hypertension and those with essential hypertension. However, these initial encouraging results have not been substantiated. In other studies, the sensitivity of the captopril test has ranged from 40% to 100%, and the specificity from 50% to 80%, with a positive predictive value of only 66% (Thibonnier et al.; Muller et al.; Wilcox et al.). This test is complicated by the fact that sodium restriction by the patient, or other drugs that may inhibit renin release, can alter the results.

Captopril Renography (Renal Scintigraphic Captopril Test)

Captopril renography is based on the finding by Wenting et al. that captopril induces a reduction in ^{99m}Tc-diethylenetriamine penta-acetic acid (DPTA) uptake and delays ^{131}I-hippurate excretion. These changes are much more marked in the stenotic than contralateral kidney. Geyskes et al. reported a high incidence of these captopril-induced changes in ischemic kidneys and concluded that the following changes could be used as criteria to identify ischemic or functionally stenotic kidneys: a fall in DPTA uptake rel-ative to the contralateral kidney, a delay in the time to the peak of the hippuran renogram, and a delay in hippuran washout. In this retrospective study, these criteria predicted the antihypertensive response to angioplasty with an 80% sensitivity and 100% specificity. Further studies have confirmed these findings (Sfakianakis et al.), and if confirmed in prospective studies, captopril renography may replace renal vein renin sampling as the test to detect functional artery stenosis. We believe that captopril renography is useful for identifying patients with critical renal artery stenosis. In patients with moderate but hemodynamically significant stenosis, captopril may not elicit a marked fall in glomerular filtration rate.

Renal Arteriography and Renal Vein Renin Ratio

Renal arteriography is performed to confirm the diagnosis of renovascular hypertension and characterize the anatomy for consideration of surgery or other therapeutic procedures. Arteriography may reveal:
1. The presence of unilateral, bilateral, or multiple stenotic lesions.
2. The location of these lesions (e.g., close to the origin of the renal artery vs. just before the bifurcation of the branches vs. in segmental branches).
3. The cause of the renovascular hypertension, i.e., atherosclerotic; renal fibromuscular dysplasia; intimal fibroplasia or periarterial fibroplasia; or extrinsic lesions resulting in compression of the renal vasculature.
4. The size of the affected kidney and the contralateral kidney.
5. The presence of collateral vascularity in the affected kidney.
6. The extent of arteriosclerosis in the abdominal aorta.

Although renal arteriography reveals the anatomy of a lesion, it does not indicate surgical curability. To determine the physiologic significance of the lesion, differential renal vein renin measurements are recommended. In a review of the literature, Marks and Maxwell and colleagues reported that of 286 patients with lateralizing ratios of 1:5–2:1 and arteriographic evidence of renal artery stenosis, 93% were cured or had significantly less severe hypertension after surgery. In this study, 126 patients with unilateral renal artery stenosis did not have lateralizing renal vein renins and 64 of these patients were cured or improved with surgery, leading to a false-negative rate of about 50%. More recent reports confirm these findings and yield a false-positive rate of 14% and a false-negative rate as high as 67%. The causes of nonlateralizing renal vein renin include bilateral renal artery stenosis, volume expansion, non-simultaneous sampling of renal vein blood, assay error, and non-significant renal artery lesion. To increase the sensitivity of the procedure, use of drugs that inhibit the secretion of renin (such as beta-adrenergic antagonist, reserpine, clonidine, methyldopa) should be discontinued three to five days before the study. Renin secretion can be further stimulated by a low-salt diet or administration of intravenous furosemide, hydralazine, or converting enzyme inhibitor, which can accentuate the differences between the two sides.

Stimulation of renin release with a single dose of captropril before the test lowers the false-negative rate (Lyons et al.), but the number of false-negative responses remains unacceptable. In this test, a single dose of oral captropril (25 mg or 1 mg/kg) is given 1 hour before sampling. A ratio of >3.0 predicts a favorable surgical outcome. The test, however, still has a false-negative rate of 40%.

The frequency of false-negative results prompted the recent recommendations in the American Heart Association's Special Report on Office Evaluation of Hypertension (Gifford et al.). This report recommended that with the advent of angioplasty, differential renal vein renins are probably not necessary and an attempt at angioplasty to increase revascularization as a diagnostic trial may be more prudent than awaiting the results of the differential renal vein renins. As discussed earlier, captopril renography may be an even better test of functional significance and because it is noninvasive, it can be used before the arteriography.

Management

Fibromuscular disease. Surgery is usually recommended for patients with fibromuscular disease. If available, a trial of percutaneous transluminal angioplasty (PTA) is warranted, with close follow-up monitoring of blood pressure, renal function, status of the lesion by DSA, and renal size by ultrasound. We consider PTA the procedure of choice for the very young patient with multiple lesions, because the probability of recurrence elsewhere after surgery is high. In young patients, PTA is technically successful in 87–100% of cases. In 80–95% of these patients, blood pressure is lowered as well as with surgical revascularization.

Atherosclerotic disease. Patients with unilateral atherosclerotic stenosis and no associated surgical risks can be treated by drugs, PTA, or surgery. The technical success rate of PTA is lower in patients with atherosclerotic disease than in those with fibromuscular disease. In nonocclusive, nonostial lesions, the success rate is 70–90%. Ostial lesions are more difficult, and the success rate of PTA is only 20%. In view of the associated problems of drug therapy (cost, compliance, inconvenience, side effects, and possible progression of disease), we favor surgery or a single trial of PTA before surgery. Even in patients with diffuse atherosclerosis (particularly involving the abdominal aorta) and with associated coronary, cerebrovascular, or pulmonary disease, we prefer a trial of PTA. Revascularization by PTA may be particularly beneficial in high-surgical-risk patients with compromised renal function. Angioplasty can be repeated once or twice, if necessary, in these patients.

High-risk patients with normal renal function may be managed with drugs. However, the patient should be monitored closely for progression of disease and evidence of renal failure or its sequelae. Surgery is usually reserved as a later option in these patients. The benefit rate (cure or improvement) in patients with unilateral focal lesions is about 90%; in those with bilateral, diffuse atherosclerotic lesions, it is 70–80%. Figure 2 summarizes our approach to evaluation and management of renovascular hypertension. The choice of a screening test depends on the institution; captopril renography may be the test of choice in centers where it is available. In patients in whom renal artery stenosis is suspected, renal arteriography may be indicated, even if screening tests are negative.

PRIMARY ALDOSTERONISM

Primary aldosteronism arises from an autonomous hypersecretion of the mineralocorticoid aldosterone from an adrenal adenoma (Conn's syndrome) or from bilateral adrenal hyperplasia. Adrenal adenoma is the more frequent cause. An excess circulating aldosterone level results in increased renal sodium retention and, usually, potassium excretion. Primary aldosteronism is a rare condition, accounting for less than 1% of the cases in unselected hypertensive patients (Lyons et al.; Weinberger et al.). It is usually associated with mild to moderate elevations in blood pres-

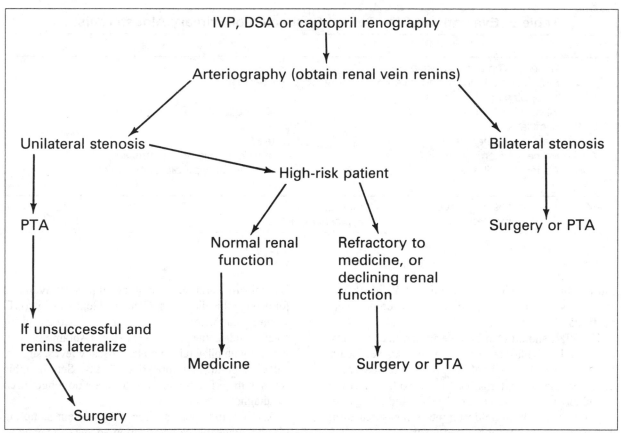

Figure 2. *Diagnosis and management of patients with renovascular hypertension. IVP = hypertensive intravenous pyelography; DSA = digital subtraction angiography; PTA = percutaneous transluminal angioplasty.*

sure but can cause severe, resistant hypertension. It is a difficult and somewhat elusive diagnosis. In its severe form, originally described by Conn, it can cause muscular weakness, polyuria, nocturia, polydipsia, tetany, parasthesia, and headache. Evaluation of primary aldosteronism is outlined in Table 6.

The usual clue for hyperaldosteronism is a low serum potassium level, usually defined as <3.5 mEq/L in a patient not taking oral diuretics, or <3 mEq/L in a patient receiving conventional diuretics for treatment of hypertension. In a prospective study of 80 patients with primary aldosteronism, all of whom had spontaneous hypertension, only 73% had spontaneous hypokalemia with normal salt intake and only 56% had provoked hypokalemia with high salt intake for three days (Weinberger et al.). Thus, about one fourth of the patients with primary aldosteronism would be missed by using only hypokalemia testing as a screening procedure.

Primary aldosteronism is diagnosed by the finding of inappropriate potassium excretion, an elevated aldosterone level, and suppressed PRA. If a patient suspected of having primary aldosteronism is receiving diuretic therapy, the therapy should be discontinued for at least two weeks. Then, if the urinary potassium level is <20 mEq/24 hr, primary aldosteronism is unlikely even though the serum potassium may be low; a nonrenal loss of potassium is more likely. The urine potassium level in cases of primary aldosteronism should be >40 mEq/24 hr. Single measurements of PRA and plasma aldosterone are not useful for screening or diagnosis. The diagnosis should be made by assessing 24-hr urinary aldosterone secretion, which should remain ≥8 μg/24 hr, with a urinary sodium level ≥250 mEq/24 hr (Gifford et al.; Weinberger et al.). To definitively test for patients with primary aldosteronism, 24-hr urinary aldosterone secretion should be measured after three days of

Table 6. Evaluation of the Patient Suspected of Primary Aldosteronism	
Tests	Positive Results
Hypertension and hypokalemia	K+ <3.5*
Stop diuretic therapy and give K+ supplement 1-2 weeks	↓ K+ persists
24-hr urine K+ excretion	>30-40 mEq/24 hr
Stimulated PRA	Suppressed
Plasma aldosterone concentration	Elevated
Saline infusion	Plasma aldosterone not suppressed
Abdominal CT scan	Bilateral adrenal hyperplasia or cortical adenoma

* Up to 10% may have a K+ 3.5-3.9 mEq/L.
CT = computed tomography; PRA = plasma renin activity.

salt loading (approximately 12 g/day) (Weinberger et al.). Nonsuppressibility of urinary aldosterone levels confirms the diagnosis.

The PRA should also be determined because very high levels of plasma renin can lead to secondary aldosteronism, which would not be suppressed by sodium loading. An alternative to oral sodium loading is sodium infusion (Kem et al.; Holland et al.). In this procedure plasma aldosterone is measured from venous blood at 8:00 a.m., before the infusion of 2 L of normal saline solution over 4 hours; plasma aldosterone is again measured at noon. Patients must discontinue antihypertensive drug therapy for two weeks before this study. It should not be performed in patients with congestive heart failure, renal failure, or a history of acute myocardial infarction or stroke in the preceding six months. In a study of normal persons, aldosterone level before infusion of saline solution averaged 30.5 ± 1.1 ng/dl; this level was reduced after saline infusion, to 3.4 ± 0.1 ng/dl. In patients with primary aldosteronism the mean aldosterone level at baseline was higher, 60.9 ± 8.8 ng/dl. The baseline aldosterone levels did overlap with values of normal subjects, so the test was not useful for identifying patients with primary aldosteronism. After the infusion of saline solution, however, patients with primary aldosteronism had a mean aldosterone value of 36.3 ± 4.2 ng/dl, with no overlap between the two groups.

Once primary aldosteronism is diagnosed, it is important to differentiate between a solitary adrenocortical adenoma and bilateral adrenal hyperplasia as the cause. The former is present in 60–85% of cases and is surgically curable. Several techniques are available for making this diagnosis. Computed tomographic (CT) scanning can identify adrenal tumors >1.0 cm in diameter and is the most useful test (Abrams et al.). Patients with bilateral hyperplasia usually reveal slightly enlarged or normal-appearing glands. Scintigraphic scans with [125]T-19-indocholesterol are no longer used for diagnostic evaluation.

Another approach is direct adrenal-vein sampling via percutaneous catheterization to measure venous aldosterone levels (Vaughan et al.). This method of localizing the tumor is accurate in more than 90% of cases. Elevated values with less than a twofold difference between the sides suggest bilateral hyperplasia; aldosterone-producing adenomas generally result in a tenfold difference between the sides. In patients with the disease, abdominal CT scanning should first be performed. If the results are inconclusive, adrenal venous sampling for aldosterone may be indicated.

PHEOCHROMOCYTOMA

Pheochromocytoma should be suspected in a patient, especially a young patient, who has a history of paroxysms of hypertension and other symptoms. The most common symptoms (in addition to labile hypertension) are paroxysms of tachycardia, headaches, palpitations, sweating, and pallor. Other symptoms include medically refractory hypertension that may at times be accelerated, weight loss, abnormal carbohydrate metabolism, and a pressor response to induction of anesthesia or other antihypertensive treatment. The most common screening test is a 24-hr urinalysis, to look for excretion of vanillylmandelic acid (VMA) or metanephrines, the latter being more reliable (Manu and Runge; Manger and Gifford). In most laboratories, a total metanephrine level >1.3 mg/24 hr or a VMA level >7 mg/24 hr is abnormal. Free catechols can also be measured in the urine, although this measurement is somewhat less reliable. Normal values in most laboratories are 100-150 µg/24 hr. The false-positive rate increases in urinary measurement with co-administration of many antihypertensive drugs (Table 7) or any endogenous stimulation of the sympathoadrenal system (Bouloux and Perret; Bravo et al. 1979).

An adjunct to measurement of 24-hour urine excretion, and perhaps a more reliable test, is measurement of plasma catecholamine levels (Bravo et al. 1979). This test has recently become more widely available and is not hindered by artifacts due to interference from drugs and angiographic contrast material, or from difficulty in 24-hr urine collections. To draw plasma catechol samples, the patient must be resting and venipuncture avoided for at least 30 minutes. In patients with pheochromocytoma, plasma catechols are usually elevated to >2,000 pg/ml. Urinary catecholamine, VMA, metanephrine and plasma catecholamine levels may overlap with normal values. Therefore, other pharmacologic tests have been devised: the clonidine suppression test (Bravo et al. 1981) and the glucagon stimulation test. In patients whose plasma catechol levels are 500–2,000 pg/ml,

the failure of 0.3 mg of clonidine given orally, or of a 25-mg bolus of phentolamine, to suppress catechols by 50% after 3 hours is a strong indication of the presence of pheochromocytoma (Gifford et al.; Bravo et al. 1981; Bravo and Gifford).

In the glucagon stimulation test (Gifford et al.; Bravo and Gifford), glucagon is administered intravenously in a dose of 1 mg to stimulate secretion of catecholamines from the tumor. A rise in plasma catechol levels to >2,000 g/L suggests pheochromocytoma.

Care must be taken in administering these pharmacologic tests because they can cause a hypertensive crisis. Phentolamine should be immediately available to counteract this event.

Once a diagnosis of pheochromocytoma is suspected, the tumor should be localized by adrenal CT scanning. The tumor can be localized in this method in 90% of the cases (Stewart et al.). The 10% of pheochromocytomas that are <1 cm in diameter (below the resolving power of CT scan) can be localized using ^{131}I-metaiodobenzylguanide scanning (Sisson et al.). False-negative results have been reported for both of these scans, and in a patient who is strongly suspected of having a pheochromocytoma, careful follow-up is indicated. In some cases selective arteriography with differential venous catheterization and measurements of regional catecholamines may be useful in localizing the tumor when all other tests are negative but the condition is strongly suspected.

Table 7. Substances Interfering with Assays for Catecholamines/Metabolites

Free catecholamines
    Increase: methyldopa, L-dopa, tetracyclines, quinidine, isoproterenol, theophylline
Metanephrines
    Increase: chlorpromazine, monoamine oxidase inhibitors
    Decrease: x-ray contrast media containing methylglucamine (e.g., Renografin, Renovist, Hypaque)
Vanillylmandelic acid (VMA)
    Increase: nalidixic acid, anileridine, nitroglycerin (slight)
    Decrease: monoamine oxidase inhibitors, clofibrate

From Ram CVS, Engelman K: Pheochromocytoma: Recognition and management. In: Harvey WP et al, eds. *Current Problems in Cardiology*. Chicago: Year Book Medical Publishers; 1979. With permission.

CUSHING'S SYNDROME

Cushing's syndrome is produced by an excess of glucocorticoid secretion by adrenal adenoma, carcinoma, or bilateral hyperplasia. Bilateral hyperplasia is often the result of an ACTH-secreting pituitary adenoma or extra-pituitary neoplasm (e.g., lung carcinoma). Hypertension is seen in patients with Cushing's syndrome; the pathogenesis of this hypertension is unclear. Glucocorticoid increases hepatic angiotensinogen production, and may, in part, increase plasma angiotensin production. Further, there is evidence of increased vascular sensitivity to vasoconstrictor hormones in affected patients. The salt-retaining effect of high glucocorticoid levels may also contribute to the development of hypertension. Only patients who have clinical stigmata of Cushing's syndrome, such as truncal obesity, buffalo hump, moon facies, and violaceous striae, should be evaluated for this form of hypertension.

A 24-hr urine cortisol excretion value is a useful screening test. The dexamethasone suppression test is a more simple alternative. This is performed by administration of 1 mg of dexamethasone at midnight; plasma cortisol is measured 8 hours later. Failure of suppression of cortisol (>5 μg/dl) warrants further investigation (Table 8). The next step is the more prolonged dexamethasone suppression test, which involves administration of dexamethasone, 0.5 mg every 6 hours for two days, followed by 2 mg every 6 hours for two more days. Urinary 17-hydroxycorticoid excretion should be measured on the second day of each dose. In patients with Cushing's syndrome, urinary 17-hydroxycorticoid levels are not suppressed to <3 mg/day with a regimen of 0.5 mg dexamethasone every 6 hours. If Cushing's syndrome is caused by an excess pituitary ACTH drive with bilateral adrenal hyperplasia, the urinary 17-hydroxycorticoid level is suppressed to $<50\%$ of the control value on the second day of a regimen of 2 mg every 6 hours. In patients whose urinary corticoid excretion is not suppressed, the ACTH level should be measured to differentiate between adrenal neoplasm and adrenal hyperplasia secondary to ACTH-producing tumor. Patients with adrenal neoplasm have normal to low ACTH levels (<50 pg/ml). Adrenal adenoma can be distinguished from carcinoma on the basis of 24-hour urinary 17-ketosteroid production. Adrenal carcinoma is associated with high urinary 17-ketosteroid excretion (>30 mg/24 hr). Metyrapone testing is also useful in differentiating adrenal tumors from adrenal hyperplasia. Patients with adrenal tumors fail to respond to metyrapone challenge with a rise in urinary 17-hydroxycorticoids. Evaluation of pituitary function by the appropriate roentgenographic and CT scanning procedures as well as a search for nonendocrine ACTH-producing tumors may be indicated. In summary, in the presence of clinical stigmata of Cushing's syndrome, the overnight dexamethasone suppression test should reliably detect and confirm the diagnosis. Further workup and management should probably be performed in consultation with an endocrinologist.

COARCTATION OF THE AORTA

Congenital narrowing of the aorta usually occurs beyond the origin of the left subclavian artery or distal to the ligamentum arteriosum. Takayasu's arteritis is an acquired form of coarctation that can also lead to hypertension. Clues from the history and physical examination usually lead to further evaluation for coarctation. Symptoms include headache, epistaxis, and bounding carotid pulsations. Claudication, stroke, and heart failure may occur. Cardiac findings include a suprasternal notch thrill, LV hypertrophy, loud A$_2$, S$_4$ gallop, and systolic flow murmur that is loudest over the left posterior thorax. A discrepancy between arm and leg blood pressure, with a delayed or absent lower extremity pulse, are classic findings. A chest x-ray film can confirm the diagnosis by the characteristic rib notching (due to large intercostal collaterals) as well as the "figure 3" sign of the descending aorta (Glancy et al.). The diagnosis is confirmed by aortography.

Patients with coarctation of the aorta have other, associated cardiac lesions; bicuspid aortic valve is seen in up to one third of adolescent and adult patients with coarctation. (See also Chapter 22.)

HYPERTENSION ASSOCIATED WITH ORAL CONTRACEPTIVES

Although blood pressure increases in most women ingesting oral contraceptives, frank hypertension develops in only 5% in five years. The incidence is three to five times higher than among those who do not use oral contraceptives. The largest increase occurs within the first year, but blood pressure continues to rise over five years (Stadel). The mechanism of oral contraceptive–related hypertension is unknown. Data indicate that plasma volume and cardiac output are

Table 8. Evaluation of the Patient Suspected of Cushing's Syndrome		
Test	Results	Conditions
Overnight dexamethasone suppression: 1 mg midnight; 8 a.m. plasma cortisol measurement	>5 µg/dl	Suspect Cushing's syndrome
Standard dexamethasone test		
a) 0.5 mg q6h × 2 days (day 1-2)	≤3 mg	Normal response
24-hr urine 17-0H corticoid	≥3 mg	Cushing's syndrome
b) 2 mg q6h × 2 days (day 3-4)	<50% control	Pituitary ACTH excess
24-hr urine 17-0H corticoid day 4	>50% control	Adrenal neoplasia, or non-endocrine ACTH tumor
Metyrapone (750 mg q4h × 14 doses) 24-hr urine 17-0H corticoid	>2 × increase	Pituitary-hypothalamic dysfunction
Plasma ACTH	<50 pg/ml	Adrenal neoplasia
	>80 pg/ml	Non-endocrine ACTH tumor or pituitary ACTH excess
24-hr urine 17-ketosteroid	>30 mg	Adrenal carcinoma
Miscellaneous: skull x-ray, chest x-ray, abdominal or brain CT scan		

increased in normal women after several months of oral contraceptive use. This may be related to the sodium-retentive effects of estrogen and synthetic progesterone. Hepatic synthesis of angiotensinogen is also stimulated by estrogen. Thus, the rate of angiotensin production increases in the plasma. Furthermore, sympathetic nervous activity may increase, as reflected by high levels of plasma dopamine-β-hydroxylase.

The hypertension is usually mild and reversible. If the blood pressure remains elevated three months after discontinuation of oral contraceptives, further workup and therapy should be initiated.

HYPERTENSION RELATED TO RENAL DISEASE

Hypertension can develop with chronic renal failure, renal parenchymal disease without renal insufficiency, acute glomerulonephritis, chronic pyelonephritis, hydronephrosis, or after bilateral nephrectomy. The mechanism of hypertension may be categorized, simplistically, as volume-dependent or renin-dependent. Volume-dependent hypertension is usually responsive to removal of sodium and fluid excess by diuretics or dialysis. Renin-dependent hypertension is usually aggravated by volume depletion and may be responsive to propranolol or alpha-methyldopa. In some cases, hypertension may be refractory to standard triple therapy. Captopril, minoxidil, and calcium blockers are effective agents for the treatment of refractory hypertension associated with renal insufficiency.

MISCELLANEOUS CONDITIONS

Secondary hypertension may be caused by excessive alcohol intake. A linear progressive increase in the level of blood pressure has been reported with increasing consumption of alcohol (Katsky et al.), as has a threshold-type effect (Jackson et al.). Obesity has been clearly shown to be associated with increases in blood pressure (Chiang et al.; Haulk et al.). For a patient who is overweight, a weight reduction program should be recommended and the blood pressure followed closely.

There are also rare endocrine causes of hypertension. Congenital adrenal hyperplasia associated with 11-hydroxylase deficiency or 17-hydroxylase deficiency is associated with hypertension. Systemic hypertension is also seen with hyperthyroidism, hyperparathyroidism, and acromegaly.

CLINICAL PRESENTATION

MALIGNANT HYPERTENSION

Because of its consequences, it is extremely important for the clinician to recognize the patient who presents with accelerated or malignant hypertension. Usually, the patient presents with a diastolic blood pressure >120 mm Hg, but the absolute level of blood pressure does not confirm the diagnosis. Headache, often severe and pulsatile, is the most common presenting complaint (Conn et al.). The headache may be accompanied by neurologic aberrations known as hypertensive encephalopathy. These include (in addition to headache) nausea, vomiting, blurred vision to transient blindness, seizures, temporary paralysis, altered mental status, and even coma. Focal neurologic deficits rarely occur, but they usually represent other central nervous system disorders that should be rigorously ruled out (Gifford and Westbrook; Bennett; Healton et al.). The cause of hypertensive encephalopathy has been attributed to a breakthrough in cerebral blood flow autoregulation, resulting in forced vasodilatation (Bennett; Healton et al.; Johansson et al.).

These pathophysiologic conditions also lead to a change in the retinal arteries. There is both obliteration and rupture of these vessels secondary to the increased blood flow in malignant hypertension. Funduscopic examination, which is essential in these patients, reveals cotton-wool exudates, representing ischemic damage to the nerve fibers, as well as flame-shaped hemorrhages due to vessel rupture (McLeod et al.; Vaziri). The increase in intracranial pressure results in papilledema, leading to blurred vision, narrowing visual field, transient visual loss, and central scotomas (Vaziri).

A major consequence of malignant hypertension is renal damage, known as malignant nephrosclerosis. Pathologically, this condition includes proliferative endarteritis, necrotizing arteriolitis, and a necrotizing glomerulitis (Vaziri; Paronetto). The clinical manifestations of these changes consist of proteinuria, microscopic and, occasionally, gross hematuria, and oliguria progressing even to azotemia (Schottstaedt). These changes may mimic an acute nephritic or vasculitic process, but are usually less severe. In rare cases a renal biopsy may be needed, especially in the patient without a history of hypertension.

Hematologic and endocrinologic abnormalities are also present. Often, a microangiopathic-hemolytic anemia may be present due to changes in the small arterioles. This anemia is often masked initially by hemoconcentration, but becomes apparent once the patient is properly hydrated. Abnormalities of the coagulation system include thrombocytopenia, increased fibrin degradation products, and increases in the concentrations of fibrinogen and factor VIII (Gavras et al.).

The endocrinologic changes are due to activation of the renin-angiotensin-aldosterone system seen in these patients. This results in hypokalemia and alkalosis, which may persist after the blood pressure has been corrected (Kahn et al.; Catt et al.). An abnormal stimulation of antidiuretic hormone, contributing to the volume-depleted state, also has been reported (Padfield and Morton).

Cardiovascular complications are not common, but acute left ventricular decompensation can occur. This is manifest by an enlarged cardiac silhouette on chest x-ray, elevated jugular venous distention, pulmonary congestion on physical exam and on the chest x-ray, and an S_3 gallop. There may also be a murmur of aortic insufficiency due to the elevated blood pressure. If an aortic insufficiency murmur is heard, the possibility of an acute aortic dissection must be considered, as it can certainly be precipitated by extreme elevations of blood pressure.

BENIGN HYPERTENSION

Few patients who present with hypertension have accelerated hypertension; most patients are asymptomatic and their chief complaint is that they were noted to have an elevated blood pressure level, which was measured for an unrelated reason. The most common complaint of symptomatic patients is headache, often described as an early morning, frontal headache. Although headache is a common complaint in normotensive patients, a number of studies demonstrate that it is more prevalent in patients with hypertension (VA 1967; Weis; Moser et al. 1962). The relationship to migraine headaches is less clear, but in at least two studies the incidence of migraines was slightly greater in patients with elevated blood pressure (Walker; Gardner et al.), although this has not been confirmed in other series (Moser et al. 1962).

Two other presenting complaints that are occasionally seen are dizziness and epistaxis. Whether these complaints are really more common in hypertensive patients is not clear (Mitchell; Shaheen); one study suggests that epistaxis is not more frequent in hypertensive patients, although it may be more severe (Shaheen).

It is clear that hypertension is usually diagnosed by screening blood pressure determination of asymptomatic patients, emphasizing the need for accurate and frequent measurement of blood pressure.

CONSEQUENCES OF HYPERTENSION

To fully appreciate the natural history of essential hypertension, it is important to examine the statistics before the advent of therapy, around 1950. In numerous studies conducted between 1913 and 1946 (Janeway; Hunter and Rogers; Bechgard), one third to two thirds of untreated patients died of heart disease, 15–40% of stroke, 5–15% of uremia, and 10–30% of intercurrent disease.

CORONARY ARTERY DISEASE

One of the major consequences of hypertension is an increased incidence of atherosclerosis, usually manifest as coronary artery disease (CAD). The Framingham Study (Kannel and Schatzbin; Castelli and Anderson) showed a striking increase in the incidence of CAD in hypertensive patients, along with smaller increases in claudication, atheroembolic stroke, and congestive failure. The individual risk of cardiovascular disease depends on the associated risk factors present in any given patient. Data from the Framingham Study also reveal the additive risks in hypertensive patients of an elevated cholesterol level, glucose intolerance, cigarette smoking, and LV hypertrophy on the ECG.

The cause of this increased risk is not clear, but there appears to be a slight positive correlation between blood pressure and cholesterol level, which may in part explain the findings. Data similar to those in the Framingham Study were reported in the Australian Risk Prevalence Study (MacMahon and MacDonald), which revealed a positive correlation between blood pressure and cholesterol levels. These data may explain a disturbing finding first noted in the Multiple Risk Factor Intervention Trial (1982) and, subsequently, in numerous other trials (Houston; O'Kelley et al.). In the 30% of hypertensive patients who had an abnormal ECG upon entry into the MRFIT trial, cardiovascular and overall mortality was higher in the special-care group than in the usual-care group. Special care included a thiazide diuretic, and this treatment resulted in an increase in plasma LDL levels.

This alteration of the lipid profile may explain the results, but this possibility has not been rigorously tested.

HYPERTENSIVE HEART DISEASE

Cardiac hypertrophy is another major cardiovascular consequence of hypertension. Classically, cardiac involvement in hypertension is separated into three stages: no clinical evidence of involvement (stage I), left atrial enlargement (stage II), and LV hypertrophy (stage III) (Frohlich et al.; Dunn et al.). Only in the final stage, when hypertrophy is present, is cardiac function impaired. These stages were originally determined using ECG criteria; with the use of echocardiography, they may have to be altered.

Numerous studies, using ECG criteria, show an increased incidence of LV hypertrophy in patients with essential hypertension (Kannel et al. 1989; Tarazi and Levy; Inouye et al.). In the Framingham population, ECG evidence of LV hypertrophy developed in 50% of patients with a systolic blood pressure >180 mm Hg (Inouye et al.). Pathologic series demonstrate that the ECG has a sensitivity of 40–50% for detection of LV hypertrophy compared with necropsy (Woythaler et al.; Reichek and Devereux; Casale et al. 1985). When M-mode echocardiography is compared to true LV weight, however, the sensitivity is 90–98% (Devereux et al.; Devereux and Reichek).

Risk factor analysis of the Framingham data shows a great increase in the prevalence of cardiac disease among patients with ECG evidence of LV hypertrophy (Kannel and Schatzbin; Castelli and Anderson; Kannel). Recent data show that echocardiographic evidence of LV hypertrophy also identifies patients at a higher risk for cardiovascular morbid events (Casale et al. 1986). In a small study with an average follow-up of only five years, seven cardiovascular morbid events were observed in 29 hypertensive patients with LV hypertrophy determined by M-mode echocardiography, and seven events in 111 patients without LV hypertrophy. Although the numbers are small, these data may indicate that echocardiography is needed to more accurately determine an individual patient's cardiovascular risk.

In the early stages of LV hypertrophy, increases in LV mass result in a decrease in LV distensibility and a resultant abnormal filling pattern during both passive and active filling (Inouye et al.; Wikstrand). Early on, there may also be an increase in cardiac output (Messerli et al. 1978, 1981). The abnormal diastolic filling has important clinical implications. Topol et al., in a study of elderly hypertensive patients, reported that among patients with concentric hypertrophy who presented with heart failure, those treated with beta blockers or calcium channel blockers did better than those treated with diuretics and vasodilators. It is hypothesized that in patients with LV hypertrophy, a small LV chamber, and normal LV systolic function, volume depletion results in further compromise of the LV cavity and, potentially, a severe hypotensive response.

Ultimately, hypertension results in cardiac failure. Hypertension is the leading cause of congestive heart failure in the United States (Kannel et al. 1972). The first studies on antihypertensive treatment, the VA Cooperative Trials (1967, 1970), demonstrated that treatment can prevent heart failure and thus reduce mortality.

NEUROLOGIC COMPLICATIONS

The Framingham data demonstrate that hypertension is a greater risk factor for cerebral damage than for cardiovascular or renal disease. This typically presents in three forms: intraparenchymal hemorrhage, large-vessel atherosclerosis presenting as ischemic strokes and small vessel disease, and lacunar infarction. The incidence of intraparenchymal hemorrhage has decreased over the last few decades, but this event still accounts for 10–14% of strokes (Mutlu et al; Wolf et al.). This condition has numerous causes, but there is a strong relationship with hypertension (Wolf et al.). Most bleeding episodes occur in the cerebral hemispheres and most patients have associated subarachnoid bleeding.

Ischemic stroke is the most common neurologic complication. Control of hypertension has played a major role in the decline in the incidence of stroke in the last two decades (Wolf et al.; Medical Research Council). Not only is the incidence of stroke increased in hypertension, but there is an increased incidence of reversible ischemic attacks. The Italian Multicenter Study (Inzitari et al.) revealed a positive correlation between systolic blood pressure and the incidence of transient ischemic attacks (TIAs), but no correlation with diastolic blood pressure. This study also found a positive correlation between systolic blood pressure and the presence of cerebral atherosclerosis. Similar data were reported in the Cooperative Study of Focal Cerebral Ischemia in Young Adults (Fieschi et al.; Gandolfo et al.). They confirmed the prominent role of hypertension as a risk factor for stroke or TIA along with cardiac disease, oral contraceptives, elevated serum lipids and smoking.

Small lacunar infarcts are a common autopsy finding in elderly hypertensive patients (Fisher 1965, 1969). These infarcts are caused by occlusion of the small penetrating arteries of the circle of Willis. They present as a variety of clinical syndromes; before the advent of hypertensive therapy, multiple lacunaes often resulted in pseudobulbar palsy with emotional instability, a slowed abulic state, and bilateral pyramidal signs.

RENAL DISEASE

Hypertension is one of the most common causes of renal insufficiency and, subsequently, the need for dialysis (Sugimoto and Rosansky). In malignant hypertension the pathology is characterized by fibrinoid necrosis, a process termed arteriolar nephrosclerosis. In essential hypertension, accelerated atherosclerosis of the small and medium resistance vessels results in progressive nephrosclerosis. This results in proteinuria, a loss in renal concentrating ability, and a decrease in creatinine clearance (Mujais et al.; Bauer et al.). The course of the disease is difficult to follow because renal damage by itself can cause hypertension. There is evidence, however, that treatment of the blood pressure protects the kidneys (Bergstron et al.).

OTHER COMPLICATIONS

In the hypertensive patient, accelerated atherosclerosis may result in an increase in peripheral vascular disease (Kannel and Schatzbin). Hypertension is the most important predisposing factor for aortic dissection (Lindsay and Hurst; Wilson and Hutchins), reported to be present in 70–90% of patients with dissections. It apparently occurs more often in distal dissections than in proximal dissections (Slater and DeSanctis). Aortic aneurysms are also reported to occur more frequently in hypertensive patients than in normotensive persons, probably as a result of the greater frequency of atherosclerosis (Cooke and Safford).

MANAGEMENT OF HYPERTENSION

In this section we discuss management of patients with essential hypertension. The specific management of renovascular hypertension has been discussed earlier. The Joint National Committee (JNC IV) recommends that patients with blood pressure >140/90 mm Hg be treated to maintain arterial blood pressure ≤140/90 mm Hg. Patients with mild hypertension (diastolic blood pressure 90–104 mm Hg) should have a repeat measurement after two months. Patients with high normal blood pressures (diastolic blood pressure 85–89 mm Hg) should be rechecked at yearly intervals. It is important to note that one retrospective study showed an increase in cardiac mortality in patients whose mean treated diastolic blood pressure was <85 mm Hg (Cruickshank et al.).

In patients with mild hypertension, a trial of non-pharmacologic therapy is recommended. This includes:

Weight reduction. There is a clear relationship between body weight, blood pressure and development of hypertension (Chiang et al.; Arisamano et al.). A reasonable goal is to be within 15% of desirable weight. Although numerous studies show that weight reduction can result in a reliable reduction in blood pressure, the likelihood of a patient achieving this goal and maintaining the reduced body weight is small (Wing and Jeffery).

Restriction of alcohol. Excessive alcohol intake can increase blood pressure both acutely and chronically (MacMahon and Norton; Kupari). Patients who drink should restrict their alcohol intake to 30 ml/day (1 oz) of ethanol, the equivalent of 60 ml (2 oz) of 100-proof whiskey, or approximately 240 ml (8 oz) of wine, or 720 ml (24 oz) of beer.

Restriction of sodium. A moderate reduction in dietary sodium intake is recommended for all hypertensive patients. It is not clear, however, whether this actually results in a substantial reduction in blood pressure (Parijs et al.; Richards et al.; Silman et al.). Studies have shown that at best, an 80–157-mmol Na^+/24 hr diet resulted in only a 7-mm Hg mean reduction in systolic blood pressure. Much of the daily sodium intake comes from prepared foods, so proper dietary counseling is important. Sodium restriction is probably best used as an adjunct to medical therapy. Recent studies reported that a large percentage of patients could reduce or discontinue their medications with moderate sodium restriction (Langford et al.; Weinberger et al. 1988).

Other. The Joint National Committee has also recommended that patients participate in regular exercise, eat a diet high in fiber and low in saturated fat, and avoid tobacco use. Regular exercise has been shown in some studies to lower blood pressure, and

a combination of these measures produces an overall reduction in cardiovascular risk (Krotkiewski et al.; Hagberg et al.).

PHARMACOLOGIC THERAPY

The principle of pharmacologic therapy is to inhibit one or several of the factors that can elevate blood pressure, including sodium and volume status, vascular tone, the renin-angiotensin system, and the sympathetic nervous system.

The National High Blood Pressure Education Program no longer recommends the step-care approach (with step one being a diuretic). The goal of therapy is still to maintain arterial blood pressure below 140/90 mm Hg, but rather than step care, the recommendation is now "individualized" step care. This approach broadens the initial choice rather than placing everyone on a diuretic at first. The recommendations are:

Step 1. Nonpharmacologic therapy: Sodium restriction, alcohol restriction, weight control, control of other cardiovascular risk factors.
Step 2. Diuretic, beta blocker, calcium channel blocker, angiotensin converting enzyme (ACE) inhibitor.
Step 3. Add a second drug from a different class, increase dose of first drug, or substitute another drug.
Step 4. Add third drug of different class or substitute second drug.
Step 5. Further evaluation and/or referral, or add third or fourth drug.

This scheme allows for individualized therapy based on the particular patient's needs, while still achieving adequate blood pressure control. Table 9 lists commonly used antihypertensive drugs, their recommended doses, and their effect on serum lipids. Every physician should become familiar with at least one agent from each of the major groups and use it when appropriate. As far as deciding which group of drugs to start with, several considerations may direct the physician: age, race, pathophysiology, associated metabolic disorders, and coexisting diseases (Tables 10-12).

The diabetic patient with hypertension requires special attention. Because diuretics can worsen hyperglycemia and beta blockers may blunt the response to hypoglycemia, these types of drugs should be avoided. Because of their proven efficacy and safety,

Table 9. Types and Examples of Antihypertensive Drugs

Agent	Dose Range (mg/day)	Frequency of Administration (times/day)	Effect on Serum Lipids*	Notes
Diuretics			↑LDL, ↓HDL, ↑TC	
Chlorothiazide	500-1,000	1-2		
Chlorthalidone	12.5-50	1-2		
Hydrochlorothiazide (HCTZ)	12.5-100	1-2		
Indapamide	2.5-5.0	1		
Furosemide	20-600	1-2		
Bumetamide	0.5-2.0	1		
Amiloride	5-10	1		
Spironolactone	25-100	1-3		
Combination diuretics			↑LDL, ↓HDL, ↑TC	
HCTZ and amiloride	1-2 tabs/day	1		Each tablet contains HCTZ 50 mg, amiloride 5 mg
HCTZ and spironolactone	2-4 tabs/day	1-2		Each tablet contains HCTZ 25 mg, spironolactone 25 mg
HCTZ and triamterene	1-4 caps/day	1-2		Each capsule contains HCTZ 25 mg, triamterene 50 mg
HCTZ and triamterene	1-2 tabs/day	1-2		Each tablet contains HCTZ 50 or 25 mg, triamterene 75 mg
Adrenergic inhibitors				
Rauwolfia derivatives				
Reserpine	0.25	1	Neutral	
Methyldopa	250-3,000	2-3	Mild ↓HDL	
Centrally acting agents				
Clonidine	0.1-2.4	2-3	↓TC, ↑HDL	
Guanabenz	8-64	1-2	↓LDL, → or ↑HDL, ↓TC	
Guanfacine	1-3	1-2	↓TC, ↓LDL, → or ↑HDL	
β-adrenergic blockers			↔ or ↑TC, ↔ or ↑LDL, ↓HDL (except for those with ISA)	
Acebutolol	200-1,200	1-2	Neutral or slight ↑HDL	Both acebutolol and pindolol have ISA
Pindolol	10-60	2	Neutral or slight ↑HDL	
Atenolol	50-100	1		
Metoprolol	100-450	2		
Nadolol	40-320	1		
Propranolol	40-640	2-4		
Timolol	20-40	1-2		
Mixed α and β blockers				
Labetalol	200-2,400	2	Neutral	
α blockers			↔ or ↓TC, ↓LDL, ↑HDL	
Prazosin	2-20	2-3		
Terazosin	2-20	1-2		

(continued)

Table 9. Types and Examples of Antihypertensive Drugs (*Continued*)

Agent	Dose Range (mg/day)	Frequency of Administration (times/day)	Effect on Serum Lipids	Notes
Vasodilators				
Nonspecific			Neutral	
Hydralazine	20-300	2-4		
Minoxidil	5-100	1-2		
Converting enzyme inhibitors			Neutral	
Captopril	50-450	2-4		
Enalapril	2.5-40	1-2		
Lisinopril	5-40	1-2		
Calcium blockers			Neutral	
Diltiazem	80-240	3-4		
Diltiazem SR	180-240	2		
Nifedipine	30-120	3-4		
Nifedipine GITS	30-90	1		
Nicardipine	30-90	3		
Verapamil	240-480	3-4		
Verapamil SR	120-480	1-2		

HDL = high-density lipoprotein; ISA = intrinsic sympathomimetic activity; LDL = low-density lipoprotein; TC = total cholesterol; SR = sustained release; GITS = gastrointestinal therapeutic system—once-a-day preparation.

*Effects of lipids are indicated for classes of drugs and do not in all cases indicate studies on individual drugs within a class.

Table 10. Demographic and Pathophysiologic Determinants of Responses to Antihypertensive Drugs

Factor	Diuretics	β blockers	α blockers	ACE Inhibitors	Ca Antagonists
Age (young/old)	More effective in older	More effective in young	Effective in both	More effective in young (?)	More effective in old (?)
Race (white/black)	More effective in black	More effective in white	Effective in both	More effective in white (?)	Effective in both
Sodium-volume	More effective	Less effective	Effective	Less effective	Effective
High renin	Less effective	More effective	Less effective	More effective	Less effective
Increased sympathetics	Less effective	More effective	More effective	Effective	Effective

Important: The effectiveness of the various drugs in different groups is *relative*, not absolute. For example, it has been shown recently that ACE inhibitors are effective in black as well as white persons, and calcium antagonists in young as well as elderly persons.

Modified from Dzau VJ: *Am J Med* 82 (Suppl IA):36, 1987.

Table 11. Effect of Antihypertensive Drugs on Concomitant Metabolic Disorders

Disorder	Diuretic	β Blocker	α Blocker	ACE Inhibitor	Ca Antagonist
Hyperlipidemia	May worsen	May worsen	No effect/ May Improve	No effect	No effect
Diabetes	May worsen	May worsen	No effect	No effect	No effect (?)
Hypokalemia	Worsens	No effect	No effect	May correct	No effect
Hyperuricemia	Worsens	No effect	No effect	No effect	No effect

Modified from Dzau VJ: *Am J Med* 82 (Suppl IA): 36, 1987.

Table 12. Effects of Antihypertensive Drugs on Coexisting Diseases

Disease	Diuretic	β Blocker	α Blocker	ACE Inhibitor	Ca Antagonist
Angina	No effect	Beneficial	No effect	Beneficial (?)	Beneficial
CHF	Beneficial	Worsens	No effect	Beneficial	± Beneficial (may worsen)
Arrhythmias	May worsen	Beneficial	No effect	No effect	Beneficial
COPD	No effect	Worsens	No effect	No effect	Beneficial (?)

CHF = congestive heart failure; COPD = chronic obstructive pulmonary disease.
Modified from Dzau VJ: *Am J Med* 82 (Suppl IA):36, 1987.

Table 13. Summary of Biochemical Effects of Antihypertensive Drugs

Drug	Potassium	Glucose	Uric Acid	Cholesterol
Thiazide diuretics	↓	↑	↑	↑
Beta blockers	↔	↔ ↑	↔	↔ ↑
Alpha blockers	↔	↔	↔	↓
Sympatholytics	↔	↔	↔	↔
ACE inhibitors	↔	↔	↔	↔
Calcium antagonists	↔	↔	↔	↔

↑ = increase; ↓ = decrease; ↔ = no change.
From Dzau VJ: *Am J Med* 82 (Suppl IA):36, 1987.

Table 14. Summary of Effects of Antihypertensive Drugs on Serum Lipid Profile

Drug	TC	LDL	HDL	Triglyceride
Thiazide diuretics	↑	↑	↔ ↓	↑
Beta blockers	↔ ↑	↔ ↑	↓	↑
Alpha blockers	↔ ↓	↓	↑	↔ ↓
Sympatholytics	↔	↓	↓	↑
ACE inhibitors	↔	↔	↔	↔
Calcium antagonists	↔	↔	↔	↔

↑ = increase; ↓ = decrease; ↔ = no change.
HDL = high-density lipoprotein; LDL = low-density lipoprotein; TC = total cholesterol.
Modified from Dzau VJ: *Am J Med* 82 (Suppl IA):36, 1987.

Table 15. Common Drug Interactions in Antihypertensive Therapy		
Drug Class	Antihypertensive Agent	Effect
Tricyclic antidepressants	Clonidine	Attenuate antihypertensive effect
	Alpha-methyldopa	As above
	Reserpine	As above
	Guanethidine	As above
	Bethanidine	As above
Sympathomimetics	Clonidine	Attenuate antihypertensive effect
	Alpha-methyldopa	As above
	Guanethidine	As above
Phenothiazines	Alpha-methyldopa	Paradoxical hypertension
	Guanethidine	Attenuate antihypertensive effect
MAO inhibitors	Guanethidine	Attenuate antihypertensive effect
	Alpha-methyldopa	Paradoxical hypertension
	Reserpine	Paradoxical hypertension
CNS depressants	Clonidine	Increase CNS depression
	Alpha-methyldopa	Increase CNS depression
		Barbiturates reduce alpha-methyldopa effect
	Reserpine	Increase CNS depression
Miscellaneous		
Digitalis	Diuretics	Hypokalemia, digitalis toxicity
Warfarin	Thiazides	Increase prothrombin time
Pyridoxine	Hydralazine	Blocks pyridoxine effects
L-dopa	Alpha-methyldopa	Interfere with L-dopa in treatment of Parkinson's disease
	Reserpine	As above
Anesthesia	Central sympatholytics	Hypotension
Digitalis, quinidine	Reserpine	Arrhythmias

CNS = central nervous system; MAO = monoamine oxidase.

first-line therapy generally includes an ACE inhibitor, a calcium channel blocker, or prazosin (Kaplan et al.). Converting enzyme inhibitors may retard renal deterioration in diabetic patients (Bjorck et al.).

A controversial topic is the magnitude and importance of the effects of antihypertensive drugs on serum lipid levels. A reduction in cardiovascular mortality in patients treated for hypertension has not been demonstrated (Houston; Zusman). Although more than 54,000 patients have been treated in antihypertensive drug trials, when the data are pooled, no consistent reduction in cardiovascular mortality is seen. This failure has been attributed to the small number of patients and short duration of the trials; the fact that in patients with preexisting coronary disease, a drop in perfusion pressure may precipitate coronary ischemia; or the adverse effects on serum lipids from the drugs used in the trials, mostly diuretics and beta blockers (Houston; O'Kelley et al.; Dzau 1989). A tradeoff between lowering one risk factor (hypertension) and raising another (serum lipid levels) may negate the beneficial effect of antihypertensive therapy. The metabolic side effects (especially involving serum lipids) of antihypertensive drugs are summarized in Tables 13 and 14.

With recent trials showing that lowering serum cholesterol reduces the frequency of coronary artery events (LRC I, II; Frick et al.), use of drugs such as beta blockers and diuretics is being reevaluated. Although it is certainly not proved that the use of drugs

Table 16. Conditions Associated with Hypertensive Crisis
Hypertensive emergencies
Malignant hypertension—eyegrounds reveal hemorrhages or exudates or papilledema
Hypertension with acute pulmonary edema
Hypertensive encephalopathy
CVA, including hemorrhage and infarction
Aortic dissection
Pheochromocytoma with severe hypertension
Hypertension following tyramine ingestion in patients taking MAO inhibitors
Severe toxemia or eclampsia
Urgent conditions associated with hypertension
Accelerated hypertension—eyegrounds reveal hemorrhage and exudates
Severe hypertension in a patient with myocardial infarction or severe angina
Occlusive stroke or transient ischemic attack in a hypertensive patient
Renal failure or significant renal impairment in a hypertensive patient
Marked hypertension associated with burns, acute glomerulonephritis or preeclampsia
Severe hypertension in patients with bleeding postoperatively
The patient with hypertension, new cardiovascular or neurologic symptoms
New patient with DBP >130 mm Hg
CVA = cerebrovascular accident; DBP = diastolic blood pressure; MAO = monoamine oxidase.

that do not adversely alter serum lipids results in a lower cardiovascular event rate, until more is known it is reasonable to use a drug that has a neutral or beneficial effect on serum lipid levels. These include ACE inhibitors, calcium channel blockers, alpha-adrenergic blockers, and beta-adrenergic blockers with intrinsic sympathomimetic activity. However, these drugs are often more expensive than the more conventional therapies.

INSULIN RESISTANCE

Studies have shown an association between hypertension and obesity with impaired glucose tolerance in humans (Chiang et al.; Jarrett et al.). Two recent studies reconfirmed this finding and showed that insulin resistance is a feature of untreated, early hypertension. Swislocki et al. looked at 16 normal and 14 untreated hypertensive patients, matched for age, weight, and lean body fat, and measured their steady-state plasma glucose and insulin concentrations achieved during the last 30 minutes of a 180-minute continuous infusion of somatostatin, insulin, and glu-

cose. Under these conditions, differences in the steady-state plasma glucose concentrations allowed comparison of the ability of exogenous insulin to stimulate disposal of an identical glucose load in various individuals. Compared with normal controls, the men with untreated hypertension had significantly elevated plasma glucose and insulin concentrations after the oral challenge, thus reconfirming the earlier observations that patients with hypertension are insulin resistant, hyperglycemic and hyperinsulinemic. Pollare et al. (1990) demonstrated similar results: they studied 143 newly detected hypertensive patients (of whom 59% were obese), using the euglycemic insulin clamp technique. They assessed insulin sensitivity by measuring both the basal insulin levels and the rate of glucose disposal after an intravenous glucose tolerance test. Hypertensive patients with normal body weight demonstrated insulin resistance, as indicated by an increased basal insulin level and decreased rate of glucose deposition.

These results may have implications for treatment of hypertension. Zavaroni et al. recently showed that healthy persons with hyperinsulinemia and normal

Table 17. Selection of Drugs for Use in Hypertensive Crises		
Type of Hypertensive Crisis	Drug of Choice (Parenteral)	Drugs to Avoid (or Use Cautiously)
Acute hypertensive encephalopathy	Diazoxide Nitroprusside Trimethaphan Labetalol	Rauwolfia Methyldopa Clonidine Guanethidine Propranolol
Intracerebral or subarachnoid hemorrhage	Nitroprusside Trimethaphan	Sympatholytics
Acute pulmonary edema with hypertension	Nitroprusside Trimethaphan Reserpine Methyldopa Furosemide Hydralazine	Diazoxide
Pheochromocytoma or MAO inhibitor with tyramines or sympathomimetics	Phentolamine or phenoxybenzamine or nitroprusside, plus propranolol	Sympatholytics
Acute glomerulonephritis or lupus nephritis crisis	Nitroprusside Diazoxide Hydralazine Methyldopa Furosemide	Trimethaphan
Dissecting aortic aneurysm	Trimethaphan Reserpine Nitroprusside Methyldopa Furosemide Labetalol	Hydralazine Diazoxide
Acute myocardial infarction	Propranolol Nitroglycerin	Hydralazine Diazoxide

Modified from Onesti G, Lowenthal DV, eds: *The Spectrum of Antihypertensive Drug Therapy.* Hahnemann College: Hahnemann Medical Proceeding, Seminar in Therapeutics; Nov. 1976, p. 106. With permission.

glucose tolerance tests have an increased risk for coronary artery disease compared with well-matched healthy controls. Since hypertensive patients have an increased incidence of insulin resistance, this may explain in part the higher incidence of coronary events in this group. It may also alter therapeutic approaches. The recent report by Pollare et al. demonstrated that hydrochlorothiazide, compared with captopril, had adverse effects on lipid metabolism,

as well as glucose metabolism. Using the euglycemic insulin clamp technique, they found that hydrochlorothiazide significantly decreased the insulin sensitivity index after 18 weeks of treatment. Captopril had no effect. These results may help explain some of the disparity between the effective control of hypertension and the lack of impact on coronary disease prevalence. The mechanisms for the increased cardiovascular risk and increased insulin resistance associated with hypertension are not well understood.

TREATMENT OF REFRACTORY HYPERTENSION

In evaluating patients with treatment-resistant hypertension, one must consider several factors:

Compliance. The most common cause of uncontrolled hypertension is patient noncompliance. This is frequently difficult to document. A careful and thorough history is important, paying particular attention to the patient's understanding of the drug regimen and a history of drug side effects. Measurements of plasma or 24-hour urine drug concentrations, and use of pill counts, have been useful in documenting patient noncompliance.

Secondary forms of hypertension. The possibility of secondary forms of hypertension should be evaluated in all patients who require step 4 drugs.

Drug interactions. Drug interactions that can result in attenuation of the effect of certain antihypertensives (e.g., tricyclic antidepressants with adrenergic blocking agents) should be excluded. A list of such drug interactions is shown in Table 15.

Inappropriate drug combinations. In evaluating drug combinations, it is helpful to separate antihypertensive agents into three broad classes: diuretics, sympatholytics, and vasodilators. Ordinarily, a second drug from the same class should not be added to a regimen because it may have little or no additional effect. For example, a patient refractory to hydrochlorothiazide, propranolol, and alpha-methyldopa should be switched to hydrochlorothiazide, propranolol, and hydralazine.

Activation of cardiovascular compensatory mechanisms. Certain drugs can activate cardiovascular compensatory mechanisms that may result in the attenuation of the primary antihypertensive action of the drug. For example, hydralazine stimulates the sympathetic nervous system (reflex tachycardia), activates the renin-angiotensin system, and promotes sodium retention. For these reasons, long-term hydralazine monotherapy is ineffective for blood pressure control.

HYPERTENSIVE CRISIS

Conditions that are hypertensive *emergencies,* requiring immediate control of blood pressure, and those that are *urgencies,* in which hypertension should be controlled over hours to days, must be differentiated. Emergencies are associated with an immediate grave prognosis if blood pressure remains uncontrolled. Rapid-acting parenteral antihypertensive agents are the agents of choice for treatment of these patients, while a rigorous regimen of oral drugs can be used in patients experiencing hypertensive urgency. Table 16 lists conditions that are classified as hypertensive emergencies and urgencies, and Table 17 lists drugs, their action, and indications for use in hypertensive crises.

Bibliography

Abrams HL, Siegelman SS, Adams DF, et al: Computed tomography versus ultrasound of the adrenal gland. A prospective study. *Radiology* 143:121, 1982.

Arisamano GG, Foster TA, Voors AW, et al: Influence of persistent obesity in children on cardiovascular risk factors: The Bogalusa Heart Study. *Circulation* 69:895, 1984.

Bauer GE, Humphrey TJ: The natural history of hypertension with moderate impairment of renal function. *Clin Sci Mol Med* 45:191s, 1973.

Bechgard P: Arterial hypertension; a follow-up study of one thousand hypertonics. *Acta Med Scand* (Suppl)172:3, 1946.

Bennett C: The syndrome of accelerated or malignant hypertension. *Cardiovasc Med* 4:1141, 1979.

Bergstron J, Alvestrand A, Bucht H, Gutierrez A: Progression of chronic renal failure in man is retarded with more frequent clinical follow-ups and better blood pressure control. *Clin Nephrol* 25:1, 1986.

Bjorck S, Nyberg G, Mulec H, et al: Beneficial effects of angiotensin-converting enzyme inhibitor on renal function in patients with diabetic nephropathy. *Br Med J* 293:471, 1986.

Bianchetti MG, Beretta-Piccoli C, Weidman P, Ferrier C: Blood pressure control in normotensive members of hypertensive families. *Kidney Int* 29:882, 1986.

Birkenhager WH, Kho TL, Schalekamp MADA, et al: Renin levels and cardiovascular morbidity in essential hypertension. A prospective study. *Acta Clin Belg* 32:168, 1977.

Bouloux PMG, Perret D: Interference of labetalol metabolites in the determination of plasma catecholamines by HPLC with electrochemical detection. *Clin Chim Acta* 150:111, 1985.

Bravo EL, Gifford RW: Pheochromocytoma: Diagnosis, localization and management. *N Engl J Med* 311:1298, 1981.

Bravo EL, Tarazi RC, Dustan HP, et al: The changing spectrum of primary aldosteronism. *Am J Med* 74:641, 1983.

Bravo EL, Tarazi RC, Fouad FM, et al: Clonidine-suppression test: A useful aid in the diagnosis of pheochromocytoma. *N Engl J Med* 305:623, 1981.

Bravo EL, Tarazi RC, Gifford RW, et al: Circulating and urinary catecholamines in pheochromocytoma: Diagnostic and pathophysiologic implications. *N Engl J Med* 301:682, 1979.

Brunner HR, Laragh JH, Baer L, et al: Essential hypertension: Renin and aldosterone, heart attack and stroke. *N Engl J Med* 286:441, 1972.

Canner PL, Berge KG, Wenger NK, et al: Fifteen year mortality in Coronary Drug Project patients: Long-term benefits with niacin. *J Am Coll Cardiol* 8:1245, 1986.

Casale PN, Devereux RB, Kligfield P, et al: Electrocardiographic detection of left ventricular hypertrophy: Development and prospective validation of improved criteria. *J Am Coll Cardiol* 6:572, 1985.

Casale PN, Devereux RB, Milner M, et al: Value of echocardiographic measurement of left ventricular mass in predicting cardiovascular morbid events in hypertensive men. *Ann Intern Med* 105:173, 1986.

Case DB, Laragh JH: Reactive hyperreninemia in renovascular hypertension after angiotensin blockade with saralasin or converting enzyme inhibitor. *Ann Intern Med* 91:153, 1979.

Castelli WP, Anderson K: A population at risk: Prevalence of high cholesterol levels in hypertensive patients in the Framingham study. *Am J Med* (Suppl 2A)80:23, 1986.

Catt KZ, Kimmet PZ, Cain MD, et al: Angiotensin II blood levels in human hypertension. *Lancet* 1:459, 1971.

Chiang B, Perlman LY, Epstein F: Overweight and hypertension: A review. *Circulation* 39:403, 1969.

Christian HA: Discussion of paper by Paullin JE. Ultimate results of essential hypertension. *JAMA* 87:931, 1926.

Conn JW: Primary aldosteronism, a new clinical syndrome. *J Lab Clin Med* 45:3, 1955.

Conn JW, Cohen EL, Lucas CP, et al: Primary reninism, hypertension, hyperreninemia, and secondary aldosteronism due to renin-producing juxtaglomerular cell tumors. *Arch Intern Med* 130:682, 1972.

Cooke JP, Safford RE: Progress in the diagnosis and management of aortic dissection. *Mayo Clin Proc* 61:147, 1986.

Cruickshank JM, Thorp JM, Zacharias FJ: Benefits of and potential harm of lowering high blood pressure. *Lancet* 1:581, 1987.

Devereux RB, Reichek N: Echocardiographic determination of left ventricular mass in man. *Circulation* 55:613, 1977.

Devereux RB, Alonso DR, Lutas EM, et al: Echocardiography assessment of left ventricular hypertrophy: Comparison to necropsy findings. *Am J Cardiol* 57:450, 1986.

Dunn FG, Chandraratna PN, de Carvalho JGR, Basta LL, Frohlich ED: Pathophysiologic assessment of hypertensive heart disease with echocardiography. *Am J Cardiol* 39:789, 1977.

Dzau VJ: Significance of vascular renin angiotensin pathways. *Hypertension* 8:553, 1986.

Dzau VJ: Recommendations of the Adult Treatment Panel of the National Cholesterol Education Program. Implications for the management of hypertension. *AHA Focus Series* 3:16, 1989.

Dzau VJ, Gibbons GH, Levin DC: Renovascular hypertension: An update on pathophysiology, diagnosis and therapy. *Am J Nephrol* 3:172, 1983.

Dzau VJ, Pratt RE: Renin-angiotensin system: Biology, physiology and pharmacology. In: Fozzard HA, Jennings RB, Haber E, Katz AM, Morgan HE. *The Heart and Cardiovascular System*. New York: Raven Press; p. 1031, 1986.

Fieschi C, Prencipe M, Carolie A, et al: Case-control study of focal cerebral ischemia in young adults. *Neurology* (Suppl)1:83, 1987.

Finnie KJC, Watts DG, Armstrong PW: Biases in the measurement of arterial pressure. *Crit Care Med* 12:965, 1984.

Fisher CM: Lacunaes: Small, deep cerebral infarcts. *Neurology* 15:774, 1965.

Fisher CM: The arterial lesions underlying lacunaes. *Acta Neuropathol* 12:1, 1969.

Frick MH, Elo O, Haapa K, et al: Helsinki Heart Study: Primary prevention trial with gemfibrozil in middle-aged men with dyslipidemia: Safety of treatment, changes in risk factors, and incidence of coronary heart disease. *N Engl J Med* 317:1237, 1987.

Frohlich ED, Grimm C, Labarthe DR, Maxwell MH, Perloff D: Recommendations for human blood pressure determination by sphygmomanometers. *Circulation* 77:592A, 1988.

Frohlich ED, Tarazi RC, Dustan HP: Clinical-physiological correlations in the development of hypertensive heart disease. *Circulation* 44:446, 1971.

Furlan AJ, Whisnant JP, Elueback LR: The decreasing incidence of primary intracerebral hemorrhage. A population study. *Ann Neurol* 5:307, 1979.

Gandolfo C, Loeb C, Moretti C, et al: Patient characteristics in the cooperative study of focal cerebral ischemia in young adults. In: Meyer JS, Lechner H, Reivich M, Ott EO, eds. Proceedings of the World Federation of Neurology 13th International Salzburg Conference. Amsterdam: Excerpta Medica, International Congress Series 736; *Cerebral Vascular Disease* 6:77, 1987.

Gardner JW, Moutain CE, Hines EA: The relationship of migraine to hypertension headaches. *Am J Med Sci* 200:50, 1940.

Gavras H, Oliver N, Aitchison J, et al: Abnormalities of coagulation and the development of malignant phase hypertension. *Kidney Int* 8:252s, 1976.

Geyskes GG, Dei HY, Puylaert CBAJ, et al: Renovascular hypertension identified by captopril-induced changes in the renogram. *Hypertension* 9:451, 1987.

Gifford RW, Westbrook E: Hypertensive encephalopathy: Mechanisms, clinical features, and treatment. *Prog Cardiovasc Dis* 17:115, 1974.

Gifford RW, Kirkendall W, O'Connor DT, Weidman W: Office evaluation of hypertension. Special report. *Hypertension* 13:283, 1989.

Glancy DL, Morrow AG, Simon AL, Roberts WC: Juxtaductal aortic coarctation—analysis of 84 patients studied hemodynamically, angiographically and morphologically after age 1 year. *Am J Cardiol* 51:537, 1983.

Hagberg J, Goldring D, Ehsani A, et al: Effect of exercise training on the blood pressure and hemodynamic features of hypertensive adolescents. *Am J Cardiol* 52:763, 1983.

Hall W: Pharmacologic therapy of hypertension in blacks. *J Clin Hypertens* 20:108S, 1987.

Haulk R, Hubert H, Fabsitz R, et al: Weight and hypertension. *Ann Intern Med* 98:855, 1983.

Healton EB, Brust JC, Feinfeld DA, Thomsom GE: Hypertensive encephalopathy and the neurologic manifestations of malignant hypertension. *Neurol* 32:127, 1982.

Helmer OM: Renin activity in blood from patients with hypertension. *J Can Med Assoc* 90:221, 1964.

Heptinstal RH: Hypertension. In: *Pathology of the Kidney*. Boston: Little Brown; 1974, p. 121.

Holland OB, Brown H, Kuhnert LV, et al: Further evaluation of saline infusion for the diagnosis of primary aldosteronism. *Hypertension* 6:717, 1984.

Hollenberg NK, Williams GH: Angiotensin as a renal, adrenal and cardiovascular hormone: Responses to saralasin in normal man and essential and secondary hypertension. *Kidney Int* 15:529, 1975.

Horne ML, Conklin VM, Ueenan RE, Varedy PD, DiNardo S: Angiotensin II profiling with saralasin: Summary of Eaton collaborative study. *Kidney Int* [Suppl]15:S1, 1978.

Houston MC: New insights and new approaches for the treatment of essential hypertension: Selection of therapy based on coronary heart disease risk factor analysis, hemodynamic profiles, quality of life, and subsets of hypertension. *Am Heart J* 117:911, 1989.

Hunter A, Rogers OH: Mortality study of impaired lives, no. 2. *Trans Acta Soc Am* 24:738, 1923.

Inouye I, Massie B, Loge D, et al: Abnormal left ventricular filling: An early finding in mild to moderate systemic hypertension. *Am J Cardiol* 53:120, 1984.

Inzitari D, Bianchi F, Pracucci G, et al: The Italian Multicenter Study of Reversible Cerebral Ischemic Attacks. IV. Blood pressure components and atherosclerotic lesions. *Stroke* 17:185, 1986.

Jackson R, Stewart A, Beaglehole R, Scruggs A: Alcohol consumption and blood pressure. *Am J Epidemiol* 122:1037, 1985.

Janeway TC: A clinical study of hypertensive cardiovascular disease. *Arch Intern Med* 12:755, 1913.

Jarrett RJ, Keen H, McCarney M, et al: Glucose tolerance and blood pressure in two population samples: Their relation to diabetes mellitus and hypertension. *Int J Epidemiol* 7:15, 1978.

Johansson B, Strandgaard S, Lassen NS: On the pathogenesis of hypertensive encephalopathy: The hypertensive breakthrough of autoregulation of cerebral blood flow with forced vasodilation, flow increase and blood brain barrier damage. *Circ Res* (Suppl)34:167, 1974.

Joint National Committee on Detection, Evaluation, and Treatment of High Blood Pressure (JNC IV): The 1988 Report of the Joint National Committee on Detection, Evaluation, and Treatment of High Blood Pressure. *Arch Intern Med* 148:1023, 1988.

Jorgensen RS, Houston BK: Family history of hypertension, personality patterns, and cardiovascular reactivity to stress. *Psychosomatic Med* 48:102, 1980.

Julius S, Weder AB, Egan BM: Pathophysiology of early hypertension: Implications for epidemiologic research. In: Gross F, Strassert T, eds. *Mild Hypertension: Recent Advances.* New York: Raven Press; p. 219, 1979.

Kahn JR, Skeggs LT, Shumway NP, et al: The assay of hypertension from the arterial blood of normotensive and hypertensive human beings. *J Exp Med* 95:523, 1952.

Kannel WB: Prevalence and natural history of electrocardiographic left ventricular hypertrophy. *Am J Med* 75:4, 1983.

Kannel WB, Schatzbin A: Risk factor analysis. *Prog Cardiovasc Dis* 26:309, 1983.

Kannel WB, Castelli WP, McNamara PM, McKee PA, Feinleib M: Role of blood pressure in the development of congestive heart failure. *N Engl J Med* 287:781, 1972.

Kannel WB, Gordon T, Offurt D: Left ventricular hypertrophy by electrocardiogram. Prevalence, incidence, and mortality in the Framingham study. *Ann Intern Med* 71:89, 1989.

Kaplan N, Rosenstock J, Raskin P: A differing view of treatment of hypertension in patients with diabetes mellitus. *Arch Intern Med* 147:1160, 1987.

Kaplan NM: Renin profiles: The unfulfilled promises. *JAMA* 238:611, 1977.

Katsky AL, Friedman GD, Armstrong MA: The relationship between alcoholic beverage use and other traits to blood pressure: A new Kaiser-Permanente study. *Circulation* 73:628, 1986.

Kem DC, Weinberger MH, Mayes DM, Nugent CA: Saline suppression of plasma aldosterone in hypertension. *Arch Intern Med* 128:380, 1971.

Kleinert HD, Harshfield GA, Pickering TG, et al: What is the value of home blood pressure measurement in patients with mild hypertension? *Hypertension* 6:574, 1984.

Korner PH: Circulatory regulation in hypertension. *Br J Clin Pharmacol* 13:95, 1982.

Krotkiewski M, Mandroukas K, Sjostrom L, et al: Effects of long-term physical training on body fat, metabolism and blood pressure in obesity. *Metabolism* 28:650, 1979.

Kupari M: Acute cardiovascular effects of ethanol: A controlled non-invasive study. *Br Heart J* 49:174, 1983.

Langford H, Blaufox MD, Oberman A, et al: Dietary therapy slows the return of hypertension after stopping prolonged medication. *JAMA* 253:657, 1985.

Levy D, Garrison RJ, Savage DD, Kannel WB, Castelli WP: Left ventricular mass and incidence of coronary heart disease in an elderly cohort. *Ann Intern Med* 110:101, 1989.

Lindsay J Jr, Hurst JW: Clinical features and prognosis in dissecting aneurysm of the aorta: A re-appraisal. *Circulation* 35:880, 1967.

Linfors EW, Feussner JR, Blessing CL, et al: Spurious hypertension in the obese patient. Effect of sphygmomanometer cuff size on prevalence of hypertension. *Arch Intern Med* 144:1482, 1984.

Lipid Research Clinics (LRC) Program: The Lipid Research Clinics Coronary Primary Prevention Trial results: I. Reduction in incidence of coronary heart disease. *JAMA* 251:351, 1984.

Lipid Research Clinics (LRC) Program: The Lipid Research Clinics Coronary Primary Prevention Trial results. II. The relationship of reduction in incidence of coronary heart disease to cholesterol lowering. *JAMA* 251:365, 1984.

Lund-Johansen P: Hemodynamic alterations in hypertension—spontaneous changes and effects of drug therapy. *Acta Med Scand* (Suppl)603:1, 1977.

Lyons DF, Streck WF, Kem DC, et al: Captopril stimulation of differential renins in renovascular hypertension. *Hypertension* 5:615, 1983.

MacGregor GA, Best F, Cam JM, et al: Double-blind randomized crossover trial of moderate sodium restriction in essential hypertension. *Lancet* 1:351, 1982.

MacMahon SW, MacDonald GJ: Antihypertensive treatment and plasma lipoprotein levels. The associations in data from a population study. *Am J Med* 80(Suppl 2A):40, 1986.

MacMahon SW, Norton RN: Alcohol and hypertension: Implications for prevention and treatment. *Ann Intern Med* 105:124, 1986.

Manger CM, Gifford RW, eds: *Pheochromocytoma.* New York: Springer-Verlag; 1977, p. 398.

Manning DM, Kuchirha C, Kaminski J: Miscuffing: Inappropriate blood pressure cuff application. *Circulation* 68:763, 1983.

Manu P, Runge LA: Biochemical screening for pheochromocytoma: Superiorlty of urinary metanephrine measurements. *Am J Epidemiol* 120:788, 1989.

Marks LS, Maxwell MH: Renal vein renin: Value and limitations in the prediction of operative results. *Urol Clin North Am* 2:311, 1975.

Marks LS, Maxwell MH, Varady PD, Lupu AN, Kaufman JJ: Renovascular hypertension: Does the renal vein ratio predict operative results? *J Urol* 115:365, 1976.

Maxwell MH, Gonick HC, Wiita R, Kaufman JJ: Use of the rapid-sequence intravenous pyelogram in the diagnosis of renovascular hypertension. *N Engl J Med* 270:213, 1964.

McLeod D, Marshall J, Kohner EM, Bird AC: The role of axoplasmic flow in the pathogenesis of retinal cotton wool spots. *Br J Ophthalmol* 61:177, 1977.

Medical Research Council Working Party: MRC trial of treatment of mild hypertension: Principal results. *Br Med J* 291:97, 1985.

Messerli FH, De Carvalho JGR, Christie B, Frohlich ED: Systemic and regional hemodyamics in low, normal, and high cardiac output in borderline hypertension. *Circulation* 58:441, 1978.

Messerli FH, Frohlich ED, Suarez DH, et al: Borderline hypertension: Relationship between age, hemodynamics, and circulating catecholamines. *Circulation* 64:760, 1981.

Mitchell JRA: Nose-bleeding and high blood pressure. *Br Med J* 1:25, 1959.

Morgan T, Gillies A, Morgan G, et al: Hypertension treated by salt restriction. *Lancet* 1:227, 1978.

Moser M, Lunn J, Materson B: Comparative effects of diltiazem and hydrochlorothiazide in blacks with systemic hypertension. *Am J Cardiol* 56:101H, 1985.

Moser M, Wish H, Friedman AP: Headache and hypertension. *JAMA* 180:115, 1962.

Mujais SK, Emmanouel DS, Kasinath BS, Spargo BH: Marked proteinuria in hypertensive nephrosclerosis. *Am J Nephrol* 5:190, 1985.

Muller FB, Dealey JE, Case DB, et al: The captopril test for identifying renovascular disease in hypertensive patients. *Am J Med* 80:633, 1986.

Multiple Risk Factor Intervention Trial: Risk factor changes and mortality results. *JAMA* 248:1465, 1982.

Mutlu N, Berry RG, Alpers BJ: Massive cerebral hemorrhage: Clinical and pathological correlations. *Arch Neurol* 8:644, 1963.

O'Kelley BF, Massie BM, Tubau JF, Szlochcic J: Coronary morbidity and mortality, pre-existing silent coronary artery disease, and mild hypertension. *Ann Intern Med* 110:1017, 1985.

Padfield PL, Morton JJ: Proceedings: Application of a sensitive radioimmunoassay for plasma arginine vasopressin pathological conditions in man (abstr). *Clin Sci Mol Med* 47:16p, 1974.

Parijs J, Joosens JV, Vader Linden L, et al: Moderate sodium restriction and diuretics in the treatment of hypertension. *Am Heart J* 85:22, 1973.

Paronetto F: Immunocytochemical observation on the vascular necrosis and renal glomerular lesions of malignant nephrosclerosis. *Am J Pathol* 46:901, 1965.

Perloff D, Sokolow M, Cowan R: The prognostic value of ambulatory blood pressures. *JAMA* 249:2792, 1983.

Pickering TG, Devereux RB: Ambulatory monitoring of blood pressure as a predictor of cardiovascular risk. *Am Heart J* 114:925, 1987.

Pickering TG, Harshfield GA, Laragh JH: Ambulatory versus casual blood pressure in the diagnosis of hypertensive patients. *Clin Exp Hypertens* A7:257, 1985.

Pollare T, Lithell H, Berne C: A comparison of the effects of hydrochlorothiazide and captopril on glucose and lipid metabolism in patients with hypertension. *N Engl J Med* 321:868, 1989.

Pollare T, Lithell H, Berne C: Insulin resistance is a characteristic feature of primary hypertension independent of obesity. *Metabolism* 39:167, 1990.

Reichek N, Devereux RB: Left ventricular hypertrophy: Relationship of anatomic, echocardiographic and electrocardiographic findings. *Circulation* 63:1391, 1981.

Richards A, Espiner E, Maslowski A, et al: Blood-pressure response to moderate sodium restriction and to potassium supplementation in mild essential hypertension. *Lancet* 1:757, 1984.

Schottstaedt MF, Sokolow M: The natural history and course of hypertension with papilledema (malignant hypertension). *Am Heart J* 45:331, 1953.

Sfakianakis GN, Bourgoignie JJ, Jaffe D, et al: Single dose captopril scintigraphy in the diagnosis of renovascular hypertension. *J Nucl Med* 28:1383, 1987.

Shaheen OH: Arterial epistaxis. *J Laryngol Otol* 89:17, 1975.

Silman A, Locke C, Mitchell P, et al: Evaluation of the effectiveness of a low sodium diet in the treatment of mild to moderate hypertension. *Lancet* 1:1179, 1983.

Simon N, Franklin SS, Bleifer KH, Maxwell MH: Clinical characteristics of renovascular hypertension. *JAMA* 220:1209, 1972.

Sisson JC, Frager MS, Valk TW, et al: Scintigraphic localization of pheochromocytoma. *N Engl J Med* 305:12, 1981.

Slater EE, DeSanctis RW: The clinical recognition of dissecting aortic aneurysm. *Am J Med* 60:625, 1976.

Sokolow M, Werdegar D, Daim HK, et al: Relationship between level of blood pressure measured casually and by portable recorders and severity of complications in essential hypertension. *Circulation* 34:279, 1966.

Stadel BV: Oral contraceptives and cardiovascular disease. *N Engl J Med* 305:672, 1981.

Stewart BH, Bravo EL, Haaga J, et al: Localization of pheochromocytoma by computed tomography. *N Engl J Med* 299:460, 1978.

Subcommittee on Definition and Prevalence of the 1984 Joint National Committee: Hypertension prevalence and the status of awareness, treatment, and control in the United States: Final report of the Subcommittee on Definition and Prevalence of the 1984 Joint National Committee. *Hypertension* 7:457, 1985.

Sugimoto T, Rosansky SJ: The incidence of treated end stage renal disease in the Eastern United States: 1973-1979. *Am J Public Health* 74:14, 1984.

Swislocki ALM, Hoffman BB, Reaven GM: Insulin resistance, glucose intolerance and hyperinsulinemia in patients with hypertension. *Am J Hypertens* 2:419, 1989.

Tarazi RC, Levy M: Cardiac responses to increased afterload. State of the art review. *Hypertension* 4(Suppl II):II-8, 1982.

Thibonnier M, Sassano P, Joseph A, et al: Diagnostic value of a single dose of captopril in renin and aldosterone dependent surgically curable hypertension. *Cardiovasc Rev Rep* 3:1659, 1982.

Topol EJ, Traill TA, Fortuin NJ: Hypertensive hypertrophic cardiomyopathy of the elderly. *N Engl J Med* 312:277, 1985.

Vaughan NJA, Jowett TP, Slater JDH, et al: The diagnosis of primary hyperaldosteronism. *Lancet* 1:120, 1981.

Vaziri ND: Malignant or accelerated hypertension. *West J Med* 140:575, 1984.

Veterans Administration Cooperative Study Group on Antihypertensive Agents I: Results in patients with diastolic blood pressure averaging 115-129 mm Hg. *JAMA* 202:1028, 1967.

Veterans Administration Cooperative Study Group on Antihypertensive Agents: Effects of treatment on morbidity in hypertension. II. Results in patients with diastolic pressure averaging 90-114 mm Hg. *JAMA* 213:1143, 1970.

Veterans Administration Cooperative Study Group on Antihypertensive Agents: Comparison of propranolol and hydrochlorothiazide for the initial treatment of hypertension. I. Results of short-term titration with emphasis on racial differences in response. *JAMA* 248:1996, 1982.

Walker CH: Migraine and its relationship to hypertension. *Br Med J* 2:1430, 1959.

Watt G, Edwards C, Hart J, et al: Dietary sodium restriction for mild hypertension in general practice. *Br Med J* 286:432, 1983.

Weinberger MH, Cohen SJ, Miller JZ, et al: Dietary sodium restriction as adjunctive treatment of hypertension. *JAMA* 259:2561, 1988.

Weinberger MH, Grimm CE, Hollifield JW, et al: Primary aldosteronism. *Ann Intern Med* 90:386, 1979.

Weis NS: Relationship of high blood pressure to headache, epistaxis, and selected other symptoms. *N Engl J Med* 287:631, 1972.

Wenting GH, Tan-Tjiong HL, Derkx FHM, et al: Split renal function after captopril in unilateral and renal artery stenosis. *Br Med J* 288:886, 1984.

Wikstrand J: Left ventricular function in early primary hypertension. Functional consequences of cardiovascular structural changes. *Hypertension* 6(Suppl III):III-108, 1984.

Wilcox C, Williams CM, Smith TB, et al: Diagnostic uses of angiotensin converting enzyme inhibition in renovascular hypertension. *Am J Hypertens* 1:3445, 1988.

Wilson SK, Hutchins GM: Aortic dissecting aneurysms: Causative factors in 204 cases. *Arch Pathol Lab Med* 106:175, 1982.

Wing R, Jeffery R: Outpatient treatments of obesity. A comparison of methodology and clinical results. *Int J Obesity* 3:261, 1979.

Wolf PA, Kannel WB, Verter J: Epidemiologic appraisal of hypertension and stroke risk. In: Guthrie GP, Kotchen TA, eds. *Hypertension and the Brain.* New York: Futura; 1984, p. 221.

Woythaler JN, Singer SL, Kwan OL, et al: Accuracy of echocardiography versus electrocardiography in detecting left ventricular hypertrophy: Comparison with postmortem mass measurements. *J Am Coll Cardiol* 2:305, 1983.

Zavaroni I, Bonora E, Pagliara M, et al: Risk factors for coronary artery disease in healthy persons with hyperinsulinemia and normal glucose tolerance. *N Engl J Med* 320:702, 1989.

Zusman RM: Alterations to traditional antihypertensive therapy. *Hypertension* 8:837, 1986.

28 Pulmonary Hypertension and Cor Pulmonale

Robert A. Kloner

PULMONARY HYPERTENSION

Pulmonary hypertension is defined as the presence of pulmonary artery (PA) systolic pressure >30 mm Hg and PA mean pressure >20 mm Hg. Normally, PA pressures are 18–25 mm Hg systolic, 6–10 mm Hg diastolic, and 12–16 mm Hg mean. Pulmonary hypertension is considered severe when PA pressures are greater than approximately 75% of systemic arterial pressures. Pulmonary hypertension may occur secondary to a variety of disorders, or it may be idiopathic.

The classification of causes of pulmonary hypertension, as recently described by Grossman and Braunwald, is shown in Table 1. Figure 1 illustrates basic mechanisms of increases in pulmonary vascular resistance including loss of pulmonary blood vessels, obstruction of blood vessels as occurs with pulmonary thromboembolism, and narrowing of the vessels due to anatomic changes or vasoconstriction. Alveolar hypoxia is a potent cause of pulmonary arterial vasoconstriction; acidosis also may cause pulmonary vasoconstriction.

The anatomic changes which have been associated with pulmonary hypertension and which were recently reviewed by Rounds and Hill include arterial smooth muscle hypertrophy and longitudinal smooth muscle proliferation (stimulated by chronic hypoxia); eccentric intimal fibrosis and web formation (associated with thromboemboli); venous intimal proliferation and fibrosis (associated with veno-occlusive disease); and plexogenic pulmonary arteriopathy (seen with primary pulmonary hypertension, in pulmonary hypertension due to cardiac shunts and in association with collagen vascular disease, liver cirrhosis, and aminorex fumarate [an appetite suppressant] ingestion). Plexogenic pulmonary arteriopathy as described by Wagenvoort consists of several pathologic findings including pulmonary arterial medial hypertrophy, intimal proliferation, concentric laminar intimal fibrosis ("onion skin" configuration), fibrinoid necrosis with or without arteritis, and dilated thin-walled side branches with endothelial proliferation (plexiform lesion). Rich and Brundage (1989) recently suggested that the abnormalities of structure and function in plexogenic pulmonary arteriopathy could inhibit endothelial derived relaxation.

Although the signs and symptoms associated with pulmonary hypertension vary to some extent depending on the associated illness, there are several common features. Patients typically complain of dyspnea, atypical chest pain, and weakness. With severe and long-standing pulmonary hypertension, symptoms of right ventricular failure emerge with peripheral edema, gastrointestinal complaints, and ascites. Marked fatigue, dizziness, and sometimes syncope occur due to low forward cardiac output. If pulmonary hypertension is secondary to cardiac disease, such as left ventricular failure or mitral valve disease, the symptoms may predominantly reflect pulmonary congestion-orthopnea, dyspnea on exertion, and paroxysmal nocturnal dyspnea. If pulmonary hypertension is secondary to chronic obstructive lung disease, symptoms are predominantly related to pulmonary disease with dyspnea, cough, and frequent episodes of bronchitis. Difficulties in sleep should prompt consideration of the sleep-apnea syndrome.

Signs of pulmonary hypertension with right ventricular pressure overload include distended jugular venous neck veins, with a prominent a-wave; a left parasternal lift due to right ventricular hypertrophy; a palpable P_2; and a palpable systolic pulsation in the second left intercostal space due to a dilated pulmonary artery. On auscultation, the second heart sound (S_2) is closely split, the pulmonic component is louder than the aortic component, and a right ventricular S_4

Table 1. Classification of Pulmonary Hypertension

Increased resistance to pulmonary venous drainage
  Elevated left ventricular diastolic pressure
    Left ventricular failure
    Reduced left ventricular compliance
    Constrictive pericarditis
  Left atrial hypertension
    Mitral valve disease
    Cor triatriatum
    Left atrial myxoma or thrombus
  Pulmonary venous obstruction
    Congenital stenosis of pulmonary veins
    Anomalous pulmonary venous connection with obstruction
    Pulmonary veno-occlusive disease
    Mediastinal fibrosis
Increased resistance to flow through pulmonary vascular bed
  Decreased cross-sectional area of pulmonary vascular bed secondary to parenchymal diseases
    Chronic obstructive pulmonary disease, restrictive lung disease
    Collagen-vascular diseases (scleroderma, systemic lupus erythematosus [SLE], rheumatoid arthritis)
    Fibrotic reactions (Hamman-Rich syndrome, desquamative interstitial pneumonitis, pulmonary hemosiderosis)
    Sarcoidosis
    Neoplasm
    Pneumonia
    Status post pulmonary resection
    Congenital pulmonary hypoplasia (Down's syndrome)
  Decreased cross-sectional area of pulmonary vascular bed secondary to Eisenmenger's syndrome
  Other conditions associated with decreased cross-sectional area of the pulmonary vascular bed
    Primary pulmonary hypertension
    Hepatic cirrhosis and/or portal thrombosis
    Chemically induced—aminorex fumarate, *Crotalaria* alkaloids
    Persistent fetal circulation in the newborn
Increased resistance to flow through large pulmonary arteries
  Pulmonary thromboembolism
  Peripheral pulmonic stenosis
  Unilateral absence or stenosis of a pulmonary artery
Hypoventilation
  Obesity-hypoventilation syndrome
  Pharyngeal-tracheal obstruction
  Neuromuscular disorders
    Myasthenia gravis, poliomyelitis, damage to central respiratory center
  Disorders of the chest wall
  Pulmonary parenchymal disorders associated with hypoventilation
Miscellaneous causes of pulmonary hypertension
  Residence at high altitude
  Isolated partial anomalous pulmonary venous drainage
  Tetralogy of Fallot
  Hemoglobinopathies
  Intravenous drug abuse
  Alveolar proteinosis
  Takayasu's disease

(Reprinted from Grossman and Braunwald. With permission. See Bibliography.)

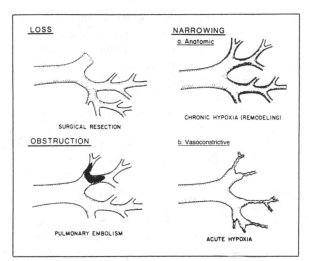

Figure 1. *Pulmonary vascular resistance can be increased if effective luminal vascular area is decreased by mechanisms illustrated in this figure (see text). (Reprinted from Rounds and Hill. With permission. See Bibliography.)*

is present. A systolic ejection click and flow murmur may be heard over the dilated pulmonary artery. As right ventricular failure occurs, peripheral edema, ascites, and hepatomegaly appear. In severe cases of pulmonary hypertension, signs of tricuspid regurgitation are present, including tall systolic regurgitant v-waves in the jugular venous pulse, a holosystolic murmur along the left sternal border that increases with inspiration, and a right ventricular S_3. A high-pitched early diastolic murmur of pulmonary regurgitation may also be heard in severe cases. With reduced cardiac output, the carotid pulse is diminished in volume, and cyanosis may develop.

The chest x-ray film in pulmonary hypertension may help reveal the underlying disorder, such as calcification of the mitral valve and enlarged left atrium in mitral stenosis. The main pulmonary artery and the right ventricle typically are enlarged. The electrocardiogram shows evidence of right ventricular pressure overload with right-axis deviation, tall p-waves suggesting right atrial enlargement, and tall R waves in V_1 and V_2, suggesting right ventricular hypertrophy.

Two-dimensional echocardiography may aid in delineating the underlying cause of pulmonary hypertension (such as mitral stenosis) by evaluating right ventricular size, hypertrophy and function. The pulmonary valve typically reveals a reduced a-wave excursion and a midsystolic notch on M-mode echocardiography. Doppler echocardiography is use-

ful for assessing the presence of tricuspid and pulmonic regurgitation. In addition, in patients with tricuspid regurgitation, this technique provides an estimate of pulmonary artery systolic pressure. Lung scans are utilized when pulmonary embolism is suspected.

Cardiac catheterization establishes the severity of pulmonary hypertension and helps determine whether the patient has a therapeutic response to oxygen or vasodilator administration. Selective pulmonary arteriography is used to help diagnose pulmonary embolism. Cardiac catheterization is also used to determine if intracardiac shunts are present.

Serologic tests may aid in determining the presence of collagen vascular disease.

Pulmonary function tests and arterial blood gas levels should be obtained in the assessment of pulmonary hypertension to help diagnose and assess the severity of pulmonary parenchymal etiologies such as chronic obstructive lung disease.

If the cause of pulmonary hypertension is unclear, some authorities recommend lung biopsy in order to determine the severity and potential reversibility of lesions as well as evidence of any active inflammatory process. Lung biopsy may also serve as a prognostic indicator.

SPECIFIC CLINICAL DISORDERS IN SECONDARY PULMONARY HYPERTENSION

CONGENITAL HEART DISEASE AND EISENMENGER'S SYNDROME

In the setting of congenital heart disease involving a left-to-right shunt, pulmonary hypertension may simply be due to increased pulmonary blood flow. This increased flow may act to secondarily cause pulmonary arteriolar vasoconstriction. If the shunt is large, with markedly increased pulmonary flow, and pulmonary hypertension is present over a long period of time, anatomic changes occur within the vascular bed. These anatomic changes initially are reversible (decreased pulmonary arteriolar cross-sectional area due to medial hypertrophy and vasoconstriction, and intimal cellular proliferation) or irreversible (necrotizing arteritis and plexiform lesions). Grading systems have been developed in order to assess the severity of morphologic alterations. Surgical correction of the shunt during the reversible phase results in an immediate reduction in pulmonary artery pressure, followed by a more gradual reduction as medial hypertrophy and intimal cellular proliferation regress.

However, as the vascular injury becomes irreversible with progressive anatomical obliteration of the pulmonary bed, there is reversal of the direction of the shunt. The term *Eisenmenger's syndrome* describes patients with congenital communications between systemic and pulmonary circulations who have irreversible pulmonary hypertension due to anatomic changes in their pulmonary vascular bed, and in whom a previous left-to-right shunt has become a right-to-left shunt. These patients have a high pulmonary vascular resistance and pulmonary arterial pressures that often approach systemic arterial pressures. Examples of congenital heart disease that may lead to Eisenmenger's complex include ventricular septal defect, patent ductus arteriosus, atrial septal defect, and transposition of the great vessels. Patients with ventricular septal defect may develop Eisenmenger's complex in their teens or late adolescent years; patients with large patent ductus arteriosus may develop it from infancy; only occasional patients with atrial septal defect ever develop Eisenmenger's physiology. Further details of these congenital heart diseases are found in Chapter 22.

Patients with Eisenmenger's syndrome typically complain of dyspnea, fatigue, syncope, hemoptysis, and atypical chest pain. Physical examination reveals cyanosis, clubbing, and signs of severe pulmonary hypertension. Polycythemia is usually present. In patients with a patent ductus arteriosus and Eisenmenger's syndrome, the cyanosis and clubbing characteristically occur in the lower extremities but not in the upper extremities. In addition to the electrocardiographic features discussed above, patients with Eisenmenger's syndrome may develop supraventricular tachyarrhythmias, including atrial tachycardia, atrial fibrillation, and atrial flutter. Chest x-ray reveals enlargement of the main pulmonary artery, proximal right and left pulmonary arteries with tapered peripheral pulmonary arteries, and an enlarged right ventricle and atrium. At cardiac catheterization, pulmonary vascular resistance is typically at least 75% of systemic vascular resistance, and arterial blood is desaturated. Cardiac catheterization rules out silent mitral stenosis and, in patients with Eisenmenger's syndrome, the pulmonary capillary wedge pressure (left atrial pressure) is usually normal. Patients with Eisenmenger's syndrome are at an increased risk of developing complications with angiographic procedures, including cardiovascular collapse and sudden death. When pulmonary vascular resistance is equal to systemic resistance, and irreversible anatomic changes in the vasculature are present, surgical closure of the intracardiac communication will fail to relieve the pulmonary hypertension and will result in severe right ventricular failure and very high risk of death. Therefore, the treatment of these patients is medical and includes salt restriction, diuretics, phlebotomy, and chronic oxygen therapy. They should receive endocarditis prophylaxis; some physicians also give chronic warfarin therapy to prevent pulmonary or paradoxical embolism. The use of vasodilators remains controversial. Pregnancy should be avoided in these patients, as it is associated with an increased risk of death. Overall prognosis is poor once Eisenmenger's syndrome develops, and most patients do not live past the fourth decade. Sudden death may occur or death may be secondary to severe heart failure, ventricular arrhythmias, pulmonary infection, thrombosis, brain abscess, endocarditis, or severe hemoptysis.

PULMONARY HYPERTENSION DUE TO MITRAL STENOSIS

Initially, the pulmonary hypertension of mitral stenosis is passive and is due to impedance of pulmonary venous drainage secondary to high left-atrial pressures. Over time, many patients develop a reactive component to their pulmonary hypertension, manifesting vasoconstriction and anatomic changes in the pulmonary vasculature. Hence, as stressed by studies of Dexter, a more proximal "second stenosis" at the level of pulmonary arterioles and small muscular arteries occurs, which results in high pulmonary artery pressures and signs of right ventricular failure. On the other hand, symptoms and signs of pulmonary congestion may actually be reduced somewhat during this stage of mitral stenosis, since the "second stenosis" is limiting blood flow to the left side of the heart. Anatomic changes that develop in the pulmonary vascular bed due to chronic venous hypertension of any cause include medial hypertrophy of small arteries and arterioles, distension of the pulmonary capillaries, swelling of capillary endothelial cells, intimal proliferation, thickening and rupture of the basement membrane of endothelial cells, transudation of red blood cells into the alveoli, distension of pulmonary lymphatics, and pulmonary hemosiderosis. In severe cases, pulmonary hemorrhage and fibrosis occur. After mitral valve surgery, pulmonary artery pressure and resistance fall within the first postoperative week with reversal of many of the antomic changes (medial hypertrophy, distension of capillaries and lymphatics, swelling of endothelial cells, intimal proliferation). Occasional patients fail to eliminate their pulmonary hypertension following mitral valve surgery and develop a progressive course.

PULMONARY HYPERTENSION IN COLLAGEN VASCULAR DISEASES

Several collagen vascular diseases are associated with pulmonary hypertension. The pathology is usually a fibrous obliteration of the pulmonary vasculature. Pulmonary hypertension is especially severe in patients with the associated CREST variant of scleroderma (calcinosis, Raynaud's phenomenon, esophagitis, sclerodactyly, and telangiectasia); it may also be severe in patients with systemic lupus erythematosus, rheumatoid arthritis, dermatomyositis, mixed connective tissue disease, and in association with Raynaud's phenomenon.

PULMONARY VENO-OCCLUSIVE DISEASE

This condition affects children and young adults and is associated with progressive fibrosis and obstruction of the pulmonary veins and venules. The etiology is uncertain but there are cases in which pulmonary veno-occlusive disease is preceded by an influenza-like illness. Symptoms include dyspnea, orthopnea and cyanosis.

PULMONARY HYPERTENSION DUE TO CHRONIC PULMONARY THROMBOEMBOLISM

While pulmonary hypertension occurs in 70–80% of patients with acute symptomatic pulmonary embolism, pulmonary hypertension also may occur in patients with chronic pulmonary thromboembolism. Clinically silent recurrent proximal emboli may lead to progressive pulmonary hypertension and cor pulmonale. Thrombotic occlusions of the pulmonary microvasculature may contribute to pulmonary hypertension, and have been associated with left-to-right intracardiac shunts and primary pulmonary hypertension. There is debate as to whether these lesions represent thrombotic versus embolic occlusion. Recent research favors thrombotic occlusion due to alterations in the endothelial cells leading to a localized procoagulant state. Antinuclear antibodies, anti-endothelial antibodies, increased levels of fibrinopeptide A, and abnormality in the clotting or lytic system have all been implicated as contributors to in situ thrombus formation.

Thrombotic occlusion of the pulmonary microvasculature is characterized by a patchy distribution of labeled albumin on lung scan and can be distinguished from the pattern of larger defects observed with proximal pulmonary emboli. Cardiac catheterization is needed to distinguish the entity of thrombi of the pulmonary microvessels from primary pulmonary hypertension and congenital heart disease. Pulmonary angiography also will localize the presence of large proximal thromboemboli. While acute proximal pulmonary emboli usually are treated with heparin and/or lytic agents, chronic proximal pulmonary thromboembolism with pulmonary hypertension will not respond to these agents and may require surgical thromboendarterectomy. This technique has been utilized in selected patients, with dramatic clinical improvement.

Patients with chronic proximal thromboemboli or microvascular thrombi should receive chronic warfarin anticoagulation to prevent further extension of the thrombi (Rich et al.).

THERAPY OF PULMONARY HYPERTENSION

The therapy of pulmonary hypertension depends on the etiology. Underlying correctable etiologies should be treated. For example, in patients with pulmonary hypertension due to mitral stenosis, surgical correction (or percutaneous balloon valvuloplasty) will result in a rapid lowering of pulmonary hypertension. Pulmonary hypertension due to left-to-right intracardiac shunts should be closed before irreversible pathology develops in the pulmonary vasculature. Thrombolysis of acute pulmonary emboli will improve pulmonary hypertension. Chronic oxygen therapy has been shown to improve pulmonary hemodynamics and, in recent studies, to improve survival of patients with pulmonary hypertension due to chronic obstructive lung disease. Anticoagulant therapy has been shown to improve survival in patients with primary pulmonary hypertension. A host of vasodilators have been used for patients with pulmonary hypertension, with variable results (Table 2). It is clear that patients' responses to vasodilators are highly variable and, therefore, the initial effects of vasodilators should be assessed preferably during cardiac

---

Table 2. Vasodilator Agents of Possible Benefit in Primary Pulmonary Hypertension

α-adrenergic blockers	*Direct smooth muscle relaxants*
Tolazoline	Hydralazine
Phentolamine	Minoxidil
	Prazosin
β-adrenergic agonists	Diazoxide
Isoproterenol	Nitroprusside
	Nitrates
Parasympathomimetics	*Calcium channel blockers*
Acetylcholine	Diltiazem
	Nifedipine
	Verapamil
Vasodilator prostaglandins	*Converting enzyme inhibitors*
Prostacylin	Captopril

(Reprinted from Rounds and Hill. With permission.)

---

catheterization with careful hemodynamic monitoring. Some studies suggest that vasodilators cause acute improvement in hemodynamics but no long-term beneficial effects. However, one recent study with very high-dose nifedipine showed long-term improvement in patients with primary pulmonary hypertension. A further discussion of such trials follows (under primary pulmonary hypertension and cor pulmonale).

The pulmonary hypertension of neuromuscular disorders such as myasthenia gravis, poliomyelitis, and kyphoscoliosis responds to improvement in ventilation and correction of hypoxia. Pharyngeal-tracheal obstruction due to hypertrophy of the tonsils and adenoids responds to tonsillectomy and adenoidectomy. Pulmonary hypertension due to obesity-hypoventilation syndrome (Pickwickian syndrome) responds to weight reduction and progesterone. Residing at high altitude may cause pulmonary hypertension, which improves with a return to sea level.

PRIMARY PULMONARY HYPERTENSION

Primary pulmonary hypertension is the term used when there is no discernible cause for the hypertension. Several possible theories have been advanced to explain primary pulmonary hypertension, including recurrent occult pulmonary emboli, development of thrombi in small pulmonary arteries, congenital abnormalities of the media of the pulmonary arteries, and persistent fetal pulmonary architecture. Other theories include the possibility that primary pulmonary hypertension is an autoimmune phenomenon, a form of collagen vascular disease, a vasculitis, or due to some genetic predisposition toward increased vasospasm of the pulmonary bed. None of these theories has been shown to be the most likely cause. The pathologic features of primary pulmonary hypertension occur in small pulmonary arteries and arterioles and include intimal thickening and fibroelastosis, producing a characteristic "onion skin" appearance to the vessel, increased thickness of the media, plexiform lesions, necrotizing arteritis, and fibrinoid necrosis with eventual thrombosis and atherosclerosis. In addition, thromboembolism without plexiform lesions has been reported in a high percentage of cases in a study from the Mayo Clinic (Fuster et al.). Rich and Brundage (1989) suggest that primary pulmonary hypertension is the result of primary damage to the pulmonary endothelium. The artery responds to the endothelial damage by developing intimal proliferation with smooth muscle hypertrophy (plexogenic pulmonary arteriopathy) or by developing intimal proliferation with superimposed thrombus (thrombotic pulmonary arteriopathy).

The age of onset of the disease is variable (3–64 years, mean age 34) and the disease is four to five times more common in women than men. Symptoms include dyspnea, fatigue, dizziness, syncope, weakness due to low cardiac output, hypoxemia, and atypical chest pain that mimics angina. In early stages of the disease these symptoms may be exercise related; in the later stages, they occur at rest. When right ventricular failure occurs, peripheral edema, abdominal discomfort, nausea, vomiting, and ascites may be present. Other symptoms that occur during the late phase of the disease include cough, hemoptysis, and palpitations due to ventricular arrhythmias. The physical findings are those typical of severe pulmonary hypertension, as discussed above. A loud second heartsound is heard in 98% of patients. Late cyanosis may be due to right-to-left shunting through a patent foramen ovale or to severely reduced cardiac output. Laboratory studies reveal arterial O_2 desaturation, polycythemia, and, with severe right ventricular failure, elevated liver enzymes. A hypercoagulable state may exist with abnormalities in fibrinolysis and platelet function. The chest x-ray film shows dilated proximal pulmonary arteries, with tapering of peripheral branches and relative oligemia of the lung fields. Right atrial and ventricular enlargement are present. The ECG reveals tall peaked p-waves and tall R waves in V_1 and V_2 (right ventricular hypertrophy). Echocardiography shows reduction of the pulmonary valve a-wave and midsystolic closure of the pulmonary valve, as well as an enlarged and hypertrophied right ventricle; Doppler echocardiography detects tricuspid and pulmonic regurgitation and provides an estimate of the severity of pulmonary artery pressure.

Cardiac catheterization delineates the severity of the pulmonary hypertension and rules out possible secondary causes of pulmonary hypertension. Some cardiologists consider cardiac catheterization mandatory, since primary pulmonary hypertension is a diagnosis of exclusion. Pulmonary artery pressure and right ventricular systolic pressure are elevated and may equal or sometimes exceed systemic arterial pressures, while left atrial and ventricular pressures are low or normal. Calculated pulmonary vascular resistance is markedly elevated. The right atrial pressure is also high, with tall a-waves; if tricuspid regurgitation is present, there may be tall regurgitant v-waves. A small right-to-left shunt may be present if the foramen ovale has become patent, due to high right-atrial pressures. Cardiac angiography may be hazardous in advanced cases of primary pulmonary hypertension, and has resulted in cardiovascular collapse and sudden death. However, if the diagnosis is unclear and there is doubt whether the pulmonary hypertension is due to a secondary cause, such as pulmonary emboli, either a perfusion-ventilation lung scan or, in some cases, cautious selective pulmonary angiography may be performed.

The prognosis of primary pulmonary hypertension is notably poor. Fuster et al. reported that only 21% of patients survived for five years. The major causes of death include right heart failure, pneumonia, and sudden death. The time from onset of symptoms to death is approximately three years.

THERAPY FOR PRIMARY PULMONARY HYPERTENSION

Fuster et al. studied 120 patients with a clinical and hemodynamic diagnosis of primary pulmonary hypertension who either did or did not receive anticoagulation over a period of three years. Patients receiving anticoagulation had an improved survival (Figure 2). At autopsy, thromboembolism without plexiform lesions was found in 57% of patients, and anticoagulation was thus recommended as standard therapy for primary pulmonary hypertension.

Numerous vasodilators have been tested in patients with primary pulmonary hypertension (Table 2). It is estimated that approximately 30% of patients respond to vasodilators; those who respond may have improved survival. In general, agents such as sublingual isoproterenol, tolazoline, phentolamine, hydralazine, and oxygen may reduce pulmonary vascular resistance and provide some symptomatic improvement initially, but as the disease progresses, these agents may have little effect. Most vasodilators have failed to achieve a prolonged and sustained reduction in pulmonary artery pressure. The data on some of the vasodilators have been conflicting. For example, Rubin and Peter showed immediate and sustained reductions of pulmonary vascular resistance with hydralazine; Packer et al. observed only minor reductions in pulmonary vascular resistance with hydralazine and the development of systemic hypotension in some patients. Packer also pointed out that vasodilators usually fail to reduce pulmonary vascular resistance selectively compared to reduction in systemic vascular resistance; thus, systemic hypotension may occur. Furthermore, calcium channel blockers may exert a negative inotropic effect on right ventricular function and exacerbate right ventricular failure. Nevertheless, a recent study by Rich and Brundage (1987) found that very high doses of calcium channel blockers (nifedipine, diltiazem) acutely reduced mean pulmonary arterial pressure by 48% and pulmonary

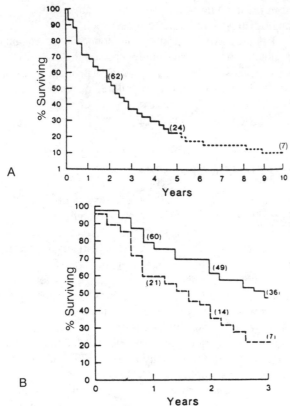

Figure 2. *Prognosis in patients with a clinical and hemodynamic diagnosis of primary pulmonary hypertension. Panel A, the observed survival for the entire group (115 patients who survived diagnostic cardiac catheterization). Panel B, the observed survival with (solid line) and without (dashed line) anticoagulant treatment in these same patients. Treatment with anticoagulants was not randomized but was based on clinical preference of the primary physician caring for the patient. As can be seen, survival was substantially better in the patients who received anticoagulants. (From Fuster et al. With permission of the American Heart Association.)*

vascular resistance by 60% in eight of 13 patients with primary pulmonary hypertension. Five patients who returned for cardiac catheterization one year later had improved symptoms, sustained reductions in pulmonary artery pressure and pulmonary vascular resistance, and evidence of regression of right ventricular hypertrophy. Additional studies will need to confirm these dramatic observations. At present, a trial of vasodilator therapy is warranted in patients with primary pulmonary hypertension; however, these agents should be initiated only under careful hemodynamic monitoring, since patients may respond unpredictably. The agents that cause the best hemodynamic response and the fewest side effects (including systemic hypotension) can be considered for chronic therapy.

Right ventricular heart failure should be treated with diuretics for control of edema and ascites. The use of digitalis remains controversial. Pulmonary hypertension is a relative contraindication to pregnancy as there is a high mortality rate in the puerperium.

Heart-lung transplantation is another potential therapy for severe pulmonary hypertension. Results at Stanford University in 40 patients showed a 57% survival rate at two years.

COR PULMONALE

Cor pulmonale, as defined by the World Health Organization, is "right ventricular enlargement resulting from disorders that affect either the structure or the function of the lungs." The right ventricle is a more compliant chamber than the left ventricle and is more suited to handling increases in preload (volume) than in afterload (pressure). Animal studies have shown that the left ventricle can maintain forward output in the setting of increased systemic pressure, whereas the right ventricle markedly reduces right ventricular stroke volume in response to small increases in pulmonary artery pressure.

There are a number of causes of cor pulmonale (Table 1). The most common cause in the United States is chronic obstructive pulmonary disease. Other causes include chronic suppurative pulmonary disease such as bronchiectasis and cystic fibrosis; restrictive lung disease including infiltrative and granulomatous lung disease, upper airway obstruction, pulmonary resection, and disorders of the neuromuscular apparatus (myasthenia gravis, poliomyelitis, Guillain-Barré syndrome); disorders of the chest wall (kyphoscoliosis, pectus excavatum); reduced ventilatory drive (obesity-hypoventilation syndrome, sleep apnea syndrome); chronic mountain sickness; and pulmonary vascular disease as outlined in the first portion of this chapter.

Cor pulmonale is a common clinical problem. In the U.S., 10–30% of hospital admissions for heart failure are due to this disease entity. The majority of such cases are associated with chronic obstructive lung disease. For cor pulmonale to develop, significant airway disease must be present. Patients with chronic bronchitis ("blue bloaters") are thus more likely to demonstrate cor pulmonale than those with primarily emphysema ("pink puffers"). However, it should be noted that in most patients with chronic obstructive lung disease, elements of chronic bronchitis coexist with elements of emphysema.

Symptoms of cor pulmonale include dyspnea, cough with syncope, peripheral edema and ascites. The symptoms of the underlying pulmonary disease also will be prominent, so that cough with sputum production, dyspnea at rest, and recurrent chest infections are common in patients with chronic bronchitis.

Physical exam will reveal abnormalities due to the underlying pulmonary disease. Patients with chronic obstructive lung disease may exhibit increased anteroposterior diameter of the thorax, cyanosis, rales, rhonchi and wheezes. The cardiac examination in cor pulmonale typically reveals distended jugular veins with prominent a- and v-waves and lack of collapse during inspiration, a right ventricular lift (due to right ventricular hypertrophy), a loud pulmonic closure sound, a right-sided S_3 (which increases during inspiration), the murmur of tricuspid regurgitation (a holosystolic murmur at the left sternal border which increases with respiration), an enlarged and pulsatile liver, peripheral edema, and cyanosis.

Laboratory tests that aid in the diagnosis of right ventricular enlargement and hypertrophy include chest x-ray, ECG, and 2D echocardiography. Single photon emission computed tomography (SPECT) with thallium has demonstrated increased activity of the right ventricular wall in right ventricular hypertrophy. Doppler echocardiography aids in the diagnosis of tricuspid regurgitation and can estimate the severity of pulmonary artery hypertension. Pulmonary function tests and blood gas analysis also should be performed.

THERAPY FOR COR PULMONALE

Therapy of cor pulmonale is aimed at treating the underlying pulmonary problem, reducing pulmonary hypertension, and improving oxygenation. Chronic obstructive lung disease is treated with bronchodilators, antibiotics for respiratory infections, supplemental oxygen, postural drainage and chest physical therapy, and, most importantly, smoking cessation therapy.

The administration of supplemental oxygen has now been found to improve survival in patients with cor pulmonale due to chronic obstructive lung disease. The Medical Research Council's study in Great Brittain randomized 87 patients with chronic obstructive lung disease to receive either oxygen therapy (about 2 liters/min by nasal prongs for 15 hours daily) or no oxygen. Nineteen of 42 patients (45%) in the oxygen-treated group died in five years, compared with 30 out of 45 patients (67%) in the control groups. In men, the beneficial effect on survival was not apparent until after 500 days. Though there were few female patients, the female control group had a high mortality rate at three years compared with those who received oxygen. Oxygen therapy also blunted an increase in pulmonary vascular resistance observed in the control group. The Nocturnal Oxygen Therapy Trial Group of the National Institutes of Health compared nocturnal oxygen (12 hours/day) with continuous oxygen therapy (24 hours/day) in patients with chronic obstructive lung disease. Within 19.3 months, this study showed improved survival in patients receiving continuous oxygen therapy (12% mean annual death rate) compared with patients receiving only nocturnal oxygen (21% mean annual death rate).

A study by Cooper et al. of patients with chronic obstructive lung disease and cor pulmonale reported that oxygen therapy for at least 15 hours/day resulted in an overall five-year survival of 62%, which is better than previous reports of control patients (five-year survival of 40%). However, 10-year survival of their oxygen-treated patients was only 26%. The investigators postulated that the fall in survival at 10 years was due to continued pathologic process affecting airway function. A poor prognostic index for these patients was an FEV_1 <450 ml.

When chronic oxygen therapy is considered, it is crucial that the physician first determine in each patient that supplemental oxygen does not worsen hypoventilation with subsequent hyprecapnia.

A recent study by Ashutosh and Dunsky suggested that the pulmonary artery pressure response to breathing oxygen for 24 hours could serve as a predictor of survival. Patients who dropped their pulmonary artery pressure by ≥ 5 mm Hg after breathing 28% oxygen had an improved three-year survival. Patients with a high peak oxygen consumption at the end of exercise also had improved survival over three years.

A host of vasodilators have been tried in patients with cor pulmonale, including nifedipine, diltiazem, nitrendipine, hydralazine, isoproterenol, phentolamine, diazoxide, and prazosin, with varying degrees of success. These agents inhibit pulmonary vasoconstriction due to hypoxia, thereby reducing afterload and improving right ventricular function. Nifedipine and hydralazine have been shown to acutely reduce pulmonary vascular resistance and increase cardiac output, while in several studies, they did not acutely reduce or only minimally reduced pulmonary artery pressure. Sturani et al. showed that nifedipine administration over eight weeks produced significant reductions in pulmonary vascular resistance. An acute reduction in pulmonary vascular resistance was related to an increase in cardiac output; a chronic reduction was due to reduced pulmonary artery pressure rather than increased cardiac output. Rubin and Moser recently reported that the calcium channel blocker nitrendipine reduced pulmonary vascular resistance and pulmonary artery pressure and increased cardiac output at six weeks.

The hazards of vasodilators include a reduction in systemic vascular resistance greater than pulmonary vascular resistance, leading to systemic hypotension; increase in venous admixture, resulting in reduced arterial oxygen tension; and the potential that calcium channel blockers might reduce right ventricular contractility.

In general, vasodilators should be used for patients with cor pulmonale only after conventional therapy with bronchodilators and oxygen has been tried. Initially, careful monitoring and blood gas analysis should be considered, due to variable responses among patients and possible adverse effects. The use of digitalis in patients with cor pulmonale remains controversial. One recent trial suggested that digitalis did not improve right ventricular function in these patients unless there was concomitant left ventricular failure. Digitalis plays a role for ventricular rate control in patients with supraventricular tachycardia. Hypoxic patients may have increased sensitivity to digitalis toxicity; also, digitalis can increase hypoxic pulmonary vasoconstriction.

Diuretics are used for treating volume overload in cor pulmonale patients. They reduce blood volume and improve symptoms of edema. However, they produce hypokalemia, which can exacerbate the arrhythmias of digitalis toxicity and exacerbate multifocal atrial tachycardia.

Sabino et al. reported the effects of the dopamine-related agent ibopamine on patients with cor pulmonale over a 12-month period. They reported a significant improvement in clinical symptoms. Additional studies are needed to confirm the usefulness of ibopamine. Vik-Mo et al. studied the effects of salbutamol, a beta$_2$-receptor agonist, in patients with cor pulmonale and observed improved cardiac performance and improvement in oxygen delivery. The beta$_2$-agonist pirbuterol was found to initially increase cardiac output without further rise in pulmonary artery pressure when administered acutely, but lost its beneficial hemodynamic effects when given over six months (Biernacki et al.).

OBESITY-HYPOVENTILATION SYNDROME ("PICKWICKIAN SYNDROME")

"Pickwickian syndrome" refers to the syndrome of obesity, somnolence, edema, and plethora and is associated with cor pulmonale. While the exact cause of this phenomenon is not known, two potential mechanisms are reduced compliance of the chest wall due to excessive obesity, and abnormal ventilatory drive due to reduced sensitivity of the central respiratory center. Treatment is weight reduction and progesterone, which has been shown to stimulate ventilation.

SLEEP APNEA SYNDROMES

Cor pulmonale can occur in patients with abnormal respiration during sleep—the sleep apnea syndrome. Typically, these patients have repetitive apneic periods during sleep with periods of hypoxemia and hypercapnia. The episodes of hypoxia result in progressive pulmonary hypertension during sleep and have been associated with both brady- and tachyarrhythmias. Patients are chronically sleep-deprived due to hypoxic arousal. In contrast to "Pickwickian syndrome" patients, sleep-apnea syndrome patients are generally not obese and have normal respirations while awake. Forms of sleep apnea include obstruction of the upper airways during sleep, a central form of apnea in which there is a cessation of all respiratory muscle effort, and a combination of both mechanisms. The obstructive form of sleep apnea has been treated with tracheostomy, continuous positive airway pressure to the nose during sleep, and surgical procedures including removal of enlarged tonsils and adenoids. Therapy for central apnea includes respiratory stimulants, phrenic nerve or diaphragmatic pacing, and use of respirators to provide ventilatory support at night. Any pharmacologic agents that may suppress ventilatory drive (such as sedatives or antihistamines) should be avoided in these patients.

Bibliography

Ashutosh K, Dunsky M: Noninvasive tests for responsiveness of pulmonary hypertension to oxygen. Prediction of survival in patients with chronic obstructive lung disease and cor pulmonale. *Chest* 92:393, 1987.

Biernacki W, Prince K, Whyte K, Macnee W, Flenley DC: The effect of six months of daily treatment with the beta-2 agonist oral pirbuterol on pulmonary hemodynamics in patients with chronic hypoxic cor pulmonale receiving long-term oxygen therapy. *Am Rev Respir Dis* 139:492, 1989.

Braunwald E, Braunwald NS, Ross T Jr, et al: Effects of mitral valve replacement on pulmonary vascular dynamics of patients with pulmonary hypertension. *N Engl J Med* 273:509, 1965.

Cooper CB, Waterhouse S, Howard P: Twelve-year clinical study of patients with hypoxic cor pulmonale given long term domiciliary oxygen therapy. *Thorax* 42:105, 1987.

Daoud FS, Reeves JT, Kelley DB: Isoproterenol as a potential pulmonary vasodilator in primary pulmonary hypertension. *Am J Cardiol* 42:817, 1978.

Dexter I: Physiologic changes in mitral stenosis. *N Engl J Med* 254:829, 1956.

Fayemi A: Pulmonary vascular disease in systemic lupus erythematosus. *Am J Clin Pathol* 65:284, 1976.

Fuster V, Steele PM, Edwards WD, et al: Primary pulmonary hypertension: Natural history and the importance of thrombosis. *Circulation* 70:580, 1984.

Grossman W, Braunwald E: Pulmonary hypertension. In: Braunwald E, ed: *Heart Disease: A Textbook of Cardiovascular Medicine*. Philadelphia: Saunders; 1988, p. 793.

Heath D, Edwards JE: The pathology of hypertensive pulmonary vascular disease: A description of six grades of structural changes in the pulmonary arteries with special reference to congenital cardiac septal defects. *Circulation* 18:533, 1958.

Heath D, Edwards JE: Histological changes in the lung in disease associated with pulmonary venous hypertension. *Br J Dis Chest* 53:8, 1959.

Himelman RB, Struve SN, Brown JK, Namnum P, Schiller NB: Improved recognition of cor pulmonale in patients with severe chronic obstructive pulmonary disease. *Am J Med* 84:891, 1988.

Hogg JC: Primary pulmonary hypertension. *Chest* 93:173S, 1988.

James TN, Frame B, Coates ED: De subitaneis mortibus. III. Pickwickian syndrome. *Circulation* 48:1311, 1973.

Jones MB, Osterholm RK, Wilson RB, et al: Fatal pulmonary hypertension and resolving immune complex glomerulonephritis in mixed connective tissue disease. *Am J Med* 65:855, 1978.

Lebrec D, Capron JP, Dhumeaux D, et al: Pulmonary hypertension complicating portal hypertension. *Am Rev Respir Dis* 120:849, 1979.

Lupi-Herrera E, Bialostozky D, Sobrino A: The role of isoproterenol in pulmonary artery hypertension of unknown cause. *Circulation* 65:645, 1982.

Lupi-Herrera E, Seoane M, Verdejo J: Hemodynamic effects of hydralazine in advanced, stable chronic obstructive pulmonary disease with cor pulmonale. Immediate and short-term evaluation at rest and during exercise. *Chest* 85:157, 1984.

McDonnell PJ, Summer WR, Hutchins GM: Pulmonary veno-occlusive disease. Morphological changes suggesting a viral cause. *JAMA* 246:667, 1981.

McFadden ER, Braunwald E: Cor pulmonale. In: Braunwald E, ed: *Heart Disease: A Textbook of Cardiovascular Medicine*. Philadelphia: Saunders; 1988, p. 1597.

McGoon MD, Vlietstra RE: Vasodilator therapy for primary pulmonary hypertension. *Mayo Clin Proc* 59:672, 1984.

MacNee W: Right ventricular function in cor pulmonale. *Cardiology* 75 (Suppl 1): 30, 1988.

Medical Research Council Working Party: Long term domiciliary oxygen therapy in chronic hypoxic cor pulmonale complicating chronic bronchitis and emphysema. *Lancet* 1:681, 1981.

Michael JR, Selinger SR, Buescher PC, Kennedy TP: Pharmacologic therapy of cor pulmonale. *Cardiovasc Clinics* 17:171, 1987.

Miller MJ, Chappel TR, Cook W, De Olazabal JR, Rubin LJ: Effects of oral hydralazine on gas exchange in patients with cor pulmonale. *Am J Med* 75:937, 1983.

Morrison EB, Ganney FA, Eigenbrodt EH, et al: Severe pulmonary hypertension associated with macronodular (postnecrotic) cirrhosis and autoimmune phenomenon. *Am J Med* 69:513, 1980.

Mookherjee S, Ashutosh K, Dunsky M, et al. Nifedipine in chronic cor pulmonale: Acute and relatively long-term effects. *Clin Pharmacol Ther* 44:289, 1988.

Nocturnal Oxygen Therapy Trial Group: Continuous or nocturnal oxygen therapy in hypoxemic chronic obstructive lung disease. A clinical trial. *Ann Intern Med* 93:391, 1980.

Newman JH, Ross JC: Primary pulmonary hypertension: A look at the future. *J Am Coll Cardiol* 14:551, 1989.

Packer M: Therapeutic application of calcium-channel antagonists for pulmonary hypertension. *Am J Cardiol* 55:196B, 1985.

Packer M: Vasodilator therapy for primary pulmonary hypertension. Limitations and hazards. *Ann Intern Med* 103:258, 1985.

Packer M, Greenberg B, Massie B, et al: Deleterious effects of hydralazine in patients with pulmonary hypertension. *N Engl J Med* 306:1326, 1982.

Reitz BA, Wallwork JL, Hunt SA, et al: Heart-lung transplantation: Successful therapy for patients with pulmonary vascular disease. *N Engl J Med* 306:557, 1982.

Rich S, Brundage BH: High-dose calcium channel-blocking therapy for primary pulmonary hypertension: Evidence for long-term reduction in pulmonary arterial pressure and regression of right ventricular hypertrophy. *Circulation* 76:135, 1987.

Rich S, Brundage BH: Pulmonary hypertension: A cellular basis for understanding the pathophysiology and treatment. *J Am Coll Cardiol* 14:545, 1989.

Rich S, Levitsky S, Brundage B: Pulmonary hypertension from chronic pulmonary thromboembolism. *Ann Intern Med* 108:452, 1988.

Rounds S, Hill NS: Pulmonary hypertensive diseases. *Chest* 85:397, 1984.

Rubin LJ, Handel F, Peter RH: The effects of oral hydralazine on right ventricular end-diastolic pressure in patients with right ventricular failure. *Circulation* 65:1369, 1982.

Rubin LJ, Moser K: Long-term effects of nitrendipine on hemodynamics and oxygen transport in patients with cor pulmonale. *Chest* 89:141, 1986.

Rubin LJ, Peter RH: Oral hydralazine therapy for primary pulmonary hypertension. *N Engl J Med* 320:69, 1980.

Ruskin JN, Hutter AM Jr: Primary pulmonary hypertension treated with oral phentolamine. *Ann Intern Med* 90:772, 1979.

Saadjian A, Philip-Joet F, Arnaud A: Hemodynamic and oxygen delivery responses to nifedipine in pulmonary hypertension secondary to chronic obstructive lung disease. *Cardiology* 74:196, 1987.

Sabino F, Bianco L, Cantoni V, et al: Treatment of heart failure following chronic cor pulmonale with ibopamine. *Respiration* 54 (Suppl 1): 114, 1988.

Salerni R, Rodman GP, Leon DG, et al: Pulmonary hypertension in the CREST syndrome variant of progressive systemic sclerosis (scleroderma). *Ann Intern Med* 86:394, 1977.

Santini D, Fox D, Kloner RA, et al: Pulmonary hypertension in systemic lupus erythematosus: Hemodynamics and effects of vasodilator therapy. *Clin Cardiol* 3:406, 1980.

Shettigar UR, Hultgren HN, Specter M, et al: Primary pulmonary hypertension: Favorable effects of isoproterenol. *N Engl J Med* 295:1414, 1976.

Sturani C, Bassein L, Schiavina M, Gunella G: Oral nifedipine in chronic cor pulmonale secondary to severe chronic obstructive pulmonary disease (COPD). Short- and long-term hemodynamic effects. *Chest* 84:135, 1983.

Vik-Mo H, Halvorsen FJ, Thorsen E, Walde NH, Rosland GA: Improved cardiac performance by salbutamol, a selective B_2-agonist, in chronic cor pulmonale. *J Cardiovasc Pharmacol* 9:129, 1987.

Wagenvoort CA: Lung biopsy specimens in the evaluation of pulmonary vascular disease. *Chest* 77:614, 1980.

Wagenvoort CA, Wagenvoort N: *Pathology of Pulmonary Hypertension*. New York: John Wiley & Sons; 1977, p. 119.

Weir EK, Archer SL, Edwards JE: Chronic primary and secondary thromboembolic pulmonary hypertension. *Chest* 93:149S, 1988.

Whyte KF, Flenley DC: Can pulmonary vasodilators improve survival in cor pulmonale due to hypoxic chronic bronchitis and emphysema? *Thorax* 43:1, 1988.

Yamaoka S, Yonekura Y, Koide H, Ohi M, Kuno K: Noninvasive method to assess cor pulmonale in patients with chronic obstructive pulmonary disease. *Chest* 92:11, 1987.

29 Pulmonary Embolism

CHAPTER

Samuel Z. Goldhaber

INCIDENCE AND RISK FACTORS

Pulmonary embolism (PE) and deep venous thrombosis (DVT) together constitute the third most common cardiovascular illness (after acute ischemic syndromes and stroke). Venous thromboembolism (VTE) accounts for approximately 300,000 hospitalizations annually in the United States (Gillum); due to underdiagnosis, the true incidence is probably several times greater. Unfortunately, during the past decade the death rate from PE has not declined (Goldhaber 1988a). This chapter summarizes recent studies that optimize strategies for detection, management, and prevention of PE.

Risk factors for VTE can be classified as primary (inherited) or secondary (acquired) (Table 1). Inherited disorders are costly to diagnose because of the large battery of tests that are required. We currently screen patients for inherited disorders of hypercoagulability with antithrombin III, protein C, and protein S levels, in addition to the lupus anticoagulant and anticardiolipin antibodies. We are probably able to diagnose only a small proportion of these inherited disorders in clinical laboratories. Furthermore, among patients with the more commonly encountered acquired disorders of hypercoagulability, many undoubtedly suffer from an underlying primary defect that cannot yet be diagnosed with our limited laboratory armamentarium.

DIAGNOSIS

A careful history is of paramount importance in the diagnosis of PE. The physician should determine whether the patient has an acquired risk factor for thrombosis, such as cancer or the postoperative state (or both). Keep in mind that about 20% of cases of PE or DVT occur in patients with a history of VTE.

Table 1. Risk Factors for Venous Thromboembolism

Inherited (primary)
   Antithrombin III, protein C, or protein S deficiencies
   Lupus anticoagulant
   Anticardiolipin antibodies
   Other disorders that have not yet been elucidated or that are not routinely evaluated in most clinical laboratories.

Acquired (secondary)
   Postoperative state
   Cancer (sometimes occult)
   Pregnancy/oral contraceptives
   Obesity
   Increasing age
   Immobilization

Search for symptoms of dyspnea, syncope, or lightheadedness. We have found that dyspnea or presyncope often denotes anatomically or physiologically massive PE. In contrast, severe pleuritic chest pain usually occurs in the setting of either a small peripheral PE that inflames the pleural lining or a nonthrombotic viral syndrome. With increasing frequency, our echocardiographers are the first to raise the possible diagnosis of PE. This occurs when patients labelled with "left heart failure" are found at echocardiography to have normal left heart function but a dilated and hypokinetic right ventricle (Goldhaber 1988b).

On physical examination, the finding of a comfortable-appearing patient may be misleading. The vital signs should be taken carefully, especially the respiratory rate. In addition, signs of right heart dysfunction should be sought. These include v-waves in the jugular veins due to tricuspid regurgitation, a left

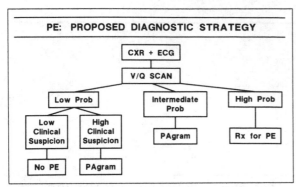

Figure 1. *Proposed diagnostic strategy for pulmonary embolism. CXR = chest x-ray; ECG = electrocardiogram; V/Q = ventilation/perfusion; PAgram = pulmonary angiogram. (Reproduced from* Hospital Medicine *25:101, 1989. With permission of Cahners Publishing Co.)*

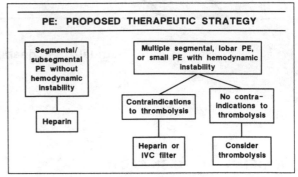

Figure 2. *Proposed therapeutic strategy for pulmonary embolism. IVC = inferior vena cava. (Reproduced from* Hospital Medicine *25:101, 1989. With permission of Cahners Publishing Co.)*

parasternal lift due to elevated right ventricular pressure, and an accentuated pulmonic heart sound due to pulmonary hypertension. Upon examination of the lungs, a pleural rub due to pulmonary infarction tends to be heard most often in patients with small peripheral PE.

In virtually all patients suspected of PE, the differential diagnosis includes pneumonia and myocardial infarction. Therefore, the proposed diagnostic strategy (Figure 1) requires a chest x-ray and electrocardiogram after completion of the history and physical examination. Note that arterial blood gases on room air should *not* be obtained, because use of the room-air PO_2 as a diagnostic screening test is more misleading than helpful. If the diagnosis of PE is still under serious consideration after a chest x-ray and ECG, a ventilation-perfusion (V/Q) scan should be obtained. If the scan is of low probability for PE in the presence of low clinical suspicion, then the diagnosis of PE can be put aside. If the lung scan is of high probability for PE, additional testing is often unnecessary unless clinical suspicion is low *or* the patient has asthma or a tumor causing compression of the pulmonary arteries (two conditions notorious for distorting the lung scan results). However, if the lung scan is of intermediate probability, or if the clinical suspicion is high despite a low-probability scan, then pulmonary angiography should usually be undertaken.

Before proceeding with pulmonary angiography, some clinicians prefer to obtain a venous ultrasound examination of the legs. If thrombus is documented, an argument can be made for terminating the diagnostic workup. However, angiography is important in most instances (pregnancy is an exception, due to the radiation exposure) to differentiate between DVT and PE. Patients with PE usually receive a longer and more intense course of Coumadin than do DVT patients. Further, the threshold for use of thrombolytic therapy is lower among PE patients than among DVT patients, because PE is more life-threatening.

Two studies support the approach of angiography for patients with low-probability scans and high clinical suspicion. A trial at McMaster University correlated "low-probability" scans with pulmonary angiograms and found that the frequency of PE in these patients ranged from 25–40% (Hull et al.). The Prospective Investigation of Pulmonary Embolism Diagnosis (PIOPED) found that, overall, about one in six patients with low-probability scans had positive pulmonary angiograms. Among patients with low-probability lung scans and high clinical suspicion, more than two in six had positive pulmonary angiograms.

By using flexible pigtail catheters with side holes instead of stiffer, antiquated catheters, the safety of pulmonary angiography has increased greatly. These features of the catheter are virtual guarantees against right ventricular perforation or catheter entrapment in the pulmonary arteries. The use of low-osmolar contrast agents has in most instances eliminated the very uncomfortable coughing and heat sensation that patients used to experience during contrast injection. In addition, these newer agents have increased the safety of pulmonary angiography for patients with pulmo-

Table 2. FDA-approved Thrombolytic Regimens for Pulmonary Embolism

Urokinase:	2,000 U/lb bolus followed by 2,000 U/lb/hr for 12-24 hr
Streptokinase:	250,000 U bolus followed by 100,000 U/hr for 24 hr

nary hypertension. Finally, we now use the lung scan as a road map and perform selective pulmonary angiography, thus avoiding hazardous injections in the main pulmonary artery.

THERAPY

After the diagnosis of PE has been established, the major choices for treatment are anticoagulation alone with heparin/Coumadin; thrombolytic therapy followed by heparin/Coumadin; or placement of an inferior vena caval filter (Figure 2). Heparin is effective for preventing additional clot from forming, but it does not dissolve clot that already exists. Heparin "buys time" for endogenous fibrinolytic mechanisms to lyse pulmonary arterial thrombus. Anticoagulation alone is adequate therapy for patients with anatomically small PE who are hemodynamically stable.

If clinical suspicion is high, initial therapy on the night of hospital admission should not be delayed in order to confirm a PE by lung scanning or angiography, unless there are absolute contraindications to the use of heparin (e.g., hemorrhagic stroke, active gastrointestinal bleeding). After scintigraphic or angiographic confirmation of PE, a five- to seven-day course of continuous intravenous heparin is administered and oral anticoagulation is initiated on the second hospital day (Second ACCP). Patients with PE should receive adequate continuous intravenous heparin to maintain a PTT at 1.5–2.5 times control.

Oral anticoagulation with Coumadin inhibits vitamin K-dependent clotting factors. For oral anticoagulation, Coumadin therapy is used to maintain the PT at 1.3–1.5 times control. Coumadin is initiated with a four to five day overlap with heparin. To minimize potential problems with bioavailability and dose adjustment, the brand Coumadin® rather than generic warfarin is preferred. If oral anticoagulants are contraindicated (e.g., pregnancy), adjusted-dose subcutaneous heparin may be used to maintain the trough PTT above the upper limit of normal (e.g., 36–40 seconds). The optimal duration of Coumadin therapy

is uncertain, but at least six months is recommended. Patients with recurrent thrombosis or a chronic risk factor such as metastatic cancer or massive obesity require indefinite anticoagulation.

For patients with anatomically large PE or PE of *any* size with hemodynamic instability, thrombolytic therapy should be considered. Agents such as streptokinase, urokinase (UK), and recombinant human tissue-type plasminogen activator (rt-PA) function by activating the endogenous fibrinolytic system (Table 2). Activation of plasminogen to plasmin causes clot lysis. Proven advantages of thrombolytic therapy include accelerated clot lysis, accelerated pulmonary reperfusion, and greater long-term improvement in pulmonary capillary blood volume compared with heparin therapy alone. Potential but not definitively proven advantages of thrombolytic therapy over heparin include reversal of right heart failure, less frequent development of chronic pulmonary hypertension, reduction in recurrent PE (because it serves as a medical embolectomy that lyses in situ residual thrombus in the pelvic and deep leg veins), and lower mortality. Ongoing trials are evaluating rt-PA, which appears especially promising (Goldhaber et al. 1986, 1987, 1988), and novel dosing regimens of UK (Goldhaber 1989) (Figure 3). A recently completed national survey of PE patients from 44 clinical centers (Terrin et al.) indicates that approximately 50% have no contraindications to thrombolysis (Table 3).

Patients with contraindications to heparin anticoagulation (e.g., recent hemorrhagic stroke or active gastrointestinal bleeding), recurrent PE despite adequate anticoagulation, or complications from heparin are candidates for inferior vena caval interruption. The most common method of interruption in the past decade has been percutaneous transvenous placement of a Greenfield filter which requires a 24F sheath. However, a new generation of filters is emerging with the advantages of smaller sheath size (9F or 12F), retrievability, and nonferromagnetic construction, so that magnetic resonance imaging scans can be obtained (Grassi and Goldhaber).

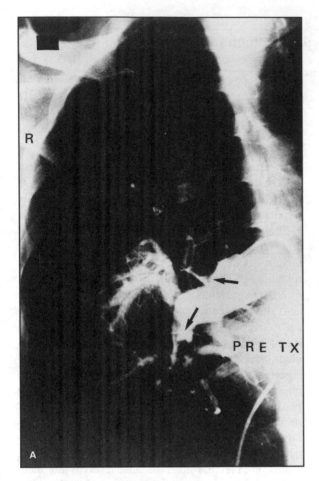

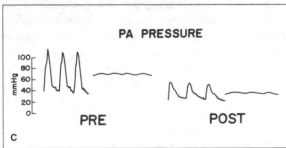

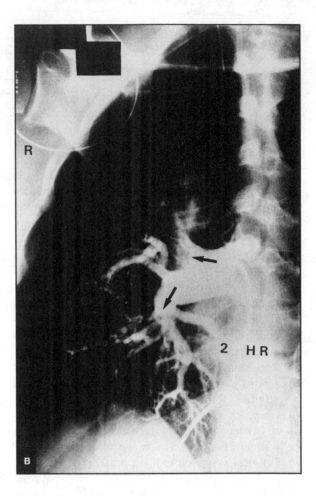

Figure 3. *Pulmonary angiograms from a 58-year-old man with a five-day history of dyspnea. (Reprinted from Goldhaber et al., 1988. With permission. See Bibliography.) A. Intraluminal clot in right upper and lower lobe arteries (arrows) before treatment. B. Clot lysis (arrows) immediately after a 2-hour course of rt-PA. C. Pulmonary artery pressures were 118/40 mm Hg (mean 65 mm Hg) before treatment and 53/19 mm Hg (mean 34 mm Hg) after 2 hours of rt-PA.*

Even when a filter is placed, most patients with PE should receive long-term Coumadin to prevent recurrent PE. Traditionally, routine plasma prothrombin times obtained from venipuncture require that the laboratory telephone the results to the physician. Then, the physician must contact the patient at home either to give reassurance about the dosing regimen or to make dosage adjustments. With the introduction of the Coumatrak, the procedure has been streamlined. This device provides the prothrombin time result in 2 minutes with a drop of whole blood obtained from a fingertip puncture (Figure 4).

PROPHYLAXIS

The rationale for employing VTE prophylaxis in most hospitalized patients is that PE is difficult to diagnose, expensive to treat, and occasionally lethal despite optimal therapy (NIH). Specific prophylactic strategies include mechanical and pharmacologic

(continued on p. 454)

Table 3. Contraindications to Thrombolytic Therapy

Absolute Contraindications
    Active or recent internal bleeding
    History of hemorrhagic stroke
    Intracranial neoplasm
    Cranial surgery or head trauma within 14 days
Relative Contraindications
    Major thoracic or abdominal surgery
    Cardiopulmonary resuscitation   } within 7-10 days
    Biopsy or invasive procedure in a location inaccessible } within 7-10 days
       to external compression
    Pregnancy
    Coagulation defects (thrombocytopenia, coagulation
       factors deficiency)
    Uncontrolled severe hypertension
    Cerebrovascular accident (nonhemorrhagic)

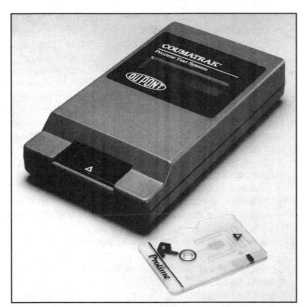

Figure 4. *The Coumatrak is a laser photometer. When a drop of whole blood is applied to the disposable plastic reagent cartridge, it is drawn by capillary action into a reagent chamber that contains a dry rabbit brain thromboplastin preparation. Coagulation begins when the blood rehydrates the thromboplastin. The reaction mixture continues flowing in the capillary channel beyond the reagent chamber before a clot develops. The laser photometer detects the cessation of blood flow (clotting) by sensing variation in light scatter caused by the movement of red blood cells.*

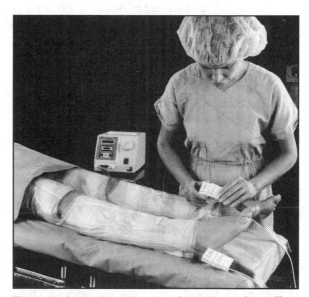

Figure 5. *Intermittent pneumatic compression utilizing the Kendall sequential compression device (SCD). The SCD provides separate compression cuffs at the ankle, calf, and thigh.*

treatment. The most commonly used mechanical approaches are graded elastic compression stockings (TEDS) to decrease venous stasis, and intermittent pneumatic compression (IPC) boots. IPC provides intermittent inflation of air-filled boots, or cuffs, which exert external leg compression and probably stimulate the endogenous fibrinolytic system (Figure 5).

Low-dose subcutaneous heparin is the most frequently used method of pharmacologic prophylaxis. Typical dosage is 5,000 U SC 2 hours preop and q8–12 hours for seven days. This regimen provides protection against development of venous thrombosis while minimizing bleeding complications (Collins et al.). Low-dose Coumadin, in combination with intermittent pneumatic compression boots, has gained increasing acceptance in prophylaxis for orthopedic surgery patients.

It is important to consider prophylactic measures in every hospitalized patient (Goldhaber 1988c). For high-risk patients, a combination of mechanical and pharmacologic measures should be employed. When absolutely no incremental blood loss is permissible (e.g., neurosurgery), IPC is the optimal modality. Those physicians who consult on preoperative patients should discuss VTE prophylaxis preoperatively with the surgeon who requested the consultation.

Clinical suspicion of PE is of paramount importance in establishing the diagnosis of PE. Recent findings from PIOPED indicate that diagnostic angiography should be employed more often. Fortunately, pulmonary angiography can be performed more safely than ever before. Advances in thrombolysis will enable us to treat effectively most of our patients with PE. During the next decade, prevention of PE will receive increased emphasis and implementation. In the 1990s, aggressive diagnosis, treatment, and prevention of PE should reduce the morbidity and mortality from this common illness.

Bibliography

Collins R, et al: Reduction in fatal pulmonary embolism and venous thrombosis by perioperative administration of subcutaneous heparin: Overview of results of randomized trials in general, orthopedic, and urologic surgery. *N Engl J Med* 318:1162, 1988.

Gillum RF: Pulmonary embolism and thrombophlebitis in the United States, 1970–1985. *Am Heart J* 114:1262, 1987.

Goldhaber SZ: Pulmonary embolism death rates. *Am Heart J* 115:1342, 1988.a

Goldhaber SZ: Optimal strategy for diagnosis and treatment of pulmonary embolism due to right atrial thrombus. *Mayo Clin Proc* 63:1261, 1988.b

Goldhaber SZ: Venous thromboembolism: How to prevent a tragedy. *Hospital Practice* 23:164, 1988.c

Goldhaber SZ: Tissue plasminogen activator in acute pulmonary embolism. *Chest* 95:282S, 1989.

Goldhaber SZ, Vaughan DE, Markis JE, et al: Acute pulmonary embolism treated with tissue plasminogen activator. *Lancet* 2:886, 1986.

Goldhaber SZ, Meyerovitz MF, Markis JE, et al. on behalf of the Participating Investigators: Thrombolytic therapy of acute pulmonary embolism: Current status and future potential. *J Am Coll Cardiol* 10:96B, 1987.

Goldhaber SZ, Kessler CM, Heit J, et al: A randomized controlled trial of recombinant tissue plasminogen activator versus urokinase in the treatment of acute pulmonary embolism. *Lancet* 2:293, 1988.

Grassi CJ, Goldhaber SZ: Interruption of the inferior vena cava for prevention of pulmonary embolism: Transvenous filter devices. *Herz* 14:182, 1989.

Hull RD, Hirsh J, Carter CJ, et al: Diagnostic value of ventilation-perfusion lung scanning in patients with suspected pulmonary embolism. *Chest* 88:819, 1985.

NIH Consensus Development Statement: Prevention of venous thrombosis and pulmonary embolism. *JAMA* 256:744, 1986.

Second American College of Chest Physicians (ACCP) Conference on Antithrombotic Therapy. *Chest* 95 (Suppl), 1989.

Terrin M, Goldhaber SZ, Thompson B, and the TIPE Investigators: Selection of patients with acute pulmonary embolism for thrombolytic therapy: The Thrombolysis in Pulmonary Embolism (TIPE) Patient Survey. *Chest* 95:279S, 1989.

30 Cardiac Disease and Pregnancy

Carl E. Orringer

Approximately 1% of the pregnancies in this country occur in women with underlying cardiac disease. Although rheumatic heart disease once accounted for about 90% of cardiac diseases during pregnancy, the incidence of rheumatic disease has fallen. Survival to childbearing age of patients operated on for congenital heart disease, and greater recognition of other types of heart disease, present the practitioner with a changing spectrum of patients with heart disease during pregnancy.

This chapter first addresses alterations in cardiovascular function and the cardiovascular signs and symptoms that accompany normal pregnancy. The majority of the remainder of the chapter is devoted to a discussion of specific cardiac disorders.

ALTERATIONS IN CARDIOVASCULAR FUNCTION DURING PREGNANCY

Pregnancy is characterized by dramatic alterations in the physiology of the cardiovascular system. Cardiac output may be substantially elevated at as early as 8–12 weeks of gestation and peaks between 20 and 24 weeks, at 30–40% above pre-pregnancy levels. During early pregnancy the elevated cardiac output is achieved primarily by increased stroke volume. In the later stages increased heart rate is the primary factor. Other factors that contribute to increased cardiac output are a diminution in afterload, largely due to the low-resistance uterine and placental circulations, and elevated estrogen levels, which increase cardiac output by expanding the blood volume and by enhancing cardiac contractility.

Maternal body position exerts a significant effect on the cardiac output. Hypotension and faintness develop in some pregnant women upon assuming the supine position; this is due to acute inferior vena cava obstruction by the gravid uterus. At term, 90% of pregnant women show complete obstruction of the inferior vena cava when they are in the supine position. Investigators have noted that cardiac output increases 31% when pregnant women turn from the supine to the left lateral decubitus position. Other characteristic physiologic changes are an expansion in maternal blood volume, averaging 40%; an increase in the resting heart rate by approximately 15 beats/min near term; an unaltered systolic, but reduced diastolic blood pressure, resulting in a widening of the pulse pressure; and no significant change in intracardiac pressures.

Up to 80% of healthy pregnant women have peripheral edema; this occurs as a result of the 8.5-L increase in total body water and the approximately 600-mEq increase in exchangeable sodium that characterizes a normal pregnancy. Uterine compression of the inferior vena cava also contributes to the edema.

Maternal hemodynamics are altered during labor, delivery, and the postpartum period. Each major uterine contraction is associated with a 10% rise in arterial pressure and an increase in the uterine blood volume of up to 500 ml. The increased venous return leads to an elevation in cardiac output of about 20% and a secondary sinus bradycardia. Each contraction also compresses the distal aorta and the common iliac arteries, resulting in an increase in blood pressure in the upper extremities and diminution of blood pressure in the lower extremities.

Anesthesia and analgesia administration may alter these values. With use of local anesthesia, the changes are virtually identical to those seen in the absence of medications during labor, delivery, and in the postpartum period. Caudal analgesia is associated with a less striking rise in the cardiac output, perhaps due to the more complete relief of pain. Cesarean section with balanced general anesthesia eliminates most of the hemodynamic changes of labor. The postpartum increase in cardiac output may also be attenuated, at least in part, by the 1,000-ml blood loss that occurs during this operation. Epidural anesthesia without epinephrine maintains maternal hemodynamic stability without significant rise in cardiac output at the time of delivery.

CARDIORESPIRATORY SYMPTOMS AND PHYSICAL SIGNS DURING NORMAL PREGNANCY

Normal pregnant women frequently have complaints which would, in nonpregnant patients, suggest cardiac or pulmonary disease. Dyspnea, diminished exercise tolerance, and easy fatigability are common. Palpitations are often reported. They may be a result of increased cardiac awareness due to the elevated stroke volume, or may be secondary to atrial or ventricular dysrhythmias. These dysrhythmias are common during pregnancy and the puerperium and are rarely of clinical importance.

On physical examination, pulses are usually full and occasionally bounding. The jugular venous pulsations are often prominent, particularly during the second and third trimesters. Venous hums are common. These continuous systolic and diastolic sounds, which are best heard in the supraclavicular fossa, are produced by the rapid downward flow of blood in the jugular veins and are of no pathologic significance. However, their tendency to be loudest during early diastole and their occasional transmission to the upper chest may lead to an incorrect diagnosis of patent ductus arteriosus or arteriovenous fistula.

On auscultation of the heart, the first heart sound is often widely split and accentuated. The second sound retains its normal phasic respiratory changes. A third heart sound, best heard at the apex, has been reported in 84% of normal pregnant women. Rarely, an early apical diastolic murmur may be heard. This sound is probably due to increased flow across the mitral valve. Systolic ejection murmurs, which occur in almost all pregnant women, are produced by a combination of the increased heart rate, blood volume and myocardial inotropy. One additional innocent murmur, the mammary souffle, may be heard over the breasts, particularly during the postpartum period. It is best heard with the patient supine and tends to diminish or disappear either with digital pressure at the site of auscultation or when the patient assumes the upright position.

ASSESSMENT OF CARDIOVASCULAR SYMPTOMS DURING PREGNANCY

The clinician who has a pregnant patient with cardiovascular symptoms should use testing procedures that offer the lowest risk to the health of the fetus and mother. Electrocardiography, echocardiography with or without Doppler studies, and 24-hour Holter monitoring can provide extensive clinical information on a wide variety of disorders, with no risk to the fetus or mother. X-ray studies should be done only when mandatory, and even then, only with appropriate shielding. Radionuclide imaging may increase the risk to the fetus that cancer will develop later in life; therefore, it should be avoided for evaluation of cardiac disease, although lung scanning may be necessary if there is a high clinical index of suspicion for the presence of pulmonary embolism. Invasive procedures, such as cardiac catheterization, coronary arteriography, or pulmonary angiography should be performed only when clinical symptoms suggest the presence of serious underlying disease, the noninvasive studies are nondiagnostic, and patient management is likely to be altered based on the results of the invasive study.

VALVULAR HEART DISEASE DURING PREGNANCY

Among pregnant patients with chronic rheumatic heart disease, 90% have pure or predominant mitral stenosis, 6–7% have predominant mitral regurgitation, and the remainder have aortic regurgitation with variable degrees of stenosis. With judicious medical management, most of these patients proceed safely through pregnancy and delivery.

Mitral stenosis is characterized by obstruction to left atrial emptying during diastole. In order to maintain cardiac output, left atrial pressure increases. Although this hemodynamic response generally serves to maintain cardiac output at or near its normal resting level, it is also associated with a concomitant rise in pulmonary capillary pressure. The increased heart rate and cardiac output of normal pregnancy result in an increased gradient across the stenotic mitral valve, and may therefore result in elevated left atrial, pulmonary venous, and pulmonary capillary pressure, leading to pulmonary congestion. The elevated left atrial pressure may also result in atrial tachyarrhythmias, particularly atrial fibrillation. Atrial fibrillation predisposes to pulmonary congestion because the loss of atrial contraction, coupled with the accompanying rapid ventricular response with its shortened diastolic filling period, increases left atrial pressure. Patients with mitral stenosis may also develop pulmonary arterial hypertension, right ventricular failure, and systemic and pulmonary embolism.

A sound therapeutic program for these patients acts to maintain a safe margin of cardiac reserve and attempts to prevent infectious complications. Cardiac reserve may be maximized primarily by adherence to a low-salt diet and by avoidance of strenuous exercise. The patient should be instructed to inform her physician promptly if palpitations, fever, or symptoms of pulmonary congestion develop. The physician should attempt to delineate the nature of the patient's palpitations by electrocardiography, ambulatory electrocardiographic monitoring, and echocardiography. Patients found to have significant left atrial enlargement or frequent paroxysmal atrial dysrhythmias should be managed with prophylactic digoxin so that the ventricular rate is controlled if the dysrhythmia becomes sustained. Patients in whom supraventricular tachycardia develops may also be treated with digoxin. Verapamil therapy may also be used, as it has not been shown to adversely affect the fetus, although it does cross the placenta. For sustained supraventricular dysrhythmias resistant to drug therapy or associated with pulmonary congestion, cardioversion may be necessary. Several reports indicate that this procedure may be performed without danger to the mother or the fetus.

Symptoms of pulmonary congestion due to dysrhythmias and refractory to salt restriction are often readily managed with small doses of oral diuretics. Complications of diuretic therapy in the newborn are rare, but include neonatal jaundice and thrombocytopenia. These drugs are generally well tolerated if the mother is carefully monitored.

In the pregnant patient with mitral stenosis, infections may have adverse hemodynamic consequences, primarily due to the tachycardia and increased cardiac output that accompanies fever. Killed influenza vaccine should be administered during pregnancy in the winter months in women with mitral stenosis, and repeated clean catch urinalyses should be performed throughout pregnancy. Women who already have small children may have increased risk of contracting streptococcal infections and should therefore receive rheumatic fever prophylaxis, preferably with penicillin.

In view of the 20% incidence of positive blood cultures that have been reported after cesarean section delivery, bacterial endocarditis prophylaxis with penicillin and an aminoglycoside should be given. Since endocarditis after spontaneous vaginal delivery is exceedingly rare, antibiotic prophylaxis is not warranted in these circumstances.

Indications for chronic anticoagulant therapy in pregnant women with mitral stenosis are the same as those in nonpregnant patients: the presence of left atrial enlargement on echocardiography or a history of atrial fibrillation or an embolic event. Warfarin (Coumadin) crosses the placental barrier, and its use is associated with embryopathy in the first trimester and neurologic defects due to fetal intracerebral bleeding in later pregnancy. Therefore, subcutaneous heparin, which does not cross the placenta, should be used. It should be administered in a dose of 10,000-20,000 units every 12 hours, as required to maintain the partial thromboplastin time 1.5 times the control value. Warfarin may once again be safely used during lactation.

Occasional pregnant patients with mitral stenosis may exhibit marked hemodynamic deterioration despite optimal medical therapy. Successful closed mitral commissurotomy during pregnancy was first reported in the United States in the 1950s, and several reviews in the 1960s reported maternal mortality rates of less than 2% and a fetal mortality rate of less than 10%. The era of open heart surgery led to mitral valve replacement using cardiopulmonary bypass in pregnant patients. There are no large series, but fetal mortality has been reported to be about 30%. The role that mitral valvuloplasty will play in the pregnant patient with mitral stenosis remains to be determined. However, in selected patients it may be an excellent temporizing measure to allow the symptomatic mother to proceed through pregnancy without the need for mitral valve surgery. Optimal candidates have mobile mitral leaflets that are not heavily calcified, minimal submitral calcification or scarring, and no or minimal concomitant mitral regurgitation.

Management of patients with mitral stenosis during labor should be directed toward maintenance of hemodynamic stability. Patients should, if possible, proceed throughout labor in the lateral recumbent position to minimize fluctuations in cardiac output. Those who exhibit hemodynamic decompensation during pregnancy should undergo arterial pressure monitoring and pulmonary artery catheterization to allow for careful and frequent assessment of oxygenation and right heart pressures.

Pregnancy in women with mechanical or bioprosthetic heart valves is becoming more common. Most of these women proceed through pregnancy without complications; the most common complications are those related to anticoagulant therapy.

The hemodynamics of aortic and mitral insufficiency generally improve with pregnancy, primarily as a result of diminished afterload; therefore, these conditions are usually not associated with symptomatic deterioration during pregnancy. Exceptions include instances of spontaneous rupture of mitral chordae tendineae or infective endocarditis involving either of these valves. Antibiotic prophylaxis is indicated for these lesions.

CONGENITAL HEART DISEASE

Although most women with acyanotic heart disease tolerate pregnancy satisfactorily, cyanotic congenital heart disease provides a major threat to both the mother and the fetus. The highest risk occurs in patients with Eisenmenger's complex, including cyanosis, pulmonary arterial hypertension, and right-to-left or bidirectional shunting. Maternal mortality is estimated to be 30–70%, and generally results from hemodynamic complications or arrhythmias either during delivery or immediately postpartum. Only 25% of fetuses reach term; therefore, the multiple complications of prematurity must be dealt with. In addition, 33% of those delivered die in the perinatal period.

Because of the high risk both to the mother and fetus, termination of pregnancy, a procedure associated with a 7% maternal mortality rate, should be considered. If termination is not elected, careful in-hospital monitoring should be undertaken and delivery should be accomplished in an intensive care unit or other location where life-threatening complications can be appropriately handled.

CARDIOMYOPATHIES

Primary myocardial disease does not usually affect pregnant patients. If it does, one of two types is likely to be seen: peripartal cardiomyopathy or hypertrophic cardiomyopathy.

Peripartal cardiomyopathy is an idiopathic congestive cardiomyopathy affecting previously healthy women during the last month of gestation or in any of the six months after delivery. No definite cause has been established, although an increased prevalence among older women and women with poor nutrition, toxemia of pregnancy, and twin pregnancies has been reported. Clinically, the patients manifest biventricular failure or embolic phenomena. Echocardiography reveals four-chamber cardiac enlargement, often with mural thrombi. Twenty-five percent to 50% of affected patients die due to emboli or heart failure, usually during the first three months postpartum. However, in those whose heart size returns to normal within six months of the onset of symptoms, the prognosis is generally good. Subsequent pregnancy is relatively contraindicated in those whose heart size has returned to normal, and is absolutely contraindicated in women with persistent cardiomegaly. Management of peripartal cardiomyopathy includes activity restriction, dietary sodium restriction, digoxin, diuretics, vasodilator therapy, and anticoagulation.

Hypertrophic cardiomyopathy sometimes becomes clinically evident for the first time during pregnancy. Affected patients exhibit left ventricular hypertrophy, often with asymmetric septal hypertrophy. The left ventricle is generally hyperdynamic and left ventricular end-diastolic pressure is often elevated. Some patients exhibit a resting gradient between the left ventricle and the aorta, while others have no gradient. The degree of left ventricular outflow tract obstruction is determined by three major factors: left ventricular end-diastolic volume; systemic vascular resistance, and the inotropic state of the left ventricle. Factors that increase the gradient include repeated Valsalva maneuvers, hypovolemia, and increased inotropy due to endogenous catecholamines produced during delivery. Clinically, these patients typically show mild functional deterioration, which resolves after delivery. Labor and delivery generally proceed well when the physician adheres to the following principles: (1) avoid digitalis glycosides; (2) avoid volume depletion and use diuretics sparingly; (3) advise the patient to maintain the left lateral recumbent position during labor to maximize venous return; (4) manage hypotension during delivery with blood replacement or pure vasoconstrictors; and (5) use intravenous beta blockers, when necessary, to improve the patient's hemodynamics.

PRIMARY PULMONARY HYPERTENSION

Idiopathic elevation of the mean pulmonary arterial pressure in the presence of normal left atrial or pulmonary capillary wedge pressure and in the absence of definable cardiac or pulmonary disease is referred to as idiopathic or primary pulmonary hypertension. As in Eisenmenger's complex, this condition is associated with a high incidence of maternal and fetal complications. The greatest risk of maternal right heart failure or death occurs during the latter part of pregnancy, at which time the hemodynamic demands are highest. Spontaneous abortions and fetal cardiac malformations are common. Termination of pregnancy is advisable. However, if this option is not chosen the patient should be hospitalized for careful monitoring. Unfortunately, no treatment has been consistently shown to alter the poor prognosis of these patients.

HYPERTENSION ASSOCIATED WITH PREGNANCY

Patients who become pregnant while taking antihypertensive drug therapy should generally continue therapy. Thiazide diuretics, methyldopa, and hydralazine have been successfully used in pregnant women, generally with good control of blood pressure and no significant fetal complications. Although there has been concern about use of beta blockers, such therapy is associated with an increased likelihood of birth of a normal infant. Angiotensin converting enzyme inhibitors reduce uterine blood flow, and therefore are not recommended during pregnancy.

Pre-eclampsia is defined as a blood pressure of 140/90 mm Hg or greater, edema, and proteinuria generally occurring after the 26th week of pregnancy. Patients with pre-eclampsia typically are young primagravida women, although an increased incidence is seen in diabetics and women with a multiple birth, and in the setting of a hydatidiform mole. This clinical picture may be distinguished from essential hypertension, which is seen earlier during pregnancy and which is often associated with higher blood pressure and evidence of end-organ involvement in a multigravid woman.

If the presence of pre-eclampsia is established, bed rest is advocated. If blood pressure is not controlled by bed rest, hospitalization and cautious antihypertensive drug therapy are warranted. Salt restriction, diuretics and sedatives should be avoided.

Pre-eclampsia–associated seizures constitute a condition known as eclampsia. Patients who exhibit eclampsia are treated with magnesium sulfate, which usually terminates the seizures. Delivery should then be postponed until the blood pressure is controlled

with use of intravenous antihypertensive therapy. This mode of therapy is associated with minimal maternal risk and excellent fetal survival. Neither pre-eclampsia nor eclampsia predisposes to chronic hypertension.

Bibliography

Brock RC: Valvulotomy in pregnancy. *Proc R Soc Med* 45:538, 1952.

Chesley LC, Annitto JE, Cosgrove RA: The remote prognosis of eclamptic women. *Am J Obstet Gynecol* 124:446, 1976.

Cooley DA, Chapman DW: Mitral commissurotomy during pregnancy, *JAMA* 150:1113, 1952.

Csapo A: Actomyosin formation by estrogen action. *Am J Physiol* 162:406, 1950.

Cutworth, R. MacDonald CB: Heart sounds and murmurs in pregnancy. *Am Heart J* 71:741, 1966.

Demakis JG, Rahimtoola SH, Sutton GC, et al: Natural course of peripartum cardiomyopathy. *Circulation* 44:1053, 1971.

Ehrenfeld EN, Brezizinski A, Braon K, et al: Heart disease in pregnancy. *Obstet Gynol* 23:363, 1964.

Golichowski A, Hathaway DR: Approach to the pregnant patient with heart disease. In: Kelley WN (ed-in-chief); Devita VT, Dupont HL, Harris ED et al., eds. *Textbook of Internal Medicine*. Philadelphia: JB Lippincott; 1988, p. 414.

Goodwin JR: Peripartial heart disease. *Clin Obstet Gynecol* 18:125, 1975.

Harken DE, Taylor WJ: Cardiac surgery during pregnancy. *Clin Obstet Gynecol* 4:697, 1961.

Hirsch J, Cade JF, Gallus AS: Anticoagulants in pregnancy: A review of indications and complications. *Am Heart J* 83:301, 1982.

Hytten FE, Leitch I: *The Physiology of Human Pregnancy*, ed 2. Oxford: Blackwell; 1971.

Hytten FE, Robertson EG: Maternal water metabolism in pregnancy. *Proc R Soc Med* 64:1072, 1971.

Hytten FE, Thompson AM: Water and electrolytes in pregnancy. *Br Med Bull* 24:15, 1968.

Kaplan NM: Systemic hypertension: Mechanisms and diagnosis. In: Braunwald E, ed. *Heart Disease. A Textbook of Cardiovascular Medicine*. Philadelphia: Saunders; 1980, p. 905.

Kaplan EL, Anthony BR, Bisno A, et al: Prevention of bacterial endocarditis. *Circulation* 56:139A, 1977.

Kolibash AJ, Ruiz DE, Lewis RP: Idiopathic hypertrophic subaortic stenosis in pregnancy. *Ann Intern Med* 82:791, 1975.

Lees MM, Taylor SH, Scott DB, et al: A study of cardiac output at rest throughout pregnancy. *J Obstet Gynecol Brit Comm* 74:319, 1967.

Logan A, Turner RWD: Mitral valvulotomy in pregnancy. *Lancet* 1:1286, 1952.

McAnulty JH, Metcalfe J, Veland K: Heart disease and pregnancy, *In*: Hurst JW, ed-in-chief; Logue RB, Rackley CE, Schlauf RC et al, eds.: *The Heart*. New York: McGraw-Hill; 1982, p. 1521.

Perloff JE: Pregnancy and cardiovascular disease. In Braunwald E, ed: *Heart Disease. A Textbook of Cardiovascular Medicine*. Philadelphia: Saunders; 1988, p. 1848.

Pritchard JA, Pritchard SA: Standardized treatment of 154 consecutive cases of eclampsia. *Am J Obstet Gynecol* 123;543, 1975

Rose DJ, Bader ME, Bader RA, et al: Catheterization studies of cardiac hemodynamics in normal pregnant women with reference to left ventricular work. *Am J Obstet Gynecol* 72:233, 1956.

Schroeder JS, Harrison DC: Repeated cardioversion during pregnancy: Treatment of refractory paroxysmal atrial tachycardia during three successive pregnancies. *Am J Cardiol* 27:455, 1971.

Snaith L, Szekely P: Cardiovascular surgery in relation to pregnancy. In: Marcus SL, Marcus CC, eds. *Advances in Obstetrics and Gynecology*. Baltimore: Williams and Wilkins; vol. I, 1967, p. 220.

Sussman HF, Duque D, Lesser ME: Atrial flutter with 1:1 conduction. *Dis Chest* 49:88, 1966.

Swan DA, Bell B, Oakley CM, et al: Analysis of symptomatic course and prognosis of hypertrophic obstructive cardiomyopathy. *Br Heart J* 33:671, 1971.

Szekely P, Snaith L: *Heart Disease and Pregnancy*. Edinburgh & London: Churchill-Livingstone; 1974.

Turner GM, Oakley CM, Dixon HG: Management of pregnancy complicated by hypertrophic obstructive cardiomyopathy. *Br Med* 4:281, 1968.

Ueland K, Akamatsu TJ, Eng M, et al: Maternal cardiovascular hemodynamics. VI. Cesarean section under epidural anesthesia without epinephrine. *Am J Obstet Gynecol* 114:775, 1972.

Ueland K, Hansen JM: Maternal cardiovascular hemodynamics. III. Labor and delivery under local and caudal analgesia. *Am J Obstet Gynecol* 103:8, 1968.

Ueland K, Hansen JM: Maternal cardiovascular hemodynamics. II. Posture and uterine contractions. *Am J Obstet Gynecol* 103:1, 1969.

Ueland K: Cardiac surgery and pregnancy. *Am J Obstet Gynecol* 92:148, 1965.

Vogel JHK, Pryor R, Blound SF Jr: Direct current defibrillation during pregnancy. *JAMA* 193:970, 1965.

Vorys N, Ullery JC, Hanusek GE: The cardiac output in various positions in pregnancy. *Am J Obstet Gynecol* 82:1312, 1961.

Zusman RM, Slater EE, Haber E: Hypertension. In: Eagle KA, Haber E, DeSanctis RW et al, eds. *The Practice of Cardiology*. Boston: Little, Brown and Co; 1989, p. 1357.

Aortic and Peripheral Arterial Disease

CHAPTER **31**

Marc A. Pfeffer

AORTIC DISEASE

As with any other viable tissue, the aorta is subject to systemic diseases, trauma, and degenerative changes, as well as congenital anomalies. Since even the grossly diseased aorta may perform the function of transmitting blood from the left ventricle to branch arteries, it is not uncommon for aortic diseases to be detected in asymptomatic persons. On the other end of the spectrum, the first clinical manifestation of aortic disease may be the catastrophic interruption in the integrity of this major arterial conduit. This chapter is concerned with diseases of the aorta that produce aneurysms and thereby threaten either rupture or the other serious manifestation of aortic disease: vascular occlusion.

The media of the large arteries have a high content of elastic fibers and smooth muscle cells. During the aging process, these cells and fibers degenerate and are replaced by fibrous tissue. This histologic change produces the well-known reduced aortic distensibility of aging and results in systolic hypertension and a greater work load on the left ventricle in elderly persons. Medionecrosis, defined as a focal loss of nuclei in the media, also has been described as an aging process of the aorta. These changes of the aorta are believed to represent injury and repair processes resulting from the continuous hemodynamic impact to which the aorta is subjected.

Another important histologic alteration of the media of the aorta is seen in idiopathic cystic medial necrosis. The histologic appearance of cystic medial necrosis is a focal loss of the normal elastic and fibromuscular elements of the media with replacement by amorphous ground substance. Although the etiology of cystic medial necrosis is truly idiopathic, the association with Marfan's syndrome has led to speculation that it is produced by a hereditary defect in elastic tissue formation. The histologic changes, whether degenerative or hereditary, are important in that they result in a weakening of the arterial wall. Such changes may result in localized dilatation of the vessel, or aneurysms. Once initiated, an aneurysm promotes its own expansion by the LaPlace relationship, in which wall tension is directly proportional to the product of the vessel radius and distending pressure. Thus, dilatation at a site of medial weakness increases wall tension, thereby promoting further expansion and thinning, which may lead to fatal rupture of a major vessel.

Aneurysms may occur at any location along the aorta, from the sinuses of Valsalva to the terminal bifurcation into the iliac arteries. The three important causes of aortic aneurysms are atherosclerosis, cystic medial necrosis, and syphilis. With the dramatic decrease in the incidence of tertiary syphilis, atherosclerotic aneurysms are now by far the most prevalent. Although atherosclerosis is an intimal process, secondary medial weakening is produced by destruction of elastic and fibromuscular support.

ATHEROSCLEROTIC ANEURYSMS

Abdominal Aortic Aneurysms

Most atherosclerotic aneurysms occur in the abdominal aorta, where over 90% of the aneurysms are caused by atherosclerosis. Typically, these aneurysms are fusiform, are located beneath the renal arteries, and may extend beyond the aortic bifurcation into the iliac arteries. Aside from the ever-present risk of rupture, these aneurysms usually contain mural thrombi and are potential sites for formation of emboli to the lower extremities.

Although patients with unruptured abdominal aortic aneurysms are usually asymptomatic, the presence

461

of dull abdominal or back pain, or awareness of an abdominal pulsation in an elderly person with other evidence of cardiovascular disease should alert the examiner to the possibility of aortic aneurysms. Physical examination may disclose a pulsatile abdominal mass, bruit, or evidence of peripheral arterial occlusive disease. In many instances, aortic aneurysms are first detected by abdominal roentgenograms performed for unrelated reasons. Not infrequently, the aneurysm is outlined by calcification of the atherosclerotic plaques. Abdominal ultrasound is a reliable method of detecting and sequentially following abdominal aortic aneurysms.

The major clinical problem with asymptomatic abdominal aortic aneurysm or with any asymptomatic aneurysm is assessing the comparative risks of operation or a life-limiting rupture. Although the actual frequency of deaths due to rupture in patients with abdominal aortic aneurysms is controversial, compilations of both autopsy and clinical studies indicate that in about one third of these patients, death was attributed to a ruptured aneurysm. One consistent conclusion is that the likelihood of rupture increased with the size of the aneurysm. The incidence of rupture of aneurysms larger than 6 cm in diameter approached 50%, whereas rupture of aneurysms less than 5 cm was considered uncommon. An autopsy series by Darling and coworkers confirmed this high rate of rupture of large aneurysms; however, the series also yielded a 23% rate of rupture of aneurysms of only 4 to 5 cm in diameter.

Although a prospective randomized study was not conducted, most available information indicates that survival after resection and graft replacement is longer than that in unoperated controls. In one particularly careful study of 480 operated and 233 untreated patients, the five-year survival of the operated group was 47%, compared with only 6% in the unoperated group. The leading cause of death in the unoperated patients was rupture of the aneurysm (45% of 174 deaths), followed by coronary atherosclerotic event (22%). Most patients surviving surgical resection eventually die from the associated cardiorespiratory problems so prevalent in this patient population.

With the progressive reduction in operative mortality, surgical treatment of the asymptomatic patient with an abdominal aortic aneurysm has become even more attractive. The operative mortality in experienced centers is 1–4% for elective resection of an abdominal aneurysm. This figure is impressive when one considers that the surgery is usually performed on elderly patients with diffuse atherosclerosis.

The clinical decision regarding resection of an aneurysm must be tailored to each patient. However, a reasonable framework is to recommend surgery for patients with aneurysms 5 cm in diameter or larger, or for symptomatic patients with even smaller aneurysms. Aneurysms 4–5 cm in diameter should not be considered benign, because there is still a definite risk of rupture. One may recommend elective resection or a more conservative course of frequent evaluation of the size of the aneurysm by ultrasound. An increase in cross-sectional diameter of 0.5 cm over three to six months is an indication for elective surgery.

In any event, the abdominal aortic aneurysm should be considered a manifestation of diffuse atherosclerosis. Patients with abdominal aortic aneurysms are at high risk of serious cardiovascular events. All efforts should therefore be directed at reducing risk factors that can be treated.

Thoracic Aortic Aneurysms

In the past half century, the etiology of the majority of the aneurysms of the thoracic aorta has shifted dramatically from syphilitic to atherosclerotic. In a large autopsy series compiled from the mid-1920s to the mid-1950s, over 80% of the aortic aneurysms were attributed to syphilis. Over 90% of these syphilitic aneurysms were located in the thoracic aorta and usually involved the ascending aorta. However, in a more recent review of 100 consecutive cases of ascending aortic aneurysms operated on by DeBakey's group, only 9% were attributed to syphilis. Secondary degenerative changes in the media produced by atherosclerosis accounted for 69% of the ascending aortic aneurysms. In 22 of the 100 patients, the ascending aortic aneurysms were believed to be due to cystic medial necrosis, and six patients demonstrated skeletal stigmata of Marfan's syndrome.

Marfan's syndrome represents an autosomal dominant transmitted disorder of connective tissue, with a constellation of musculoskeletal, ocular, and cardiovascular abnormalities. These patients are usually tall, with long extremities (span exceeds height) and with elongated fingers and toes (arachnodactyly). High arched palate, pectus excavatum, and kyphoscoliosis are other musculoskeletal abnormalities associated with the syndrome. Lax ligaments, including the suspensory ligament of the lens, may result in subluxation of the lens (ectopia lentis). The cardiovascular abnormalities, which may include "floppy" redundant mitral valves and degenerative changes in the media of the major vessels, account for most of the premature deaths in affected persons. The medial degeneration characteristically involves the aortic ring and sinuses. Aortic regurgitation or rupture, and/or medial dissection of the aorta arc grave consequences of the focal loss of elastic and fibromuscular elements in the aortic wall. The terms *anuloaortic ectasia* and *idiopathic cystic medial necrosis* are often used to describe similar aortic conditions without other musculoskeletal stigmata of Marfan's syndrome.

The clinical approach to aneurysms of the thoracic aorta, whether atherosclerotic, luetic, or cystic medial necrotic, should be directed to the basic clinical question: whether the aneurysm poses such a threat to survival that surgical resection should be undertaken.

As with abdominal aortic aneurysms, several associated factors appear to greatly reduce the five-year survival rate of persons with thoracic aortic aneurysms. A vessel diameter of 6 cm or larger, associated atherosclerotic disease manifested in other regions, hypertension, and the presence of symptoms all appear to adversely alter the natural history of thoracic aortic aneurysms.

Thoracic aneurysms are more likely to produce symptoms than abdominal aneurysms. Pain described as a deep throbbing or aching sensation was the presenting symptom of 18 of the 107 patients with aneurysms of the thoracic aorta reported by Joyce et al. Other presenting symptoms include cough and dyspnea from compression of the tracheobronchial tree, dysphagia from extrinsic compression of the esophagus, and hoarseness from involvement of the recurrent laryngeal nerve. Symptoms in patients with ascending aortic aneurysms may also reflect the commonly associated aortic regurgitation due to dilatation of the aortic ring.

In patients with ankylosing spondylitis, very limited aortic involvement may lead to severe aortic insufficiency. In this relatively benign rheumatologic condition, a very limited area of aorta behind the sinuses and into the leaflets may be involved by an adventitial infiltrate clustering around the vasa vasora, as in syphilitic aortitis. Because of the critical location of this limited aortic involvement, severe aortic regurgitation may be produced which, when present, is the leading cause of cardiovascular morbidity in this otherwise benign disease.

Advances in prosthetic valves and synthetic grafts and in cardiopulmonary bypass procedures have reduced the mortality and morbidity rates of even complex aortic reconstruction by experienced thoracic surgeons. Surgical intervention is urgent in patients with large symptomatic aneurysms. In patients who have smaller asymptomatic aneurysms but who do not have aortic insufficiency, the risk of surgery must be weighed against the risk of the continued presence of the aneurysm. In patients with Marfan's syndrome, prophylactic repair of asymptomatic ascending aortic aneurysms of 6 cm or greater is recommended.

Aortic Dissection

Perhaps the most catastrophic of all diseases of the aorta is acute dissection. A compilation of almost 1,000 untreated patients revealed a 50% mortality rate within 48 hours after the onset of pain. Before effective treatment was available, 90% of the patients died within three months of acute aortic dissection. During the past quarter of a century, advances in radiologic, medical, and surgical practices have so altered this grim prognosis that one can now expect to save 70–80% of patients presenting with acute aortic dissections.

The fundamental pathologic lesion in aortic dissection is a cleavage of the aortic media by a dissecting hematoma. Degenerative changes in the media of the aorta, whether from congenital defects or changes produced by aging and hypertension, are the predisposing factors for aortic dissection. With each cardiac contraction, the ascending aorta and the aorta just distal to the left subclavian are flexed by the sudden installation of the volume of blood into the arterial tree. In some patients, these forces produce an intimal tear, permitting blood to enter the weakened media. Once initiated, the dissecting hematoma may propagate rapidly, involving a variable length of the aorta. The aortic media is cleaved into a thin outer wall surrounding a false channel. This thin outer wall is all that protects the aorta against fatal rupture and extravasation of blood. The propagation of the dissecting hematoma has been shown in experimental animals to depend on the rate of rise of arterial pressure (dP/dt) and the level of blood pressure. Untreated, a dissecting hematoma almost invariably progresses to rupture and death. Hemopericardium with cardiac tamponade and hemothorax are the most frequent fatal complications. Aside from outright rupture, the medial hemorrhage may distort the aortic annulus and produce aortic regurgitation. Occlusion of a major branch artery is yet another major complication of aortic dissection. The false channel may so compress the lumen of the true channel as to produce arterial insufficiency of the region supplied by the branch vessel. In aortic dissection, renal, splanchnic, cerebral, and even coronary ischemia may be encountered as a consequence of compression of the vital arteries.

As with other catastrophic disease processes, a rapid and accurate diagnosis is essential so that life-sustaining therapy can be immediately instituted. Severe pain is the outstanding clinical feature that should alert the physician to the possibility of aortic dissection. The pain is usually characterized as sharp and tearing; however, it may mimic the pain of a myocardial infarction. It may be localized in the anterior chest, interscapular region, and, particularly in distal dissections, may occur simultaneously in several regions both above and below the diaphragm. In some instances, because of an altered state of consciousness, pain is not perceived, and therefore is not a presenting symptom. Neurological symptoms indicative of cerebral ischemia represent an ominous presentation of aortic dissection.

Patients with acute aortic dissection characteristically appear in overt distress. Arterial pressure is usually elevated at the time of presentation. Hypotension is suggestive of proximal dissection or aortic rupture. Occlusion of an arterial branch of the aorta by compression of the true lumen produces the reduced or absent arterial pulse found in about one third of the patients with aortic dissections. Therefore, careful examination of carotid, brachial, radial, and femoral arteries is important.

A murmur of aortic regurgitation is detected in about one third of the patients with aortic dissection. It usually indicates proximal dissection with loss of annular support.

The electrocardiogram is usually abnormal, but nonspecific. Left ventricular hypertrophy with or without evidence of strain or ischemia is common. Severe chest discomfort without electrocardiographic evidence of myocardial necrosis should raise the suspicion of aortic dissection.

Plain films of the chest often provide findings suggestive of aortic dissection. The most common abnormalities are in the region of the aortic knob. In one study of patients with aortic dissection, findings of an increased aortic diameter, double density as a result of posterior aortic enlargement, or deviation of the trachea to the right were reported in more than half the cases of aortic dissection. Mediastinal widening or displacement of calcified intima by more than 1 cm was noted in only 11% and 7%, respectively, of the plain films of patients with confirmed dissections. In this study, the plain chest films were not suggestive of aortic diseases in 20% of the patients with confirmed aortic dissection.

Transesophageal echocardiography may provide an accurate method of diagnosing aortic dissection, but experience with this technique is limited.

Aortography is required to confirm the diagnosis of aortic dissection. The objectives of the procedure are to determine the origin of the dissection and to define the extent of the dissecting hematoma. The most common angiographic finding is opacification of the false channel, creating a double lumen.

Treatment of aortic dissection has progressed dramatically in the past 25 years. In 1955, DeBakey and co-workers reported a surgical approach to dissecting aneurysms. By the mid-1960s, they reported a 74% survival rate in an extensive series of patients with dissections. Based on this experience, DeBakey defined specific surgical approaches to aortic dissection according to the origin and extent of the dissection. Type I dissections begin at the ascending aorta and extend to the abdominal aorta; type II dissections are localized to the ascending aorta and aortic arch; and type III dissections begin just distal to the left subclavian artery and extend to below the diaphragm. The results of other surgical series are not as impressive as those of DeBakey's group.

Wheat and co-workers reported encouraging results with intensive medical therapy in patients with acute aortic dissection. They reasoned that the complications of aortic dissection were produced by progression of the medial hematoma and not the initial intimal tear itself. Hydrodynamic forces in the arterial system, particularly the rate of rise of arterial pressure, as well as the level of blood pressure, are the major factors determining the propagation of the hematoma to rupture and death. Pharmacologic attempts to halt progression of the medial hematoma, therefore, are directed at reducing the steepness of the pulse wave (dP/dt) and reducing arterial pressure. By the late 1960s, Wheat had treated more than 50 patients using medical therapy, with survival rates as impressive as in DeBakey's surgical series.

By the early 1970s, as more experience was gained with both surgical and medical therapies, it was apparent that neither blanket surgical nor medical strategies provided optimal management of patients with aortic dissection. The Stanford group introduced a new classification that is of therapeutic and prognostic importance: type A dissections originate in the ascending aorta (DeBakey I and II) and type B dissections begin after the left subclavian artery (DeBakey III). Roughly two thirds of aortic dissections are type A and one third are type B.

Recent results compiled from six centers indicate that surgery is the treatment of choice for proximal (type A) aortic dissections. Of the 46 patients with acute dissection originating in the ascending aorta who were treated medically, only 12 patients (26%) survived. In contrast, of the 71 patients with type A dissections who were treated surgically, 50 (70%) survived. With ascending aortic involvement, the potential for retrograde dissection and fatal pericardial tamponade is great and prompt surgical intervention is indicated.

In contrast, patients with type B, or dissecting hematoma distal to the left subclavian artery not involving the ascending aorta, have a slight advantage with medical therapy. In this same report from six centers, 62 patients with type B dissections were treated medically and 50 (81%) survived. In patients with distal dissection, the surgical survival was not as good as in the medically treated group. Of the 40 patients with distal dissections undergoing surgical intervention, only 20 (50%) survived. Therefore, in the uncomplicated distal dissection, medical therapy has an advantage over surgical intervention.

Using recent carefully documented experiences, a unified plan can be suggested that will provide for the optimal management of patients with acute aortic dissection. Patients suspected of having an aortic dissection should be treated immediately to halt progression of the dissecting hematoma. This therapy should reduce arterial pressure to the lowest level commensurate with organ perfusion and reduce the rate of rise of arterial pressure. The ganglionic blocker trimethaphan has been used effectively for this purpose. Alternatively, use of the vascular smooth muscle dilator nitroprusside in combination with a beta-adrenergic blocking agent such as propranolol provides therapy designed to arrest the progression of the dissecting hematoma.

Once the patient's pain and blood pressure are controlled, aortography should be performed promptly. The aortogram should confirm the diagnosis and determine whether the dissecting hematoma involves the ascending aorta. The distal circulation should be defined to determine if the dissection is producing an occlusion of a major branch of the aorta. Identification of a proximal dissection provides an urgent indication for surgical therapy.

Distal dissections not involving the ascending aorta do somewhat better with medical therapy. If no complications are encountered in patients with type B dissections, intravenous antihypertensive agents can be replaced by an oral therapy, which should include a beta-adrenergic blocking agent. If a patient with distal dissection receiving intensive medical therapy has complications, surgical intervention is required. Indications for surgical intervention in patients with distal dissection are: evidence of continued propagation of the hematoma, continued pain, new aortic insufficiency murmur, and signs of occlusion of a major branch of the aorta, such as new neurologic findings, loss of an arterial pulse, or inability to control pressure. Indications of impending rupture of the dissecting hematoma, such as increasing size of the aneurysm and blood in the pleural space or pericardium, are other indications for surgical intervention, even in patients with type B acute dissections.

If a medically or surgically treated patient has survived the acute phase of dissection, careful follow-up evaluations should be performed. Impressive five-year survival rates have been reported for both medically and surgically treated patients who have survived the acute phase of the aortic dissection.

In summary, in the past 25 years, much progress has been made in the management of acute aortic dissection. One can now expect a 70–80% survival rate for a condition that was once almost always fatal.

OCCLUSIVE DISEASES OF AORTA AND PERIPHERAL VESSELS

Atherosclerosis is the cause of chronic occlusive disease of arteries in 95% of the cases. The infrarenal abdominal aorta and its iliac branches are the common sites of extensive atherosclerosis that produces chronic ischemia of the lower limbs. A dynamic state exists between progressive occlusive disease and development of collateral channels. As with coronary artery disease, ischemia is a result of an imbalance between oxygen delivery and utilization.

Intermittent claudication, the discomfort in the limbs that occurs with exercise and is relieved by rest, is usually the first symptom of chronic occlusive arterial disease. This ischemic pain is usually indicative of severe multisegmental occlusive disease. With severe occlusive disease, nonobstructing factors that reduce oxygen delivery, such as reduced cardiac output, relative hypotension, and anemia, may enhance peripheral ischemia. In the patient awakened by an aching numbness from a distal limb, the slight increase in arterial inflow produced by the gravitational effect of hanging the extremity over the edge of the bed may be sufficient to relieve the ischemic pain. In its most severe form, chronic occlusive arterial disease may present as ischemic ulcers with gangrene as an end stage. The hallmark of the physical examination of patients with chronic occlusive arterial disease is diminished peripheral pulses. Bruits may or may not be heard. Postural color changes such as pallor on elevation and rubor on dependency of the extremity are indicative of moderate to severe arterial insufficiency. Nutritional atrophy of skin and nails should be noted.

Noninvasive assessment of the arterial inflow to the extremity provides a more standardized diagnostic assessment. A pressure index of Doppler-determined systolic pressures in tibial and brachial arteries provides quantitative assessment of the degree of chronic occlusive arterial disease.

In consideration of therapeutic courses, both the patient and physician must be aware that intermittent claudication does not alter life expectancy. The limitation of activity imposed by the exercise-induced pain may be acceptable to the patient. However, the intermittent claudication may so disable the patient that elective revascularization to improve the quality of life may be desired. Also, revascularization may be urgently recommended to avoid the possible loss of a limb.

A detailed medical evaluation is most important in all patients considered for arterial reconstructive surgery. Patients with symptoms of atherosclerosis in the extremities usually have coexisting cardiac and respiratory disease. In obtaining a cardiac history from these patients, the physician must be aware that the functional limitations produced by the peripheral vascular disease may mask significant coronary artery disease. Indeed, it is our practice to perform exercise tests for ischemic cardiac changes before vascular reconstructive surgery even though the test is usually limited by claudication. If there is clinical evidence of impressive myocardial ischemia at low exercise levels, coronary angiography is recommended.

Patients with chronic occlusive arterial disease should be instructed to provide meticulous care and avoid trauma to ischemic extremities. It is not uncommon for urgent bypass surgery or even amputation to be required in a person considered a relatively poor operative risk because of avoidable injury to the ischemic extremity. Cigarette smoking is strongly contraindicated, as evidenced by the 10–fold increase in amputation rate of patients with chronic occlusive arterial disease who continue to smoke compared with those who stop. Vasodilator therapy is generally ineffective. Pentoxifylline, by making red blood cells more deformable and thereby increasing post-stenotic blood flow, purportedly prolongs time to onset of leg pain during exercise testing in patients with intermittent claudication. However, the subjective clinical responses to this therapy have not been impressive.

Arterial reconstructive surgery then should be considered in suitable candidates to improve a disabling lifestyle, relieve pain at rest, or—the most urgent indication—prevent tissue necrosis and amputation.

Percutaneous transluminal angioplasty in appropriate patients provides an excellent alternative to reconstructive surgery. Long-term patency appears better for iliac than for femoral angioplasty, with approximately 80% and 60% three- to five-year patency rates, respectively. Experience with the newer atherectomy catheters and laser probe is too recent to determine long-term outcome.

Takayasu's Arteritis

Takayasu's arteritis, or pulseless disease, is a rare, nonspecific inflammatory process of unknown etiology affecting segmental areas of the aorta and its main branches. The disease process results in a marked thickening of the arterial wall, which eventually produces occlusions of major branches of the aorta. Takayasu's arteritis has been linked to rheumatic fever, syphilis, and tuberculosis; however, the evidence for each of these associations is sketchy. It is far more prevalent among women; the female to male ratio is 9:1. Unlike giant cell (temporal) arteritis, which usually afflicts elderly men, Takayasu's arteritis is a disease of young persons. Although typically described as a disease of young Oriental women, Takayasu's arteritis has a worldwide distribution.

Several classifications of regional involvement of the aorta and major branches have been described. The most common areas of the arterial tree to be involved with the proliferative process are the aortic arch, including the origins of the brachiocephalic arteries, and the thoracoabdominal aorta, including the renal arteries.

The symptoms and signs of arterial occlusive disease are usually preceded by an initial systemic illness presenting with fever, weight loss, arthralgias, and fatigue. In the chronic phase, the young patient presents with cardiovascular and neurologic symptoms related to arterial obstruction. Absent pulses and vascular bruits are almost always found. Hypertension was reported in 72% of a recent series of 107 patients with Takayasu's arteritis (Lupi-Herrera et al.). Renal artery involvement caused hypertension in the majority of cases. The clinical course of this devastating arteritis is unpredictable. At present, therapy is directed only at the manifestations of the disease process: steroids for constitutional symptoms; antihypertensive therapy; possible anticoagulation therapy; and surgical vascular bypass procedures to reconstruct flow to vital organs.

Bibliography

Coffman JD: New drug therapy and peripheral vascular disease. *Med Clin North Am* 72:1, 1988.

Cooke JP, Safford RE: Progress in the diagnosis and management of aortic dissection. *Mayo Clin Proc* 61:147, 1986.

Darling RC, Messina CR, Brewster DC: Autopsy study of unoperated abdominal aortic aneurysms. The case for early resection. *Circulation* 56 (Suppl 2):II–161, 1977.

Gott VL, Pyeritz RE, Magovern GJ, Cameron DE, McKusick VA: Surgical treatment of aneurysms of the ascending aorta in the Marfan syndrome. Results of composite-graft repair in 50 patients. *N Engl J Med* 314:1070, 1986.

Joyce JW, Fairbairn JF II. Kincaid OW, et al: Aneurysms of the thoracic aorta. *Circulation* 29:176, 1964.

Lindsay J Jr, Hurst JW: *The Aorta.* New York: Grune & Stratton; 1979.

Lupi-Herrera E, Sánchez-Torres G, Marcushamer J, et al: Takayasu's arteritis. Clinical study of 107 cases. *Am Heart J* 93:94, 1977.

Mannick JA: Surgical treatment of aneurysms of the abdominal and thoracic aorta. *Prog Cardiovasc Dis* 16:69, 1973.

Perdue GD, Smith RB III: Chronic aortoiliac occlusion. *In:* Lindsay, Hurst, eds: *The Aorta.* New York: Grune & Stratton; 1979, p. 189.

Pyeritz RD, McKusick VA: The Marfan syndrome: Diagnosis and management. *N Engl J Med* 300:772, 1979.

Roberts WC: Aortic dissection: Anatomy, consequences, and causes. *Am Heart J* 101:195, 1981.

Wheat MW Jr: Acute dissecting aneurysms of the aorta: Diagnosis and treatment—1979. *Am Heart J* 99:373, 1980.

Widlus DM, Osterman FA: Evaluation and percutaneous management of atherosclerotic peripheral vascular disease. *JAMA* 261:3148, 1989.

32 Cardiovascular Problems in Patients With Primarily Noncardiac Diseases

Joel S. Landzberg
James D. Marsh

The internist or cardiologist is frequently asked to see patients who have primarily noncardiac disorders but are suspected of having some cardiovascular complication arising from their primary disease or its therapy. Many disorders have secondary manifestations that involve the pericardium, myocardium, epicardium, valves, great vessels, coronary arteries or the neurohumoral regulation of the heart and circulation. This chapter discusses the recognition and management of cardiovascular manifestations of primarily noncardiac diseases.

RHEUMATOID AND BONE DISORDERS

Paget's Disease

Paget's disease (osteitis deformans) is a skeletal abnormality that afflicts between 1% and 3% of the United States population over age 40 years. Cardiac manifestations of Paget's disease can include high-output congestive heart failure and metastatic calcification of the cardiac skeleton, producing varying degrees of conduction abnormalities. For many years arteriovenous fistulas were believed to be present in the bone marrow of patients with this disorder. However, radiolabeled macroaggregated-albumin studies show that there are no true AV fistulas present. Instead, cutaneous and soft tissue vasodilatation frequently accounts for increased flow to an extremity. In some patients, the blood flow through the involved extremity is nine times the normal level.

Paget's disease most frequently presents in elderly patients. However, the most frequent causes of congestive heart failure in Paget's disease patients are also the usual causes in an elderly population, such as ischemic heart disease or hypertensive heart dis-

ease, and not high-output heart failure. High-output symptoms respond well to a pulse of steroids such as prednisone, 60 mg/day. Hemodynamic improvement is usually evident within three or four days.

Rheumatoid Arthritis

Involvement of cardiac structures in rheumatoid arthritis is very common but usually subclinical (Table 1). Nodular granulomas are the characteristic pathologic lesions involving the myocardium, endocardium, and valves. Granulomas sometimes involve the conduction system and produce varying degrees of heart block. The most frequent electrocardiographic abnormality in patients with rheumatoid arthritis is first-degree atrioventricular (AV) block. Rheumatoid granulomas may involve the cardiac valves, but very rarely cause enough distortion of the valve structure to cause regurgitation or stenosis of any hemodynamic significance. Myocarditis and coronary arteritis may be present at necropsy but they rarely cause clinical symptoms.

In approximately 30% of patients with rheumatoid arthritis, the pericardium is involved at necropsy or on echocardiographic study. However, pericarditis is clinically evident in only about 5% of patients with rheumatoid arthritis and usually follows a benign course, responding to moderate doses of steroids. Rarely, pericarditis is severe, producing either constriction or tamponade. Needle pericardiocentesis is often technically difficult to perform because of the markedly thickened pericardium and the tendency for loculation of pericardial effusions. When pericardial fluid is obtained, complement levels and glucose are frequently depressed, as they are in fluid from other serous spaces in rheumatoid arthritis.

Table 1. Cardiovascular Manifestations of Rheumatoid Diseases

	Pericarditis	Fibrosis	Myocarditis/ Endocarditis	↑ BP	Valves Involved	Conduction Abnormalities	Granulomas
Rheumatoid arthritis	+ +	+	+		AoV MV	+	Nodular granulomas
SLE	+ + + +	+ +	+ + +	+ +	AoV MV	+	Microvasculitis
Periarteritis nodosa		+ +		+ + + +			Necrotizing vasculitis
Scleroderma	+ +	+ + + +	+	+ + + +		+ + +	Vascular fibrosis

AoV = aortic valve; BP = blood pressure; MV = mitral valve; SLE = systemic lupus erythematosus.

Systemic Lupus Erythematosus

Cardiac manifestations of systemic lupus erythematosus (SLE) are numerous (Table 1). The underlying pathologic abnormality is diffuse microvasculitis. Cardiac involvement is very common at necropsy, although clinical cardiac involvement is present in only about half of cases. Systemic lupus erythematosus produces pancarditis with involvement of the pericardium most evident clinically. Approximately 30% of all patients with SLE have clinical symptoms of pericarditis and another substantial proportion may have findings of pericarditis on auscultation or electrocardiography. Inflammation of the pericardium may be pronounced, involving the epicardium and occasionally even the sinoatrial (SA) and AV nodes, with destruction of conducting fibers and resulting arrhythmias and conduction blocks. Pericardial constriction or tamponade occurs in a small but important number of patients. Corticosteroids usually control the symptoms of pericarditis. No compelling evidence shows that administration of steroids prevents progression to constriction. Patients with refractory pericardial symptoms may rarely require pericardiectomy.

The myocarditis of SLE is due to segmental arteritis of the small arteries in the myocardium. Subclinical myocarditis is common. It produces fibrinoid necrosis in small vessels, although actual necrosis of myocardial cells is rare. In SLE, arteritis of the major coronary arteries leading to a clinical myocardial infarction is a very rare event. However, the incidence of atherosclerotic coronary artery disease may be somewhat higher in patients with SLE. In these patients, clinical myocardial ischemia or necrosis is far more likely to be due to typical large-vessel coronary artery disease than to arteritis. Thus, patients with signs of myocardial ischemia are best treated with conventional measures rather than with a pulse of steroids as a first approach.

Libman-Sacks endocarditis is observed at necropsy in 50% of cases of SLE. These verrucous excrescences on valve leaflets are comprised of degenerating valve tissue. A prospective echocardiographic study found that 18% of patients with SLE had abnormalities of their heart valves. Those with Libman-Sacks vegetations had a relatively benign course, whereas 80% of those with rigid, thickened valves required surgery over a five-year period. In view of the frequent valve abnormalities in SLE patients, and the frequency of immunosuppressive therapy with steroids, antibiotic prophylaxis for endocarditis is recommended.

Children born to mothers with SLE are at risk for congenital complete heart block, due to transplacental transfer of maternal antibodies.

Periarteritis Nodosa

Necrotizing vasculitis of muscular arteries is the pathologic hallmark of periarteritis nodosa (Table 1). Gross nodularity of the involved vessels is apparent at necropsy. The vasculitis may produce infarction of an involved organ and, when coronary arteries are involved, as they frequently are, myocardial necrosis may occur. Clinically recognized acute myocardial infarction caused by periarteritis nodosa is uncommon, although clinically unrecognized events are frequent, as patchy fibrosis of the myocardium is common and contributes to the dilation of the left ventricle that frequently occurs. Small aneurysms of coronary arteries are present, particularly at bifurcations; on occasion, they may rupture and produce hemopericardium. Pericarditis is uncommon in the disorder, as is endocarditis.

The clinical picture of cardiac involvement with periarteritis nodosa is most frequently dominated by the effects of hypertension resulting from renal involvement. Indeed, congestive heart failure secondary to hypertension and renal involvement is a very common cause of death.

Scleroderma (Progressive Systemic Sclerosis)

In this systemic fibrosing disease, visceral rather than skin involvement is the main determinant of the clinical course. There is gradual obliteration of small vessels with extensive fibrosis and scarring. Progressive systemic sclerosis often involves the heart pathologically, although clinical involvement is less often appreciated (Table 1). A pancarditis is produced, with pericarditis common but often asymptomatic, myocarditis common, and endocardial thickening unusual. Intimal sclerosis of small intramural coronary arteries produces ischemia and focal areas of myocardial necrosis and fibrosis. Focal fibrosis frequently causes conduction abnormalities; if fibrosis is extensive, cardiomyopathy may result. Direct cardiac involvement is often overshadowed by cardiac effects of both pulmonary and systemic hypertension. Both right and left ventricular failure are common. If congestive heart failure develops, due either to hypertension or to direct myocardial involvement, the prognosis is poor. Conduction abnormalities usually indicate primary myocardial involvement.

Specific treatment is not entirely satisfactory. Corticosteroids have a beneficial effect on pericarditis in scleroderma, and there have been reports of calcium channel blockers improving myocardial and pulmonary blood flow. Conduction disturbances occasionally require management with a permanent pacemaker. Aggressive management of hypertension in scleroderma is essential.

Ankylosing Spondylitis

Dilatation of the aortic root and fibrosis of the aortic valve cusps produce incompetence of the aortic valve in approximately 10% of patients with ankylosing spondylitis. Fibrosis usually occurs at the base of the valves but can extend into the conduction system, causing conduction defects. Aortic regurgitation may become severe and valve replacement may be necessary.

Dermatomyositis

Dermatomyositis involves primarily the skin and the skeletal muscles. Clinical cardiovascular manifestations are unusual, although pathologic abnormalities are frequently present. Degeneration and fibrosis occur primarily in the conduction system and occasionally in scattered areas of myocardium. While usually asymptomatic, arrhythmias and heart block have been observed and repolarization abnormalities are frequently present on the electrocardiogram.

Kawasaki Syndrome (Mucocutaneous Lymph Node Syndrome)

Kawaski syndrome is an idiopathic acute febrile illness of children associated with fever, rash, peripheral edema, dry fissured lips, strawberry tongue, conjunctival congestion, cervical lymphadenopathy and cardiac involvement. Coronary artery aneurysms develop in approximately 20% of children and thrombosis of the coronary arteries is the major cause of death. Two-year follow-up coronary arteriography in children with aneurysms shows resolution in half of the cases. Randomized studies show that therapy with intravenous gamma globulin plus aspirin significantly reduces the incidence of coronary artery abnormalities when administered early.

Marfan's Syndrome

Cardiovascular manifestations of Marfan's syndrome are prominent and frequently determine the fate of patients with the syndrome (Table 2). Cystic medial necrosis is present in the aorta, with degeneration of the elastic elements. The ascending aorta is frequently dilated, as is the aortic annulus. Sinuses of Valsalva may become grossly enlarged; frequently, the proximal pulmonary artery is dilated. Chronic aortic dissection and tears with dissection are frequently found. Dilatation of the aortic valve annulus leads to chronic aortic regurgitation, with left ventricular dilatation and hypertrophy as a consequence. The mitral valve may have intrinsic abnormalities as well, with redundancy of the mitral valve leaflets often seen by echocar-

Table 2. Cardiovascular Manifestations of Connective Tissue Disorders

Syndrome	AoV	MV	Ascending Aorta	Peripheral Arteries	Cardiac Chambers
Marfan's	+ + + +	+ + +	+ + + +		
Osteogenesis imperfecta	+ + +	+ +	+ + +		
Ehlers-Danlos		+	+ +	+ + +	
Pseudoxanthoma elasticum	+ +	+ + +		+ + + +	Restriction
Hurler's	+ +	+ +			Dilation

AoV = aortic valve involvement; MV = mitral valve involvement.

diography. The chordae tendineae are often elongated, and occasionally there is frank fenestration of the mitral valve leaflets.

In patients with Marfan's syndrome, death from a cardiac cause is very common, with aortic dilatation, dissection, or rupture in most patients. Mitral regurgitation may be the dominant clinical feature, although somewhat less frequently than aortic regurgitation. Because of markedly altered hemodynamics and turbulent blood flow, endocarditis may be a complication. Ventricular conduction abnormalities have also been reported.

The cardiovascular management of a patient with Marfan's syndrome is directed toward minimizing the hemodynamic stress in the arterial tree. To this end, beta-adrenergic blockers are frequently used. Replacement of the ascending aorta with a Dacron graft-valve conduit before severe dilatation and aortic regurgitation evolve appears to improve the prognosis in patients with progressive aortic root dilatation (>6 cm in diameter). (See also Chapter 31.)

Miscellaneous Connective Tissue Disorders

All of the connective tissue disorders, not surprisingly, affect the heart and vascular system (Table 2). Due to valvular involvement, endocarditis prophylaxis is generally recommended.

Osteogenesis imperfecta affects type 1 collagen, which is responsible for structural support. The spectrum of cardiac manifestations is similar to that of Marfan's syndrome except that clinical cardiac involvement is much less frequent and severe.

Ehlers-Danlos syndrome is characterized by defective collagen synthesis, leading to weakness in arterial walls, cardiomegaly and valvular heart disease.

Affected patients have a high incidence of aortic and peripheral vascular dissection and rupture, both spontaneously and secondary to minimal trauma. Therefore, arterial catheterization, including placement of radial arterial lines, should be avoided.

Pseudoxanthoma elasticum is characterized by dysplasia of the elastic tissue with an increase in elastic fibers that are structurally abnormal and have a propensity to calcify. This results in abnormally calcified and thickened vessels, causing coronary artery disease, peripheral vascular disease, and hypertension (renal artery involvement). Endocardial involvement results in restriction to filling, with congestive heart failure and valvular abnormalities ensuing.

Hurler's syndrome is due to abnormal mucopolysaccharide metabolism producing abnormal collagen fibers. Cardiac chambers may be dilated, valves and chordae thickened, and coronary arteries narrowed.

MUSCULAR DYSTROPHIES

Cardiac involvement may be seen with the hereditary familial muscular dystrophies. In *Duchenne's X-linked muscular dystrophy,* there is selective necrosis and fibrosis of the posterobasal and lateral left ventricle, accounting for the characteristic electrocardiographic pattern of tall R waves in the right precordial leads, with an increased R/S ratio and deep Q waves in the lateral leads. Affected patients may develop arrhythmias (usually atrial) and congestive heart failure, which is rapidly progressive.

Myotonic muscular dystrophy is an autosomal dominant disease whose cardiac manifestations are due primarily to involvement of the His-Purkinje system. Conduction block, which may be life-threatening, may develop. The electrocardiogram shows prominent Q waves in the anterior precordial leads. Myocardial involvement is usually clinically silent.

Friedreich's ataxia is an autosomal recessive disorder that may be associated with a wide spectrum of cardiac abnormalities. On the basis of electrocardiographic and echocardiographic studies, 95% of patients have cardiac involvement. Electrocardiographic abnormalities include right-axis deviation (40%), a tall R wave in lead V_1 (20%), abnormal inferior Q waves (14%), and left ventricular hypertrophy (16%). Twenty percent of patients have echocardiographic evidence of left ventricular hypertrophy and 7% have globally decreased left ventricular function.

HEMATOLOGIC/ONCOLOGIC DISEASES

Sickle-Cell Disease

Cardiac manifestations of sickle-cell disease are principally the sequelae of chronic anemia and chronic hypoxemia. Pulmonary arterial thrombosis in situ occurs frequently in patients with sickle-cell anemia, with resulting arteriovenous shunting and systemic desaturation. Cardiovascular findings are principally those of a hyperdynamic circulation. However, the additional burden of arterial desaturation for any given hemoglobin concentration produces auscultatory and hemodynamic findings that are more prominent than in other forms of anemia.

At necropsy, most hearts are found to have cardiac hypertrophy and ventricular dilatation. The right and left ventricle generally remain compensated in a high cardiac output state until the appearance of an intercurrent problem, at which time symptoms of congestive heart failure may develop.

Although pulmonary infarction is common and frequently causes a painful crisis, pulmonary hypertension is infrequent, and the incidence of cor pulmonale is not increased in patients with sickle-cell disease. Myocardial infarction due to sickling and thrombosis in situ is exceedingly rare, although it has been reported to occur. Chest pain in painful crises may mimic the pain of myocardial ischemia, and repolarization abnormalities are very common on the electrocardiogram. Nevertheless, this frequent clinical picture very rarely represents myocardial infarction.

Neoplastic Disease

Pericardial metastases are seen most often in patients with lymphoma, leukemia, carcinoma of the lung and carcinoma of the breast. Distinguishing metastatic disease from radiation-induced pericarditis may be difficult.

Radiation therapy can affect the entire heart, although the most common complication is pericarditis. The risk of pericarditis is related to the dose of radiation and quantity of heart within the radiation field. The incidence of pericarditis peaks at approximately six months, although symptoms may occur up to 10 years later. Less common complications of radiation therapy include constrictive pericarditis, endocardial fibrosis, and accelerated coronary artery disease.

The chemotherapeutic agents with the greatest cardiac effects are the anthracycline drugs doxorubicin (Adriamycin) and daunorubicin (Cerubidine). Early cardiotoxicity manifestations include arrhythmias and nonspecific electrocardiographic changes, occurring in approximately 10% of patients, as well as rare idiosyncratic episodes of myocarditis and acute left ventricular dysfunction. Late cardiotoxicity is characterized by a dose-dependent cardiomyopathy that occurs after receiving doses >500 mg/m^2. Concomitant use of radiation therapy or cyclophosphamide increases the risk of cardiotoxicity.

Multiple myeloma is associated with amyloid deposits in the myocardium, leading to a restrictive cardiomyopathy. A high cardiac output syndrome in multiple myeloma has been described as well. The etiology of the high-output state remains obscure. The cardiac output can be elevated to two to three times normal in patients at rest, a degree of elevation in cardiac output that is greater than that which can be ascribed to the concomitant anemia.

CEREBROVASCULAR DISEASE

Not only does the heart play a role in the pathogenesis of cerebrovascular disease, but it also frequently reflects active intracerebral processes. The manifestations are principally disturbances of cardiac conduction and rhythm. In 90% of patients with cerebrovascular accidents who have been carefully monitored for the first 3 days, electrocardiographic abnormalities are present. Sinus bradycardia may be present; at times, it may be symptomatic and require pharmacologic or pacemaker intervention. Sinus tachycardia, atrial fibrillation, atrial flutter, supraventricular tachycardia, ventricular tachycardia and conduction abnormalities are also frequently reported. Perhaps the most characteristic electrocardiographic changes of cerebrovascular disease are caused by subarachnoid hemorrhage or spontaneous intracranial hemorrhage. These changes may closely simulate acute myocardial ischemia, with ST elevation and symmetric T-wave inversion. The classic "cerebral T waves" occur in these disorders and are manifest by deep and markedly symmetric T-wave inversion. Frequently, prominent U waves are present and there is QT prolongation. The etiology of the repolarization abnormalities is not clear, but it is not simply related to increased cerebrospinal fluid pressure. One common cardiac sign of increased intracerebral pressure is the Cushing reflex: elevation of blood pressure and bradycardia, at times marked.

Intrinsic cardiac disease is often involved in the pathogenesis of cerebral events. Cerebral emboli frequently occur in patients with abnormal valves (prosthetic valves, rheumatic heart disease, and bacterial and marantic endocarditis), atrial fibrillation, left atrial myxomas, left ventricular aneurysms, recent myocardial infarction, and from paradoxical emboli from the venous system and right heart. In a young person with an unexplained embolic stroke, it is not rare that an intraatrial shunt, due either to a previously unsuspected atrial septal defect or patent foramen ovale, is present. Affected patients warrant very careful examination by Doppler and contrast echocardiography. Surgical closure of the shunt may be indicated if the shunt is implicated in an embolic event.

In evaluating a patient with a recent cerebrovascular accident, one must be aware that 12-30% of these patients have had a recent myocardial infarction. Coincidence of myocardial infarction and stroke is particularly common in patients over age 65. The diagnosis of recent myocardial infarction in this setting is sometimes subtle, since an accurate history frequently is not available and the clinician may be inclined to attribute electrocardiographic abnormalities to the cerebral event. However, elevation of the MB fraction of the serum creatine kinase level may be helpful in making the diagnosis.

PSYCHOTROPIC DRUGS

Tricyclic Antidepressants

Tricyclic antidepressants (TCAs) are very effective in the management of certain types of depression. These drugs block reuptake of catecholamines from the synaptic clefts of central neurons, compensating for a relative deficiency of the neurotransmitters. This relative augmentation of neurotransmitters available at postsynaptic receptors is not limited to the central nervous system and is partially responsible for the vascular and cardiac side effects of TCAs. In addition to the sympathomimetic action of TCAs, their pharmacologic effects include anticholinergic action (tachycardia), alpha-adrenergic blockade (hypotension), and quinidine-like effects (arrhythmias and conduction abnormalities).

Resting heart rate increases to some extent in nearly all patients receiving TCAs. A degree of postural hypotension is almost universal, and in 24% of cardiac patients receiving TCAs the hypotension causes marked symptoms. This is particularly common in patients with congestive heart failure. Postural hypotension is often attenuated after the first several days of therapy. TCAs have, in varying degrees, properties of a type IA antiarrhythmic. This may be manifest by suppression of ventricular premature beats and, in higher doses, conduction abnormalities and depression of myocardial contractility. Electrocardiographic changes include prolongation of the PR, QRS and QT segments, T-wave abnormalities, and development of AV block. Patients with preexisting AV block are at increased risk for conduction abnormalities. TCAs may also exacerbate atrial and ventricular arrhythmias, analogous to the potential proarrhythmic effect of all antiarrhythmic agents.

When starting patients on a TCA, the clinician should obtain a baseline ECG and then a follow-up ECG to monitor for conduction abnormalities (particularly in patients with preexisting AV block), and for QTc prolongation >0.50 sec, which, if present, should prompt a reduction in dosage.

Widening of the QRS interval is the most reliable marker for complications of TCA overdose, with seizures occurring only in patients with QRS durations of ≥0.10 sec, and ventricular arrhythmias occurring only in patients with QRS duration ≥0.16 sec. Acidosis potentiates the toxicity of TCAs and adminstration of sodium bicarbonate to correct the acidosis is the first line of treatment for cardiovascular complications. Management of TCA toxicity includes use of the anticholinesterase physostigmine for atrial tachyarrhythmias, lidocaine for ventricular arrhythmias, and fluid boluses and alpha-adrenergic agonists such as norepinephrine for profound hypotension.

Monoamine Oxidase (MAO) Inhibitors

This class of antidepressants commonly produces some degree of postural hypotension. Conversely, a hypertensive crisis is a major hazard with MAO inhibitors. This can be induced by ingesting food containing tyramine or from administration of sympathomimetic amines. The management of a hypertensive crisis for patients taking MAO inhibitors is administration of an alpha-adrenergic blocker such as prazosin. Intravenous sympathomimetic amines (such as dopamine) should be assiduously avoided in patients taking MAO inhibitors, as these drugs can markedly potentiate the pressor effect of vasoactive amines. Monoamine oxidase inhibitor therapy must be discontinued well in advance of any surgical procedure in which the use of pressors might be required.

Antipsychotics

The cardiovascular effects of antipsychotic medications are similar to those of TCAs. Prominent among the effects are alpha-adrenergic blockade producing orthostatic hypotension, anticholinergic effects causing tachycardia, and a quinidine-like effect on the heart. Haloperidol should be considered for agitated patients with cardiac disease requiring an antipsychotic agent. Haloperidol has fewer anticholinergic and alpha-blocking effects than thioridazine (Mellaril), which should be avoided. In addition, a specific toxic cardiomyopathy has been reported for phenothiazines. Management of toxic effects of phenothiazines is similar to that for TCAs. In patients with TCA and phenothiazine toxicity, use of type IA antiarrhythmics should be avoided, as they may worsen conduction abnormalities.

Lithium

Lithium carbonate is frequently very effective for management of manic depressive illnesses. It has minimal important cardiotoxicity and minimal blood pressure effects. Lithium can cause electrocardiographic abnormalities that appear similar to those of hypokalemia, as it partially displaces intracellular potassium. Flattening and inversion of the T wave may be seen. Patients with congestive heart failure are at increased risk of lithium toxicity due to decreased renal clearance, and increased plasma levels caused by thiazide diuretics. In these patients, serum lithium concentrations must be closely monitored.

Sedative-Hypnotic Drugs

In therapeutic doses, sedative-hypnotic drugs have minimal cardiovascular effects. Intentional overdos-

ing with them can result in hypotension and pulmonary edema due to increased capillary permeability.

Narcotics

Narcotic overdose produces centrally and peripherally mediated increases in vagal tone and decreases in sympathetic tone, causing bradycardia and hypotension in addition to the triad of decreased mental status, meiosis and respiratory depression. The specific narcotic antagonist naloxone is an important first line of therapy. As with the sedative-hypnotic class of drugs, noncardiogenic pulmonary edema can occur with narcotics.

Stimulants

Amphetamines, cocaine, phencyclidine and marijuana have similar cardiovascular effects, although their basic pharmacologic properties differ substantially. Excessive use of these agents may produce hypertension and tachyarrhythmias.

With recent widespread usage of cocaine, the potential for life-threatening cardiac complications from the drug has been increasingly recognized. Cocaine blocks the reuptake of norepinephrine and dopamine, with resultant vasoconstriction, hypertension, tachycardia and a predisposition to arrhythmias. Cocaine has been associated with myocardial infarction in patients with known coronary artery disease (increased myocardial demand) and in patients with normal coronary arteries (spasm). Arrhythmias due to cocaine are treated with beta blockers, with recent evidence suggesting that calcium channel blockers may also be effective. Acute aortic rupture has also been associated with cocaine usage, secondary to acute increased systemic arterial pressure.

RENAL AND ELECTROLYTE ABNORMALITIES

Renal disease and cardiac function are inextricably linked, as the kidneys ultimately determine extracellular fluid volume and intravascular volume. The heart must circulate the volume of fluid that the kidneys have regulated.

Acute Renal Failure

Three principal aspects of acute renal failure have cardiovascular sequelae: altered fluid volume, hypertension, and metabolic abnormalities. Fluid overload in acute renal failure may usually be managed by zealous attention to fluid intake and use of potent loop diuretics. Occasionally, ultrafiltration may be required.

Hypertension is often "volume-dependent," with blood pressure exquisitely responsive to reduction in intravascular volume status. Methyldopa, propranolol, hydralazine and calcium channel blockers may be used in usual doses because they do not critically depend on renal function for their clearance.

Recognition and management of electrolyte abnormalities in acute renal failure is critically important because electrolyte abnormalities in this setting may produce life-threatening arrhythmias and conduction abnormalities (see following discussion of electrolytes).

Chronic Renal Failure

End-stage renal disease presents a panoply of cardiovascular complications, and indeed, success or failure in management of the cardiovascular complications of renal disease often determines the patient's survival. Hypertension is a significant problem in most patients with end-stage renal failure. As in acute renal failure, the hypertension is frequently "volume dependent." A subset of patients with end-stage renal failure have exceedingly high plasma renin activity and alterations of intravascular volume make little difference for blood pressure control. In some patients with chronic renal failure, baroreceptor function is altered significantly. Nonetheless, with the addition of angiotensin converting enzyme inhibitors, hypertension can be controlled subsequent to control of intravascular volume and judicious use of other antihypertensive medications.

Accelerated atherogenesis is common in patients with end-stage renal disease. This process is multifactorial, with probable contributions by the elevated triglyceride levels and decreased high-density lipoprotein levels found in these patients; by hypertension; and by diabetes mellitus.

Pericarditis is a common complication of both acute and chronic renal failure. Echocardiography frequently reveals a small asymptomatic effusion in patients with chronic renal failure. Clinically, pericarditis may be diagnosed by characteristic symptoms of positional pleuritic precordial pain and by the presence of a precordial friction rub. Characteristic electrocar-

diographic abnormalities include ST elevation without reciprocal ST depression. In patients undergoing dialysis, one suggestive sign of some degree of constriction or pericardial tamponade is marked hypotension as intravascular volume is reduced. The pericardial effusion tends to be fibrinous and hemorrhagic, and systemic heparinization for dialysis may augment hemorrhage into the pericardium and lead to tamponade. Therefore, in patients with active pericarditis, regional heparin administration may help to prevent this problem. When an effusion does produce tamponade, pericardiocentesis can rapidly relieve the symptoms; often, catheter drainage of the pericardium is needed. With vigorous dialysis, the size of the effusion can usually be reduced, and pericardiectomy is not usually required.

Dialysis introduces additional demands on the cardiovascular system. At initiation of dialysis, extracellular potassium concentration often rapidly decreases, extracellular ionized calcium concentration rapidly increases, and transient hypoxemia develops, with a decrease in PO_2 of 10–15 mm Hg. Dialysis patients are frequently receiving digoxin, and this combination of electrolyte and metabolic alterations sets the stage very effectively for signs and symptoms of digitalis toxicity despite "normal" serum digoxin levels. This can best be managed by very cautious use of digoxin in these patients, maintenance of a relatively high potassium level in the dialysis bath at the initiation of dialysis, and supplemental oxygen if indicated. Most patients undergoing chronic hemodialysis have one or more arteriovenous fistulas or shunts for circulatory access. In patients with symptoms of congestive heart failure who no longer require their arteriovenous shunt, closure of the shunt is often beneficial. The presence of vascular access for dialysis also increases the incidence of infectious endocarditis due to shunt or fistula infections.

Partially because of the hemodynamic ravages of chronic renal failure as well as the rapid progression of atherosclerosis, chronic renal failure patients may occasionally benefit from cardiac valve replacement or coronary artery bypass grafting. When scrupulous attention is paid to electrolyte balance, fluid replacement, and arrhythmias, these procedures can be undertaken with only modestly higher risk of morbidity and mortality over that expected for the general population. Surgical correction of these important cardiac lesions may make subsequent clinical management substantially smoother.

Table 3. Electrocardiographic Manifestations of Electrolyte Abnormalities

	Interval			T wave	U wave	Atrial Activity	VPB Frequency
	PR	QRS	QT				
↑K	↑	↑		↑		↑ or ↓	↓
↓K		↑	↑*	↓	↑		↑
↑Ca++	↑	↑	↓				
↓Ca++	↓	↓	↑				

* QU prolongation. VPB = ventricular premature beat.

Electrolyte Abnormalities

Abnormalities of potassium balance may have critical cardiac manifestations. The presence of congestive heart failure itself alters potassium balance, as there is enhanced exchange of sodium for hydrogen and potassium ions in the renal distal tubule under the influence of excess aldosterone associated with heart failure. In addition, many diuretics increase sodium delivery to the distal tubule, thereby enhancing potassium wasting. Potassium replacement in congestive heart failure should be in the form of potassium chloride because potassium excretion is augmented and accompanied by alkalosis.

Hyperkalemia may have catastrophic cardiac effects. The earliest electrocardiographic effects of hyperkalemia (Table 3) are peaked symmetric T waves, followed by broadening of the QRS and prolongation of the PR interval. This can occur with a serum potassium level >6.5 mEq and is usually present when levels are >8 mEq. As the serum potassium level increases, atrial excitability is suppressed, followed by complete AV dissociation, ventricular fibrillation, or asystole. These electrocardiographic and electrophysiologic changes are potentiated by hyponatremia or hypocalcemia. Mild elevations in the potassium level decrease the rate of spontaneous diastolic depolarization of all pacemaker fibers; ectopic pacemakers are more sensitive than the SA node, with the resulting antiarrhythmic effect of mild hyperkalemia. When hyperkalemia has abolished atrial activity, broadened the QRS, and altered repolarization so that the electrocardiogram has developed a sine wave pattern, a true medical emergency exists. Ten to 20 ml of 10% CaCl$_2$ should be administered intravenously while the electrocardiogram is continuously monitored. This helps to correct some of the electrophysiologic abnormalities produced by hyperkalemia, but does not lower the serum potassium levels. Administration of NaHCO$_3$ (1–2 ampules, 44–88 mEq), followed by 50 ml of D50W and 10 units of regular insulin, lowers extracellular potassium concentrations within 15 minutes; the effect lasts for a few hours. However, total body potassium level is not altered by this regimen. Sodium polystyrene sulfonate (Kayexalate), a cation exchange resin, should be administered orally or by rectum in a dose of 50 g. When it is administered orally, it should be combined with sorbitol to avoid gastrointestinal inspissation. This resin will bind potassium (1 mEq/g resin), effectively lowering total body stores.

Hypokalemia has important cardiac effects as well, although by itself it is less life-threatening than hyperkalemia. A low potassium level has a mild negative inotropic effect. On the electrocardiogram, T waves are flattened or inverted and U waves may become more prominent. TU fusion produces pseudo-QT prolongation. The correlation between the serum potassium level and electrocardiographic findings for both hypo- and hyperkalemia is rough, and may vary with the acuity of the change in serum levels. Hypokalemia increases arrhythmogenicity, in particular the digitalis-toxic arrhythmias, and should be particularly avoided in patients receiving cardiac glycosides.

Chronic elevations in serum calcium level may produce ectopic calcification of the cardiac skeleton and produce varying degrees of heart block. The electrophysiologic effects of hypercalcemia include augmented contractility, shortened systole and decreased automaticity. The electrocardiographic manifestations are a slight increase in the PR and the QRS intervals and shortening of the QT interval. Hypercalcemia can be managed in the short term by sodium chloride infusion and furosemide administration. Hypocalcemia may prolong the QT interval and shorten the PR and QRS intervals.

Elevated serum magnesium levels in experimental preparations decrease cardiac conduction and ventricular irritability. There are no diagnostic electrocardiographic findings of hypermagnesemia. Hypomagnesemia may be associated with atrial and ventricular arrhythmias and correction of hypomagnesemia may be an effective strategy for control of arrhythmias.

Alterations in serum pH have no direct electrocardiographic effects but are associated with alterations in potassium and calcium concentrations. Marked acidosis has an important negative inotropic effect, decreases ventricular response to epinephrine, and lowers the ventricular fibrillation threshold. Correction of acidosis is frequently critical in cardiac defibrillation.

Hypophosphatemia depresses cardiac contractility, and repleting phosphate stores has a rapid positive inotropic effect. The mechanism is uncertain, although hypophosphatemia may be related to depressed intracellular high-energy phosphate concentrations.

In any patient with new arrhythmias, electrolyte levels should be checked in a search for a readily reversible precipitating cause. In particular, patients with torsades de pointes should have serum potassium, calcium and magnesium levels checked because low concentrations are associated with prolongation of the QT interval.

ENDOCRINOLOGIC ABNORMALITIES

Hyperthyroidism

Cardiovascular signs and symptoms are common in hyperthyroidism and can be found even in "apathetic hyperthyroidism." Palpitations, dyspnea, tachycardia, and hypertension occur in about 30% of these patients.

Supraventricular arrhythmias, particularly atrial fibrillation, occur in approximately 20% of hyperthyroid patients. Echocardiographic or radionuclide assessment of ventricular function reveals hyperdynamic ventricles. In general, symptoms of coronary artery disease or congestive heart failure are due to underlying cardiac disease. Rarely, these symptoms may be due to hyperthyroidism alone. Symptoms of congestive heart failure may be due to a high output state and relative myocardial ischemia.

One physical finding helpful in making the diagnosis of hyperthyroidism is the minimal diminution in heart rate while the patient sleeps. Patients may also have a midsystolic scratch present at the left upper sternal border, believed to be secondary to hyperdynamic rubbing of the pericardial and pleural surfaces.

Pharmacologic management of cardiovascular signs and symptoms may be difficult until the underlying hyperthyroid state is treated. Patients are relatively refractory to the effects of digoxin. Thirty percent of patients in atrial fibrillation rendered euthyroid will convert to sinus rhythm. Indeed, treatment of the hyperthyroidism may be dramatically effective for most cardiovascular symptoms. In the short term, beta-adrenergic blockade may ameliorate many of the signs of a hyperdynamic circulation. The combination of beta blockers and digoxin often is effective in regulating the ventricular response in atrial fibrillation, while avoiding toxic effects of either medication.

Hypothyroidism

In studies of hypothyroid animals, myocardial contractility is decreased. In severe, long-standing hypothyroidism there is myofibrillar swelling with interstitial fibrosis and the heart may become grossly dilated. It is uncommon for hypothyroidism to be prolonged and severe enough to produce symptoms of congestive heart failure. It is believed that the mild reduction in myocardial contractility in hypothyroid patients is compensated for by the decreased demands placed on the heart. The presence of effusions more likely represents altered capillary permeability rather than myocardial failure. One third of patients with myxedema have pericardial effusions, only rarely leading to tamponade.

Electrocardiographic findings include bradycardia, prolongation of the QT interval, decreased electrical voltage, and a threefold increased incidence of conduction disturbances.

Serum cholesterol and triglyceride levels are often elevated in hypothyroid patients. This may contribute to the increased incidence of atherosclerosis in these patients. Evaluation of chest pain in a hypothyroid patient can be perplexing, as hypothyroidism itself can cause modest elevations in serum creatine kinase level.

Hypothyroidism frequently occurs in elderly patients, who may have underlying ischemic heart disease or other important cardiac disorders. Therefore, thyroid replacement therapy must proceed cautiously so as not to induce severe angina or myocardial necrosis. Should severe medically refractory angina develop during thyroid replacement, coronary artery bypass surgery may be performed.

Oral Contraceptives

The use of oral contraceptives is associated with a threefold increased risk of myocardial infarction. Platelet adhesiveness is increased, concentrations of clotting factors increase and levels of antithrombin III decrease; all of these changes increase the risk of thromboembolic disease. Once oral contraceptive therapy is discontinued, the risk reverts to baseline.

ACQUIRED IMMUNODEFICIENCY SYNDROME

Infection with the human immunodeficiency virus (HIV) leads to immune dysfunction, resulting in opportunistic infections and Kaposi's sarcoma. While pulmonary, neurologic and gastrointestinal involvement produces most of the clinical complications, cardiac involvement is common, with myriad findings. Reports have included pericardial effusion, tamponade, myocarditis, marantic endocarditis, and right and left ventricular dysfunction. Autopsy studies show a 50% incidence of cardiac involvement. Myocarditis is common, with the etiology histologically suggestive of viral infection in most cases (see Chapter 18). Myocarditis results in biventricular dilatation in 20% of cases and clinical congestive heart failure in 10%. Pericardial effusions are often seen by echocardiography, and a high clinical suspicion of cardiac tamponade must be maintained in patients with hemodynamic compromise.

Bibliography

Anderson DW, Virmani R, Reilly J, et al: Prevalence of myocarditis at necropsy in the acquired immunodeficiency syndrome. *J Am Coll Cardiol* 11:792, 1988.

Benowitz NL, Rosenberg J, Becher CE: Cardiopulmonary catastrophes in drug overdosed patients. *Med Clin North Am* 63:267, 1979.

Boehnert MT, Lovejoy FH: Value of the QRS duration versus the serum drug level in predicting seizures and ventricular arrhythmias after an acute overdose of tricyclic antidepressants. *N Engl J Med* 313:474, 1985.

Bonfiglio T, Atwater EC: Heart disease in patients with seropositive rheumatoid arthritis. *Arch Intern Med* 124:714, 1969.

Child JS, Perloff JK, Bach PM, et al: Cardiac involvement in Friedreich's ataxia: A clinical study of 75 patients. *J Am Coll Cardiol* 7:1370, 1986.

Chung KJ, Fulton DR, Lapp R, Spector S, Sahn DJ: One year follow-up of cardiac and coronary artery disease in infants and children with Kawasaki disease. *Am Heart J* 115:1263, 1988.

Criscitiello MG, Ronan JA, Besterman EMM, et al: Cardiovascular abnormalities in osteogenesis imperfecta. *Circulation* 31:255, 1965.

deDeuxchaisnes CN, Krane SM: Paget's disease of bone: Clinical and metabolic observations. *Medicine* 43:233, 1964.

Dimant J, Grob D: Electrocardiographic changes and myocardial damage in patients with acute cerebrovascular accidents. *Stroke* 8:448, 1977.

Fisch C: Relation of electrolyte disturbances to cardiac arrhythmias. *Circulation* 47:408, 1973.

Fletcher GF, Hurst JW, Schlant RC: Electrocardiographic changes in severe hypokalemia. *Am J Cardiol* 20:268, 1967.

Furfar JC, Muir AL, Sawers SA, et al: Abnormal left ventricular function in hyperthyroidism: Evidence for a possible reversible cardiomyopathy. *N Engl J Med* 307:1165, 1982.

Galve, E, Candell-Riera J, Pigrau C, et al: Prevalence, morphologic types, and evolution of cardiac valvular disease in systemic lupus erythematosus. *N Engl J Med* 319:817, 1988.

Gerry JL, Bulkley BH, Hutchins GM: Clinicopathologic analysis of cardiac dysfunction in 52 patients with sickle cell anemia. *Am J Cardiol* 42:211, 1978.

Gott VL, Pyeritz RE, Magovern GJ, et al: Surgical treatment of aneurysms of the ascending aorta in the Marfan syndrome. *N Engl J Med* 314:1070, 1986.

Hart RG, Miller VT: Cerebral infarction in young adults: A practical approach. *Curr Concepts Cerebrovasc Dis* 17:110, 1982.

Himelman RB, Chung WS, Chernoff DN, Schiller NB, Hollander H: Cardiac manifestations of human immunodeficiency virus infection: A two-dimensional echocardiographic study. *J Am Coll Cardiol* 13:1030, 1989.

Holsinger DR, Osmundson PJ, Edwards JE: The heart in periarteritis nodosa. *Circulation* 25:610, 1962.

Ikaheimo MJ, Niemela KO, Linnaluoto MM, et al: Early cardiac changes related to radiation therapy. *Am J Cardiol* 56:943, 1985.

Isner JM, Estes NAM, Thompson PD, et al: Acute cardiac events temporarily related to cocaine abuse. *N Engl J Med* 315:1438, 1986.

Jackson WK, Roose SP, Glassman AH: Cardiovascular toxicity of antidepressant medications. *Psychopathology* 20(Suppl 1):64, 1987.

Lamberti JJ, Cohn LH, Collins JJ: Cardiac surgery in patients undergoing renal dialysis or transplantation. *Ann Thorac Surg* 12:135, 1975.

Lechat P, Mas JL, Lascault G, et al: Prevalence of patent foramen ovale in patients with stroke. *N Engl J Med* 318:1148, 1988.

McBride W, Jackman JD, Gammon RS, Willerson JT: High-output cardiac failure in patients with multiple myeloma. *N Engl J Med* 319:319, 1988.

Newberger JW, Takahashi M, Burns JC, et al: The treatment of Kawasaki syndrome with intravenous gamma globulin. *N Engl J Med* 315:341, 1986.

Rhodes BA, Greyson ND, Hamilton CR, et al: Absence of anatomic arteriovenous shunts in Paget's disease of the bone. *N Engl J Med* 287:686, 1972.

Stampfer MJ, Willett WC, Colditz GA, et al: A prospective study of past use of oral contraceptive agents and risk of cardiovascular diseases. *N Engl J Med* 319:1313, 1988.

Tilkian AG, Schroeder JS, Kao JJ, et al: The cardiovascular effects of lithium in man. *Am J Med* 61:665, 1976.

VanderArk GD: Cardiovascular changes with acute subdural hematoma. *Surg Neurol* 3:305, 1975.

Varat MA, Adolph RJ, Fowler NO: Cardiovascular effects of anemia. *Am Heart J* 83:415, 1972.

33 Noncardiac Surgery in the Cardiac Patient

Lee Goldman
Thomas H. Lee

Although cardiology consultants are frequently asked to "clear" a patient for surgery, their role is considerably more complex. The consultant should be prepared to assess the individual patient's risk of cardiac complications; determine whether specialized testing may be appropriate to refine this risk assessment; recommend risk reduction strategies; and participate in postoperative medical management. This chapter addresses these specific tasks and reviews approaches to common perioperative problems.

ASSESSMENT OF RISK

The aging of the population has led to an increase in the prevalence of chronic diseases (e.g., diabetes, ischemic heart disease) in surgical patients. Despite this trend toward higher-risk patients, the overall risk of cardiac complications with noncardiac surgery remains low and has probably decreased over the last 20 years. The risk of perioperative myocardial infarction (MI) is now only about 0.1% and cardiac deaths occur in only about 0.04% of general surgical patients.

These risks are not homogeneous, however, and identification of higher-risk candidates who may warrant special management strategies should be based upon a preoperative cardiac evaluation that includes a history, physical examination, chest x-ray, electrocardiogram, and a serum chemistry evaluation of renal function. This general database is intended to identify conditions associated with an increased risk of anesthesia and surgery.

Coronary Artery Disease

The most important predictor of cardiac complications remains ischemic heart disease, with recent acute MI carrying an especially high risk. Analysis of pooled data from the 1960s and 1970s showed that recurrent MI or cardiac death occurred in about 30% of patients who underwent noncardiac surgery within three months after acute MI and about 15% of patients who underwent surgery within three to six months (Table 1). Complication rates were stable, about 5%, if more than six months had elapsed after acute MI. However, more recent data indicate that this risk has fallen, and with careful patient selection and perioperative invasive hemodynamic monitoring, reinfarction rates of 6% within the first three months after an MI and 2% at three to six months have been reported. Patients with a non-Q-wave infarction have complication rates similar to those of patients with Q-wave infarctions.

Because elective noncardiac surgery is usually deferred in postinfarction patients, a much more common and difficult challenge for the cardiology consultant is assessing perioperative risk for patients with stable angina. This risk is low if the patient's ischemic symptoms are truly stable, but physicians may be misled by self-reported histories of the frequency of angina, because patients may voluntarily reduce their activity levels to avoid cardiac or noncardiac symptoms. Some clinicians have advocated aggressive evaluation of the extent of coronary disease, including angiography and possible bypass graft surgery for every operative patient with angina or a history of MI. They cite nonrandomized data demonstrating that patients with New York Heart Association class I or II anginal symptoms have higher mortality rates with noncardiac surgery if they have not undergone previous coronary artery bypass graft surgery. However, the operative mortality risk of elective coronary artery bypass graft surgery would erase any potential benefit of this strategy in patients with mild stable angina. Thus, instead of routine

Table 1. Risk of Reinfarction with Noncardiac Surgery In Patients After Acute Myocardial Infarction		
	Reinfarction Risk	
Months after initial MI	Before 1976 (pooled data)	Rao et al. (1983)*
0-3	31%	6% (3/52)
4-6	15%	2% (2/86)
>6	5%	1.5% (9/595)
*See Bibliography.		

angiography, evaluation of patients with stable angina should focus on assessment of the threshold at which ischemia is induced. This assessment sometimes requires the use of specialized cardiac tests (see later).

Data on patients with unstable angina who undergo noncardiac surgery are scanty, but unstable angina is known to be a poor prognostic factor for patients undergoing coronary artery bypass graft surgery, and its impact on noncardiac surgical mortality is also deleterious. Therefore, elective surgery should be postponed until ischemic symptoms are stabilized, and noninvasive and invasive testing should be considered in the interim. If the operation cannot be delayed, the patient should undergo the procedure with full hemodynamic monitoring to reduce volume shifts that may induce ischemia.

Congestive Heart Failure

Because anesthesia and surgery are associated with rapid changes in the volume status, patients with preoperative congestive heart failure are clearly at increased risk for a postoperative exacerbation or other cardiac events. The new onset of pulmonary edema occurs in about 16% of patients whose signs or symptoms of congestive heart failure persist up to the time of operation, with even higher risk (23–35%) among patients who have jugular venous distention or an S_3 gallop at the time of the preoperative evaluation, or have a history of pulmonary edema. Patients who have a history of heart failure but are not in failure at the time of surgery have about a 6% risk of pulmonary edema, which suggests that treatment of manifestations of heart failure before surgery may reduce complication rates. However, because many anesthetic agents cause arterial and venous vasodilation, over-diuresis may lead to hypotension; thus, diuretic

therapy should probably be withheld if patients demonstrate orthostatic changes in blood pressure and heart rate. New onset of pulmonary edema or heart failure is rare in patients with no history of heart failure, and, when it occurs, is related to a postoperative MI in about 30% of cases.

Valvular Heart Disease

Patients with preoperative valvular heart disease have about a 20% risk of new or worsened heart failure developing in the perioperative period; these patients are often candidates for preoperative noninvasive cardiac testing. The most important lesion to diagnose is severe aortic stenosis, a lesion which is increasing in prevalence as the population ages and which has historically been associated with risks of perioperative mortality as high as 13%. Evaluation and management of patients with suspected aortic stenosis is evolving, however, because echocardiography with Doppler analysis allows reliable noninvasive diagnosis of this lesion, and aortic balloon valvuloplasty offers an alternative to aortic valve replacement for patients in whom cardiac surgery may be too risky or inappropriate. Noncardiac surgery has been performed with careful hemodynamic monitoring in small series of selected patients with critical aortic stenosis, without major sequelae; thus, it is preferable to embark on surgery without aortic valve replacement or balloon valvuloplasty if the patient does not have symptoms from the aortic valve disease, and even in some patients with symptoms. In patients with advanced symptoms, however, an aortic valve procedure should be strongly considered before noncardiac surgery.

In patients with mitral stenosis, supraventricular tachyarrhythmias may develop and precipitate congestive heart failure and ischemia. Digitalis administration, which may not prevent atrial tachyarrhythmias but may decrease the rate of ventricular response should one occur, can be started preoperatively in patients who have mitral stenosis and are in sinus rhythm; alternatively, atrial arrhythmias can be treated when they arise with intravenous administration of drugs that slow conduction through the atrioventricular node. In patients with chronic aortic and mitral regurgitation, the left ventricle is subjected to high volume loads that may impair contractility. These patients are not as sensitive to small shifts in hemodynamic status as are those with critical aortic stenosis, and they can often be managed without hemodynamic monitoring during the perioperative period if they are not in congestive heart failure at the time of the preoperative evaluation.

Patients with any of these valvular abnormalities or with prosthetic valves should receive appropriate antibiotic prophylaxis before procedures that are associated with bacteremia (see Chapter 25). In addition, patients with prosthetic valves who receive chronic anticoagulation therapy may require special management strategies (see later).

Arrhythmias

Patients with preexisting rhythm disorders are at increased risk for cardiac complications, but much of this increased risk is due to underlying cardiomyopathies and ischemic heart disease. Thus, patients with ventricular arrhythmias and myocardial dysfunction are at higher risk for perioperative congestive heart failure and cardiac death, and there are no data that suggest that prophylactic antiarrhythmic therapy lowers these risks. Arrhythmias and conduction abnormalities that occur in these patients during the perioperative period can usually be managed as they arise, and pharmacologic interventions or pacemakers should be reserved for cases in which patients meet indications for these therapies. In general, in patients without evidence of structural heart disease, ventricular premature contractions are not associated with increased risk of cardiac death or morbidity, and their prognostic importance in the perioperative setting is probably also limited.

Other Risk Factors

The risk of cardiac complications increases in an almost linear fashion with age, so that the risk of peri-

operative cardiac death is about 10 times higher for patients over age 70 than for patients below 70. The increase in perioperative risk among the elderly persists even after adjustment for their higher prevalence of cardiac disease and other conditions. Risk assessment may be hindered by inability of many elderly patients to undergo treadmill exercise testing. Because the risk of cardiac complications is highest in patients who cannot exercise, alternative tests for evaluating inducibility of ischemia may be especially appropriate.

The type and timing of the surgery are also major correlates of perioperative cardiovascular risk. Major intraabdominal, intrathoracic or aortic procedures are associated with higher risks than other types of operations, probably because of several factors, including the prevalence of underlying coronary artery disease; the seriousness of the surgery; the degree of respiratory compromise and postoperative pain; and the fluid and electrolyte shifts associated with these procedures. The risk of any operation increases fourfold if it is performed emergently instead of electively, probably because of general medical problems that cannot be corrected before emergency operations. Abnormalities such as hypoxia, carbon dioxide retention, acidosis, hypokalemia, elevated liver function enzyme levels, and evidence of renal failure are all associated with increased risk.

Multivariate Assessment of Risk

Integrating the impact of the presence of more than one of these factors into a single overall risk estimate can be performed using a multivariate index of cardiac risk in noncardiac surgery that was derived from data on 1,001 patients at a single hospital in the mid-1970s. Nine independently important factors were identified (Table 2). Points were assigned to each factor that can be used to place patients into approximate risk classes (Table 3). In the original series of patients, more than half of all patients were placed into risk class I, and the risk of life-threatening or fatal cardiac complications in such patients was less than 1%. In risk classes II and III, the rate of complications increased, but only 2% of patients died perioperatively. Only 18 patients were in risk class IV, but more than 50% died of cardiac causes.

In prospective testing at other institutions in varying patient populations, this index has been shown to separate patients reliably into risk groups (Table 4), although recent data indicate that mortality rates as

Table 2. Multifactorial Index of Cardiac Risk in Noncardiac Surgery

Parameter	Points
History	
Myocardial infarction within six months	10
Age over 70 years	5
Physical examination	
S_3 or jugular venous distention	11
Important aortic stenosis	3
Electrocardiogram	
Rhythm other than sinus or sinus plus APBs on last preoperative electrocardiogram	7
More than five premature ventricular beats/min at any time preoperatively	7
Other factors	
Poor general medical status*	3
Intraperitoneal, intrathoracic, or aortic surgery	3
Emergency operation	4
TOTAL	53

APB = atrial premature beat.
*Electrolyte abnormalities (potassium <3.0 mEq/L or HCO_3 <20 mEq/L); renal insufficiency (blood urea nitrogen >50 mg/dl or creatinine >3.0 mg/dl); abnormal blood gases (pO_2 <60 mm Hg or pCO_2 >50 mm Hg); abnormal liver status (elevated serum aspartate transaminase or signs on physical examination of chronic liver disease); or any condition that has caused the patient to be chronically bedridden.
Adapted from Goldman et al., 1977. With permission.

low as 8% can be achieved in risk class IV patients through patient selection and hemodynamic monitoring. Because the risk index may underestimate the rate of cardiac complications in certain higher-risk populations such as patients undergoing abdominal aortic aneurysm surgery, some authors suggest that the index be used in a Bayesian manner that takes into consideration the patient's prior probability of complications. Other suggested refinements include adding factors to account for prior histories of class III or IV angina, remote MI, and pulmonary edema.

SPECIALIZED TESTS FOR RISK ASSESSMENT

Patients with evidence of ischemia during exercise tolerance testing have higher rates of cardiac complications with noncardiac surgery, but whether exercise test results add information to data from a careful history is unclear. Patients with stable angina usually do well if angina is their only risk factor, and patients with severe symptoms of ischemic heart disease at a low level of exertion are candidates for catheterization and consideration of revascularization with angioplasty or bypass graft surgery. However, the clinician must determine whether patients with apparently stable angina are active enough to increase cardiovascular work to a level similar to that of surgery. If the patient's threshold for inducibility of ischemia is uncertain, an exercise test, with or without thallium scintigraphy, may provide important information.

Many patients cannot undergo adequate treadmill exercise testing due to poor conditioning or noncardiac disorders, but two new techniques are being investigated for their ability to predict perioperative cardiac complications in these patients. Dipyridamole-thallium scintigraphy uses intravenous or oral

Table 3. Prospective Performance of the Cardiac Risk Index

Class (Points)	No. of patients		Life-threatening complications*		Cardiac death	
	MGH	Toronto	MGH	Toronto	MGH	Toronto
I (0-5)	537	590	<1%	<1%	<1%	<1%
II (6-12)	316	453	5%	2%	2%	1%
III (13-25)	130	74	12%	11%	2%	4%
IV (>25)	18	23	22%	4%	56%	26%

MGH = Original series at Massachusetts General Hospital (Goldman et al. 1977).
Toronto = Prospective evaluation by Zeldin in Toronto (*Can J Surg* 27:402, 1984).
* Documented intraoperative or postoperative myocardial infarction, pulmonary edema, or ventricular tachycardia without progression to cardiac death.

dipyridamole to increase flow in areas perfused by nonstenotic coronary arteries; myocardium supplied by stenotic arteries should receive its usual flow, although flow sometimes diminishes because of a coronary "steal" syndrome or peripheral vasodilatation. These differences in flow can be detected with the radionuclide thallium, which will be present in lower concentrations in areas of the heart in which flow does not increase. The dipyridamole-thallium test enhances the preoperative cardiac risk assessment of

patients undergoing major vascular surgery and can be expected to be applied more widely if intravenous dipyridamole is approved for distribution (see Chapter 5).

Ambulatory ischemia monitoring uses electrocardiographic monitoring equipment similar to that frequently used for arrhythmia detection. The electrocardiographic tracings for a 24-hour period are reviewed with the assistance of a computer for evidence of ischemia. Preliminary studies of this tech-

Table 4. Use of the Multifactorial Cardiac Risk Index in Patient Subgroups with Different Baseline Risks of Cardiac Complications

Patient Type	Approximate Baseline Risk: Major Cardiac Complications	Adjusted Cardiac Complication Risk Using Multifactorial Index			
		I	II	III	IV
Minor surgery	1%	0.3%	1%	3%	19%
Unselected consecutive patients >40 years old who have major noncardiac surgery	4%	1.2%	4%	12%	48%
Patients undergoing abdominal aortic aneurysm surgery or who are >40 years old and have high-risk characteristics that generally generate medical consultations before major noncardiac surgery	10%	3%	10%	30%	75%

Adapted from Goldman 1987. With permission.

nology in vascular surgery patients suggest that it may become a valuable test for patients who cannot walk on a treadmill and who have normal ST segments on their baseline electrocardiograms (see Chapter 6).

Few data are available on the value of tests of left ventricular function in assessing perioperative cardiac risk. Patients undergoing vascular surgery who have a low ejection fraction detected by radionuclide angiography have higher complication rates, but whether this test adds information beyond that available through a clinical assesment is unclear.

All of these tests are expensive and may be difficult to arrange on short notice before surgery. Risk assessment for most patients can be performed on the basis of readily available information from the history, physical examination, and routine laboratory data.

RISK REDUCTION STRATEGIES

Several of the factors associated with increased cardiac risks in noncardiac surgery may be "controlled." For example, delaying an operation until three to six months after MI may decrease the risk of perioperative cardiac complications. However, emergent and urgent operations (e.g., resection of a possibly malignant lesion) often cannot be delayed. Therefore, clinicians are often required to weigh the risks of surgery against nonsurgical management.

Although no controlled trials have studied this issue, some data suggest that preoperative control of congestive heart failure reduces the risk of postoperative pulmonary edema or worsened congestive heart failure. Because both general and spinal anesthetic agents may induce intraoperative hypotension if the patient is volume-depleted, preoperative diuresis must not result in dehydration. Such over-diuresis can be avoided by monitoring the patient's blood urea nitrogen and creatinine levels and by carefully assessing postural blood pressure and pulse changes.

Because of the potential hemodynamic consequences of small volume shifts in patients with critical aortic stenosis, suspicious murmurs must be evaluated preoperatively with a careful history and physical examination, and if the data are consistent with aortic stenosis, echocardiography should be performed. Echocardiography supplemented by Doppler analysis can usually identify critical aortic stenosis; only rarely is cardiac catheterization required. Determining whether patients with aortic stenosis have symptoms as a result of the lesion may be more difficult, because noncardiac conditions may limit ex-

ertional capacity. Therefore, detailed questioning about the patient's ability to perform specific tasks should be conducted.

The value of coronary angiography followed by revascularization with percutaneous transluminal coronary angioplasty or coronary artery bypass graft surgery in patients with stable angina pectoris is uncertain. However, there is general agreement that patients with unstable or crescendo angina should not undergo noncardiac surgery until the angina is controlled, unless immediate surgery is imperative.

Effective treatment of a patient's general medical problems is also likely to decrease operative risk by reducing cardiac stress. The consulting cardiologist may recommend that surgery be delayed until such problems can be corrected.

Although hypertension is not an independent risk factor for perioperative cardiac complications, hypertensive patients are more likely to have labile blood pressures during anesthesia and surgery. At one time, it was felt that this lability might be reduced by discontinuing antihypertensive medications several days before surgery or by aggressively controlling blood pressure before surgery. More recent data suggest, however, that neither of these two extremes is correct, and that perioperative blood pressure lability is independent of the degree of preoperative blood pressure control as long as the diastolic blood pressure is not greater than about 110 mm Hg. Thus, antihypertensive medications may be continued until surgery, and surgery need not be delayed in patients with moderate persistent hypertension until better control is achieved. The cardiology consultant should follow the patient postoperatively, however, to ensure that he or she is receiving an effective antihypertensive regimen.

Anesthesiologists are usually more familiar than internal medicine physicians with the risks and benefits of various agents and techniques, so the cardiology consultant rarely plays a major role in these choices. Data suggest that the advantages of local or spinal anesthesia may be limited to patients with very severe congestive heart failure, probably because these agents do not share the myocardial depressant action of general anesthetic agents. Spinal anesthesia causes as much peripheral vasodilation and subsequent hypotension as does general anesthesia. Furthermore, any anesthetic technique that does not effectively eliminate pain will be associated with markedly increased cardiac demands. Therefore, spinal anesthesia seems preferable from a cardiac standpoint only in patients in whom preexisting class IV congestive heart failure is the overwhelming preoperative risk factor (although newer general anesthesia techniques may be just as good as spinal anesthesia even in such patients). Spinal anesthesia may also be preferable for patients with important pulmonary disease in whom postoperative hypoxia or other pulmonary problems might increase cardiac demands.

The selection of general anesthetic agents is not nearly as critical as formerly believed. Halothane, which causes both myocardial depression and peripheral vasodilation, is the agent most frequently associated with hypotension, and it should be used cautiously in patients who have other risk factors for intraoperative hypotension. In patients with hypertrophic cardiomyopathy (idiopathic hypertrophic subaortic stenosis) or with right-to-left shunts, peripheral vasodilation during anesthesia may be especially hazardous. Ketamine, which has a sympathomimetic effect, is often recommended for such patients; alternatively, an alpha-adrenergic agent may be used to increase systemic vascular resistance.

COMMON PERIOPERATIVE QUESTIONS AND COMPLICATIONS

One of the major roles of the cardiology consultant is to anticipate common problems that may develop in the perioperative period. The delineation of such problems and the description of contingency plans are often of more help to surgical and anesthesia colleagues than calculations of overall perioperative risk.

Ischemic Heart Disease

For both the postinfarction patient and the patient with angina, a key determinant of surgical risk is functional status. In general, patients who are in functional class I or early class II (which implies that they can do exercise equivalent to carrying two grocery bags up a flight of stairs) can achieve a heart rate and blood pressure equivalent to what would be expected with general anesthesia and surgery. If such an activity level can be achieved, the risk of perioperative infarction is probably no higher than 1-4%, with a risk of perioperative cardiac death of ≤2%. In such patients, the two principal approaches, which are continued medical management versus "prophylactic" coronary artery bypass grafting, have apparently equivalent morbidity and mortality risks. Thus, unless percutaneous transluminal coronary angioplasty

is shown to be a more efficacious management strategy, routine revascularization appears to be of no benefit for patients with stable coronary symptoms.

If the patient's functional status can be determined accurately by a good medical history, exercise testing is not routinely necessary. If the history is not definitive, exercise testing is helpful in determining functional status. In such cases, decisions about the safety of surgery should depend more on the patient's ability to exercise than on the magnitude of ST-segment depression, since perioperative risk is probably more related to physiologic status than to the underlying coronary anatomy per se (although the latter may be an important long-term prognostic factor). In patients who cannot exercise, dipyridamole-thallium scintigraphy or ambulatory electrocardiographic monitoring are alternative strategies for determining the patient's level of ischemia and for determining risk. However, current data are not sufficient to mandate that patients who have positive results on either of these two tests must have preoperative coronary arteriography and revascularization.

Patients who have more severe angina should routinely be considered for coronary arteriography before undergoing elective noncardiac surgery. The physician should, as noted earlier, concentrate more on the patient's functional status than on the frequency of angina, since very active patients may have relatively more-frequent angina whereas patients with angina on very minimal activity may so curtail their exertion that their angina decreases in frequency.

Premature Ventricular Contractions

Patients with ventricular arrhythmias have an increased risk of cardiac complications with surgery, but most of these complications are related to ischemia and congestive heart failure rather than to uncontrolled ventricular arrhythmias. Therefore, therapeutic interventions in patients with arrhythmias should usually be directed toward the underlying coronary artery disease or cardiomyopathy, and antiarrhythmic therapy should be reserved for patients who meet criteria for chronic antiarrhythmic therapy.

Accordingly, prophylactic lidocaine is usually recommended for patients with a history of symptomatic ventricular arrhythmias, a history of cardiac arrest, or very high-grade degrees of asymptomatic ventricular arrhythmia. Patients with less severe ventricular arrhythmias may be given lidocaine intraoperatively if arrhythmias compromise cardiac function. Because many ventricular arrhythmias during surgery result from inadequate anesthesia, hypoxia, myocardial ischemia, or fluid and electrolyte imbalance, the identification and correction of such problems is more appropriate than is reliance on the antiarrhythmic effects of drugs such as lidocaine. It should be remembered that anesthesia may obscure the usual neurologic warnings of lidocaine overdose.

Patients Taking Beta-adrenergic Blocking Agents

Concerns that beta-adrenergic blocking agents blunt sympathetic responses during the perioperative period have been allayed by recent data that suggest that patients taking propranolol usually respond appropriately to surgical stresses and that supplemental isoproterenol can be used to overcome the negative inotropic and chronotropic effects of these drugs. Thus, patients being treated with beta-adrenergic blockers for hypertension or angina can usually be maintained on their medications until the morning of surgery. Perioperative hypotension or bradycardia in these patients should not be treated with alpha-adrenergic agents or catecholamines with mixed alpha- and beta-adrenergic effects (e.g., epinephrine), since unopposed alpha-adrenergic effects may lead to a hypertensive crisis.

In patients who must discontinue use of beta-adrenergic blocking agents, the risk of a symptomatic rebound in sympathetic activity after abrupt cessation is small, but patients may be hypersensitive to sympathetic stimuli after the drug is discontinued. The timing of this hypersensitivity varies with different beta-adrenergic blocking agents, with longer half-lives leading to delays in the withdrawal phenomenon. Thus, in many patients, oral therapy can be resumed before the drug is cleared completely. Only an unusual patient requires intravenous propranolol, given as a 1-mg test dose followed by 1 mg every 5-10 minutes to control hypertension or tachycardia, and then by either 1 mg every 20-60 min or a constant infusion of about 0.01-0.05 mg/min. An alternative is esmolol, a short-acting beta-adrenergic blocking agent, which can be given with a loading infusion of 500 μg/kg/min for 1 minute followed by a 4-minute maintenance infusion of 50 μg/kg/min. If the desired therapeutic effects have not been achieved, this maintenance infusion can be increased to 100-200 μg/kg/min.

Prophylactic Digitalis

Patients who develop new perioperative supraventricular tachyarrhythmias during digitalis administration do so at a lower rate than that seen in patients who have not taken digitalis. Therefore, preoperative initiation of digitalis is often considered in patients who are at risk of these arrhythmias, including elderly patients undergoing pulmonary surgery, patients with valvular heart disease, and patients who have congestive heart failure. However, intravenous calcium channel blocking agents that slow conduction through the atrioventricular node (e.g., verapamil, 5-10 mg given as an intravenous bolus over 2 minutes) provide an acute alternative that can be reserved for when tachyarrhythmias occur.

Digitalis is the only routinely available oral inotropic agent, and it has been shown to prevent the myocardial depression caused by general anesthetic agents. However, prophylactic digitalis is not useful for prevention of perioperative heart failure in patients at risk for this complication.

Anticoagulant Therapy

Management of patients receiving chronic anticoagulant therapy is determined by the indication for anticoagulation. Patients taking prophylactic anticoagulants for prevention of systemic emboli in the setting of atrial fibrillation or rheumatic heart disease or for the prevention of deep venous thrombosis can usually discontinue warfarin therapy several days preoperatively, allowing the prothrombin time to decline to normal, and then have anticoagulation restarted several days postoperatively. Patients who undergo anticoagulation because of prosthetic heart valves can follow a similar regimen, except that heparin should be started 48 hours postoperatively and continued until warfarin has resulted in an appropriate prothrombin time.

Patients who have caged-disk valves (e.g., Harken prostheses) have an especially high risk of thromboembolism, even with brief discontinuation of anticoagulant use. In such cases, the patient may be admitted two to three days before surgery and receive intravenous heparin while the prothrombin time decreases. If a long preoperative hospitalization is not possible, the effect of warfarin may be reversed pharmacologically about 24 hours preoperatively, and low-dose heparin may be initiated at the same time; then, full-dose heparin can be started 12-24 hours postoperatively and continued until the patient can resume oral warfarin. It is always easier to reverse heparin rapidly (with protamine) than to reverse the effects of oral vitamin K antagonists.

Pacemakers

Prophylactic temporary pacemakers are usually indicated only in patients who meet criteria for placement of a permanent pacemaker. Patients with asymptomatic bifascicular or trifascicular block are at risk for development of complete heart block, but such events rarely occur during the perioperative period unless the patient has a new MI. When autonomic instability associated with intubation and surgery leads to second- or third-degree heart block or hemodynamically significant sinus bradycardia, intravenous atropine usually restores normal conduction and rate.

If implantation of a permanent pacemaker is indicated, it can be implanted before the operation if the planned surgery is elective. If the operation is urgent or emergent, a temporary pacemaker can be used. If the planned procedure may lead to a bacteremia, a temporary pacemaker may be used perioperatively to avoid contamination of a permanent device.

An exception to this conservative approach to the use of temporary pacemakers may be made for patients with preoperative left bundle branch block who are undergoing placement of a pulmonary artery catheter. This procedure is associated in about 5% of cases with the transient development of right bundle branch block, which, superimposed on a left bundle branch block, could lead to complete heart block. Thus, a method of ventricular pacing should be readily available before right heart catheterization in this patient population.

A potentially fatal intraoperative problem for patients with permanent pacemakers is inhibition of demand pacemakers by electrocautery. If electrocautery is used, frequency and duration should be limited to 1-second bursts 10 seconds apart, and the ground plate should be placed as far from the pacemaker pulse generator as possible. Placing a magnet over many types of pacemakers switches them into a mode in which the heart is paced at a fixed rate, but because programming of more sophisticated devices may vary, it is important to determine before surgery the pacemaker type and model number, its response to electrical interferences, and reprogramming methods.

During periods of electrocautery, the electrocardiogram may be useless for monitoring heart rhythm, and an alternative such as direct palpation of the radial pulse should be used.

Prophylactic Antibiotics

Patients with valvular heart disease, prosthetic valves, many forms of congenital heart disease, and arterial abnormalities such as arteriovenous shunts should receive appropriate high-dose antibiotic prophylaxis for the type of bacteremia that might be expected based on the site of surgery. In general, antibiotic prophylaxis should begin 6-24 hours preoperatively and be continued for no more than about 48 hours postoperatively.

Speed and Extent of Surgery

After adjusting for the type of operation, there is no correlation between the length of surgery and the development of cardiac complications. Thus, there is no evidence that planned operations should be shorter in patients with cardiac disorders, although it is sometimes appropriate to choose a less ambitious procedure (e.g., a cholecystotomy instead of a cholecystectomy) in the patient with acute cardiac decompensation. Most cardiac complications occur when patients are experiencing postoperative pain, fluid shifts, hypoxia, and other stresses. Thus, intraoperative management should be planned to minimize these postoperative risks.

Intraoperative Monitoring

Because marked changes in blood pressure or volume status contribute to the development of myocardial ischemia and other cardiac complications, careful intraoperative monitoring is important in the management of patients with cardiovascular disease. A pulmonary artery catheter or a radial artery catheter may be helpful in patients with substantial left ventricular dysfunction, recent preoperative MI or other unstable coronary artery disease syndromes, aortic stenosis, or other high-risk factors.

Intraoperative Bradycardia

Intraoperative bradycardias are usually the result of vagal stimulation, and if arrhythmias such as sinus bradycardia or nodal rhythms do not cause hypotension, ischemia or inadequate perfusion, no therapy is necessary. Otherwise, these arrhythmias can be treated with changes in anesthetic technique, small doses of intravenous atropine, or, occasionally, small doses of beta-adrenergic agents. Such arrhythmias are almost always benign and short-lived and do not correlate with more serious perioperative cardiac complications.

Perioperative Hypertension

Perioperative hypertension, defined as a systolic blood pressure of ≥200 mm Hg or an increase in systolic pressure of ≥50 mm Hg, occurs in about 5% of patients without a preoperative history of hypertension and in about 25% of patients with a preoperative history of hypertension. These hypertensive episodes are common during intubation, during periods of inadequate anesthesia and in the recovery room as the patient begins to wake up. Although cardiology consultants may recommend adjustments in the antihypertensive regimen if preoperative blood pressure control is not satisfactory, the risk of perioperative hypertension is not definitely reduced by such measures. Episodes can usually be reversed when they occur by changes in anesthetic technique in the operating room or by correcting the hypoxia, fluid overload, or inadequate postoperative analgesia that has precipitated the hypertension.

If these measures fail, antihypertensive agents may be administered. Intravenous nitroprusside is the best means of controlling hypertension gradually and effectively, and it can be administered in the recovery room or intensive care unit setting. Labetalol, a newer antihypertensive agent that has alpha- and beta-adrenergic blocking effects, may be given as a 20-80 mg intravenous bolus every 10 minutes or as a 2 mg/min infusion, and can be expected to take effect within 5-10 minutes. Intravenous methyldopa, an older but effective alternative, is usually given as 500 mg every 6 hours; it will not manifest its pharmacologic effects for about 6 hours, but is often enough to control moderate blood pressure elevations. Hydralazine, a vasodilator that can be given intramuscularly or intravenously, is an effective antihypertensive drug, but it often precipitates supraventricular tachycardia; hence it should not be used unless other measures have failed, and it should usually be combined with small doses of intravenous propranolol (1 mg every 5-10 minutes) to control tachycardia.

Valvular Heart Disease

Careful perioperative fluid control is especially important in patients with valvular heart disease because of their increased risk of congestive heart failure. In addition, in patients with mild-to-moderate mitral stenosis who are asymptomatic, pulmonary edema may develop if marked tachycardia develops during the perioperative period, making adequate anesthesia essential in these patients.

Hypertrophic Obstructive Cardiomyopathy

Patients with hypertrophic obstructive cardiomyopathy (formerly idiopathic hypertrophic subaortic stenosis, or IHSS) develop hypotension if they become volume depleted, receive beta-adrenergic agents, or develop tachyarrhythmias. Intravenous propranolol or verapamil can be used to reduce left ventricular outflow obstruction and to improve diastolic filling of the left ventricle. Diuretics may worsen outflow obstruction and hence worsen congestive heart failure.

Mitral Valve Prolapse

There is no evidence that patients with mitral valve prolapse are at increased risk for cardiac complications with surgery. Patients whose prolapse is accompanied by an audible murmur of mitral regurgitation should receive prophylactic antibiotic therapy, but antiarrhythmic or other therapy should be administered only if the patient meets routine indications for them.

POSTOPERATIVE MEDICAL MANAGEMENT

Recent studies show that most perioperative MIs occur within 48 hours of surgery, but postoperative complications such as congestive heart failure and hypertension frequently occur three to five days after surgery, when extravascular fluid returns to the intravascular space, thus increasing cardiac preload and work. Consequently, cardiology consultants should follow patients for at least five days after major surgery. During this postoperative period, the consultant can assist with the management of any acute postoperative complications and help to plan chronic therapy for conditions such as hypertension, congestive heart failure, or arrhythmias.

Postoperative Myocardial Ischemia and Infarction

Because of anesthesia and noncardiac postoperative pain, only about half of postoperative infarctions are accompanied by a complaint of chest pain. Nevertheless, most postoperative MIs are associated with some symptoms or signs: decreased blood pressure, congestive heart failure, arrhythmias, or a change in mental status. Electrocardiograms may reveal asymptomatic ischemia, but their interpretation may be complicated by the high prevalence of ST-segment or T-wave changes of doubtful significance in postoperative patients. ST-T wave changes are probably more likely to reflect ischemia if they are prolonged in duration.

Similarly, cardiac enzyme levels may be difficult to interpret because the trauma of surgery can be expected to lead to abnormalities of creatine kinase (CK), lactate dehydrogenase (LDH), and LDH isoenzyme levels. CK-MB is usually unaffected by noncardiac surgery if measured in its usual serial manner, but the definitive diagnosis of MI may still be difficult in many cases. Some investigators recommend that a combination of enzymatic and electrocardiographic criteria be used.

Postoperative Heart Failure

Congestive heart failure is often precipitated by postoperative surgical problems that increase myocardial demands, but some uncomplicated patients develop mild heart failure about 12-36 hours postoperatively, when mobilization of intraoperative fluid begins. Diuretic therapy is usually sufficient to manage these volume shifts, but all patients with postoperative heart failure should be evaluated carefully to determine whether a perioperative MI may have contributed to their failure.

Postoperative Arrhythmias

The new onset of supraventricular tachyarrhythmias or the development or worsening of ventricular arrhythmias in the postoperative period may be due to increased sympathetic tone in response to surgery, but may also reflect coexisting medical problems. New supraventricular tachyarrhythmias are associated with other cardiac disorders in about 50% of cases, but other major disorders that must be considered include infection, anemia, metabolic abnormalities, hypoxia, and new intravenous medications.

In general, new postoperative supraventricular tachyarrhythmias do not require cardioversion, because most resolve either with continuation of the patient's chronic cardiac medications or with treatment with intravenous verapamil or digitalis. Electrical cardioversion should be used only if cardiac output is compromised or evidence of ischemia develops.

Bibliography

Charlson ME, MacKenzie CR, Ales KL, et al: The postoperative electrocardiogram and creatine kinase: Implications for diagnosis of myocardial infarction after noncardiac surgery. *J Clin Epidemiol* 42:25, 1989.

Eagle KA, Coley CM, Newell JB, et al: Combining clinical and thallium data optimizes preoperative assessment of cardiac risk before major vascular surgery. *Ann Intern Med* 110:859, 1989.

Gerson MC, Hurst JM, Hertzberg VS, et al: Cardiac prognosis in noncardiac geriatric surgery. *Ann Intern Med* 103:832, 1985.

Goldman L: Multifactorial index of cardiac risk in noncardiac surgery: Ten-year status report. *J Cardiothorac Anesth* 1:237, 1987.

Goldman L, Caldera DL: Risks of general anesthesia and elective operation in the hypertensive patient. *Anesthesiology* 50:285, 1979.

Goldman L, Caldera DL, Nussbaum SR, et al: Multifactorial index of cardiac risk in noncardiac surgical procedures. *N Engl J Med* 297:845, 1977.

Goldman L, Wolf MA, Braunwald E: General anesthesia and noncardiac surgery in patients with heart disease. In: Braunwald E, ed. *Heart Disease. A Textbook of Cardiovascular Medicine*. Philadelphia: W.B. Saunders; 1988, pp. 1693–1705.

Goldman L, Caldera DL, Southwick FS, et al: Cardiac risk factors and complications in noncardiac surgery. *Medicine* 57:357, 1978.

Raby KE, Goldman L, Creager MA, et al: Correlation between preoperative ischemia and major cardiac events after peripheral vascular surgery. *N Engl J Med* 321:1296, 1989.

Rao TLK, Jacobs KH, El-Etr AA: Reinfarction following anesthesia in patients with myocardial infarction. *Anesthesiology* 59:499, 1983.

CHAPTER 34

Perioperative Evaluation of the Cardiac Surgical Patient

Gilbert H. Mudge

Cardiology is the most surgically oriented of all medical subspecialties. The properly trained cardiologist is always assessing the timing of surgical intervention in patients with valvular heart disease, is reappraising medical therapy and symptomatic status in patients with angina pectoris, and must be critical of potential benefits and pitfalls of emergency operative intervention for acute ischemia. A firm working relationship between the cardiologist and cardiothoracic surgeon is mandatory so that patients receive expeditious surgical intervention when so indicated, and so that common cardiologic problems can be easily addressed postoperatively. This chapter reviews certain aspects of the perioperative care of patients undergoing both valvular replacement and coronary artery bypass grafting. Subtleties of perioperative care that enhance the cardiologist's contribution to postoperative management are emphasized.

PERIOPERATIVE EVALUATION

It is assumed that the cardiologist is satisfied with the preoperative cardiac evaluation that has led to the decision for surgical intervention. Cardiac examination of patients with surgical valvular heart disease or coronary artery disease, with or without left ventricular dysfunction, is not emphasized here. However, several aspects of the general physical examination must not be overlooked during final preoperative evaluation.

In a patient being considered for valve replacement, a careful oral examination is required, and carious teeth must be removed. Since one of the most serious complications of prosthetic valve replacement is superimposed bacterial endocarditis, all necessary dental procedures should be completed before surgical intervention; a full mouth extraction and complete healing of the gum may be required before elective valve replacement in cases of severe tooth decay.

Patients undergoing coronary artery bypass surgery or mitral valve replacement should be carefully examined for evidence of aortic insufficiency. One of the most severe complications that can occur during institution of cardiopulmonary bypass is significant distention of the left ventricle during the period of ventricular fibrillation. If such distention is not attended to, extensive subendocardial damage may ensue. Patients with hemodynamically insignificant aortic insufficiency may have such ventricular distention when they are placed on bypass, for central aortic perfusion will distend the left ventricle. Accordingly, the surgeons should be advised when such insufficiency is suspected.

The peripheral circulation should be scrutinized preoperatively. Blood pressure should be assessed in both arms and peripheral pulses assessed in all extremities. A complete history for transient cerebral ischemia should be recorded. Patients with asymptomatic carotid bruits should undergo noninvasive evaluation of their carotids, with digital subtraction angiography or carotid angiography if so indicated. Because patients are often perfused at a nonpulsatile pressure of 50 mm Hg while on cardiopulmonary bypass, uncertainties about the carotid circulation must be clarified. Carotid endarterectomy followed by cardiopulmonary bypass can be effectively and safely performed in patients with high-grade symptomatic carotid disease who require cardiac surgical intervention (Graver et al.). If not performed, major neurologic insult may occur following the hypotension required for cardiopulmonary bypass. The role of carotid surgery in the asymptomatic patient who is to undergo cardiac surgery is debatable.

The abdominal aorta should be examined for bruits, and the competency of the iliofemoral system checked. This is particularly important in patients who may require transient intraaortic balloon counterpulsation after surgery. Significant peripheral vascular disease may preclude femoral artery cannulation for initiation of cardiopulmonary bypass. Women who have undergone radical mastectomies, especially a left radical mastectomy, may not be candidates for utilization of the internal thoracic arteries as conduits; compromised thoracic arterial blood supply may prevent adequate sternal and wound healing.

A careful gastrointestinal, renal, and neurologic history and examination is likewise required; the latter is particularly important should any question regarding alteration in neurologic status arise after surgery. Venous status should be examined carefully in patients who are to undergo aortocoronary artery bypass surgery. A history of venous ligation or remote history of thrombophlebitis should be underscored in the admitting note. If arm veins are to be used as conduits, they should not be used preoperatively for intravenous therapy. Patients with tinea pedis may have recurrent lower-extremity cellulitis after revascularization surgery that uses saphenous veins.

Conventional laboratory studies are mandatory in preoperative evaluation. Patients with chronic obstructive lung disease or a long-term history of cigarette smoking should have a pulmonary function test; this will help in planning postoperative extubation and pulmonary care. The conventional indices of hepatic function should be carefully scrutinized in patients with advanced right heart failure. Thyroid studies should be performed for patients with underlying atrial fibrillation. Stool guaiacs for occult blood are mandatory because they may help direct the choice of prosthetic valve. Chronic renal failure with hemodialysis is not a contraindication to cardiopulmonary bypass, but compromised renal function that has not yet required hemodialysis may be reason for reconsideration of surgery; hypotension and nonpulsatile blood flow that occur during cardiopulmonary bypass may exacerbate renal dysfunction. There is preliminary evidence that a cardiopulmonary bypass machine capable of pulsatile blood flow will help in preserving borderline renal function.

Patients who are to undergo elective surgery may be candidates for autologous blood donations. While policies vary from blood bank to blood bank, patients with chronic stable angina can make such donations under careful supervision; saline replacement may be necessary. Patients with unstable ischemia, recurrent congestive heart failure, tight aortic stenosis or critical left main coronary artery disease are usually not considered acceptable candidates for autologous donations.

The results of cardiac catheterization must be carefully reviewed before the final decision regarding surgery. In patients with severely compromised left ventricular function with high left ventricular end-diastolic pressure and pulmonary capillary wedge pressure, the elevation of pressures can be expected to persist during the early postoperative stages.

Two other aspects of the results of cardiac catheterization should be emphasized. First, right atrial pressure should be noted as a rough approximation of right ventricular function and estimation of the degree of tricuspid regurgitation before coronary artery bypass surgery. Many patients with significant right coronary artery disease have sustained subclinical right ventricular infarctions. Right ventricular dysfunction may be exacerbated in the early postoperative stages, especially if pulmonary function findings are abnormal. A right atrial pressure greater than 10 mm Hg should alert the cardiologist that right ventricular dysfunction and tricuspid regurgitation is present and that enhanced volume may be required during the first 48 hours after surgery. This need can obviously be further assessed with Doppler echocardiography.

Second, pulmonary artery pressure should be noted. In many patients with mitral valve disease and pulmonary hypertension, pulmonary artery pressures are persistently elevated during the first postoperative days. Such fixed pulmonary vascular resistance is identified by a pulmonary artery diastolic pressure that exceeds the mean pulmonary capillary wedge pressure by 10 mm Hg. In this case, severe pulmonary hypertension may continue through the early postoperative days. This condition not only necessitates extremely high right atrial filling pressures, but may also be exacerbated by hypoxia. These patients must be well oxygenated, and a pulmonary vasodilator, such as isoproterenol, should be considered in their early pharmacologic regimen. Patients with severe pulmonary hypertension whose pulmonary artery diastolic pressure equals pulmonary capillary wedge pressure usually have rapid resolution of such pulmonary hypertension when the pulmonary capillary wedge pressure is reduced after mitral valve replacement.

Most medications can be safely continued right up until the time of surgery. Some centers administer digoxin during the last preoperative day, not only for inotropic support but also to control atrial fibrillation should it occur postoperatively (Burman; Selzer and Walter). Diuretic therapy can also be continued, bearing in mind that many patients receiving long-term diuretic therapy have relative total-body potassium depletion although serum potassium levels are normal. Since hypokalemia may account for many early postoperative ventricular arrhythmias, additional potassium supplementation should be considered in the final preoperative days for patients receiving large doses of diuretics.

A beta-adrenergic blocking agent is usually administered to patients about to undergo coronary artery revascularization. In most patients with a left ventricular ejection fraction >0.40, beta-adrenergic blocking therapy can be continued until the time of surgery (Caralps et al.). By so doing, "rebound" is avoided. In patients with compromised left ventricular function, beta-adrenergic blocking agents are best discontinued for at least 24 hours before surgery, as long as the patient's activity is curtailed and adequate nitrate administration is maintained to protect against recurrent ischemia.

There is no current contraindication to continued use of calcium channel blocking agents up to the time of surgery. This is mandatory if part of a patient's clinical presentation is coronary artery vasospasm superimposed upon a high-grade fixed obstructive lesion. Sudden withdrawal of a calcium channel blocking agent can exacerbate coronary artery vasospasm, provoking a preoperative myocardial infarction (Muller and Gunther). Since one of their potential pharmacologic effects is to uncouple myocardial excitation from subsequent contraction, calcium channel blocking agents may have profound negative inotropic effects during the early hours after cardiopulmonary bypass in patients with severe left ventricular function. Indications for use of diltiazem and high-dose beta blocking therapy should be questioned preoperatively by the clinician. The negative chronotropic effects of both agents may be compounded by hypothermia as the patient is weaned from cardiopulmonary bypass; junctional heart rates of 25–30 beats/min are frequently seen in this setting and are often unresponsive to isoproterenol infusion or atropine; pacing may be required for 24–36 hours postoperatively.

Conventional anticoagulation with warfarin obviously must be discontinued so that the prothrombin time and partial thromboplastin time return to normal before surgery. Patients with absolute indications for anticoagulation must be switched to heparin. Aspirin is associated with significant postoperative bleeding and should not be administered for at least 72 hours before surgery. The safety of other antiplatelet agents in the final preoperative hours is unclear. In a recent investigation, dipyridamole was administered preoperatively to patients undergoing myocardial revascularization, without resulting in excessive postoperative bleeding (Chesebro et al.).

Most conventional oral antiarrhythmics can be continued up to the time of surgery, and replaced with intravenous preparations if needed, as determined by the anesthesiologist. Amiodarone has substantial clinical and subclinical pulmonary toxicity, and its administration has been associated with persistent and prolonged hypoxia after cardiopulmonary bypass. The indications for its use should be carefully reviewed with the surgeons before surgical interventions. The indications for other antiarrhythmic agents with potent negative inotropic effects should also be reassessed perioperatively.

INTRAOPERATIVE CONSIDERATIONS

The choice of anesthetic agents is best deferred to the anesthesiologist. Inhalation anesthetics may be used in patients undergoing low-risk procedures. Morphine sulfate is a safe and effective anesthesia when used in conjunction with nitrous oxide. The dose of morphine may vary from 1 to 3 mg/kg. Its primary benefit is the absence of myocardial depression (Lowenstein et al.). Major disadvantages to morphine anesthesia are its vasodilating capacity and the prolonged postoperative intubation required. Because morphine may reduce both preload and afterload, patients may often require enhanced volume administration early postoperatively. Such anesthesia may be dangerous in patients whose cardiac output is dependent on their preload status, such as patients with critical aortic stenosis whose left ventricular stroke volume depends on left ventricular filling volume. In patients with significant right-to-left shunts, the shunt can be exacerbated if peripheral vascular resistance is precipitously reduced during induction of anesthesia. Both patient populations—those with critical aortic stenosis and those with right-to-left shunts—should be vigorously treated with both volume expansion and administration of pressor agents. Morphine anesthesia also requires prolonged intubation, usually 12–18 hours after the patient has left the operating room. This is often unnecessary after uncomplicated surgery.

While the cardiologist's presence may not be required during surgery, he or she must be thoroughly familiar with the techniques of thoracotomy, of placing the patient on the pump oxygenator, of the surgical procedure itself, and of weaning the patient from cardiopulmonary bypass. The sternotomy and cardiac dissection must be done with extreme care in any patient undergoing reoperation and who has a patent vein graft or internal thoracic artery to the left anterior descending artery; interruption of this conduit may be disastrous. The aortic arch is usually cannulated to receive the arterial input from the pump oxygenator, but the femoral artery can be used. Femoral artery cannulation is often indicated in patients with severely compromised left ventricular function so that partial cardiopulmonary bypass support may be given during sternotomy. Femoral artery cannulation may also be required if the surgery involves the aortic arch itself. Cannulation of the aortic arch saves time by avoiding groin dissection, but it must be done with extreme care, particularly in elderly patients with fragile calcified aortas. Dissection from a proximal aortic cannulation usually has dire consequences. The venous return to the oxygenator is usually obtained from the vena cava via the right atrium. Once venous and arterial cannulas are in place, the patient may be cooled to approximately 28°C, with supplemental topical cardiac hypothermia applied during the time that the aorta is cross-clamped. Left ventricular distention must be prevented during the time of aortic cross-clamp; a left ventricular vent may be required to decompress the left ventricle during this time. The cardiologist should also be familiar with the technique that the surgeon uses to remove air from the left heart and aorta before resumption of left ventricular ejection is permitted. The pump oxygenator usually maintains a blood flow of 2.0-2.5 L/min/m², which generates a mean nonphasic blood pressure of 50-60 mm Hg. Lower blood flows are permitted with more intense cooling, and total circulatory arrest may be feasible for brief periods at 20°C.

When the surgical procedure is complete, monitoring lines are inserted before the patient is weaned from cardiopulmonary bypass. The exact line used will often depend on the preference of the anesthesiologist or surgeon. Percutaneous pulmonary artery catheters are always feasible; direct left atrial lines inserted to the posterior aspect of the left atrium via the pulmonary veins provide a precise definition of hemodynamics for the first 48 postoperative hours. These can be brought out easily through a small skin incision and pulled before the chest tubes are removed. Right atrial lines may be similarly inserted by the surgeons, with minimal complications during their removal. Once both right and left heart pressures

are measured, the surgeon weans the patient from cardiopulmonary bypass. Anterior and posterior mediastinal chest tubes are then inserted; additional chest tubes may be required if the pleural cavities have been entered. The pericardium is usually left open. Atrial and ventricular pacing wires are attached and brought out through the skin. The former wires are particularly helpful in the postoperative management of patients with hypertrophy, in noncompliant ventricles that require pacing, and in diagnosis and treatment of postoperative supraventricular tachycardias. The sternum is then reapproximated, the skin is closed, and the patient is returned to the recovery room intubated, with need for continued ventilatory support.

POSTOPERATIVE CARE

Hemodynamic Monitoring and Support

The presence of an arterial line, potential right and left atrial lines, and perhaps a pulmonary artery catheter simplifies the close hemodynamic monitoring required for patients after cardiopulmonary bypass. The right atrial line may be a venous access; the left atrial line must never be so used, to avoid systemic arterial embolization.

Postoperative hypotension is the most common hemodynamic problem in the first hours after surgery. Pharmacologic inotropic support usually does not need to be added to the patient's intravenous regimen until adequate right and left atrial filling pressures are achieved. During the first hours after coronary artery bypass surgery, patients may have enormous volume requirements. Such enhanced fluid requirements are most often due to systemic venous vasodilation; a less likely reason is transient right ventricular dysfunction. During the final phases of cardiopulmonary bypass, with a body temperature of 28°C, there is a significant vasoconstriction with increased systemic vascular resistance. As the patient's temperature returns to normal, vasodilatation increases volume requirements. Patients with normal left ventricular function and an uncomplicated postoperative course often require 6–7 L of fluid before their condition stabilizes. The choice of type of volume is made in conjunction with the surgeons; the patient should receive any blood from the pump oxygenator. Daily weights during the first postoperative week and comparison to preoperative weight constitute an important means of assessing fluid balance.

Hypotension associated with high left atrial filling pressures should be treated with inotropic support. Many patients may have inappropriately high systemic vascular resistance with depressed left ventricular function and borderline hypotension; combined inotropic support with afterload reduction in such patients is justified. During the first 24 hours after surgery, intravenous nitroprusside and dopamine are often adequate. Patients should be closely monitored for arrhythmias, which may be precipitated by inotropic agents such as dopamine and epinephrine. There is some evidence that dobutamine has equal positive inotropic effect with greater afterload reduction capability; these characteristics may justify single drug therapy in patients with severely depressed left ventricular function (DiSesa et al.).

Significant hypertension after coronary artery bypass surgery is reported to occur in 30–50% of patients undergoing myocardial revascularization (Viljoen et al.; Salerno et al.). Hemodynamic studies indicate that this is related to an increase in total peripheral vascular resistance without a significant change in cardiac output; an increase in resting alpha-adrenergic vasoconstrictor tone is postulated as the mechanism. Plasma epinephrine and norepinephrine levels are documented to increase significantly in the early postoperative course; the renin-angiotensin system has also been incriminated, and converting enzyme inhibitors have been used successfully to control blood pressure (Niarchos et al.). There is no significant correlation with history of hypertension or previous propranolol dosage. Most patients become significantly hypertensive within 2 hours after surgery, the hypertension abating 48–72 hours later. Aggressive therapy of this acute hypertension is indicated for several reasons. Not only does myocardial oxygen consumption increase significantly as a result of the enhanced blood pressure, but the degree of postoperative bleeding, both from the aortic cannulation site and from saphenous vein graft anastomosis, can be related to the blood pressure. Chest tube drainage often resolves when postoperative hypertension is controlled. Because postoperative hypertension is a transient hemodynamic phenomenon during the first 48 postoperative hours, intravenous therapy with sodium nitroprusside is often indicated to lower the systolic pressure to 120 mm Hg. This therapy can be easily tapered as the hypertension resolves. Should blood pressure elevation persist for more than 48 hours postoperatively, nifedipine, captopril, or a beta-blocking agent may be administered. Almost all patients who are nor-

motensive during preoperative evaluation can be tapered off antihypertensive medication before hospital discharge.

Postoperative bleeding should be carefully monitored by the anterior and posterior mediastinal chest tubes. Adequate protamine sulfate should be administered to reverse the effects of heparin given when the patient was on the pump oxygenator. Protamine sulfate may produce peripheral vasodilatation and hypotension, thus enhancing the initial postoperative volume requirements. Platelet count should also be carefully monitored. In most patients with a normal preoperative platelet count, that count will drop to 60,000–70,000 secondary to destruction from the pump oxygenator. Platelet transfusions may be rarely required. Some surgeons will control mediastinal bleeding with positive end-expiratory pressure from the respiratory ventilator. If bleeding continues at 200–300 ml/hour for 4 hours after initial chest closure, surgical reexploration is usually required.

Cardiac Arrhythmias

Significant ventricular arrhythmias often occur after valvular or revascularization surgery (Angelini et al.). Such dysrhythmias have many causes: direct trauma to the ventricle, hypoxia, depressed left ventricular function, anesthetic agents, endogenous or exogenous catecholamine stimulation, electrolyte or acid-base abnormality, and, more often, the underlying disease process itself. Since maximal depression of left ventricular function does not occur for 18–24 hours after cardiopulmonary bypass, all significant ventricular premature contractions occurring more frequently than 10 per minute should be treated with intravenous therapy, after correcting transient causes such as hypoxia, hypokalemia, acidosis, or alkalosis. The possibility of digitalis toxicity must not be overlooked. Lidocaine is often preferred as the initial intravenous antiarrhythmic agent, because depression of myocardial contractility and peripheral vasodilatation are far less severe than with equivalent doses of procainamide or the newer parenteral antiarrhythmic agents. If a patient is refractory to lidocaine administration, intravenous procainamide can be administered, and the patient can then be switched to an oral preparation if needed. Diphenylhydantoin, bretylium tosylate, or amiodarone may also be considered as intravenous agents should patients have refractory high-grade and life-threatening ventricular ectopic activity. A patient with persistent life-threatening ventricular ectopic activity for more than 72 hours postoperatively must be aggressively treated. Full electrophysiologic testing may be required in the late postoperative course, but is probably not justified in the first 24–48 hours postoperatively, because many of the early arrhythmias are secondary to the transient and correctable causes mentioned above (Garan et al.).

All patients who require intravenous antiarrhythmic therapy for ventricular ectopic activity should receive 24 hours of continuous monitoring in the final postoperative days before discharge. Significant ventricular ectopic activity, including couplets, multiform ventricular premature beats, or brief ventricular tachycardia, is usually suppressed by oral therapy for at least six weeks after surgery, although the value of this practice is unproved except in patients suspected of having a perioperative myocardial infarction.

Supraventricular tachycardias are also common after valvular or coronary bypass surgery. Atrial premature beats are typical, and transient atrial flutter or fibrillation is reported to occur in as many as 30% of patients who were in normal sinus rhythm preoperatively. Most of these atrial dysrhythmias can be easily converted and controlled with conventional antiarrhythmic therapy. Cardioversion is rarely needed. The atrial electrode should be used if the diagnosis of any supraventricular tachycardia is equivocal; the atrial wire can be connected to the precordial lead of an electrocardiogram and atrial activity recorded. Causes of recurrent supraventricular tachycardia in the early postoperative course must be carefully considered. Hypoxia, persistent pulmonary infiltrates, pericarditis, gastric dilatation, anemia, fever, or right or left atrial cannulas are often the cause. Rapid supraventricular tachycardias that cause hemodynamic embarrassment should be immediately treated by cardioversion. Little additional anesthesia is usually required in the first 12 postoperative hours; 5–10 mg of intravenous diazepam is usually adequate. Supraventricular tachycardias in patients who have undergone valve replacement should be treated with either quinidine or procainamide. Among patients who have such dysrhythmia after coronary artery bypass surgery, low-dose beta-adrenergic blockade or verapamil are extremely effective and safe (Mohr et al.).

Atrial flutter with rapid ventricular response may severely compromise the patient's condition. Rapid atrial pacing is safe and atraumatic in this condition and can be considered if an atrial wire is in place (Waldo et al.). The atrial rate should be increased to 125% of the rate of the underlying arrhythmia. When pacing is abruptly terminated, normal sinus rhythm or atrial fibrillation often follows, the latter more easily controlled than atrial flutter with intravenous digoxin or verapamil. In patients with postoperative atrial fibrillation who were in normal sinus rhythm preoperatively and maintain normal sinus rhythm for five to six weeks after surgery, antiarrhythmic therapy can be discontinued.

Many patients with mitral valve disease and chronic atrial fibrillation preoperatively may have normal sinus rhythm postoperatively. In these patients, the left atrium has been inspected for the presence of thrombi. While most of these patients may revert to their atrial dysrhythmia during the first postoperative week, antiarrhythmic therapy should be administered to try to maintain a sinus mechanism. In patients with an aortic porcine heterograft, maintenance of normal sinus rhythm may obviate the need for long-term anticoagulation.

The possibility of digitalis toxicity should always be considered as a cause of arrhythmias and digoxin levels should be checked when clinically indicated. This is particularly important after quinidine therapy is instituted.

Third-degree heart block is a rare complication of open heart surgery, more common after repair of ventricular septal defect and endocardial cushion defect. In adults, debridement of a heavily calcified aortic valve may produce complete heart block by disrupting the conduction system below the noncoronary cusp. This is often recognized in the operating room and treated with ventricular wires. In patients with evidence of bifascicular conduction abnormalities preoperatively or a complete heart block on the operating table, a permanent epicardial wire can be brought down to a subcutaneous subxiphoid pouch. These can easily be retrieved and attached to a pacemaker if normal conduction is not spontaneously restored after surgery. Nodal rhythms are a common conduction abnormality, particularly after mitral valve and aortic valve replacement. Nodal rhythms are usually well tolerated if the rate is adequate, but can always be treated with overdrive pacing or isoproterenol infusion. Such nodal rhythm disturbances usually last 48–72 hours and resolve spontaneously.

Myocardial Infarction

Intraoperative myocardial infarction is a complication that must be addressed within the first 48 hours after surgery. The appearance of new Q waves should be interpreted as evidence of infarction, with little clinical emphasis placed on the changes in ST segment or T-wave contour. There can be marked ST-segment elevation and T-wave inversion that do not represent myocardial ischemia. Such ST-segment elevation may resolve when the anterior and posterior mediastinal chest tubes are removed. Post-pericardiotomy ST-T wave abnormalities may persist for six months after surgery. Conventional myocardial enzyme levels are often elevated following cardiac surgery; a CK of 600-800 IU/L is not unusual and may be associated with trace elevation of the CK-MB fraction. The CK-MB isoenzyme is frequently found in patients who have required direct conversion of ventricular fibrillation to sinus rhythm in the operating room with paddles placed upon the heart. An SGOT >100 IU/L coupled with a CK >1,000 IU/L with more than 10% CK-MB should be considered evidence of subendocardial myocardial infarction.

The incidence of perioperative myocardial infarction after coronary artery bypass surgery is 10–12%. Most such infarctions are subendocardial and do not cause major hemodynamic compromise, and the patients can usually be ambulated and managed late postoperatively without undue complication. Perioperative infarction with major hemodynamic compromise should be treated with conventional therapy, including proper inotropic support, and intraaortic balloon counterpulsation if necessary. Patients with perioperative infarction are usually not considered candidates for emergency repeat revascularization and can certainly not receive thrombolytic therapy.

Pre- and Post-discharge Care

Patients are usually slowly ambulated 48–72 hours after surgery. If the postoperative course is uncomplicated, discharge can be anticipated on the seventh to tenth postoperative day. In patients who have undergone coronary artery bypass surgery, the leg incisions are often the primary source of discomfort. The physical examination should be directed toward evidence of congestive heart failure, pulmonary consolidation, atelectasis, pericardial rub, pericardial tamponade (evidence of pulsus paradoxus should be sought), and thrombophlebitis. The incidence of post-pericardiotomy syndrome is low, about 5% in most series. Unexplained fever, chest pain, and pericardial rub are indications for treatment with nonsteroidal anti-inflammatory agents, but renal function should

be carefully monitored if these agents are used. Other postoperative complications include wound infection, pulmonary embolism, cerebrovascular accident, urinary tract outlet obstruction, complications from use of intraaortic balloon pump, and hepatitis resulting from transfusion.

Indefinite anticoagulation is required for all mechanical prosthetic valves. A porcine xenograft valve placed in the aortic position does not require anticoagulation therapy, but a patient with a porcine xenograft in the mitral position and normal sinus rhythm usually receives anticoagulation for six weeks after surgery. If normal sinus rhythm is maintained, then anticoagulation therapy can be discontinued without undue risk of thromboembolic complications (Cohn et al.). Patients with chronic atrial fibrillation should receive anticoagulation indefinitely, irrespective of the type of valve used. Anticoagulation can be started 48 hours after surgery, once the chest tubes and atrial cannulae have been removed.

Early evidence suggests that aggressive antiplatelet therapy should be initiated in patients with coronary artery disease. Studies of sulfinpyrazone therapy (Baur et al.) and of combined aspirin/dipyridamole therapy (Chesebro et al.) showed that graft closure rate can be reduced to 3–4% after coronary artery revascularization; patients who received placebo therapy had a graft closure rate of 9–10%. In the study with aspirin/dipyridamole, dipyridamole was initiated before surgery and aspirin instituted as soon as mediastinal bleeding ceased. Initiation of antiplatelet therapy during the first 48 hours before surgery may be critical for its success.

The VA Cooperative Study showed little additional benefit with dipyridamole over aspirin alone. When one takes this study into account with the recent studies on unstable angina (Fuster et al.) and the natural history of coronary artery disease (Steering Committee of the Physicians' Health Study Research Group), it seems reasonable to suggest that after surgical revascularization all patients should receive enteric aspirin therapy unless it is specifically contraindicated.

Before discharge, the patient's physical examination should be carefully noted in the record; a post-operative echocardiogram evaluating prosthetic valve function has been advocated as a baseline control observation. The physician should check the stability of the sternum, placing fingers on either side of the incision and asking the patient to cough. Patients must be instructed regarding the complications of anticoagulation and prophylaxis for subacute bacterial endocarditis as so indicated. In patients with significant left ventricular dysfunction, the diuretic regimen and sodium intake must be carefully adjusted.

Patients are encouraged to slowly increase their daily activity as comfort and energy permit. Most patients continue to experience variable degrees of fatigue for four to six weeks after surgery, with residual leg and sternal discomfort; resumption of normal activity usually is not recommended until eight weeks postoperatively. An active rehabilitation program may not be practical until discomfort is fully resolved, and evaluation of operative success by exercise tolerance study is of little benefit until the surgically induced ST-segment and T-wave abnormalities have resolved and the patient is completely comfortable. Stress thallium studies may be indicated if surgically induced ST-segment abnormalities prevent precise electrocardiographic analysis.

Most patients should be seen at least once a year by a cardiologist after open heart surgery. Those with valve replacement must be carefully followed for evidence of paravalvular leaks or primary valve dysfunction. Recognizing that coronary artery bypass surgery is a palliative procedure, such patients should be carefully followed for evidence of recurrent myocardial ischemia. Risk factors that contribute to the development of coronary artery disease cannot be ignored. Cigarette smoking must cease, blood pressure must be controlled, and lipid level elevations must be lowered when possible.

CARDIAC TRANSPLANTATION

One-year survival after cardiac transplantation exceeds 85% in some large transplant centers. Morbidity from immunosuppressive regimens has been reduced by combination therapy with cyclosporine, prednisone, and azothioprine, and use of monoclonal OKt3 antibodies to treat acute rejection. With expanding capabilities for cardiac transplantation to treat the terminally ill patient, the procedure must be primarily limited to patients with end-stage congestive heart failure. Refractory angina with inoperable coronary artery disease or life-threatening ectopic activity is not an accepted indication for such intervention. The dilemma confronting cardiac transplantation in the 1990s is that this procedure has become a standard form of therapy for end-stage congestive heart failure, and the number of potential recipients is greater than the number of potential donors.

Whatever the cause of the patient's terminal illness, symptoms of congestive heart failure should be refractory to conventional medical therapy, limiting the patient with ordinary daily activity or at rest, to consider transplantation. Simple documentation of advanced left ventricular dysfunction is not an indication, for some patients may be very well compensated for years before presenting with a terminal condition. Circulating catecholamines (Levine et al.) and serum sodium (Packer et al.) are poor prognostic indicators, as is poor exercise capacity (Engler et al.). The age of the patient is a consideration; most transplant centers are reluctant to evaluate patients over 60 years of age. Patients at the upper limit of age consideration must be carefully screened for comorbid conditions. Many younger patients are physiologically over 60; many individuals approaching 60 are physiologically much younger.

Secondary medical conditions may serve as general exclusion criteria. Patients with an active infectious process cannot receive the intense immunosuppressive therapy required after transplantation. Those with clinically significant cerebral and peripheral vascular disease may have limited rehabilitation potential after cardiac transplantation. Insulin-dependent diabetes with secondary retinopathy or nephropathy is a relative contraindication to cardiac transplantation. Most cardiac transplant centers recognize that simple glucose intolerance, without other organ involvement, can be easily managed; it often becomes initially manifest when the patient is placed on high-dose steroid therapy.

The presence of pulmonary embolism with residual scar formation predisposes patients to cavitation at the site of infarction, and serves as a relative contraindication to cardiac transplantation. Clinically active chronic obstructive pulmonary disease, including chronic bronchitis and bronchiectasis, will only be exacerbated with aggressive immunosuppressive therapy. The differentiation between advanced obstructive or restrictive pulmonary disease and severe congestive heart failure is not often easily established by pulmonary function studies; severe congestive heart failure may simulate restrictive physiology. Patients with an FEV_1/FVC ratio $< 45\%$ of predicted value are at relatively high risk for post-transplant pulmonary problems. When such patients are being considered for transplantation, pulmonary function studies while a patient is in congestive heart failure must be compared with those that might have been obtained before the clinical presentation of congestive heart failure (Thompson et al.).

Clinically active peptic ulcer disease will certainly be exacerbated with high-dose drug administration, and serves as a relative exclusion criterion, as does the presence of any other coexisting systemic illness that might limit life expectancy. Preexisting malignancy should not be an absolute contraindication to cardiac transplantation if such malignancy might be cured. This consideration becomes particularly germane to patients who die of adriamycin cardiotoxicity, having been cured of the primary neoplastic disease by conventional clinical guidelines.

Psychosocial support is an important consideration, as is the patient's ability to follow a complicated medical regimen. In persons with active and continued alcohol or drug abuse, poor compliance makes the complicated postoperative follow-up impossible. Intensive counseling is mandatory in any patient with a history of such abuse.

All potential recipients are screened for preformed antibodies to potential donors lymphocytes. The presence of such antibodies predicts a high likelihood of acute rejection at the time of cardiac transplantation. A candidate who has high titer of such preformed antibodies may be very difficult to match with potential donors.

Potential recipients require careful right heart catheterization six months before transplantation. Pulmonary hypertension, with a pulmonary vascular resistance of 480–600 dynes-sec-cm^{-5}, is an absolute contraindication to conventional orthotopic cardiac transplantation. With high pulmonary vascular resistance, the new heart can be expected to develop acute right ventricular failure; this complication accounts for approximately 5% of all intraoperative deaths. In patients who have an elevated pulmonary vascular resistance, this condition must be further assessed with acute afterload reduction with nitroprusside or oxygen therapy at the time of cardiac catheterization. Patients whose pulmonary vascular resistance can decrease are usually suitable for orthotopic transplantation.

While most clinicians will not become actively involved in the day-to-day decisions on immunosuppressive therapy after cardiac transplantation, their involvement before transplantation is mandatory. Once a patient is listed at a cardiac transplant center, he or she must be meticulously followed. (Twenty percent to 30% of all potential recipients die before a suitable heart is identified.) All patients should receive anti-coagulant therapy to reduce the risk of venous and arterial embolization.

While most patients can be satisfactorily managed at home, a small percentage require intermittent inotropic support or prolonged hospitalization. Intraaortic balloon counterpulsation may be required, but probably only should be undertaken at the cardiac transplant center, where the patient can be monitored for complications and suitability as a potential recipient can be reassessed on a day-to-day basis. Use of a left ventricular assist device or total artificial heart as a bridge to cardiac transplantation has received limited attention; the complications of these devices often preclude cardiac transplantation. The overall results when such bridge devices are used are less impressive than those achieved when the transplant patient is in a more stable condition. This particular dilemma raises many ethical issues about the suitability of using a scarce and limited resource in patients with a hopeless prognosis.

Other logistical issues that the clinician should consider include preservation of the right internal jugular vein; thrombosis of this access site may limit options for endomyocardial biopsy. In addition, the potential recipient should receive blood transfusions only when absolutely necessary; frequent transfusions may alter antibody levels, making a suitable match more difficult. Moreover, there is no compelling evidence that repeated transfusions alter rejection episodes for cardiac transplant recipients, as is also suggested in the literature for renal transplantation.

Post-Transplantation Follow-up

Postoperative follow-up is primarily directed toward immunosuppressive requirements. Endomyocardial biopsy is mandatory because it is the only reliable means of diagnosing early rejection. Rejection that is diagnosed by noninvasive techniques or hemodynamic compromise is often far advanced, and may not adequately respond to aggressive changes in immunosuppressive regimens.

Patients receiving cyclosporine therapy as part of their immunosuppressive regimen will have little myocardial edema when they have fulminant rejection. They may be asymptomatic. Hence, there may be no gallop rhythms and no elevation of right or left ventricular diastolic pressures. Endomyocardial biopsy is the only means of detecting such rejection.

Acute histologic rejection is usually treated with Solu-Medrol (methylprednisolone) therapy; more advanced rejection is treated with either OKt3 monoclonal antibody or antilymphocyte serum. Chronic immunosuppressive regimens almost always include prednisone, azothioprine, and cyclosporine. The prednisone dosage is usually tapered to 0.1 mg/kg over six months after cardiac transplantation; cyclosporine is adjusted to achieve serum concentrations of 100–125 ng/ml; and azothioprine is administered at a rate of 1.5–2 mg/kg; the white count should not fall below 4,500. These guidelines are of course arbitrary, for there is a wide variation in the histologic response of patients with cardiac transplantation. Each immunosuppressive regimen must be individualized.

Patients are often placed on pneumocystis prophylaxis, usually Bactrim DS® (trimethoprim/sulfamethoxazole). Aspirin or dipyridamole is usually prescribed after cardiac transplantation in an effort to prevent the development of graft atherosclerosis, although the clinical evidence to support this therapy is lacking. Patients are usually maintained on antacids to reduce the possibility of duodenal ulcers. Since cyclosporine therapy is associated with a high renin state, antihypertensive agents are frequently required.

After cardiac transplantation, the patient has a denervated heart and the clinician must be aware of certain limitations with this deficit. First and foremost, the post-transplantation patient never has anginal pain. If secondary graft atherosclerosis, a chronic form of rejection, develops, the patient does not have traditional symptoms of angina. Accordingly, symptoms of transient left ventricular dysfunction must be aggressively pursued. The patient complaining of paroxysmal exertional dyspnea must be screened for obstructive coronary disease. Because of such graft atherosclerosis, each recipient requires yearly coronary arteriography. Stress thallium studies are also important in long-term follow-up of these patients.

With a denervated heart, the compensatory response to enhanced physiologic demands may be slower. Hypotension cannot be met with rebound tachycardia. Any heart transplant recipient in whom peripheral vasodilation suddenly develops must be treated with aggressive fluid administration; the most frequent clinical settings are septic shock and general anesthesia for noncardiac surgery. In this latter situation, at least 1 L of volume replacement should be administered before induction of general anesthesia.

Bibliography

Angelini P, Feldman MI, Lufochanowski R, et al: Cardiac arrhythmias during and after heart surgery: Diagnosis and management. *Prog Cardiovasc Dis* 16:649, 1974.

Baur HR, Van Tassel RA, Purach CA, et al: Effects of sulfinpyrazone on early graft closure after myocardial revascularization. *Am J Cardiol* 49:420, 1982.

Burman SO: The prophylactic use of digitalis before thoracotomy. *Ann Thorac Surg* 14:359, 1972.

Caralps JM, Julet J, Wienhe HR, et al: Results of coronary artery surgery in patients receiving propranolol. *J Thorac Cardiovasc Surg* 67:526, 1974.

Chesebro JH, Clements IP, Fuster V, et al: A platelet inhibitor drug trial in coronary artery bypass operations: Benefit of perioperative dipyridamole and aspirin therapy on early postoperative vein graft patency. *N Engl J Med* 307:73, 1982.

Cohn LH, Mudge GH, Pratter F, et al: Five to eight year follow-up of patients undergoing porcine heart-valve replacement. *N Engl J Med* 304:258, 1981.

DiSesa V, Brown E, Mudge GH, et al: Hemodynamic comparison of dopamine and dobutamine in the postoperative volume-loaded, pressure-loaded, and normal ventricle. *J Thorac Cardiovasc Surg* 83:256, 1982.

Engler R, Ray R, Higgins CB, et al: Clinical assessment and follow-up of functional capacity in patients with chronic congestive cardiomyopathy. *Am J Cardiol* 48:1832, 1982.

Fuster V, Cohen M, Halperin J: Aspirin in the prevention of coronary disease. *N Engl J Med* 321:183, 1989.

Garan H, Ruskin JN, DiMarco JP, et al: Electrophysiologic studies before and after myocardial revascularization in patients with life-threatening ventricular arrhythmias. *Am J Cardiol* 51:519, 1983.

Graver JM, Murphy DA, Jones EL, et al: Concomitant carotid and coronary artery revascularization. *Ann Surg* 195:712, 1982.

Harris D, Segel N, Bishop JM: The relationship between pressure and flow in the pulmonary circulation in normal subjects and in patients with chronic bronchitis and mitral stenosis. *Cardiovasc Res* 1:73, 1968.

Levine TB, Francis GS, Goldsmith SR, et al: Activity of the sympathetic nervous system and renin-angiotensin system assessed by plasma hormone levels and their relationship to hemodynamic abnormalities in congestive heart failure. *Am J Cardiol* 49:1659, 1982.

Lowenstein E, Hallowell P, Levine FH, et al: Cardiovascular response to large doses of intravenous morphine in man. *N Engl J Med* 281:1389, 1969.

Mohr R, Smolensky A, Goor DA: Prevention of supraventricular tachyarrhythmia with low dose propranolol after coronary bypass. *J Thorac Cardiovasc Surg* 81:840, 1981.

Muller JE, Gunther S: Nifedipine therapy in Prinzmetal's angina. *Circulation* 57:137, 1978.

Niarchos AP, Roberts AJ, Case DB, et al: Hemodynamic characteristics of hypertension after coronary artery bypass surgery and effects of converting enzyme inhibitor. *Am J Cardiol* 43:586, 1979.

Packer M, Medina N, Ushak M: Relation between serum sodium concentration and the hemodynamic and clinical responses to converting enzyme inhibition with captopril in severe heart failure. *J Am Coll Cardiol* 3:1035, 1984.

Salerno TA, Henderson M, Keith FM, et al: Hypertension after coronary operation. *J Thorac Cardiovasc Surg* 81:396, 1981.

Selzer A, Walter RM: Adequacy of preoperative digitalis therapy in controlling ventricular rate in postoperative atrial fibrillation. *Circulation* 34:119, 1966.

Steering Committee of the Physicians' Health Study Research Group: Final report on the aspirin component of the ongoing Physicians' Health Study. *N Engl J Med* 321:129, 1989.

Thompson ME, Kormos RL, Zerke A, Hardesty RI: Patient selection and results of cardiac transplantation in patients with cardiomyopathy. In: Shaver JA, ed. *Cardiomyopathies: Clinical Presentation, Differential Diagnosis and Management.* Philadelphia: FA Davis; 1988.

Viljoen JF, Estafanous FG, Tarazi RC: Acute hypertension immediately after coronary artery surgery. *J Thorac Cardiovasc Surg* 71:548, 1976.

Waldo AL, MacLean WAN, Karp RB, et al: Continuous rapid atrial pacing to control recurrent or sustained supraventricular tachycardia following open heart surgery. *Circulation* 54:245, 1976.

35

Effect of Exercise Training on Cardiovascular Physiology and the Process of Cardiac Rehabilitation

Damian A. Brezinski
Peter H. Stone

It is estimated that 66 million Americans suffer from manifestations of cardiovascular disease and hypertension. More than 1.5 million Americans have a myocardial infarction (MI) each year, 45% of whom are under age 65. With an average length of hospital stay of 7.6 days for acute MI and more than 32 million office visits each year, cardiovascular disease is estimated to cost $88.2 billion annually. Progress has indeed been made, as reflected by the 12.3% decrease in the age-adjusted mortality and morbidity rates from 1979 to 1987, but clearly more is required to reduce further the effect of cardiovascular disease on the population. Cardiac rehabilitation is a means of maximizing function and performance of patients with cardiovascular disease. If rehabilitative efforts are successful, the time and money spent for hospitalization and rehospitalization for these patients may decrease and the rehabilitated patients may return more rapidly to a productive and satisfying existence.

Before discussing the design of cardiac rehabilitation programs and their record of performance, we will first review briefly the physiologic effects of immobilization and exercise.

PHYSIOLOGIC EFFECTS OF IMMOBILIZATION

The sequence of the pathologic changes after MI was described by Mallory et al. in 1939. They noted that a period of six to eight weeks is required for the major portion of the necrotic myocardium to be removed and organized. The concept of bed rest for six weeks to allow for full healing originated from this information, and the concept became widely accepted. As early as 1941, however, Tinsley Harrison questioned the wisdom of prolonged bed rest after MI. Controversy surrounded early mobilization after acute MI until a series of investigations, mostly by Levine and Lown, advocated the "armchair regimen" for early MI patients. This concept was gradually accepted and further advanced to advocate rapid mobilization, early exercise, and rapid discharge of patients after uncomplicated acute MI.

Much of the impetus for early mobilization of post-MI patients came from an understanding of the deleterious effects of prolonged bed rest. For example, the classic study by Saltin and co-workers showed that physical work capacity strikingly decreased after immobilization. Healthy normal volunteers were kept at bed rest for three weeks, and a 20-25% decrease in maximal oxygen uptake was seen during exercise testing. At least three weeks of training were required to restore the pretest physical work capacity. The current understanding of the effects of immobilization has come from investigations on astronauts in preparation for aerospace efforts. These studies confirm that the most marked alteration after immobilization at bed rest is a decrease in physical work capacity and maximal oxygen uptake.

The physiologic effects of immobilization are shown in Table 1. Immobilization causes a decrease in circulating blood volume of 700-800 ml, causing significant tachycardia and orthostatic hypotension. The plasma volume decreases to a greater extent than does the red blood cell mass; these changes are independent of changes in serum erythropoietin levels and may predispose to thromboembolism by increasing blood viscosity. A negative nitrogen and protein balance has also been demonstrated. Recent microscopic studies in animal models show that prolonged immobilization is associated with a decrease in cardiac protein synthesis. Structural changes associated with prolonged bed rest include increasing dilation of the sarcoplasmic reticulum and homogenization of mi-

Table 1. Effects of Immobilization

Physiologic effects
    Decreased physical work capacity and
       maximal oxygen uptake
    Decreased circulatory blood volume
    Plasma volume decrease > RBC mass
       decrease
    Decrease in lung volume and vital capacity
    Negative nitrogen and protein balance
    Decrease in skeletal muscle mass,
       contractile strength and efficiency

Myocardial effects
    Dilated sarcoplasmic reticulum of cardiac
       myocytes
    Homogenization of cristae of cardiac
       myocytes
    Possible decrease in cardiac protein
       synthesis

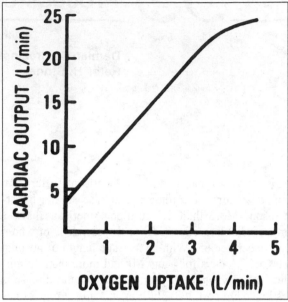

Figure 1. *The linear relationship between cardiac output and oxygen uptake. The data were collected from 23 adult men and women. (From Hammond HK, Froelicher VF: The physiologic sequelae of chronic dynamic exercise. In: Goldberg L, Elliot DL, eds. Med Clin North Am Vol 69, No. 1. Philadelphia: W.B. Saunders Co.; 1985, pp. 21–39. With permission.)*

tochondrial cristae. These changes may be significant in the healing phases of MI. A decrease in skeletal muscle contractility and muscle mass also occurs with bed rest. The contractile strength may diminish by as much as 10-15% after the first seven to 10 days of immobilization. Inefficiently contracting muscle during immobilization demands more oxygen for the same amount of work to be performed, imposing a greater stress on the heart in patients with recent MI.

Based on these extensive data concerning the effects of bed rest, gradually progressive, low intensity, early ambulation programs were designed to avert or lessen the deleterious effects of prolonged immobilization.

PHYSIOLOGIC RESPONSE TO EXERCISE

In contrast to strength exercise of the isometric type, which results in hypertrophy of the muscle cells, "endurance" exercise does not result in muscle hypertrophy or an increase in strength. Instead, it brings about an increase in the capacity for aerobic metabolism. The most accepted physiologic index of total body fitness is oxygen uptake at maximal exercise, or VO_2 max, which is determined by collecting the expired air at the individual's maximal exercise effort and measuring its volume per minute and percentage of oxygen extracted. This capacity to take up oxygen is related not only to the effectiveness of the lungs,

but also to the ability of the heart and circulatory system to transport oxygen and to the ability of the peripheral tissues to metabolize it. The VO_2 max is reproducible; it increases and decreases directly with the degree of physical conditioning. The relationship between cardiac output and oxygen uptake is almost linear (Figure 1).

Generally, the increase in VO_2 max after endurance exercise comes equally from cardiac factors, such as an increase in cardiac output, and from peripheral factors, such as an increase in peripheral tissue extraction of oxygen (i.e., widened arteriovenous oxygen difference) (Table 2). The resting cardiac output of a normal adult is about 5.6 L/min; at maximal exercise in a well-trained athlete, cardiac output may increase to about 36 L/min. This dramatic augmentation results from cardiovascular mechanisms, such as an increase in heart rate, stroke volume, and contractility, and from a marked net decrease in peripheral vascular resistance. The heart rate progressively increases to a predetermined amount with exercise, and it then cannot accelerate further. If the subject

Table 2. Cardiovascular Responses to Exercise

Cardiac factors
  Increased cardiac output
  Increased stroke volume
    Increased venous return
    Increased myocardial contractility
  Decreased heart rate at rest and any given
    work load
  Decreased myocardial oxygen consumption
    and blood pressure at rest and at any
    given work load

Peripheral factors
  Decreased peripheral vascular resistance
  Enhanced capacity for aerobic metabolism
  Increased serum high-density lipoprotein
    cholesterol concentration
  Decreased serum total cholesterol concen-
    tration
  Decreased serum low-density lipoprotein
    cholesterol and triglyceride concentration

continues to exercise, however, and the peripheral tissues require more oxygen than the heart can provide, lactate and other metabolites rapidly accumulate and soon render the cardiovascular system incapable of functioning. There is a direct linear relationship between the percent VO_2 max and percent maximal heart rate, and this relationship is a convenient means of comparing submaximal levels of exercise in a wide range of individuals regardless of their state of cardiovascular fitness.

Stroke volume progressively increases with exercise, but it levels off somewhat before the maximal pumping capacity is achieved. The increased stroke volume is due both to an increase in venous return and to an increase in myocardial contractility. Immediately after the onset of exercise there is a reflex-mediated increase in venous tone that enhances venous return to the heart. Additionally, the exercising leg muscles serve as a pump, which further augments venous return. The increase in blood return causes an increase in myocardial fiber stretch. This increase in myocardial fiber stretch is believed to cause an increase in myocardial contractility and stroke volume through the Frank-Starling mechanism. Prolonged endurance conditioning leads to a progressive increase in stroke volume; the stroke volume of conditioned athletes may be 50–75% higher than that of sedentary

persons. This response enables those who are conditioned to satisfy the oxygen requirements of the body at a slower heart rate.

In addition to the cardiac responses that enable the heart to pump more blood, peripheral factors also enhance myocardial pump function (Table 2). First, the increase in cardiac output is facilitated by a marked net decrease in peripheral vascular resistance. This unloading allows for a greater increase in cardiac output than is possible with increased heart rate and stroke volume alone. Systemic vascular resistance decreases primarily because of vasodilation in the exercising muscle areas, while a concomitant decrease in blood flow to the splanchnic bed and nonworking muscles provides a shunt to the areas of demand. As a result of the increased cardiac output and decreased systemic vascular resistance, systolic blood pressure increases while diastolic blood pressure changes little or decreases slightly, creating a physiologic situation characteristic of an increased volume load. Another major peripheral effect of endurance exercise is an increase in the capacity for aerobic metabolism due to alterations in the biochemical content of skeletal muscle. When skeletal muscle adapts to endurance, it becomes more like cardiac muscle in that its content of mitochondria and its capacity to generate ATP from oxidation of pyruvate and fatty acids increases. Increases in both the size and number of mitochondria cause the increase in total mitochondrial protein. Myoglobin content of skeletal muscle also increases as physical conditioning progresses. Because very little adaptive enhancement of carbohydrate metabolism occurs with exercise training, it appears that physical conditioning shifts the metabolic emphasis toward enhanced utilization of fatty acids, initiating a glycogen saving effect. The fundamental contractile properties of skeletal muscle, however, are not altered by chronic exercise.

Coronary blood flow increases proportionately with the increased myocardial demands during exercise in normal persons. Unlike the peripheral tissues, which can increase their oxygen extraction from the blood in response to exercise, the cardiac muscle extracts the maximal amount of oxygen from the blood at rest. The resting arteriovenous oxygen difference across the coronary circulation is therefore much wider than that across the peripheral vascular beds. Since the myocardium cannot increase oxygen extraction during exercise, the only means of providing more oxygen to the myocardium is an actual increase in coronary blood flow. In normal persons, coronary blood flow is autoregulated by myocardial oxygen demand; coronary flow therefore increases in an almost linear fashion as myocardial oxygen demand or consumption increases.

Myocardial oxygen demand (MVO$_2$) or consumption depends on a variety of factors, many of which can be noninvasively measured. Noninvasive measurements are helpful in quantitating cardiac performance in patients with coronary disease. The principal determinants of MVO$_2$ are heart rate, contractility, and ventricular wall tension, the last being in turn determined by peak ventricular systolic pressure (afterload) and ventricular volume (preload). Measurements of MVO$_2$ are helpful in patients with ischemic heart disease because MVO$_2$ reflects the limitations of the diseased coronary arteries to provide increased flow during stress. The rate-pressure product (the product of the heart rate and the peak systolic blood pressure) is widely accepted as a useful approximation of the MVO$_2$.

Chronic dynamic exercise can also alter serum lipoprotein levels, which may affect the atherosclerotic process. In patients with normal or elevated cholesterol levels, exercise training has little effect on total cholesterol (-0.5%), but increases HDL by 8% and lowers triglyceride levels by 6%. In patients with hypertriglyceridemia, the effects of exercise are more marked: total cholesterol is reduced by about 7%, HDL is increased by about 23%, and triglycerides are reduced by about 37%.

EFFECT OF EXERCISE IN PATIENTS WITH ISCHEMIC HEART DISEASE

An understanding of these physiologic responses to exercise is particularly germane for management of the cardiac patient. These physiologic mechanisms indicate how the patient with ischemic heart disease and myocardial dysfunction may be limited in the ability to exercise; equally important, they provide an understanding of the potential role of physical rehabilitation for the cardiac patient.

Figure 2 illustrates the effect of intensive physical training on VO$_2$ max in patients with ischemic heart disease. After training, there is a dramatic 55% increase in VO$_2$ max in these patients, although at any given submaximal work load, it is the same in trained and untrained patients. These benefits in physiologic conditioning are progressively increased with prolonged periods of training (Figure 3). Also, since

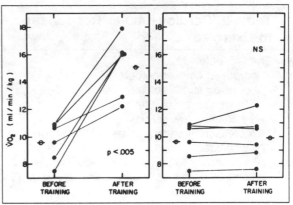

Figure 2. *Effects of training on total body oxygen consumption. The left panel shows values obtained at the highest level of exercise that could be attained before the onset of angina. In the right panel, points to the left represent the values obtained during the highest level of exercise that could be attained without angina before training; points to the right represent values obtained after training when patients exercised at the identical pretraining exercise load. Mean values are represented by the barred circles. (Reproduced with permission from Redwood et al. See Bibliography.)*

trained patients have increased their VO$_2$ max, they can exercise for much longer periods (Figure 4).

The effects of exercise training on the major determinants of MVO$_2$ are shown in Figure 5. At submaximal workloads, heart rate, systolic blood pressure, and rate-pressure product are significantly lower after a period of physical training than the values before conditioning. The MVO$_2$, therefore, is less at any given workload after training. The physiologic benefit of physical conditioning is thus similar to that obtained from antianginal medications. Physical conditioning leads to a decrease in MVO$_2$ by decreasing the determinants of heart rate and blood pressure; antianginal medications decrease MVO$_2$ generally by decreasing heart rate, blood pressure, preload, or contractility. Collateral blood flow to the ischemic myocardium is also enhanced by physical training.

A recent disturbing report from Jugdutt and colleagues indicated that a low-level exercise program starting 15 weeks after a moderate-sized anterior Q-wave MI led to significant exacerbation of left ventricular cavity distortion, an increase in asynergy, and a decrease in ejection fraction compared to values in a group of nonrandomized control patients who did

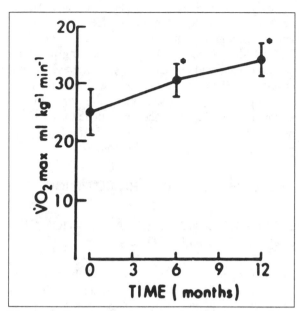

Figure 3. *Progressive increase in response to 12 months of high-intensity exercise training in patients with ischemic heart disease (p <0.01) (trained vs. untrained state). (Reproduced with permission from Ehsani 1987.)*

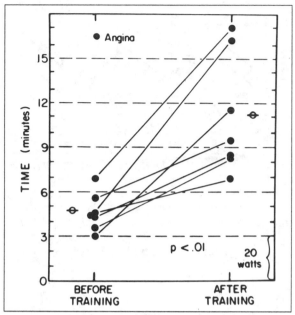

Figure 4. *Effect of training on exercise capacity. Closed circles indicate the time at which angina occurred; barred circles indicate mean values. Dashed lines represent the intervals at which the work load was increased by 20 watts. (Reproduced with permission from Redwood et al.)*

not exercise after infarction. The authors suggested that exercise training might be deleterious in patients with an extensive transmural infarct that has not healed completely. More information is needed in a larger group of patients to confirm these results and to identify the patients who may be at greatest risk from the stresses of physical exercise.

ORGANIZATION OF CARDIAC REHABILITATION

With this background of exercise physiology, the organization of the cardiac rehabilitation process can be considered. Cardiac rehabilitation involves all efforts designed to restore and maintain the cardiac patient at an optimal level of function, and therefore attention is directed toward the physiologic, psychosocial, educational, and vocational areas of rehabilitation. Although this review concentrates primarily on the physiologic aspects of cardiac rehabilitation, equally important to the cardiac patient are the nonphysiologic elements of rehabilitation, that is, those elements that help restore the sense of well-being and optimism. Physical therapists, social workers, occu-

pational therapists, and dietitians have a central role in the operation of a complete rehabilitation program.

STRUCTURE OF A FORMAL EXERCISE PROGRAM

The process of cardiac rehabilitation is generally separated into three phases. Phase I is the in-hospital phase, which begins during the patient's hospitalization for the acute cardiac event (MI or cardiac surgery). Patients qualify for the rehabilitation program only if they have had an uncomplicated hospital course, that is, they don't have recurrent angina, arrhythmias, or congestive heart failure. Phase II begins when the patient leaves the hospital, and continues for about three months. This is the hospital-based early outpatient rehabilitation phase and involves close medical supervision. Phase III is the maintenance rehabilitation phase that continues indefinitely and generally requires only intermittent supervision and safety checks.

The exercise tolerance test (ETT) provides the objective basis for serial determination of the patient's

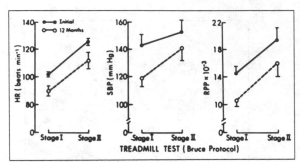

Figure 5. *Effects of endurance training on heart rate (HR), systolic blood pressure (SBP) and rate-pressure product (RPP) at absolute work rate (stages I and II of the Bruce protocol). All the variables after training (open circles) were significantly (p <0.01) lower than those before training (circles). (Reproduced with permission from Ehsani et al. 1982.)*

physical condition, as well as the safety monitor to ensure that a particular degree of activity can be performed safely. If the acute MI is uncomplicated, a low-level ETT is generally performed before hospital discharge. Usually, an arbitrary endpoint of completion of stage I of the modified Bruce protocol (5 METs) or achievement of a target heart rate of 130 beats/min is used to terminate the test. The patient who tolerates this degree of exercise well is discharged and given an exercise prescription for phase II. After one or two months of phase II training, a maximal symptom-limited ETT is performed; if that is safely tolerated, the patient progresses to phase III of rehabilitation. Exercise tolerance tests are then performed at six- and 12-month intervals to assess safety and the degree of conditioning.

In order for physical conditioning, defined as an increase in VO_2 max, or aerobic capacity, to take place, exercise must be of a certain intensity, duration, and frequency. To make the greatest improvement in aerobic capacity with minimal risk, 70–80% of maximal heart rate should be reached. The risk of complications from this degree of exercise is negligible. Exercise should generally last for 20-30 minutes at each workout. Workouts should be performed at least three times, and preferably four or five times, per week.

Sample recommendations for an exercise prescription for cardiac patients are shown in Table 3. During phase I, the patient should exercise two or three times a day, with a target heart rate of about 20 beats/min over the resting rate. Physical activity should be closely

supervised, especially during the acute hospitalization, to ensure that no untoward effects such as angina, arrhythmias, or congestive failure develop. Activity should last 5–20 minutes. During phase II, the frequency and intensity of the exercise do not change, but the duration increases to 20–40 minutes. During phase III, in order to maximize conditioning, as noted earlier, exercise should be three to five times per week, with a heart rate of 70–85% of maximal predicted heart rate, for 30–60 minutes.

VALUE OF CARDIAC REHABILITATION

EFFECT OF CARDIAC REHABILITATION ON MORBIDITY AND MORTALITY

The long-term benefits of cardiac rehabilitation are controversial. Table 4 lists representative international studies of the effects of exercise training on recurrence of MI, total death rate, and cardiac death rate for patients after acute MI. Participants in these exercise programs had an acute MI and then became active in rehabilitation programs. Exercise training took place in a supervised setting, with target peak heart rates of about 70–85% of maximum predicted for age. Although some trends exist favoring a program of structured exercise activities, the benefits do not achieve statistical significance. Furthermore, the statistical interpretation of some reports is invalidated by the nonrandom selection of patients and uncertainties regarding duration of exercise and the average follow-up period. The control groups, for example, have often consisted of arbitrarily selected populations, including patients not wishing to participate in an exercise class or those attending clinics that do not recommend exercise therapy.

Another major problem in assessing the benefit of organized cardiac rehabilitation is the lack of compliance to the exercise program. Experience from a number of large clinical investigations indicates that the dropout rate varies between 30% and 85% over a period of about four years. In addition, 10–35% of patients may develop medical contraindications to continued participation in an exercise program. It is obviously difficult to draw meaningful conclusions from a study when only 20–50% of the original cohort continues to participate.

In the United States, the National Exercise and Heart Disease Project (Shaw) is one of the most closely controlled and well-executed randomized studies to

Table 3. Guidelines for Exercise Prescription for Healthy Adults and Cardiac Patients

	Frequency	Intensity	Duration (min)	Mode
Healthy adult	3–5 times/wk	60–80% VO$_2$ max	15–60	Aerobic activities, weights, games
Angina	3–5 times/wk	70–85% anginal threshold	15–60	Walk, jog, bike
MI/CABG				
Phase I	2–3 times/day	HR rest + 20	5–20	Range of motion, ambulation, stairs
Phase II	3–4 times/wk	HR rest + 20 or 50–70% VO$_2$ max	15–60	Range of motion, walk, bike, arm ergometry
Phase III	3–4 times/wk	50–80% VO$_2$ max	30–60	Range of motion, walk, jog, bike, swim, games, weights
PTCA	Same as phase III			
Transplants (outpatient)	3–4 times/wk	RPE 12–14	15–60	Range of motion, walk, bike, arm ergometry
Fixed HR pacemaker	3–4 times/wk	60–80% systolic BP range	15–60	Walk, jog, bike, swim, games

BP = blood pressure; CABG = coronary artery bypass graft; HR = heart rate; MI = myocardial infarction; PTCA = percutaneous transluminal coronary angioplasty; RPE = relative perceived exertion. (From Ward et al. See Bibliography.)

evaluate the effects of exercise in post-MI patients. The study was a three-year, multicenter trial of 651 men who were randomized to a supervised program or to routine post-MI care. In the intervention group, overall mortality was reduced by 37%, cardiovascular deaths by 29%, nonsudden cardiovascular deaths by 56%, and all MIs by 24% (Figure 6, Table 5). Unfortunately, none of the differences in the study achieved statistical significance, perhaps because of relatively small sample sizes. The investigators concluded that exercise rehabilitation after acute MI appeared to be valuable, but suggested a large-scale trial to provide definitive confirmation. Such a study may not be performed because of prohibitive costs; however, O'Connor and colleagues performed an exhaustive meta analysis of all randomized trials of cardiac rehabilitation after acute MI (n = 4,554 patients) and concluded that exercise indeed significantly reduced the risk of death by 20%. The reduced risk of cardiovascular mortality and fatal MI persisted for at least three years after the index event, whereas the reduction in sudden death was only present in the first year after MI. No benefit was observed for nonfatal recurrent MI.

EFFECT OF CARDIAC REHABILITATION ON RISK FACTORS

The effect of exercise on risk factors is important to consider, since the benefits of exercise, if any, may be due more to a decrease in risk factors than to actual enhancement of cardiorespiratory fitness. A composite of recent data indicates that the change in risk factors from exercise training programs may be small. Over a three-year period of observation, changes in body weight and skinfold thickness are negligible. Rest systolic blood pressure shows a small decrease, possibly associated with increased habituation to the test laboratory, but maximal systolic pressure tolerated during exercise actually increases as myocardial contractility improves.

Changes in serum lipid levels observed in the trials of cardiac rehabilitation have not been striking. Cholesterol values remain essentially unchanged. However, the multicenter Lipid Research Clinics North American Prevalence Study (Goor et al.) indicated that strenuous exercise may increase the protective plasma HDL levels. Although neither treadmill exercise test duration nor heart rate response to sub-

Table 4. Estimate of the Value of Exercise to Reduce Morbidity and Mortality After Myocardial Infarction

1st Author (year)	n	Intervention	Follow-Up (mo)	Exercise Group			Control Group		
				Recurrent MI Rate (%/yr)	Death Rate (%/yr)	Cardiac Death Rate (%/yr)	Recurrent MI Rate (%/yr)	Death Rate (%/yr)	Cardiac Death Rate (%/yr)
Carson (1982)	303	Supervised exercise 2×/week	25	3.5	3.8	–	3.2	6.7	–
Hedback (1987)	305	Supervised exercise 2×/week	60	3.5	5.9	5.4	6.7	6.3	6.1
Kentala (1972)	158	Supervised exercise 2–3×/week	24	7.8	14.3	11.6	4.9	13.6	12.3
Palatsi (1976)	380	Daily home exercise	29	4.9	4.6	4.2	6.0	6.9	5.8
Rechnitzer (1983)	199	Daily home exercise	24	1.5	3.8	3.8	5.5	9.4	9.4
Roman (1983)	193	Supervised exercise 3×/week	108	3.6	3.6	2.8	5.0	5.8	5.2
Sanne (1979)	1026	Home exercise	48	6.6	3.8	2.9	12.5	8.8	8.3
Shaw (1981)	651	Supervised exercise 3×/week	36	1.5	1.5	1.4	1.1	2.4	2.0
Wilhelmsen (1975)	315	Supervised exercise 3×/week	48	8.4	4.4	3.6	10.0	5.6	5.3

maximal exercise was significantly related to HDL cholesterol levels, participants who reported strenuous physical activity at home had higher HDL cholesterol levels than those who reported none. Although triglyceride levels decrease, they often decrease almost equally in the control groups. The significance of decreased triglyceride levels is unknown. The percentage of cigarette smokers is also a little lower in exercised than in nonexercised groups of post-MI patients, although in some studies, more than a third of the exercising patients who continued to smoke claimed to have made substantial reductions in their cigarette consumption. Although exercise itself may contribute relatively little to an improved risk factor profile in

coronary patients, other components of the cardiac rehabilitation program, including dietary modification, stress management, cessation of cigarette smoking, and close control of hypertension and hyperlipidemia, may have a major impact on secondary prevention.

EFFECT OF CARDIAC REHABILITATION ON PSYCHOSOCIAL STATUS

The psychologic effects of exercise training are important to explore, since exercise rehabilitation programs may be justified if the patients' sense of well-being and employment activities are improved even

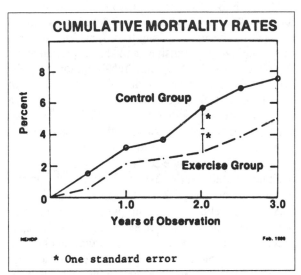

Figure 6. *Cumulative mortality of National Exercise and Heart Disease Project. (Reproduced with permission from Shaw.)*

if true physiologic benefits cannot be documented. The psychological benefits from rehabilitation, however, do not appear to be major. For example, psychological factors seem to play a relatively minor role

in whether coronary patients return to work. Most studies that have investigated the typical course of return to vocational function in coronary patients suggest that 80% generally resume their pre-illness level of activity. Psychological factors contribute only to a small degree. In a recent study, 46% of patients followed after discharge from a coronary care unit failed to return to work as soon as one might expect, but only 10% of these patients (5% of the total sample) listed anxiety as the primary reason (Gentry). Other investigators estimate that psychological problems after MI are responsible for only 3–12% of the patients not returning to work. Therefore, the possible benefits of exercise to make patients psychologically better able to return to work appear to be small. Several investigations suggest that a program of physical exercise leads to a significant reduction in self-reported anxiety and, to a somewhat lesser degree, in depression. It also appears to increase self-esteem and perception of one's health, providing reinforcement and increased motivation for further adherence to the rehabilitation regimen. In perhaps the best study of this type, Ibrahim and associates investigated the effect of group psychotherapy on post-MI patients during the first 18 months after MI. Most patients were eager and faithful participants in this type of rehabilitation

Table 5. Mortality of Participants by Study Group and Estimates of Effectiveness of the Exercise Program

Events Counted	Control Group (n = 328) n	%	Exercise Group (n = 323) n	%	Comparison Statistics χ^2	p	Estimates of Effectiveness of Program (%) Minimum (C_L)	Observed (E)	Maximum (C_u)
All deaths	24	7.3	15	4.6	1.62	0.22	−15	37	68
Cardiovascular deaths									
Acute myocardial infarction	8	2.4	1	0.3	3.96	0.047	22	87	98
Other definite*	6		5						
Subtotal	14	4.3	6	1.9	2.42	0.13	−5	56	84
Sudden deaths†	6		8						
Total	20	6.1	14	4.3	0.70	0.40	−33	29	66
Indeterminate cause	4		1						

*Includes six deaths from arrhythmias, two from congestive cardiac failure, one from cardiogenic shock and two from cerebrovascular accidents.
† Within 1 hour.
C_L = lower 95% confidence limit; C_u = upper 95% confidence limit; p = probability.
Reproduced with permission from Shaw.

program. Results suggested that patients receiving such therapy experienced less social alienation after MI than patients receiving no therapy. Patients receiving psychotherapy also showed a decrease in levels of competition and in the exaggerated sense of responsibility. However, such effects were short-lived, in that most of the post-MI patients returned to their pre-illness levels of stressful behavior within six months after the end of therapy.

Many experienced investigators remain skeptical of the psychological benefits of cardiac rehabilitation. They note that almost all of the participants in their training programs say that they feel better as a result of exercising. Yet these changes are difficult to demonstrate objectively by formal psychological testing. In the few randomized controlled studies of psychosocial improvement during cardiac rehabilitation, the effect of exercise on well-being is unimpressive. Shephard noted that after 12–15 months of rehabilitation, as many as a third of the cohort showed the neurotic triad on the Minnesota Multiphasic Personality Inventory: high scores for hysteria and hypochondriasis and very high depression scores. Over four years of rehabilitation, the investigators observed some favorable changes in those who complied with the prescribed exercise regimen. Gains were relatively small, however, even in those who trained themselves to the point of participating in marathon events. On the basis of the most recent studies, expected improvements in psychosocial well-being cannot justify enrollment in cardiac exercise rehabilitation after myocardial infarction.

SUMMARY

A long-term program of intensive physical training enables cardiac patients to perform more work with a decreased physiologic expenditure. Cardiac patients can perform their daily activities, therefore, with fewer symptoms and less disability. Recent studies and pooled analyses suggest that exercise may prolong life and decrease reinfarction in patients after MI but the few controlled clinical trials of long-term exercise training, using relatively small sample sizes, do not support that concept. The effects of exercise itself on coronary risk factors are slight, but a more definitive program of cardiac rehabilitation including dietary modification and control of hypertension and hyperlipidemia may have a major impact on secondary prevention.

Many investigators in the field of cardiac rehabilitation acknowledge that a more definitive study of the possible benefits of long-term rehabilitation may be prohibitively expensive, and that a judgment on the overall value of cardiac rehabilitation may be needed. The Health and Public Policy Committee of the American College of Physicians recently issued a position paper on cardiac rehabilitation services that concluded that the value of formal programs appears to be slight. They suggest that the common practice of offering 30–60-minute supervised sessions per week beginning within four weeks of hospital discharge and continuing for up to 12 weeks can be considered a maximal guideline for patients who qualify for participation. Supervision beyond this relatively short program is not generally considered worthwhile.

It is reasonable and appropriate to explain clearly the actual benefits and the limitations of cardiac rehabilitation to cardiac patients and to offer the appropriate options. Cardiac rehabilitation programs may enable interested patients to live a more active, comfortable, and fruitful life.

Bibliography

Carson P, Philips R, Lloyd M, et al: Exercise after a myocardial infarction: A controlled trial. *J R Coll Physicians* (London) 16:147, 1982.

Ehsani AA, Martin WH, Heath GW, Coyle EF: Cardiac effects of prolonged and intense exercise training in patients with coronary artery disease. *Am J Cardiol* 50:246, 1982.

Ehsani AA: Cardiovascular adaptations to endurance exercise training in ischemic heart disease. *Exer Sport Sci Rev* 15:53, 1987.

Gentry W: Psychosocial concerns and benefits in cardiac rehabilitation. In: Pollack ML, Schmidt DH, eds. *Heart Disease and Rehabilitation*, 2nd edition. Boston: Wiley; 1986.

Goor R, Hosking JD, Dennis BH, et al: Nutrient intake among selected North American populations in the Lipid Research Clinics Prevalence Study: Comparison of fat intake. *Am J Clin Nutrition* 41:299, 1985.

Health and Public Policy Committee, American College of Physicians. Position Paper. Cardiac Rehabilitation Services. *Ann Intern Med* 109:67, 1988.

Hedback B, Perk J: 5-year results of a comprehensive rehabilitation programme after myocardial infarction. *Eur Heart J* 8:234, 1987.

Ibrahim MA, Feldman JG, Sultz HA, et al: Management after myocardial infarction: A controlled trial of the effect of group psychotherapy. *Int J Psychiatric Med* 5:253, 1974.

Jugdutt BI, Michorowski BL, Kappagoda CT: Exercise training after anterior Q-wave myocardial infarction: Importance of regional left ventricular function and topography. *J Am Coll Cardiol* 12:362, 1988.

Kavanagh T, Shephard RJ, Qureshi S, et al: Prognostic indexes for patients with ischemic heart disease enrolled in an exercise-centered rehabilitation program. *Am J Cardiol* 44:1230, 1979.

Kentala E: Physical Fitness and Feasibility of Physical Rehabilitation after myocardial infarction in lieu of working age. *Ann Clin Res* 4 (Suppl 9):1, 1972.

Leon AS: Physical activity levels and coronary heart disease. *Med Clin North Am* 69:3, 1985.

Levine SA, Lown B: The chair treatment of acute coronary thrombosis. *Trans Assoc Am Physicians* 64:316, 1951.

Laslett L, Paumer L, Armstrong E: Exercise training in coronary artery disease. *Cardiol Clin* 5:211, 1987.

Mallory GK, White PD, Salcedo-Salgar J: The speed of healing of myocardial infarction: A study of the pathologic anatomy in 72 cases. *Am Heart J* 18:647, 1939.

O'Connor GT, Buring JE, Yusuf S, et al. An overview of randomized trials of rehabilitation with exercise after myocardial infarction. *Circulation* 80:234, 1989.

Oldridge NB, Donner AP, Buck CW, et al. Predictors of dropout from cardiac exercise rehabilitation. *Am J Cardiol* 51:70, 1983.

Palatsi I: Feasibility of physical training after myocardial infarction and its effect on return to work, mobility, and mortality. *Acta Med Scan* 399 (Suppl):7, 1976.

Pollock ML, Schmidt DH, eds: *Heart Disease and Rehabilitation*. 2nd ed. Boston: Wiley; 1986.

Rechnitzer PA, Cunnigham DA, Andrew GM, et al: Relation of exercise to the recurrence rate of myocardial infarction in men. *Am J Cardiol* 51:65, 1983.

Rechnitzer PA, Pickard HA, Paivio A, et al: Long-term follow-up study of survival and recurrent rates following myocardial infarction in exercising and control subjects. *Circulation* 45:853, 1972.

Redwood DR, Rosing DR, Epstein SE: Circulatory and symptomatic effects of physical training in patients with coronary artery disease and angina pectoris. *N Engl J Med* 286:959, 1972.

Rogers MA, Yamamoto C, Hagberg JM, Holloszy JO, Ehsani AA: The effect of 7 years of intense exercise training on patients with coronary artery disease. *J Am Coll Cardiol* 10:321, 1987.

Roman O, Guitierez M, Lusic I, et al: Cardiac rehabilitation after myocardial infarction: 9 year controlled follow-up study. *Cardiology* 70:223, 1983.

Saltin B, Blomqvist G, Mitchell JH, et al: Response to exercise after bed rest and after training. *Circulation* 38(Suppl VII):78, 1968.

Sanne H: Risk factor modification studies in Europe. In: Pollock ML, Schmidt DH, eds. *Heart Disease and Rehabilitation*. Boston: Houghton Mifflin; 1979, p. 352.

Shaw LW: Effects of a prescribed supervised exercise program on mortality and cardiovascular morbidity in patients after a myocardial infarction. The National Exercise and Heart Disease Project. *Am J Cardiol* 48:39, 1981.

Shepard J: Evaluation of earlier studies. In: Cohen LS, Mock MB, Rengqvist I: *Physical Conditioning in Cardiovascular Rehabilitation*. New York: Wiley; 1981, pp. 271–288.

Superko HR, Haskell WH. The role of exercise training in the therapy of hyperlipoproteins. *Cardiol Clinics* 5:285, 1987.

Ward A, Molloy P, Rippe J: Exercise prescription guidelines for normal and cardiac populations. *Cardiol Clin* 5:197, 1987.

Wilhelmsen L, Sanne H, Elmfeldt D, et al: A controlled trial of physical training after myocardial infarction. *Preventive Med* 4:491, 1975.

CHAPTER 36 Cardiopulmonary Resuscitation

Richard F. Wright

Resuscitation has been performed for thousands of years, but only in the last century has it been performed with any measure of success. Despite reports of success with external chest compression and artificial ventilation in the late nineteenth century, direct internal cardiac massage remained the standard mode of resuscitation until the value of external chest compression was redescribed in 1960. Basic cardiopulmonary resuscitation has changed little since then.

Each year, more than 500,000 people die suddenly from cardiac causes in the United States. Prompt institution of resuscitative efforts could save many of these lives. Reported success rates for cardiopulmonary resuscitation vary from 10% to 90%. In general, the success rate is low among critically ill patients and when institution of resuscitation is delayed; the success rate is high among patients in whom primary ventricular fibrillation is rapidly identified and treated. In out-of-hospital victims of ventricular fibrillation, resuscitation is successful less than 40% of the time.

External chest compression and mouth-to-mouth ventilation are temporizing measures, designed to prevent irreversible ischemic deterioration while the patient awaits more definitive therapy. Although no absolute rules predict the success of resuscitation, the success rate is very low if basic resuscitation is instituted beyond 4–5 minutes. If more advanced resuscitative efforts are delayed by 7–8 minutes, chances of survival are even lower. In certain causes of cardiac arrest, particularly hypothermia, these guidelines do not apply and patients may be successfully revived after much longer delays. In general, however, time is the most important predictor of successful resuscitation.

CAUSES OF CARDIAC ARREST

The most common causes of sudden death are ventricular tachycardia and ventricular fibrillation. Other tachyarrhythmias, such as atrial fibrillation in the patient with accelerated atrioventricular conduction, may occasionally cause sudden death. Bradyarrhythmias are less common precipitating events; ischemia-induced sinus arrest or complete heart block are the usual causes.

Other causes of sudden death include primary respiratory arrest; electromechanical dissociation (absence of effective mechanical systole despite persistent electrical complexes); and acute mechanical lesions, such as massive pulmonary embolism, acute disruption of the cardiac valves or great vessels, pericardial tamponade, and myocardial rupture. Regardless of the cause of cardiac arrest, the initial approach to the victim is the same.

MECHANISMS OF BLOOD FLOW DURING RESUSCITATION

The success of cardiopulmonary resuscitation depends, in large part, on achieving adequate blood flow to the heart and brain. External chest compression was initially described as "closed-chest cardiac massage," implying that resuscitation-induced blood flow was a result of the heart being squeezed between the sternum and spine, mimicking the action of internal cardiac compression and propelling blood forward by increasing intracardiac pressure above aortic pressure. However, recent work by many investigators casts doubt on the validity of this proposed mechanism. It is now apparent that cardiac output during sternal compression may be due at least in part to an increase in intrathoracic pressure during each compression. According to this hypothesis, the heart acts as a conduit for blood flow rather than as a pump. When intrathoracic pressure is elevated by chest compression, blood is squeezed out of the thorax. Retrograde flow is prevented by the cardiac and systemic venous valves, and possibly by collapse of the systemic veins as they exit from the thorax. Thus, as intrathoracic pressure rises, blood is forced from the lungs, through the heart, and into the aorta. As pressure on the sternum is released, blood flows back into the pulmonary vascular bed from the systemic veins. Flow from the aorta back into the heart is prevented by the aortic valve.

Evidence for such a flow pattern was originally based on clinical observations. Patients with flail chests, in whom the unstable chest segment precludes attainment of positive intrathoracic pressure with sternal compression, were at times revived only after stabilization of the chest wall. Emphysematous patients were not more difficult to resuscitate despite the increased distance between their sternum and spine. Coughing, which substantially increases intrathoracic pressure, was noted to generate remarkable cardiac output in the absence of cardiac systole; in fact, repetitive coughing maintains consciousness in humans with ventricular fibrillation. Recent attempts to duplicate the physiology of the cough, by increasing abdominal pressure (with binding, for example) and by inflating the lungs simultaneously with sternal compression, have resulted in demonstrable increases in forward blood flow during resuscitation.

Hemodynamic data also support a role for the "chest pump" hypothesis. Measured pressures in the great vessels and the intracardiac chambers can be equal during sternal compression; if forward blood flow were due to direct squeezing of the heart, intracardiac pressures should exceed pressures elsewhere in the thorax. In addition, angiographic and two-dimensional echocardiographic views show that some patients exhibit flow through open mitral and aortic valves during sternal compression. However, some investigators have reported evidence for direct cardiac compression during resuscitation, at least in dogs. In some patients, either or both proposed mechanisms of flow could occur.

Supplemental maneuvers, such as abdominal binding, interposed abdominal compression, and simultaneous lung inflation-chest compression, can further increase intrathoracic pressure and carotid blood flow during sternal compression in some studies. However, these techniques have not been shown to improve the success rate of resuscitation and cannot be recommended for general use.

TECHNIQUE OF CARDIOPULMONARY RESUSCITATION

Figure 1 is a diagram of the process of resuscitation.

VENTILATION

Once a patient is determined to have had a cardiac arrest, a patent airway must be established. This is accomplished most quickly by placing the patient supine and tilting the head back while simultaneously pulling the jaw forward and opening the mouth slightly. These maneuvers preclude airway obstruction by the tongue and pharynx and allow inspection of the pharynx if ventilatory difficulties indicate upper airway obstruction.

Mouth-to-mouth resuscitation at a rate of about 12 breaths/min can then be instituted. Adequate ventilation may be gauged by the presence of chest expansion and the sounds of the victim's exhalations. Mouth-to-mouth ventilation is a temporizing measure, as the fractional inspired oxygen so administered is only 0.17. In a prolonged resuscitation, this will usually be insufficient to achieve adequate arterial oxygenation. Therefore, the use of a respirator bag and a tight-fitting mask, esophageal airway, or endotracheal tube is necessary to administer 100% oxygen if initial attempts at restoring spontaneous ventilation are unsuccessful. Endotracheal intubation also provides a route for drug administration if intravenous cannulation is unavailable.

Adequacy of ventilation should be monitored by arterial blood gas determinations. Hyperventilation is frequently necessary to compensate for the metabolic acidosis often seen in the patient with cardiac arrest. Arterial pH should be maintained at 7.30–7.45. Hypoxia is invariably present because of intrapulmonary shunting; therefore, 100% oxygen should always be administered. Use of high levels of oxygen for brief periods is not dangerous.

Arterial blood gas levels are poor indicators of tissue acid-base status and oxygenation during resuscitation. Arterial blood gas determinations are necessary to assess the adequacy of ventilation and pulmonary gas exchange, but mixed venous blood gas levels and end-tidal carbon dioxide levels are much better measures of tissue perfusion. This disparity is due to the poor cardiac output achieved during resuscitation. Such low flow leads to poor delivery of carbon dioxide to the lungs, with a resultant striking degree of hyper-

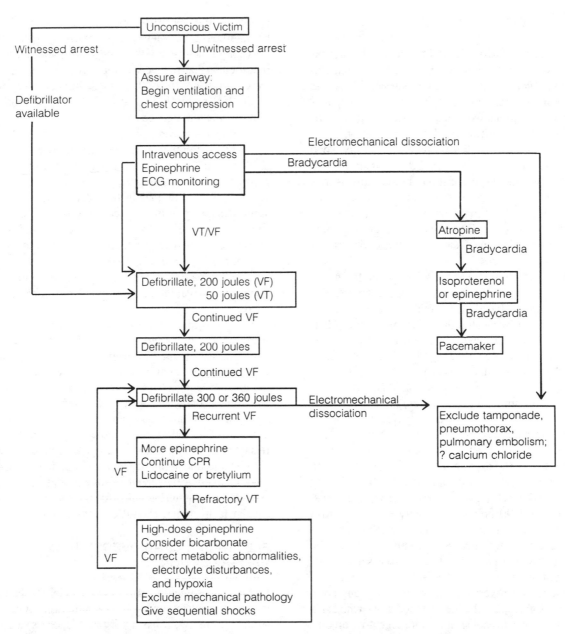

Figure 1. *The steps instituted during a typical cardiopulmonary resuscitation. If the electrocardiogram reveals ventricular tachycardia, a chest thump may be attempted. See text for further discussion of the use of the chest thump. See text for dosages and dosing intervals.*

capnia and acidosis in the tissues and in venous blood. In such situations, arterial blood gases give insufficient and potentially misleading information regarding the adequacy of tissue perfusion and usually mask the severity of tissue ischemia.

Upper airway obstruction due to foreign body aspiration, as in the so-called cafe coronary syndrome,

caused by aspiration of food, may be treated successfully by use of the Heimlich maneuver. The rescuer stands behind the victim with the fists clenched beneath the victim's xiphoid and delivers a swift thrust upward and inward. This usually drives the diaphragm up and expels the blocking agent from the airway.

CIRCULATION

Adequate circulation must be achieved simultaneously with restoration of effective ventilation. External chest compression usually produces 25% or less of the normal cardiac output. This reduced output is directed predominantly cephalad and is often sufficient to perfuse the brain, at least temporarily. Myocardial perfusion is much less optimal. Coronary blood flow during resuscitation may be less than 10% of normal. Insufficient myocardial blood flow is frequently the cause of inability to achieve stable cardiac rhythm. This suboptimal flow is due to the low diastolic blood pressure (and thus a poor driving force for coronary artery perfusion) attained during resuscitation.

Proper chest compression is important for maximizing blood flow during resuscitation. The rescuer kneels or stands beside the victim and places his interlocked hands, one atop the other, on the lower half of the sternum. The exact position is not critical as long as the hands are above the xiphoid process (pressure on the xiphoid may result in ineffective thoracic compression and/or hepatic lacerations). If sternal placement is impossible, positioning of the hands anywhere on the thorax can be effective. For instance, one hand can be placed on each hemithorax. Each compression is accomplished by depressing the sternum 4–6 cm. This is most easily done by locking the elbows and leaning over the victim's chest, thereby transmitting the weight of the upper torso to the hands. A force of 60–90 pounds is usually needed. A firm surface beneath the patient makes the job easier and more effective, but successful compressions can be performed with a patient in bed, if necessary.

The optimal rate, force, and velocity of chest compression is controversial. Although early observers noted no significant change in blood flow with rates of 40–120 compressions/min, more recent reports indicate a rise in output over this range. For this reason, a rate of 80–120 compressions/min is recommended. The duration of compressions may be important: 50–60% "down-time" results in improved flow compared to briefer periods of compression during slow rates, but this variable appears to be less important at faster compression rates. Recent data show that "high impulse" compression, in which the velocity of initial chest compression is increased, achieves higher systolic and diastolic pressures. Chest compression force is also an important variable: increased force results in higher cardiac output. Ventilations should be interposed between every fourth or fifth compression; if a rescuer is alone, this pattern can be modified so that two ventilations are administered between every 12–15 compressions. In sum, a regimen of 80–120 forceful, high-velocity compressions per minute is recommended.

Internal cardiac massage results in demonstrably better cardiac output than sternal compression but is used infrequently because it is an invasive technique. Nevertheless, it is indicated in certain cases of penetrating cardiac trauma; in the postoperative cardiac surgical patient; in mechanical lesions such as aortic stenosis; in the patient with a grossly unstable chest; in some patients with prosthetic valves (external pressure applied over prosthetic valve rings may cause cardiac trauma during chest compression); and in patients who have failed to respond to more routine measures.

The precordial thump has a low success rate and therefore is no longer recommended in the unwitnessed arrest. It may be useful for the patient with witnessed ventricular tachycardia, in which a single thump may convert the patient to sinus rhythm, or with severe bradycardia, in which repetitive thumps may induce spontaneous cardiac contractions. From a height of 20–30 cm above the victim's chest, the fleshy portion of the fist is used to deliver a swift blow to the midsternum. Conscious patients will not like this maneuver, and alternative modes of therapy, such as intravenous lidocaine for the patient with ventricular tachycardia, should be considered.

ELECTRICAL CARDIOVERSION AND DEFIBRILLATION

Direct-current electrical defibrillation is by far the most useful element in successful resuscitation. When instituted promptly, it has a very high success rate in a variety of dysrhythmias. Defibrillators deliver a monophasic depolarization of several thousand volts over a period of about 10 msec. The delivered energy can be varied up to a maximum of 360 joules (watt-seconds) on most defibrillators.

The optimal power setting for external cardiac defibrillation has been debated. Advocates of high-energy shocks maintain that body weight is a variable in determining the power requirements for successful defibrillation, but this has not been borne out by clinical studies. High-energy shocks result in increased electrical injury to the myocardium and a higher incidence of post-shock asystole and atrioventricular block. Current evidence indicates that 200 joules is optimal for initial attempts at defibrillation; much less energy (10–50 joules) is usually required for conversion of ventricular tachycardia.

The technique of defibrillation is straightforward. The machine is set to the desired power level and the paddles are charged. Exact paddle placement is less critical than ensuring that adequate electrode paste (or saline pads) and firm paddle pressure are used, as these simple maneuvers will maximize the amount of energy delivered to the victim. One paddle is placed just below the right clavicle; the other is placed just lateral to the cardiac apex (or below the left scapula, when a flat posterior paddle is used). When everyone stands clear of the patient and the bed, the shock is delivered. Additional shocks of 200–360 joules are administered if needed, usually in prompt succession.

In the monitored patient with witnessed ventricular tachycardia or ventricular fibrillation, electrical therapy, if immediately available, must *not* await initiation of chest compression and ventilation. There is no reason to delay the delivery of the definitive treatment for these arrhythmias. In the unwitnessed arrest, cardiopulmonary resuscitation and pharmacologic intervention are often used for 1–2 minutes before countershock is attempted. This may increase the likelihood of successful conversion; however, even in an unwitnessed arrest a rapidly administered shock may be life-saving and must be delivered as soon as possible.

Some patients have recovered even after several hours of ventricular fibrillation and cardiopulmonary resuscitation; therefore, attempts at defibrillation should continue until irreversible cardiac asystole appears. If several attempts at defibrillation fail, more intensive pharmacologic therapy, closer attention to metabolic abnormalities, and higher-energy shocks may be useful. Rapid sequential shocks, spaced a few seconds apart, occasionally are of benefit as the first shock lowers skin impedance and allows a higher delivery of energy by the second shock.

Asystole has the poorest prognosis of any arrhythmia and is rarely responsive to cardioversion. Although successful shocks have been reported in cases of asystole, ventricular fibrillation was probably present in these patients. If asystole appears on the electrocardiographic monitor, the monitor's gain should be increased and the electrical leads should be changed

to obtain a configuration perpendicular to the first lead. This ensures that the tracing is not actually ventricular fibrillation, which occasionally may be isoelectric in a particular lead.

PHARMACOLOGY OF RESUSCITATION

Effective restoration of circulation often depends on pharmacologic manipulation (Table 1). Rapid placement of an intravenous line is crucial. Any vein can be used but a vein above the diaphragm is preferred. Blood flow during chest compression may be preferentially directed cephalad; infusion into the saphenous or femoral veins may therefore result in delayed entry of instilled medications into the central circulation. If an arm vein is palpable, it should be used. Frequently this is not possible due to the marked venospasm that may accompany cardiac arrest. In this situation, the external or internal jugular vein should be cannulated. The subclavian vein also may be used, but this approach carries a higher incidence of potentially serious complications and the vein may be difficult to cannulate while the patient is undergoing chest compression.

If technical problems preclude rapid intravenous access, epinephrine, atropine, and lidocaine can be safely instilled into the tracheobronchial tree via an endotracheal tube, in doses equal to initial intravenous doses. Sodium bicarbonate should not be instilled into the lungs.

Except during open-chest massage, intracardiac injection of medications is indicated only if intravenous or intratracheal administration is unavailable. Potentially serious complications of this route include coronary artery laceration, intramyocardial injection, and pericardial tamponade. Epinephrine is inherently no more effective when administered by the intracardiac route. When intracardiac administration is indicated, the subxiphoid approach is preferable to the parasternal approach.

Volume expansion with 1–2 L of normal saline or other volume expander is often helpful in elevating blood pressure during resuscitation in the volume-depleted patient, but is not usually useful in the normovolemic patient.

EPINEPHRINE

The most useful and important drug for resuscitation is epinephrine. Experimental evidence clearly shows

Table 1. Drugs Frequently Used During Cardiopulmonary Resuscitation

Drugs	Dose	Route	Mechanism of Action	Comments and Precautions
Epinephrine	≥1.0 mg every 5 min or continuous infusion (1 ampule = 1 mg)	IV, ET, IC	Increases blood pressure and heart rate	Drug of choice for resuscitation; inactivated by sodium bicarbonate
Sodium bicarbonate	After initial 5–10 min, 1 mEq/kg, then 0.5 mEq/kg as needed (1 amp = 44.6 or 50 mEq)	IV	? Helps prevent acidosis	May result in alkalemia, hypernatremia, hyperosmolar state; inactivates epinephrine; precipitates with calcium
Calcium chloride	250–1,000 mg (1 amp = 1 g)	IV, IC	Increases contractility ? Helps electromechanical dissociation	Precise role undefined. Intracardiac injection may cause severe bradycardia; precipitates with bicarbonate; contraindicated in digitalis toxicity
Atropine	0.5–1.0 mg every 5 min up to 3 mg (1 amp = 1 mg)	IV, ET, IC	May reverse bradycardia or heart block	Low doses may cause paradoxical bradycardia
Lidocaine	100–300 mg in 50–100 mg boluses; then 1–4 mg/min		May prevent ventricular fibrillation	High doses may cause central nervous system toxicity
Bretylium	5 mg/kg every 10 min up to 30 mg/kg; then 1–2 mg/min		May prevent or convert ventricular fibrillation; lowers threshold for successful cardioversion	Can cause hypotension

IV = intravenous; ET = endotracheal route; IC = intracardiac.

that administration of epinephrine enhances survival in cardiac arrest, but this potentially life-saving drug is frequently underutilized. Since epinephrine has both alpha- and beta-adrenergic agonist activity, in doses given during resuscitation it increases both peripheral vasoconstriction (alpha effect) and cardiac rate and contractility (beta effect). This enhancement of peripheral vasoconstriction results in higher rates of successful resuscitation, presumably due to augmented myocardial blood flow resulting from an increase in diastolic blood pressure. Other alpha agonists, such as methoxamine, phenylephrine, and norepinephrine, may also be effective in this regard, but are less frequently used and less readily available than epineph-

rine. An alpha-adrenergic agonist should be administered as soon as possible during cardiac resuscitation. Epinephrine, 1 mg or more intravenously at least every 4–5 minutes throughout the duration of the resuscitation or as a continuous infusion, is the usual choice, but the optimal dose is unknown; doses 10-fold higher than this have dramatically improved survival rates in several animal studies. Frequent administration is necessary due to the rapid metabolism of this drug. If intravenous access is unavailable, epinephrine should be given endotracheally by diluting the desired dose in 10 ml of fluid and instilling this into the endotracheal tube. In animals, the success rate of resuscitation is unaffected by beta-adrenergic stimulation. For this reason, other beta agonists, such as isoproterenol and dobutamine, usually have no role in the initial phase of cardiac resuscitation. However, these agents may be of value in the patient with bradycardia.

SODIUM BICARBONATE

Sodium bicarbonate is frequently used during resuscitation, but its role in resuscitation is extremely controversial. Although valuable for the temporary correction of metabolic acidosis, premature or excessive use of this drug may result in hypernatremia, the hyperosmolar state, severe arterial alkalemia, or possible excessive CO_2 production peripherally and centrally, thus potentially worsening intracellular and cerebral acidosis. These conditions may be dangerous and may preclude successful resuscitation. Sodium bicarbonate is not proved to beneficially affect the outcome of resuscitation. Therefore, this drug must be administered cautiously. In the witnessed arrest, it usually does not need to be given for the first 10 minutes of resuscitation if the patient is being adequately ventilated and metabolic acidosis did not precede the arrest. In the unwitnessed arrest and in the patient with known metabolic acidosis, correction of arterial acidosis may in part be accomplished by hyperventilation-induced hypocarbia. Sodium bicarbonate may still be necessary, usually at an initial dose of 1 mEq/kg. Subsequent doses should be gauged by monitoring the arterial or central venous pH. If blood gas determinations are unavailable, half of the initial dose can be administered empirically every 10–15 minutes until spontaneous circulation reappears. Sodium bicarbonate inactivates epinephrine and precipitates with calcium chloride; therefore, these drugs should not be administered concurrently through the same intravenous line.

CALCIUM

Although calcium is necessary for myocardial contraction, few data indicate that calcium salts are therapeutically useful in cardiac resuscitation. Studies have failed to demonstrate a beneficial effect of calcium administration during resuscitation in asystole or electromechanical dissociation. Calcium overload may aggravate postischemic injury. Therefore, it should be given with caution, if at all, during resuscitation. Appropriate uses for calcium administration include hypocalcemic states, such as after transfusion with large quantities of citrated blood, and hyperkalemia. Calcium administration is contraindicated in patients with digitalis toxicity due to possible aggravation of ventricular dysrhythmias.

ATROPINE

Atropine, a parasympatholytic drug, is occasionally useful in transiently reversing sinus bradycardia and high-degree atrioventricular block due to excessive vagal tone. It has little role in the initial stages of resuscitation unless bradycardia is identified as the initial rhythm. The usual dose is 0.5–1.0 mg every 5 minutes as needed, to a total of 3 mg. Smaller doses, 0.2 mg or less, should be avoided because they may cause a paradoxical increase in vagal tone.

ISOPROTERENOL

Isoproterenol is sometimes effective in accelerating the heart rate of patients who remain bradycardic despite atropine and in patients with complete heart block. The usual dose is 1–10 μg/min, titrated down to the smallest dose capable of maintaining adequate heart rate. Epinephrine has similar chronotropic efficacy and is often preferable, but neither agent is as effective as artificial pacing.

ANTIARRHYTHMIC AND OTHER DRUGS

Antiarrhythmic agents can be valuable adjuncts in maintaining sinus rhythm after successful defibrillation. These drugs do not usually directly contribute to restoring sinus rhythm and may occasionally raise the threshold for successful cardioversion. Therefore, antiarrhythmics need not be administered during the initial stage of resuscitation of the patient with ventricular fibrillation. If ventricular tachycardia or ventricular fibrillation is persistent or recurrent, lidocaine (50–75 mg IV every 5 minutes for three doses, followed by a continuous infusion at 1–4 mg/min), or bretylium (5 mg/kg loading dose IV repeated in 10–15 minutes if necessary, to a total dose of 30 mg/kg, followed by a continuous infusion at 1-2 mg/min, if needed) may be useful. These drugs are often used in this sequence. Bretylium may have the unique effect of lowering the defibrillation threshold, but has potentially serious side effects and is not usually recommended as a first-line drug.

Morphine, beta blockers, corticosteroids, diuretics, nitrates, and calcium channel antagonists have no proven role in basic cardiac resuscitation.

MECHANICAL AND ELECTROMECHANICAL SUPPORT

Emergent use of a transcutaneous external pacemaker or placement of a pacing wire is often useful in the symptomatic bradycardic patient, but is unlikely to resuscitate the asystolic patient. Transvenous pacers are preferable to transthoracic wires, as the latter are less often effective and can be associated with serious complications.

The antishock garment (MAST suit) directs blood flow toward the central circulation and thus may have a role in cardiac resuscitation; its exact place remains to be defined. Mechanical devices to compress the sternum are effective when properly used and can administer external chest compression more reliably than manual compression.

WHEN RESUSCITATION IS FAILING

When resuscitative efforts fail, often little can be done to avert death. However, potentially treatable causes do exist. Ventilation may be ineffective, perhaps because of improper endotracheal tube placement or tension pneumothorax. Unreliable intravenous access is often a problem; during frenetic resuscitation efforts, subcutaneous infiltration of an intravenous line may go unnoticed. Severe metabolic abnormalities, such as hyperkalemia, may be present. Volume depletion may be unsuspected and may need empiric treatment if suspicion warrants. Pericardial tamponade may be present; in such instances, pericardiocentesis may result in dramatic hemodynamic improvement. Emergency two-dimensional echocardiography is extremely useful in these differential diagnoses. Resuscitation should not be abandoned until all potentially reversible causes are investigated.

CEREBRAL PROTECTION AND RESUSCITATION

Despite successful cardiac resuscitation, many patients suffer severe and irreversible ischemic encephalopathy after cardiac arrest. This is due to long periods of cerebral ischemia and to delayed cranial reperfusion after successful restoration of spontaneous circulation. Despite early hopes for effective cerebral protection utilizing high-dose barbiturates, phenytoin, corticosteroids, anticoagulation, hypothermia, and a variety of other measures, there is little evidence that these interventions are beneficial after resuscitation. More recent data indicate that calcium channel antagonists may have a role in this setting, but further studies are needed before these drugs can be recommended for routine use.

Bibliography

Adrogue HJ, Rashad MN, Gorin AB, et al: Assessing acid-base status in circulatory failure. *N Engl J Med* 320:1312, 1989.

American Heart Association: Standards and guidelines for cardiopulmonary resuscitation (CPR) and emergency cardiac care (ECC). *JAMA* 255:21, 1986.

Brown CG, Werman HA, Davis EA, et al: The effects of graded doses of epinephrine on regional myocardial blood flow during cardiopulmonary resuscitation in swine. *Circulation* 75:491, 1987.

Criley JM, Niemann JT, Rosborough JP, et al: Modifications of cardiopulmonary resuscitation based on the cough. *Circulation* 74 (Suppl IV): IV-42, 1986.

Falk JL, Rackow EC, Weil MH: End-tidal carbon dioxide concentration during cardiopulmonary resuscitation. *N Engl J Med* 318:607, 1988.

Feneley MP, Maier GW, Gaynor JW, et al: Sequence of mitral valve motion and transmitral blood flow during manual cardiopulmonary resuscitation in dogs. *Circulation* 76: 363, 1987.

Feneley MP, Maier GW, Kern KB, et al: Influence of compression rate on initial success of resuscitation in dogs. *Circulation* 77:240, 1988.

Guerci AD, Chandra N, Johnson E, et al: Failure of sodium bicarbonate to improve resuscitation from ventricular fibrillation in dogs. *Circulation* 74 (Suppl IV): IV-75, 1986.

Jaffe AS: Cardiovascular phamacology I. *Circulation* 74 (Suppl IV): IV-70, 1986.

Kouwenhoven WG, Jude JR, Knickerbocker GG: Closed chest cardiac massage. *JAMA* 173:94, 1960.

Olson DW, Thakur R, Stueven HA, et al: Randomized study of epinephrine versus methoxamine in prehospital cardiac arrest patients with refractory ventricular fibrillation. *Ann Emerg Med* 18:250, 1989.

Otto CW: Cardiovascular pharmacology II: The use of catecholamines, pressor agents, digitalis, and corticosteroids in CPR and emergency cardiac care. *Circulation* 74 (Suppl IV): IV-80, 1986.

Rudikoff MT, Maughan WN, Effron M, et al: Mechanisms of blood flow during cardiopulmonary resuscitation. *Circulation* 61:345, 1980.

Stueven HA, Thompson BM, Aprahamian C, Tonsfeldt DJ, Kastenson EH: The effectiveness of calcium chloride in refractory electromechanical dissociation. *Ann Emerg Med* 14:626, 1985.

Swenson RD, Weaver WD, Niskanen RA, et al: Hemodynamics in humans during conventional and experimental methods of cardiopulmonary resuscitation. *Circulation* 78:630, 1988.

Thompson BM, Stueven HS, Tonsfeldt DJ, et al: Calcium: Limited indications, some danger. *Circulation* 74 (Suppl IV): IV-90, 1986.

Werner JA, Greene HL, Janko CL, et al: Visualization of cardiac valve motion in man during external chest compression using two dimensional echocardiography. *Circulation* 63:1417, 1981.

INDEX

An f following entry indicates a figure is included in the reference; a t indicates a table is included.